CLINICAL GENETICS
A SHORT COURSE

D0557893

CLINICAL GENETICS

A SHORT COURSE

GOLDER N. WILSON, M.D., Ph.D.

Mary McDermott Cook Distinguished Professor of Pediatric Genetics
Department of Pediatrics
University of Texas Southwestern Medical Center

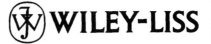

A John Wiley & Sons, Inc., Publication

New York ■ Chichester ■ Weinheim ■ Brisbane ■ Singapore ■ Toronto

For ordering and customer service, call 1-800-CALL-WILEY.

Library of Congress Cataloging-in-Publication Data:
Wilson, Golder.
    Clinical genetics : a short course / Golder N. Wilson
        p.   cm.
    Includes bibliographical references and index.
    ISBN 0-471-29806-9 (paper : alk. paper)
    1. Medical genetics.   I. Title.
    [DNLM: 1. Hereditary Diseases.   2. Genetics, Medical.   QZ 50
W748c 2000]
RB155.W552   2000
616′.042—dc21
DNLM/DLC
for Library of Congress   99-40663

Printed in the United States of America.

10 9 8 7 6 5 4 3 2 1

To my teachers:

Harris W. Wilson, C. Fred Fox, Roy D. Schmickel, and Charles M. Ginsburg.
I particularly thank Roy for introducing me to the practice of
clinical genetics, the wonders of DNA, and the
ennobling care of children with disabilities.

CONTENTS

PREFACE

This book provides an overview of clinical genetics by using case presentations and patient-oriented problems to illustrate important genetic principles. The first 10 chapters are drawn from traditional medical genetic coverage as presented in our genetics course to first-year medical students at the University of Texas Southwestern Medical Center. The last 6 chapters are more unique among medical genetic texts and emphasize genetic diagnosis and management in the areas of pediatrics (Chapters 11,12), surgery (Chapter 13), medicine (Chapter 14), obstetrics (Chapter 15), and allied health (Chapter 16). The first two parts of the book should therefore be useful for first- or second-year medical genetics courses, with the last section useful for subsequent clinical clerkships and medical practice. The clinical emphasis and broad approach should also be useful for nurses, therapists, social workers, and counselors who frequently encounter patients with genetic disorders.

Each chapter begins with learning objectives and one or more illustrative cases. The reader can scan these introductory materials to determine if the chapter contains relevant information. The increasing importance of ethics in clinical genetics is also acknowledged by discussion in many chapters. After each chapter, a problem set is provided to test retention of the learning objectives. Answers are listed for quick reference, followed by more detailed solutions that reinforce or expand upon the learning objectives. Space limitations have required that many problems and some basic information be placed on a companion website. The companion website also has links to internet resources in genetics, from sites on genome mapping to those listing parent support groups.

Another unique feature of the book is the use of McKusick numbers as references to particular medical diseases. Every genetic or potentially genetic disease has been assigned a six-digit number that begins with 1 for autosomal dominant, 2 for autosomal recessive, and 3 for X-linked disorders. The McKusick number provides rapid access to additional information about a disease by using the on-line (http://www3.ncbi.nlm.gov/omim) or text (McKusick, 1994) reference.

■ ACKNOWLEDGMENTS

The author would like to thank Colette Bean, Medical Editor, Wiley-Liss, Inc., for her persistence, insight, and encouragement.

ROSTER OF CASES

Part I

INHERITANCE AND PREDISPOSITION

INTRODUCTION TO CLINICAL GENETICS: GENES, TRAITS, AND PEDIGREES

■ LEARNING OBJECTIVES

1. Genetic diseases occur in 10–12% of individuals and will be encountered by all health professionals.
2. Recognition of genetic disease and risk factors is crucial for providing counseling and management.
3. A family history can be helpful in discovering inherited disease and is represented as a standardized diagram called a pedigree.
4. Pedigrees and knowledge of genetic principles allow visualization and tracking of alleles.
5. Probabilities for allele transmission can be converted to probabilities for genotypes in offspring (recurrence risks).

Case 1: *In Sickness and in Health*

A young couple request counseling regarding their reproductive risks. The man appears thin and fragile with atrophied lower limbs that confine him to a wheelchair. He has been diagnosed with a neurologic disorder called Friedreich ataxia (229300), which causes loss of coordination, speech defects, heart disease, and a shortened life span. The husband is quiet and withdrawn during the interview, but his wife is smiling and holding his hand. She speaks eloquently about her love for her husband and their wish to have a family. Their minister and their parents have urged them to adopt, saying that it would be a sin to propagate so severe a disease.

■ 1.1. WHAT IS GENETIC? DEFINITIONS AND THE ROLE OF FAMILY HISTORY

The word *genetic* derives from the Greek root *gen*, meaning to become or grow into something. Genetics is thus an appropriate discipline for the beginning health professional, and its focus on emerging character applies to all stages of life and to all manner of disease. At the core of the genetic approach are the ideas of anticipation and prevention that are essential

3

for modern medical practice. If one can anticipate disease based on individual characteristics or a family history, then measures to prevent the disease or its complications can be set in motion.

"Genetic" and its related terms *congenital* and *familial* usually arise when discussing particular characteristics or *traits* of an individual. Examples include eye color, hair patterns, or the peculiar nose that may appear in the family photograph album. Families assume that certain traits are genetic because they are passed down (exhibit *vertical transmission*) from parent to child. These intuitive concepts of *inheritance* and *genetic transmission* are well entrenched in lay parlance, as are fallacies that require education.

Congenital refers to a trait that is present at birth, whereas *familial* means that the trait appears in more than one family member. It is important to understand that neither term defines a trait as genetic. Fetal bleeding due to maternal platelet antibodies is congenital but not genetic, and infectious diseases that spread to several family members by *horizontal transmission* can appear familial. On the other hand, diseases like albinism may be congenital and genetic without any family history. The idea of a genetic disorder without a family history often seems paradoxical to families, and it is important to explain the relationship between disease and family pattern. Such distinctions are introduced during the educational process of *genetic counseling.*

> *Case 1 Follow-up:* The fact that the potential father is affected with Friedreich ataxia led to the false conclusion by certain family members and clergy that this genetic disease would be inherited by all of his children. Knowledge that genetic risks vary according to the type of disease and the degree of relationship would prompt referral for accurate genetic counseling.

■ 1.2. CATEGORIES OF GENETIC AND CONGENITAL DISEASES—INCIDENCE AND IMPACT IN MEDICINE

Health professionals may not realize that at least 10% of conceptions and 2–3% of live-born infants have a genetic or congenital disease. At the other end of the life cycle, common diseases such as heart attacks, breast cancer, or prostate cancer include genetic factors in their causation and/or diagnosis. Although individual genetic diseases may be rare, their aggregate frequency makes them an inescapable part of medicine. An estimated 10–12% of all live-born individuals will develop a genetically influenced disease in their lifetime (Table 1.1).

■TABLE 1.1. Categories of genetic or congenital disease

Disease Category[2]	Number of Diseases	Aggregate Frequency[b]	Shortened Lifespan	Major Handicap
Mendelian	> 4500	1	++[c]	+++
Chromosomal	> 100	0.5	++++	++++
Multifactorial	> 100	5–10	++	+++
Metabolic errors	> 500	0.3	+++	++++
Syndromes	> 1000	0.7	+++	++++
Isolated anomalies	> 200	2–3	+	++
Total	> 5000	10–12	++	+++

[a]Some diseases appear in more than one category (e.g., some syndromes exhibit chromosomal or Mendelian inheritance; many isolated birth defects are multifactorially determined).

[b]Percentage of individuals that manifest or will eventually manifest the disease.

[c]Estimated impact on + to ++++ scale: as an example, 60% of Mendelian disorders cause a shortened lifespan, 80% a major handicap, and > 95% of chromosomal disorders cause major handicaps (Wilson, 1992).

Mendel's rules of inheritance apply to more than 4000 disorders that have an aggregate frequency of about 1% in the population. When a disorder exhibits *Mendelian inheritance,* the alteration (*mutation*) of a single gene is implied as the cause of the disorder. Every disorder that is known or suspected to exhibit Mendelian inheritance has been assigned a six-digit number and catalogued by Victor McKusick (1994). An on-line version of this catalogue of Mendelian diseases can be accessed at http://www3.ncbi.nlm.nih.gov/omim, providing a valuable resource. When a Mendelian disorder is mentioned in this book, the corresponding McKusick number follows in parentheses so interested readers can obtain information about the disease. Among the Mendelian disorders are those that lead to enzyme deficiencies with consequent alterations in metabolism. The reference of Scriver et al. (1995) is a comprehensive resource for these metabolic diseases.

Other genetic disease categories include multifactorial disorders (e.g., cleft palate, diabetes mellitus) or chromosomal disorders (e.g., Down syndrome), with more than 100 individual disorders in each category (Table 1.1). Usually congenital and often genetic are patterns of abnormalities called *syndromes,* including more than 1000 recognized entities. Comprehensive references for multifactorial (Rimoin et al., 1995), chromosomal (Schinzel, 1984), and syndromal (Jones 1997; Gorlin et al. 1990) diseases are also available to supplement their discussion in this book. New causes of genetic disease are also being discovered using the techniques of molecular biology. These causes can be grouped together by their atypical inheritance, as summarized in Chapter 10. Because genetic diseases may arise de novo as *sporadic* or isolated cases, extreme or unusual presentations should always be suspected of genetic etiology, even in the absence of affected relatives. The text of Strachan and Read (1996) provides a comprehensive overview of human molecular genetics that is also accessible through the wiley.com website.

Genetic diseases are individually rare, but sufficiently common in aggregate to impact every phase of the human life cycle. Some chromosomal disorders or genetic syndromes disrupt embryonic or fetal life, resulting in spontaneous abortions or stillbirths. An example is the Mendelian disorder called incontinentia pigmenti (308300) that produces streaks of pigment in affected females and abortion of affected males. Metabolic or chromosomal disorders can cause death or disability in early childhood, while others can disrupt puberty or reproductive function. Examples include Turner syndrome that results when females are missing an X chromosome. Mendelian disorders like Marfan syndrome (154700) can present in childhood, but usually become manifest in late adolescence or adulthood with alterations of the eye or heart. Sudden death can occur due to rupture of the aorta in Marfan syndrome, and the tragedies of certain athletes dramatize the adverse consequences that can result from genetic disease.

■ 1.3. THE GENETIC APPROACH IN MEDICINE

The approach to the patient with genetic disease is similar to that in other areas of medicine and is summarized in Figure 1.1. First and most important is the initial contact with a symptomatic individual or family. This first contact should initiate a counseling process that proceeds in parallel with medical management. The first phase of counseling is *supportive,* meaning that a general outline of the problems and management plan are provided without detailed diagnostic or recurrence risk information. Medical concerns are explained in lay language, and the involvement of relatives or clergy is encouraged to bolster the family during their crisis. The example of Case 1 illustrates that these family or religious contacts may require education about genetic principles along with the affected individuals. Because a period of denial, anger, and/or grief often accompanies the presentation of a genetic disease, the family may not be ready to comprehend factual information. This delay in family acceptance often corresponds to a delay in obtaining the precise diagnosis, allowing the process of supportive counseling to parallel the process of medical evaluation as shown in Figure 1.1.

Once the plan for evaluation has been outlined in a supportive way, the medical history assumes its usual importance. For neonates, particular attention to the gestational history is needed and for adults, records or photographs from their childhood may be extremely helpful. The family history is always an essential component but may not be revealing when new genetic changes (*mutations*) or environmental causes are involved. The steps in taking a fam-

ily history and in constructing a pedigree are discussed later in this chapter (section 1.6).

The physical examination often has special aspects when a genetic disorder is being considered. Examples include the unusual appearance or subtle anomalies that occur in syndromes, the odors or rashes that occur in metabolic diseases, or the elastic skin, lax joints, and abnormal scarring that occur in adults with genetic defects of connective tissue. These and other physical findings are reviewed in Part III. Expertise in the physical examination is one reason for involving a genetic specialist, but the primary care provider must

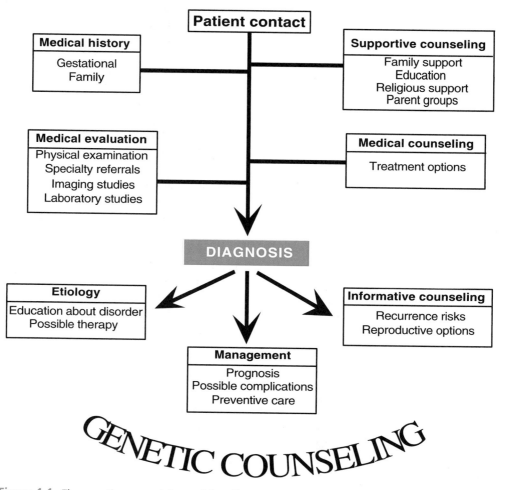

Figure 1.1. The genetic approach in medicine, illustrating parallel stages of diagnosis and counseling. The diagnostic, educational, and management aspects of this approach are encompassed by the process known as genetic counseling.

be familiar enough with signal findings to initiate the referral. After the history and physical are analyzed to construct a differential diagnosis, then a medical evaluation utilizing radiographic or laboratory testing may be necessary to discriminate among the possibilities. Medical counseling to the patient and/or family should parallel the medical evaluation, and families should be informed about options for testing or treatment (Fig. 1.1). A specific diagnosis is always the goal of the genetic approach. Without a definitive diagnosis, informative counseling about the prognosis, management, recurrence risk, and options for prenatal diagnosis is not possible. The stages of supportive, medical, and informative counseling, including patient education and dialogue, contribute to the complex process known as *genetic counseling*. Genetic counseling is an integral part of the genetic approach, and every health professional should be comfortable with its supportive and educational aspects.

Case 1 Follow-up: Upon hearing of this couple's reproductive concerns, the primary care provider should ensure that the husband has had a valid diagnosis. If the physician/counselor is not a neurologist qualified to confirm the diagnosis of Friedreich ataxia, then he or she should ensure that medical records are available that document this diagnosis. Until diagnostic results are available, supportive counseling can be provided that outlines the need for accurate diagnosis and counseling.

■ 1.4. TRAITS IN MEDICINE

Individuality is a striking feature of biology. Even simpler organisms such as bacteria or fruit flies exhibit individual differences when observed with the appropriate tools. Mendel's great insight was to focus on individual differences among pea plants, differences he called *unit characters*. Now these unit characters are called traits, and the collection of traits that defines an individual organism is called the *phe-notype*. Figures 1.2 and 1.3 illustrate examples of human traits that are important in clinical genetics.

Traits occur at every level of the medical enterprise, from surface differences noted on physical examination to the peculiarities of tissue type, cell count, or protein size noted in the laboratory. In clinical genetics, the terms "trait" or "phenotype" can refer to any individual characteristic of interest. Many traits are *qualitative,* defined by alternative states that can be distinguished subjectively. Examples include components of diseases—illustrated by the scalp defect (Fig. 1.2A), cleft lip (Fig. 1.2B), cloudy cornea (Fig. 1.2C)—or an entire pattern of disease (Fig. 1.2D), called a *syndrome*. The child in Figure 1.2D has a pattern of changes in the face and sheleton due to Hunter Syndrome (309900). Qualitative traits include the normal or absent iris (*aniridia*) in Figure 1.3A, the multiple discrete eye colors shown in Figure 1.3B, or biochemical markers such as the ABO blood types. A population can be subdivided into discrete groups according to which qualitative traits they possess as in Figure 1.3D.

Quantitative traits refer to measurements rather than to subjective characteristics. Examples of quantitative traits include a height of 6 ft 7 in, a systolic blood pressure of 115 ml of mercury, a mean red cell volume of 81 fl, or an interpupillary distance of 3 cm as shown in Figure 1.3C. In populations, quantitative traits have a distribution of values, as shown for interpupillary distance in Figure 1.3E. A qualitative trait like hypertelorism or widely spaced eyes (Figure 1.3C) can be viewed as an extreme of this distribution that is easily perceived in individuals like Jackie Kennedy Onassis. The inheritance of quantitative traits is usually determined by complex interactions of multiple genes and the environment. When quantitative traits cross certain thresholds, like the higher values for interpupillary distance that are perceived as hypertelorism, they may become qualitative traits—for example, tall or short, bright or dumb, fat or thin. The inheritance of quantitative traits, including their

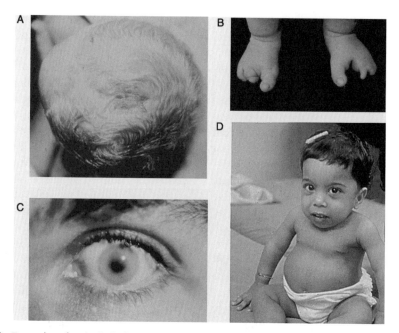

Figure 1.2. Examples of traits include *A*, scalp defect with absent skin typically seen in children with trisomy 13; *B*, missing toes typical of autosomal dominant ectrodactyly (cleft hands and feet,183600); *C*, cloudy cornea typical of children with mucopolysaccharide storage disease; *D*, child with dwarfism (spondyloepiphyseal dysplasia, 120140) illustrating a narrow chest.

ability to be converted into qualitative traits by the phenomena of thresholds, is discussed in Chapter 3.

The frequency and context of traits often determines whether they are viewed as *benign variants* or *polymorphisms* versus signs of disease. Polymorphisms (literally, multiple shapes) refer to variable traits at the morphologic or molecular level that do not cause harm to the individual. A pouch of intestine called the Meckel diverticulum occasionally causes bowel obstruction and requires surgery, but is an incidental finding at autopsy in 2–3% of people who have led long and normal lives. Since a population frequency of 1% or greater may be used as the arbiter of variant versus disease, Meckel diverticulum usually qualifies as a variant or harmless trait.

Sometimes the environmental or societal context determines whether a trait is harmless, indicated by the healthy status of individuals with sickle trait at normal altitudes. However, those with sickle cell trait at high altitudes may develop painful obstruction of the blood vessels as occurs in people with sickle cell anemia (141900). Sickle trait may also be a disadvantage for marriage in certain social contexts due to risks for offspring with sickle cell anemia. The frequency and context of traits is an important factor to consider when taking a family history. Some traits occur frequently among various family members and are not mentioned unless specifically asked about. As illustrated in the case of sickle cell anemia, medical use of the term "trait" often connotes harmless variation rather than disease.

The concept of polymorphism provides an important perspective on traits or phenotypes as they are encountered in medicine. Human variation is extensive, and it is the functional context of the variation that determines whether it is abnormal—that is, whether it is termed a disease. Variation in shape of the external ears among individuals is easily ob-

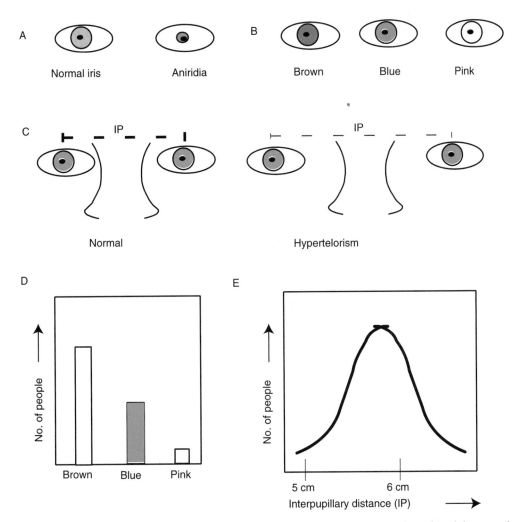

Figure 1.3. Qualitative traits exemplified by normal iris versus small or absent iris (aniridia, *A*), by several types of eye color (*B*), by normal or widely spaced eyes (hypertelorism, *C*). Qualitative traits form multiple categories in a population (*D*), while quantitative traits form a distribution illustrated by interpupillary distance (IP, *E*). Some qualitative traits like hypertelorism (*C*) can be viewed as subjectively perceived extremes on a quantitative distribution (*E*).

served, but only variations with cosmetic or functional significance would be called a disease. Individual differences in chromosomal, protein, or deoxyribonucleic acid (DNA) structure are commonly detected by laboratory methods, but it is the context of gene structure and expression that determines whether a DNA nucleotide variation is a disease mutation or a polymorphism. The use of higher frequency to distinguish polymorphism from dis-

ease phenotype is readily understood, because variations associated with disease are less likely to be transmitted to offspring.

In summary, biological variation extends from the molecular to the anatomic level and provides a kaleidoscope of traits or phenotypes. Qualitative traits are descriptions such as "eyes are blue"; quantitative traits are numbers, such as 5 ft 2 in. Traits that impact function become rare and are known as disease; benign variations are common and are described as traits, variants, or polymorphisms.

> *Case 1 Follow-up:* The couple can be reassured that the diagnosis of Friedreich ataxia does not imply that the husband is genetically "defective" and therefore should not reproduce. A perspective on disease as a quality of the particular allele rather than of the individual is helpful to many couples.

■ 1.5. CORRELATING TRAITS WITH GENES: THE NATURE OF GENETIC INFORMATION

In 1886, Mendel deduced that certain unit characters (traits or variants) were determined by invisible factors (genes). He made this important discovery by breeding parents with different traits (*crosses*) and noting the ratio of parental traits in offspring. Mendel attributed the appearance or phenotype of each offspring to the types of parental factors it received (genotype); offspring genotypes were reconstituted from parental genotypes by separation (*segregation*) and reassortment (*recombination*) of parentally transmitted genes. He recognized that parental genes must occur as alternative forms (*alleles*), and that certain alleles were crucial (*dominant*) in the determination of phenotype. In modern language, each pea plant trait that Mendel studied was determined by alternative alleles at a single genetic *locus*. The ratio of phenotypes in offspring could be predicted if the parental genotypes were known. These ratios were simple enough (e.g., 1:1, 3:1) that each parental genotype was likely to consist of two alleles at each locus. This mechanism is now referred to as *Mendelian inheritance.*

The invisible factors that Mendel deduced are now known as *genes:* linear segments of DNA within a longer strand called a *chromosome.* The mechanisms of gene action and gene segregation are illustrated on the supplementary website for this book (see Preface) and should be consulted by students unfamiliar

with the following synopsis. The position (*locus*) of the gene is constant for a particular organism, but its DNA sequence can vary to produce different alleles. Genetic information is encoded by the sequence of nucleotides in DNA, flows from gene to ribonucleic acid (RNA) to protein within each cell, and produces phenotypes by the action of RNA or proteins on cell functions. In *diploid* organisms, genes are transmitted from cell to cell by *mitosis,* and from parent to child by *haploid* gametes that are produced during *meiosis.* Abnormal mitotic or meiotic divisions can produce chromosomal abnormalities in tissues or offspring, whereas abnormal DNA replication can produce mutant alleles that cause genetic disease. Chromosomal or genetic diseases can be tracked in families using diagrams called *pedigrees.* Clinical genetics is thus the study of gene/chromosome action and segregation that produces human disease phenotypes.

■ 1.6. PEDIGREES AND PATTERNS OF TRANSMISSION

A *pedigree* is a scientific genealogy that takes advantage of special symbols. Family relationships have been diagrammed in many ways as illustrated in Figure 1.4*A*, but the use of symbols and organized generations facilitates the analysis of inheritance mechanisms (Fig. 1.4*B*). The word *pedigree* derives from *pied de gris* or crow's feet in French, which reflects the early custom of drawing multiple symbols off a central family axis. Note the special symbols for male, female, mating, marriage, divorce, relatedness (*consanguinity*), twinning, abortion, and death in Figure 1.5, and the use of filled symbols for affected individuals in Figure 1.4*B*.

The starting point of the pedigree is usually the affected individual who has prompted evaluation. This key person is called the *proband or propositus (proposita for females)* according to gender and is highlighted by an arrow on the diagram (Figs. 1.4*B*, 1.5). In prenatal clinics, a person other than those affected may be

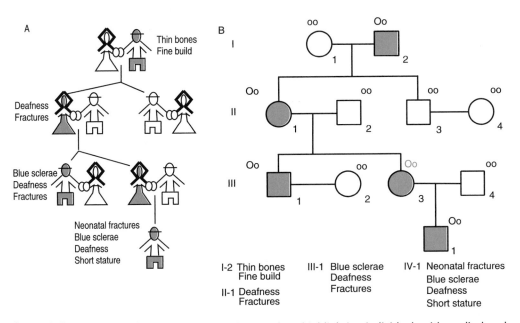

Figure 1.4. Constructing a pedigree. *A*, family genealogy highlighting individuals with medical problems by filled symbols; *B*, standardized pedigree of the same family, showing genotypes where O is the allele causing osteogenesis imperfecta and o is the normal allele.

the patient who seeks genetic and reproductive advice. In these cases, the arrow may identify that individual as the *consultand.* The frame of reference provided by the proposita or consultand gives focus to the family history and centers the pedigree diagram.

The diagram and pedigree in Figure 1.4 concern a family in which several individuals have a complex phenotype that includes fine bones, recurrent fractures, blue *sclerae* (whites of the eyes), and deafness. The occurrence of affected individuals over four generations makes it likely that this phenotype has a genetic causation. In Figure 1.4*B*, Mendelian inheritance is postulated by assuming a normal allele o and an abnormal allele O. Since humans are diploid, each individual has two chromosomes containing the locus for this brittle bone disease and possesses two alleles. If abnormal allele O is dominant to the normal allele o, then individual genotypes listed above the pedigree symbols in Figure 1.4*B* correlate nicely with the family transmission and disease status displayed in the pedigree. A disease called osteogenesis imperfecta (166240) fits

with the symptoms and inheritance pattern displayed in Figure 1.4*B*. The pedigree becomes a useful document for explaining the pattern of transmission in this family (inheritance pattern), and for predicting risks for various family members to have offspring with disease (*recurrence risks*).

Although a family history should be obtained on every new patient, a pedigree is not always indicated. Even when a genetic disease is considered likely, some preliminary questions are helpful to ascertain whether a pedigree is useful and how many individuals/ generations it should include. For the family in Figure 1.4*B*, preliminary knowledge that four generations were involved allowed appropriate spacing rather than compression of key symbols near the margin. If a student or health professional takes the trouble to construct a pedigree, it is helpful to provide a clear document that can be placed in the medical record.

For pedigrees with complex information, each generation and individual may be numbered as shown in Figure 1.4*B*, with pertinent information summarized below the diagram.

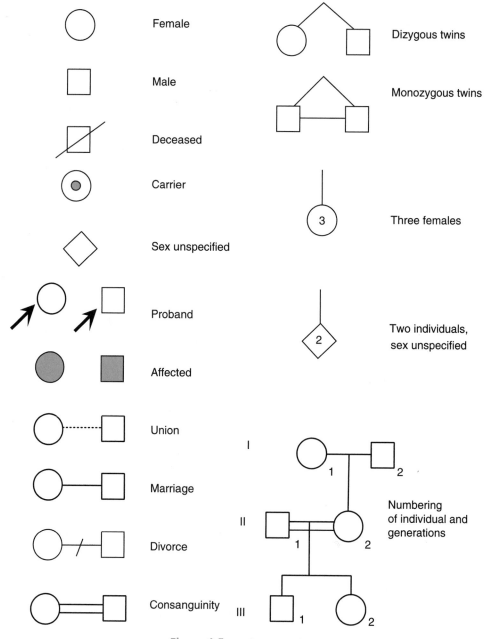

Female

Male

Deceased

Carrier

Sex unspecified

Proband

Affected

Union

Marriage

Divorce

Consanguinity

Dizygous twins

Monozygous twins

Three females

Two individuals,
sex unspecified

Numbering
of individual and
generations

Figure 1.5. Pedigree symbols.

This strategy prevents clutter around the pedigree symbols and facilitates the interpretation of phenotypes and pedigree patterns. By using the convention of filled pedigree symbols to indicate affected individuals, the pedigree in Figure 1.4*B* clearly shows a vertical pattern.

Chapter 2 discusses the correlation between pedigree patterns and particular mechanisms of inheritance.

The family represented in Figure 1.4 illustrates two final points about traits that are important for clinical genetics. First, as illustrated in Figure 1.2*D*, diseases may be *syndromic* with multiple signs and symptoms produced by a single etiology. It is important to recognize that the thin bones, deafness, and blue sclerae described in Figure 1.4 are all parts of a complex phenotype that may represent an inherited disease. Second, affected individuals in a family may exhibit different severity of disease. This phenomenon is known as *variable expressivity,* and is discussed further in Chapter 2. As illustrated by the fable of the blind men and the elephant, the scoring of signs such as thin bones or blue sclerae as independent findings rather than parts of the disease phenotype called osteogenesis imperfecta would obscure the vertical pattern of transmission demonstrated in Figure 1.4*B*.

Case 1 Follow-up: It is important to recognize that the depression, limb atrophy, and muscle wasting exhibited by the husband are components of a single disorder called Friedreich ataxia, and that these findings are all manifestations of the same abnormal allele. Consultation of the McKusick catalogue (Online Mendelian Inheritance in Man) reveals that the Friedreich ataxia phenotype (229300) is the result of alleles at a single genetic locus. OMIM indicates further that Friedreich ataxia is *autosomal recessive,* which implies that the abnormal allele f will not cause problems when the normal allele F is present. The affected husband will therefore have an ff genotype, and his normal wife an Ff or FF genotype.

■ 1.7. PREDICTING GENETIC RISK FROM PROBABILITIES OF ALLELE SEGREGATION

The Mendelian model of inheritance leads directly to the prediction of traits in offspring. During *gametogenesis* (the formation of eggs or sperm), the parental alleles are separated by the process known as *segregation.* Haploid gametes containing single alleles then reunite during fertilization to produce diploid offspring with one allele from each parent. If it is assumed that each parental allele is transmitted to gametes with equal probability, then the expected ratios of genotypes in the diploid offspring can be predicted. The basis for these simple calculations are now reviewed, saving discussion of the mechanics of allele segregation for chapter 3.

Probabilities are fractions or percentages that estimate the likelihood for a particular result to occur. In general, the probability of occurrence is the number of possibilities that yield the result divided by the total number of possibilities. A standard deck of playing cards offers a good illustration of probabilities: The odds for drawing the ace of spades are 1 result out of 52 possibilities or a probability of 1/52 ($\cong 2\%$). The odds of drawing an ace of any suit would be 4 positive results out of 52 possibilities, or a probability of 1/13 (7.7%).

In clinical genetics, a particular result is often a combination of events, meaning that several individual events must occur to yield the final result. Three types of compound events occur: additive, joint, or conditional. For event A and event B, their *additive probability* is represented by P{A + B}: the likelihood that event A, event B, or both will occur. *Joint probabilities* estimate the chance of several events to occur together, expressed for two events as P{AB}. *Conditional probabilities* express the probability of one event given that the other has already occurred—that is, P{A/B}, or the chance of A given B. Hartl (1980) provides a nice review of probability as it is used in genetics.

Returning to the card model, the odds of drawing an ace could be rephrased as the additive probability P{A + B + C + D}, equal to the sum of individual probabilities for the ace of spades P{A} = 1/52, ace of hearts P{B} = 1/52, and so forth, to yield {1/52 + 1/52 + 1/52 + 1/52} = 4/52 or 1/13. For drawing an ace of spades, the alternative to knowing there are 52 different cards in the deck would be to calculate the joint probability P{AB} = the probability of being an ace P{A} = 1/13 times the probability of being a spade P{B} = 1/4 to yield $(1/13)(1/4) = 1/52$. If it is known that an ace has been drawn (result B), then the conditional probability of its being an ace of spades (result A) is $P\{A/B\} = 1/4$.

Probabilities are applied to human reproduction by realizing that each allele in a diploid organism has a 1/2 or 50% probability of being transmitted to an offspring. If the parental genotypes are known, then the likelihood for any given genotype in offspring can be calculated by combining the probabilities for individual results. In Figure 1.5B, individual I-1 can transmit only allele o (probability of 1), while individual I-2 has a 1/2 probability of transmitting allele O and a 1/2 probability of transmitting allele o. The probability for an oo genotype in their offspring is thus the joint probability $P\{AB\} = P\{A\}P\{B\} = (1)(1/2) = 1/2$; the probability for an Oo genotype is also 1/2. Since the O allele has already conferred the phenotype of osteogenesis imperfecta on individual I-2, the 50% probability for an Oo genotype in his offspring can be described as a *recurrence risk.*

For a grandchild of individual I-2, the chance to have osteogenesis imperfecta (the Oo genotype) would again be a joint probability. The child would have a probability of 1/2 to receive the O allele from parent I-2, and the grandchild would have a 1/2 probability to receive the O allele from the child II-1, yielding a joint probability of $(1/2)(1/2) = 1/4$. This calculation assumes that the child's spouse was not affected with osteogenesis imperfecta, an assumption made realistic by its 1 in 20,000 population frequency. If two people with osteogenesis imperfecta did marry, then the probability to have an offspring (Oo genotype) would be the additive probability of 1/2 (from father) plus 1/2 (from mother) minus the joint probability that both would transmit the O allele. The final probability is thus $1 – (1/2)(1/2) = 3/4$, assuming that the phenotype of OO individuals is the same as Oo individuals. Figure 1.6 illustrates a useful way to visualize these probabilities that is known as a *Punnett square.* Parental alleles are assigned columns in a grid, and the possible genotypes of off-

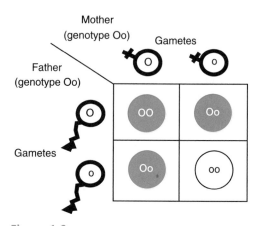

Figure 1.6. Visualization of genotype ratios using the Punnett square. Two people with osteogenesis imperfecta (genotype Oo) will produce gametes with alleles O and o in equal proportions, combining to produce a ratio of 1 OO, 2 Oo, and 1 oo genotypes in offspring. Assuming that genotypes OO and Oo both produce osteogenesis imperfecta, the recurrence risk is 75%.

spring are deduced as events within the grid. The probability of any particular genotype can then be read directly as a proportion of all genotypes on the grid.

■ 1.8. RISK ASSESSMENT AS A PART OF GENETIC COUNSELING

As introduced in Section 1.1, *genetic counseling* is an educational and medical process that provides parents with information. For phenotypes that relate directly to single genetic alleles, knowledge of segregation and probability allows the provision of *recurrence risks.* Such information can be extremely helpful for families, but recurrence risk counseling is subject to two pitfalls. The first concerns errors in genetic interpretation, and the second concerns emotional bias in parental understanding.

A common misconception about genetics, illustrated by the ill-informed advice in Case 1, might be called the *all-or-none fallacy.* The assumption is made that persons affected with a genetic disease will transmit it to all of their offspring. As illustrated by the allele segregation diagrammed in Figure 1.6, the odds of genetic transmission are rarely 100%. This fallacy was one of several that led to the eugenics movement at the beginning of the twentieth century, and its implications are extremely negative for individuals with genetic disease. Eugenics led to the forced sterilization of thousands of individuals with mental retardation in the United States (Gould, 1981) and influenced the horrors of Nazi Germany. A sobering statistic from the latter episode is that 50% of German physicians became members of the Nazi party (Müller-Hill, 1988) and that some participated directly in genocide (Parent and Shevell, 1998).

A second fallacy of eugenics relevant to counseling concerns the *reductionist* assumption that complex human traits are determined by single genetic alleles. Complex phenotypes like mental retardation or cerebral palsy have many different causes that may be genetic and/or environmental. Only when a definitive genotype has been assigned is a counselor able to provide specific recurrence risks. Laboratory testing offers the most solid ground for defining genotypes, with DNA testing for specific alleles constituting the gold standard. If DNA testing is not available for a disorder, then the measure closest to the gene level— enzyme, protein, cell, organelle, or chromosome—should be sought to confirm impressions based on the external phenotype. Specific laboratory diagnoses avoid the complexities of phenotypic variability illustrated by the family with osteogenesis imperfecta in Figure 1.4.

When knowledge of the genotype allows the calculation of accurate recurrence risks, counseling is still complicated by the difference between *genetic risk* and *genetic burden*. This difference is illustrated by the strategy of drawing to an inside straight in poker: The odds are 1 in 11, but the level of tension accompanying the outcome depends on the amount of money wagered. Another example of burden is the exaggerated fear some people have of air travel despite the low risk (about 1 in 635,000) compared to a 1 in 3700 risk for a fatal car accident (Murphy and Chase, 1975).

Because of fear or genuine experience, the burden of genetic disease often has great influence on the perception of recurrence risks. The background risk of 2–3% for congenital anomalies in the average pregnancy may be unacceptable to some families, while others may accept a 50% risk with calm resolve. Assumptions about burden by the counselor may be unfounded, as illustrated by some couples with dwarfism who are ambivalent about having a "normal" or average-sized child. Because their home and car have been designed for short stature, the parents may not desire an average-sized child.

Some studies have concluded that the burden of genetic disease is more of a factor in reproductive decisions than actual recurrence risk (Leonard et al., 1972). The pivotal role of burden in genetic counseling is illustrated by the reflections of selected families:

Concerning a child with Down syndrome:

> I'd never known a child with Down syndrome. I had worked a little with adults with Down syndrome, and it was horrible. They were very poorly functioning individuals. No speech, minimal comprehension of receptive speech or language, just very low functioning. But those people were institutionalized since birth. . . . We had a geneticist who knew what could happen, that a child could function very well or very poorly, and explained the need for early intervention right from the beginning. I think we need more health professionals who are educated to push parents in this direction. (Stray-Gunderson, 1986)

Concerning a child with trisomy 18, a severe chromosomal syndrome with an average survival of 8 months:

> It's getting harder and harder to get to the hospital twice a day to feed him and let him know we care about him. He had learned to nipple and was taking one ounce every three hours. Everything went fine for two weeks. Then he developed congestive heart failure again . . . he was kept there in ICU [intensive care unit] for four days. We did not enjoy our stay there. Everyone went

out of their way to be kind and helpful, but it just wasn't home! Anthony has not been the same since then. I feel he is giving up . . . maybe he's just plain tired. He's back on the gavage tube again. This time, for good they tell me. Even with the tube he will only accept two ounces every four hours. If I try to give him more, he vomits shortly afterward. (Support Organization for Trisomy 13, 18, and Related Disorders, 1989)

Concerning a father who learns that his child has progeria (176670), a severe and often lethal disease with rapid aging:

How does one handle news like that? I was a young, inexperienced rabbi, not as familiar with the process of grief as I would later come to be, and what I mostly felt that day was a deep aching sense of unfairness. It didn't make sense. I had been a good person. I had tried to do what was right in the sight of God. More than that, I was living a more religiously committed life than most people I knew, people who had large, healthy families. I believed that I was following God's ways and doing His work. How could this be happening to my family? If God existed, if He was minimally fair, let alone loving and forgiving, how could He do this to me? (Kushner, 1981)

The foregoing statements indicate the dual agenda inherent in a genetic counseling session. There are first the objective facts of disease—signs, symptoms, diagnoses, recurrence risks, options. Equally important, and often more amenable to intervention, are the interpretations of medical facts by patients and their relatives. Without proper understanding and integration of medical information, follow-up care and compliance may be negated. For genetic counseling in particular, time and effort are required to ascertain the family's understanding of the genetics and their frame of reference for approaching the relevant decisions. Underlying this approach is the avoidance of *parentalism* or, in genetic terms, the provision of nonjudgmental or *nondirective* counseling.

Case 1 Follow-up: Although it was stated that the wife's genotype could be Ff or FF, it is much more likely that she is FF because of the rarity of the abnormal Friedreich allele. Chapter 4 illustrates the use of the Hardy-Weinberg law to calculate the likelihood of Ff or FF genotypes. If the wife's genotype is FF and the husband's ff, then the risk for offspring to have Friedreich ataxia is virtually 0%. Although the burden of disease plus the demands of normal children should still be discussed with the couple, the low recurrence risk offers strong rebuke to the warnings against reproduction. The wife was overjoyed after hearing this information and left the room with tears of happiness. She symbolizes the powerful benefits that can accrue from genetic counseling and the accessibility of simple genetic reasoning to all health professionals.

◼ 1.9. LABORATORY ASPECTS OF GENETICS (THE GENETIC HIERARCHY)

Genetics is probably best known for the laboratory advances that have led to chromosomal, biochemical, and DNA testing. It is thus somewhat paradoxical when generalists or lay people discover that confirmatory laboratory testing is unavailable for many genetic diseases. In particular, there is no "gene screen" that covers all DNA mutations in the way that a karyotype can screen for most chromosomal abnormalities. Awareness of the strengths and limitations of genetic testing requires knowledge of the *genetic hierarchy* extending from DNA segments (genes, genotypes) to organ structure and personal appearance (phenotypes). Figure 1.7 diagrams this genetic hierarchy and illustrates the ways that gene and gene product testing interface with organ imaging and cell studies (tissue biopsy, tissue culture) to provide laboratory diagnoses in various fields of medicine. A more detailed view of the genetic hierarchy and of genetic laboratory methods is presented in Part II.

An appreciation of the possibilities for genetic testing requires understanding of the lev-

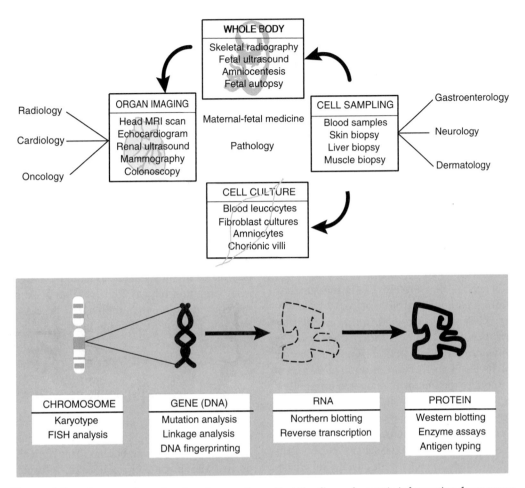

Figure 1.7. Laboratory investigations in genetics reflect the flow of genetic information from genes (DNA segments on chromosomes) through RNA and protein (lower diagram). Diagnostic testing of genes (DNA) or gene products (RNA, proteins) interfaces with organ imaging, biopsy, and cell culture (upper diagram).

els from gene to individual that are detailed in Chapter 6. Humans, like all biologic organisms, are clusters of cells that acquire different shapes and functions during embryogenesis through the process of *differentiation*. Every cell derives from the fertilized egg (*zygote*), which is in turn constructed by fusion of maternal (egg) and paternal (sperm) gametes. Each parent contributes one-half of their genetic material to offspring, producing a zygote with 22 paired *autosomes* and one pair of sex chromosomes. Each chromosome is a chain of

DNA with about 10,000 individual links (DNA segments) that comprise individual genes. Genes act according to the regulatory instructions laid down during embryogenesis, making RNA and protein or remaining silent according to their cell type.

Genetic testing can be performed at various levels in the genetic hierarchy, often combining several levels in the diagnostic process. Whole body studies include physical measurements and radiography of the entire skeleton for adults or various ultrasound studies for the fetus. Radiologic imaging of the brain, heart, or kidneys can be accomplished before or after birth, and these imaging techniques can guide tissue sampling for the study of cells in the laboratory. *Chorionic villus sampling* or *amniocentesis* are usually employed to obtain fetal cells; blood sampling, skin, liver or muscle biopsy provide tissue samples from children or adults after birth.

At the cellular level (Fig. 1.7, lower portion), chromosomes can be counted to construct a *karyotype,* or probed with fluorescent DNA segments (*fluorescent in situ hybridization = FISH* analysis) to search for small chromosomal deletions. The steps by which a gene (DNA segment) encodes *RNA* and then protein are accompanied by corresponding levels of molecular testing. Proteins can be measured by *Western blotting, enzyme* assay, or *antigen* typing; RNA by *northern blotting* or *reverse transcription,* and DNA by *Southern blotting* or the *polymerase chain reaction.* Enzymes control the levels of small molecules (*metabolites*) in the cell, so measurement of altered metabolites in cells, blood, or urine (*metabolic testing*) may point to a defective gene or protein.

It can be seen that some tests like skeletal radiography or chromosome studies are very general in nature, screening for any and all abnormalities in a particular structure. Other tests, like those for genes or enzymes, are disease-specific and yield only a normal/abnormal result for the disease in question. Assays of galactose enzymes must be performed to diagnose galactosemia (230400), and measurement of hemoglobin proteins or genes must be made to diagnose sickle cell anemia (141900). Methods to screen individuals for any possible gene or protein alteration, and thus for all possible Mendelian diseases, are far from being realized.

Case 1 Follow-up: A DNA test is now available for Freidreich ataxia, examining the frataxin gene on chromosome. This disorder is one of several caused by unstable triplet repeats that may expand or contract with each generation.

■ 1.10. ETHICAL ISSUES IN GENETICS: A PREVIEW

A heartening advance in medicine has been the recognition of ethics as a formal component of health care. Hospitals now have ethics committees, and health professional students are usually given training in ethics as part of their introduction to clinical medicine. Ethical concerns in genetics may be general as befits the ubiquity of genetic disease, or specific arising from advances in genetic technology. General medical ethics is covered in the texts by Ahronheim et al. (1994) or by Beauchamp and Childress (1994), while specific genetic concerns are addressed in subsequent cases and problem sets. Common ethical conflicts that arise in genetic medicine are summarized here as a preview of subsequent discussions.

Autonomy Versus Parentalism

A fundamental principle of health care concerns the patient's right to select among diagnostic and management options. This right underlies the medical principle of informed consent, where procedures or treatments with risk to the patient must be explained and consented to. It is sometimes tempting for healthcare providers with greater medical understanding to interfere with patient autonomy by dictating or directing patient decisions (*parentalism*). Prenatal counselors may have negative feelings about mental disability and describe the quality of life for people with Down syndrome in very negative terms. Children with familial risk for cancer may be advised to have genetic tests, even they are not mature enough to provide informed consent. Although this conflict is inevitable in certain areas, nondirective or unbiased counseling is the standard of care in medical genetics. As stated by Sheldon Reed (1980): "[T]he counselor should not drive the family car, but ride along and share the view."

Autonomy/Confidentiality Versus Beneficence

Most health workers choose their professions with some consideration for benefiting their patients and society at large. When patient choices compromise another individual (e.g., child abuse) or society (e.g., continued sex after positive HIV testing), then the care provider's higher goal of beneficence comes in conflict with patient autonomy. Regarding individuals, a genetic diagnosis may dispose the health care provider to mandate lifestyle changes or to inform at-risk relatives. Regarding society at large, genetic tests may have implications for employment, health insurance, or life insurance. Examples of this ethical conflict pertain to children with genetic obesity (e.g., Prader-Willi syndrome) whose parents choose not to enforce life-saving calorie restriction, individuals with chromosome translocations who choose not to inform family members of their potential risks, or employees with genetic diseases that can negatively affect their job performance or insurance status. In most medical situations, well-intentioned actions to promote individual or societal beneficence are prohibited by principles of autonomy (patient choice or guardianship) and confidentiality (release of medical information only with patient permission).

Autonomy/Confidentiality Versus Nonmaleficence

Advances in DNA diagnosis have allowed the identification of genetic predisposition before the actual presentation of disease. Examples include Huntington chorea (143100), a neurodegenerative disease of middle age, and certain forms of breast cancer. A fundamental medical principle, included in the Hippocratic oath, is to do no harm. The imperative to do no harm (nonmaleficence) may conflict with the patient's desire to know her future or her children's future as determined by genetic testing. Because presymptomatic diagnosis of diseases like Huntington chorea have resulted in major

lifestyle changes or suicides, elaborate protocols have been devised to assess patient mental status prior to genetic testing. Although such protocols provide the health professional some recourse in declining to offer testing (e.g., to individuals with depressive illness or to minors in the case of Huntington disease), the right of patients to information is usually considered paramount. Physicians are obligated to outline the options for testing and to report the results of testing even if knowledge of these results may harm the patient.

Case 1 Follow-up: The autonomy of the couple's reproductive decision was, from the view of their family and clergy, in conflict with beneficence to their prospective children who might be affected with Freidreich ataxia. Resolution of this apparent conflict was possible through application of genetic principles, providing a satisfying outcome. In many genetic case examples, the conflict between reproductive autonomy and adverse consequences to children remains as a difficult issue for couples and health professionals.

PROBLEM SET 1
Genetics in Medicine

Select the single most appropriate answer to the following questions:

1.1. At her first obstetric visit, a woman tells you she has a brother with mental retardation. She asks what the risk for mental retardation will be for her current pregnancy. You reply:

    (A) Mental retardation is a complex phenotype that is rarely genetic.

    (B) Mental retardation fits into the polygenic category with a low recurrence risk.

    (C) It is imperative to establish a more specific diagnosis before counseling can be provided.

    (D) It is imperative to perform a karyotype on her brother before counseling can be provided.

    (E) The risk is significant but there is no prenatal diagnosis for mental retardation.

1.2. An individual with genotype Aa at a genetic locus will produce:

    (A) Only gametes with genotype Aa

    (B) Only gametes with genotype a

(C) Only gametes with genotype aa
(D) Half of gametes with genotype A and half with genotype a
(E) Only gametes with genotype AA

1.3. If allele B causes disease and allele b is associated with a normal phenotype, what is the chance that a baby born to a Bb mother will have the disease? Assume that the father has a bb genotype and that there is no variable expressivity.

(A)	100%	(D)	25%
(B)	75%	(E)	Less than 1%
(C)	50%		

1.4. The allele for normal hemoglobin is represented as A, and that for sickle hemoglobin as S. A man with sickle cell trait (genotype AS) marries a woman who is also sickle trait. What are their chances to have a child with sickle cell anemia (genotype SS)?

(A)	100%	(D)	25%
(B)	75%	(E)	Less than 1%
(C)	50%		

Match the following questions with one or more correct answers:

Questions 1.5–1.7. A man learns that he has an abnormal allele Z for a particular type of liver disease that is extremely rare in the general population. If his genotype is Zz, what are the chances for the following relatives to have the Z allele? Assume that no mutations have occurred.

(A)	3/4	(D)	1/8
(B)	1/2	(E)	1/16
(C)	1/4		

1.5. His son

1.6. His first cousin

1.7. His grandson

For the following questions, draw the pedigrees, derive genotypes or probabilities for different genotypes in probands and their primary relatives (sibs, parents), and calculate recurrence risks as specified:

1.8. A couple brings their son and younger daughter for evaluation because of possible cystic fibrosis (219700) and request genetic counseling. Review of the sweat test results show that their son is affected and their daughter is normal. The father of these children has one sister and the mother has one brother. The paternal grandmother and the maternal grandmother are sisters and the only children of the great-grandparents. A person affected with cystic fibrosis has two abnormal alleles (genotype cc), while normal people have genotypes Cc or CC.

1.9. A 23-year-old woman and her fiancee request genetic counseling regarding a family history of brittle bones. The woman has blue sclerae, deafness, and a history during childhood of more than 30 fractures, which ceased after puberty. This description and her Xrays suggest the bone disease called osteogenesis imperfecta (166200), which occurs in individuals with an Oo genotype but not those with an oo genotype (see Fig. 1.4*B*). The woman's mother also had blue sclerae and fractures as a child, as did her maternal grandfather. She had one brother who presented in childhood from multiple fractures, and another brother who has no medical problems. Her sister had a mental breakdown, and a sister of her father had Down syndrome.

Respond to the following question with a short answer:

1.10. A middle-aged couple brings their 22-year-old daughter to clinic for reproductive counseling. The daughter has been mildly mentally retarded since childhood, with an overall IQ estimated at 70. She has graduated from special education high school and is currently working as a janitor and living with her parents. Although she has three normal siblings and the family history reveals no other family members with mental retardation, the parents have been told that the mental retardation is genetic and wish you to perform a tubal ligation on their daughter so that she will not have mentally retarded children. What genetic and ethical issues should be considered in your response?

PROBLEM SET 1
Answers

	1.3. C	1.6. D
1.8.–1.10. See Solutions	1.2. D	1.5. B
	1.1. C	1.4. D	1.7. C

PROBLEM SET 1
Solutions

1.1. Specific recurrence risks cannot be given for general categories like mental retardation.

1.2. The paired alleles in diploid cells segregate during gametogenesis to produce eggs or sperm with single alleles. Diploid individuals with genotype Aa will produce equal numbers of gametes with haploid genotype A and haploid genotype a.

1.3. The Punnett square in Fig. 1.8A illustrates the 50% probability for a Bb genotype in offspring.

1.4. The Punnett square in Fig. 1.8B illustrates the 25% probability that the offspring will have an SS genotype (sickle cell anemia).

1.5. to **1.7.** The segregation of diploid alleles implies that children, sibs, or parents have a 1/2 chance to possess an abnormal allele that is present in the individual. In Fig. 1.8C, the chances for individuals to have the abnormal Z allele are diagrammed on the pedigree. In Chapter 4, the chances of shared alleles are correlated with degrees of relationship.

1.8. The pedigree (Fig. 1.8D) shows that both parents have the Cc genotype with a 25% recur-

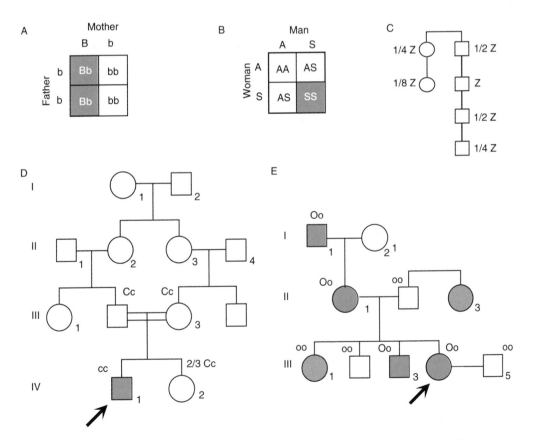

Figure 1.8. Answers for problems 1.3 (*A*), 1.4 (*B*), 1.5–1.7 (*C*), 1.8 (*D*), and 1.9 (*E*).

rence risk for cystic fibrosis in their next child. The normal sister has a 2/3 chance to be genotype Cc and a 1/3 chance to be genotype CC.

1.9. The pedigree (Fig. 1.8*E*) indicates that the proband (III-4) is affected with osteogenesis imperfecta (genotype Oo), so that her recurrence risk is 50%.

1.10. A first step in counseling would be to inform the parents that mental retardation is not always genetic. If the daughter did have a genetic form of mental retardation, her recurrence risks might be low. From the genetic perspective, more information about the disorder is required before assuming there is a high recurrence risk that justifies sterilization. From the ethical perspective, major issues are parentalism, informed consent, and beneficence. The woman is no longer a minor, and an involved process of establishing guardianship would be required for the parents to give legal consent for a sterilizing operation. Their parental authority must be balanced against autonomy for their daughter and her ability to give informed consent. The physician must also consider beneficence (protection from unwanted pregnancy, menstrual inconvenience) versus parentalism (compromise of patient autonomy, lack of informed consent). In most cases, permanent sterilization of minors or of persons with mental retardation is not performed.

BIBLIOGRAPHY

General References for Clinical Genetics

Ahronheim JC, Moreno J, Zuckerman ID. 1994. *Ethics in Clinical Practice.* New York: Little, Brown.

Beauchamp T, Childress J. 1994. *Principles of Biomedical Ethics,* 4th ed. New York: Oxford.

Gorlin RJ, Cohen MM Jr, Levin LS. 1990. *Syndromes of the Head and Neck,* New York: Oxford.

Jones KL. 1996. *Smith's Recognizable Patterns of Human Malformation.* Philadelphia: WB Saunders.

McKusick VA. 1994. *Mendelian Inheritance in Man,* 11th ed. Baltimore: Johns Hopkins; online at http://www3.ncbi.nlm.nih.gov/omim.

Reed S. 1980. *Counseling in Medical Genetics,* 3rd ed. New York: Alan R. Liss.

Rimoin DL, Emery AEH, Pyeritz R. 1995. *Principles and Practice of Medical Genetics.* Edinburgh: Churchill Livingstone.

Schinzel A. 1984. *Catalogue of Unbalanced Chromosome Aberrations,* 2nd ed. Berlin: de Gruyter.

Scriver CR, Beaudet AL, Sly WS, Valle D. 1995. *The Metabolic and Molecular Bases of Inherited Disease,* 7th ed. New York: McGraw-Hill.

Shepard TH. 1995. *Catalog of Teratogenic Agents.* Baltimore: Johns Hopkins University Press.

Strachan T, Read AP. 1996. *Human Molecular Genetics.* New York: Wiley-Liss.

Weaver DD. 1992. *Catalogue of Prenatally Diagnosed Conditions,* 2nd ed. Baltimore: Johns Hopkins University Press.

General Texts and Articles

Gould SJ. 1981. *The Mismeasure of Man.* New York: WW Norton.

Hartl DL. 1980. *Principles of Population Genetics.* Sunderland, MA: Sinauer Associates.

Müller-Hill B. 1988. *Murderous Science.* New York: Oxford University Press.

Murphy EA, Chase GA. 1975. *Principles of Genetic Counseling.* Chicago: Year Book Medical Publishers.

Reed S. 1980. *Counseling in Medical Genetics.* New York: Alan R. Liss. p.19.

Specific References

Cohen, MM Jr. 1987. The elephant man did not have neurofibromatosis. *Proc Greenwood Genet Center* 6:187–192.

Kushner HS. 1981. *When Bad Things Happen to Good People.* New York: Schocken Books.

Leonard CO, Chase GA, Childs B. 1972. Genetic counseling: A consumers view. *New Engl J Med* 287:433–439.

Parent S, Shevell M. 1998. The 'first to perish.' Child euthanasia and the Third Reich. *Arch Pediatr Adolesc Med* 152:79–86.

Support Organization for Trisomy 13, 18, & Related Disorders. 1989. *The Soft Touch.* September, vol. 11.

Stray-Gunderson K. 1986. *Babies With Down Syndrome. A New Parents Guide.* Baltimore: Woodbine House.

Wilson GN. 1992. The genomics of human dysmorphogenesis. *Am J Med Genet* 43: 187–196.

2

MENDELIAN INHERITANCE

■ LEARNING OBJECTIVES

1. Mendelian inheritance concerns alternative alleles at single genetic loci, while polygenic inheritance mechanisms concern alleles at multiple genetic loci.
2. Distinctive pedigree patterns are associated with autosomal dominant, autosomal recessive, X-linked dominant, and X-linked recessive inheritance.
3. The interpretation of pedigree information, together with knowledge of Mendelian inheritance mechanisms, allows the calculation of recurrence risks for family members.

■ 2.1. MENDELIAN PRINCIPLES AND THEIR CLINICAL APPLICATION

In the early 1900s, the laws of inheritance deduced by Mendel some 40 years earlier were applied to human disease. Alkaptonuria (203500), named for the black diapers caused by an abnormal metabolite in urine, and brachydactyly (112500), named for the shortened fingers of affected individuals, were among the first diseases explained by the same genetic "factors" that Mendel recognized in peas (see Fig. 2.1). Soon the classic Mendelian patterns of autosomal dominant, autosomal recessive, and X-linked recessive inheritance were defined. Although Mendel had not encountered X-linked inheritance in peas, his model by which traits were related to paired "factors" or alleles was readily extended to humans with one X versus two X chromosomes (i.e., males versus females).

Because Mendelian inheritance relates traits directly to transmission of alternative alleles at a genetic locus, recognition of a particular Mendelian pattern leads directly to recurrence risks. These two skills are the focus of this chapter: recognition of classical Mendelian patterns in pedigrees and, once recognized, prediction of recurrence risks for various members of the family. By using simple rules for pedigree recognition and probability, the health professional student can acquire sufficient knowledge to provide genetic counseling for more than 4000 human diseases that exhibit Mendelian inheritance. Each medical condition that may exhibit Mendelian inheritance is listed in the catalogue assembled by McKusick (1994), and the six-digit McKusick number is used here as a quick reference that allows the reader to access a brief summary about the dis-

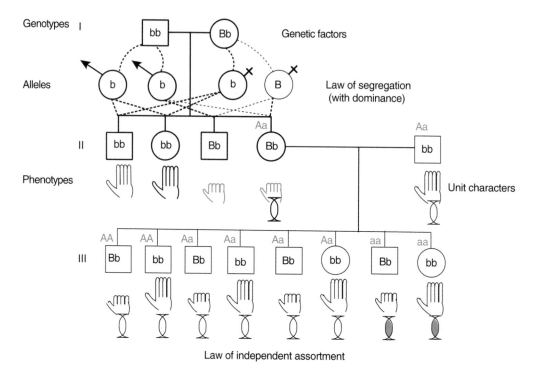

Figure 2.1. Mendel's insights. A hypothetical pedigree involving the traits brachydactyly (short fingers) and alkaptonuria (black urine) illustrates Mendel's concepts of genetic "factors" (genes), unit characters (traits), dominance, and the laws of segregation and dominance. The dominant brachydactyly trait requires the heterozygous Bb genotype for expression, while the recessive disease alkaptonuria (evidenced by ochronosis or black cartilage) requires a homozygous aa genotype for expression.

order. Mendel's classic experiments in peas serve as a reminder that Mendelian genetics has universal application to plants and animals and that its explanatory power extends beyond our particular focus on medicine.

In Figure 2.1, Mendel's insights (right of diagram) are reviewed using the examples of brachydactyly (112500) and alkaptonuria (203500) cited previously. Modern terminology (left of diagram) recognizes the Mendelian view that phenotypes depend on genotypes (pairs of alleles), and that segregation of alleles to reconstitute genotypes in offspring can explain ratios of particular traits. Brachydactyly is an example of dominance whereby one allele (B) can overide the action of its partner allele b. A normal man and brachydactylous woman (generation I in Fig. 2.1) will thus have a 1:1 ratio of brachydactylous and normal children (generation II in Fig. 2.1), reflecting seg-

regation of paternal B and b alleles. This segregation ratio translates to a 50% chance for each offspring of the couple to receive the B allele and have shortened fingers. In other words, there is a 50% recurrence risk for brachydactyly in each offspring of the brachydactylous parent.

Mendel also recognized that two genetic loci may segregate randomly with regard to their inheritance by offspring (law of independent assortment). Generations II and III in Figure 2.1 illustrate the independent segregation of brachydactyly (B, b) and alkaptonuria (A, a) alleles to produce offspring with various phenotypes. Those who receive two copies of the recessive a allele at the alkaptonuria locus will have black urine and black cartilage as shown in the diagram; those who receive the dominant B allele will have short fingers. Independence of the brachydactyly and alkaptonuria alleles is demonstrated by the random combination of these phenotypes in generation III offspring. An exception to independent assortment occurs if the two loci are located close together on the chromosome and exhibit genetic linkage. Mendel was unaware of this possibility and was fortunate to choose pea traits that were controlled by loci on separate pea chromosomes.

The British physicians Julia Bell and Archibald Garrod who demonstrated the Mendelian inheritance of brachydactyly and alkaptonuria catalyzed an enormous surge of activity involving the recognition of Mendelian diseases. As with many trends, almost every phenotype was then assumed to be Mendelian, a fallacy that led to the eugenics movement early in the twentieth century. Only later would it be realized that many phenotypes are caused by the interaction of multiple genes and the environment (multifactorial determination, see Chapter 3) rather than the single "factors" recognized by Mendel.

■ 2.2. AUTOSOMAL DOMINANT INHERITANCE

Case 2A: A Child with Heart Disease
A 5-year-old child (propositus in Fig. 2.2A) with a chest concavity, dislocated lenses of the eye, and a heart murmur is diagnosed with Marfan syndrome (154700). The family history (Fig. 2.2B) is normal for the mother, but shows numerous relatives with heart problems on the father's side. The father (individual III-2) is not unusually tall (5' 10″) and has no eye or heart problems. However, the father's brother (individual III-1) developed aortic dilation and insufficiency at age 39, was 6' 5″ tall, and had a lean build with flat feet and inguinal hernias.

Diseases that can be attributed to the presence of one or more abnormal alleles at a single genetic locus exhibit Mendelian inheritance. A disease exhibits autosomal dominant inheritance when one abnormal allele at an au-

tosomal locus is sufficient to cause the disease phenotype. Note that autosomes denote chromosomes 1–22 that are paired in all somatic cells (see Chapter 7).

The basis of autosomal dominant inheritance is diagrammed in Figure 2.3. In Figure 2.3A, alternative D or d alleles are shown to reside at an equivalent position (locus) on the chromosome. Since the D locus is autosomal, each parent has a pair of chromosomes that segregate during meiosis to produce gametes containing D or d alleles. The possible genotypes in offspring that can be generated by joining of D or d gametes at fertilization are listed below the diagram in Figure 2.3A. Another way of visualizing the potential gametes in offspring is shown via the conventional pedigree diagram in Figure 2.3B. The presence of an abnormal trait (shaded symbol) is correlated with the presence of the abnormal D allele. Because each parent gives one of their paired autosomes to each child, a new pair of alleles is created with a Dd or dd genotype. The probability that this mating will produce an abnormal Dd genotype in an offspring is 50%, as can be directly visualized using the Punnett square (Fig. 2.3C). The Punnett square lists parental alleles on each side, allowing possible offspring genotypes to be entered within each portion of the square. The proportion expected for any one genotype (i.e., Dd) is then represented by its number of squares (2) relative to the total number (4 for 2 parents with 2 alleles, yielding a probability for Bb of 2/4 = 50%—Fig. 2.3C).

The ability of one abnormal allele at an autosomal locus to produce a medical illness is associated with a characteristic pedigree pattern shown in Figure 2.3B. Because individuals with abnormal alleles manifest the disease and have a high probability (50%) to transmit it, pedigrees involving autosomal dominant diseases exhibit a vertical pattern with approximately equal numbers of affected males and females. There is also transmission from affected males or females, with approximately equal numbers of affected or unaffected offspring. Unaffected individuals would not have

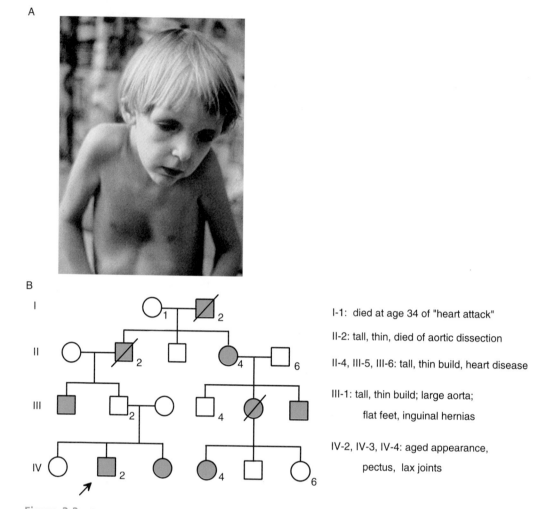

Figure 2.2. Case 3A. *A*, a 4-year-old child with Marfan syndrome illustrating the aged appearance, lax skin, and pectus. *B*, pedigree typical of autosomal dominant inheritance illustrating variable expressivity of the abnormal fibrillin allele that produces Marfan syndrome (154700).

abnormal alleles, so they should not transmit the disease. These characteristics of autosomal dominant inheritance are listed in Table 2.1.

As with most rules, exceptions to these generalizations about autosomal dominant inheritance do occur and are listed in Figure 2.4. Prominent among them are individuals who transmit the disorder without being affected. If there is no sign or symptom of disease by all available measures, then these individuals are said to exhibit incomplete penetrance (Fig. 2.4A). Other individuals may exhibit mild symptoms of disease by comparison to rela-

tives with severe symptoms. Such families are said to show variable expression of the abnormal allele, and the overall phenomenon is known as variable expressivity (Fig. 2.4B). Spontaneous mutations also produce exceptions to the rule for autosomal dominant inheritance. Despite a long history of normal generations, a family member may be the first to have an autosomal dominant disease because one of their two alleles at a locus has mutated to become abnormal (Fig. 2.4C). Much less commonly, the mutation may occur during gametogenesis to produce a fraction of ova or

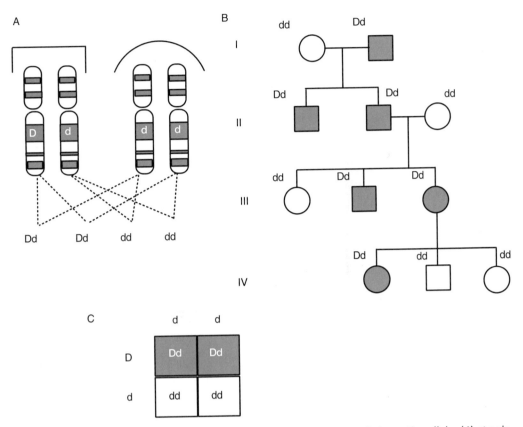

Figure 2.3. Autosomal dominant inheritance produced by segregation of alternative alleles (A) at a single autosomal locus (B) as predicted using a Punnett square (C).

sperm that carry the mutant allele. Individuals with germinal or germ-line mosaicism can thus be unaffected but have several affected offspring (Fig. 2.4D). The possibility that such individuals represent new mutations with incomplete penetrance can only be eliminated by direct analysis for the abnormal allele in germinal and somatic cells. Although germ-line

■ **TABLE 2.1.** Characteristics of Mendelian Inheritance Mechanisms

Characteristic	Autosomal Dominant	Autosomal Recessive	X-Linked Recessive
Pedigree pattern	Vertical	Horizontal	Oblique
Sex of affecteds	Males = Females	Males = Females	Males > > Females
Transmitted through	Affecteds, males or females	Carriers, males or females	Carrier females or affected males
Probability of transmission	50% for affecteds 0% for unaffecteds	25% for carrier parents	25% for carrier females 0% male to male
Associated phenomena	New mutations Germinal mosaicism Incomplete penetrance Variable expressivity	Consanguinity	New mutations Nonrandom X inactivation

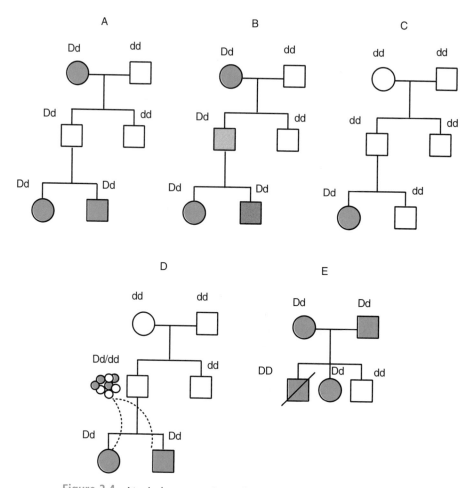

Figure 2.4. Atypical presentations of autosomal dominant inheritance.

mosaicism was assumed to be very rare, molecular analyses have demonstrated frequencies up to 6% in the case of unaffected parents and affected children with osteogenesis imperfecta (166200). Finally, there are rare occasions when two individuals with the same autosomal dominant disorder marry. They then have a 25% risk to transmit both abnormal alleles to offspring, producing a homozygous abnormal genotype (Fig. 2.4E). In most cases, as with the autosomal dominant disorder achondroplasia (100800), the homozygous abnormal individuals have more severe disease than do heterozygous affected individuals. Homozygosity for achondroplasia is lethal in the newborn period, and this concern is significant because matings of achondroplasts is more

common than imagined due to their participation in organizations such as Little People of America (see assortative mating in Chapter 4).

The usual and exceptional characteristics of autosomal dominant inheritance are combined in Table 2.1. It should be obvious that individual pedigrees like those in Figure 2.2B may not give sufficient evidence to conclude that a disorder exhibits autosomal dominant inheritance. Sometimes studies of multiple families are required to prove that a disorder exhibits autosomal dominant inheritance, and rare disorders may not provide enough patients to discriminate this inheritance pattern from other Mendelian or multifactorial mechanisms. It can be imagined that high rates of new mutations, the inability of affected individuals to reproduce, or large numbers of individuals with mild symptoms due to variable expressivity would hinder recognition of autosomal dominant inheritance. Recent application of molecular techniques has demonstrated that many sporadic disorders (i.e., those with no family history) are in fact new mutations that produce one abnormal allele at an autosomal locus. Often these mutations delete a copy of the gene from one autosome, a dominant mechanism known as *haploinsufficiency* (see Section 7.9). Additional examples of autosomal dominant inheritance are provided in the problems at the end of this chapter.

Case 2A Follow-up: Recognition that the child, father, and various paternal relatives have phenotypes that are variations on a theme establishes a vertical pedigree pattern with male-to-male transmission. Autosomal dominant inheritance with variable expressivity fits with the pedigree and with the established inheritance pattern for Marfan syndrome. A recurrence risk of 50% can then be provided to the parents of individual IV-2, even though the father exhibits incomplete penetrance without signs of Marfan syndrome (Fig. 2.2). Preventive management for affected individuals includes regular eye and heart examinations, with possible β-adrenergic antagonists (e.g., propranolol) for individuals with dilated aortas. DNA diagnosis is potentially available for Marfan syndrome, because it is caused by mutations in the fibrillin gene on chromosome 15 (see Section 11.4).

■ 2.3. AUTOSOMAL RECESSIVE INHERITANCE

Case 2B. A Family with Vision Loss
A 14-year-old boy is referred for genetic counseling because of an eye disorder known as retinitis pigmentosa (propositus in Fig. 2.5). He experienced deteriorating vision at age 10 and is now virtually blind. He has a younger brother, age 7, who has noted visual prob-

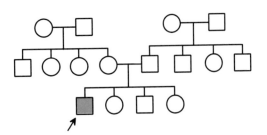

Figure 2.5. Case 3B pedigree illustrating autosomal recessive inheritance of retinitis pigmentosa (268000), a condition associated with blindness.

lems the past year. Two younger sisters, ages 8 and 3, and the rest of the family are normal. The parents ask their risk for future children to have retinitis pigmentosa, and their affected son's risk to transmit the disease. They also ask if they or their normal children are at risk to develop the disease.

Autosomal recessive inheritance implies that both alleles at a single genetic locus must be abnormal before there is expression of the disease trait. Figure 2.6 illustrates the usual circumstance of autosomal recessive inheritance where heterozygous Rr parents produce a homozygous rr offspring. In contrast to the uppercase letters used to represent dominant alleles, lowercase letters are used by convention to represent recessive alleles. The potential genotypes of offspring result from segregation of the parental chromosomes at meiosis, producing gametes with alleles R or r according to which chromosome is retained (Fig. 2.6A). The joining of gametes during fertilization restores the paired chromosomes, producing three possible genotypes in offspring (RR, Rr, or rr). The possible offspring genotypes are diagrammed under a conventional pedigree in Fig. 2.6B, and their probability of occurrence is shown by the Punnett square in Fig. 2.6C. Because each parent possesses one abnormal r allele at the locus but shows no abnormal findings, each is said to be a carrier. The probability that each carrier parent will transmit its abnormal r allele to offspring is 1/2, so the joint probability that an offspring will receive an r allele from each parent is 1/2 × 1/2 = 1/4. This 1/4 or 25% probability of genotype rr in off-

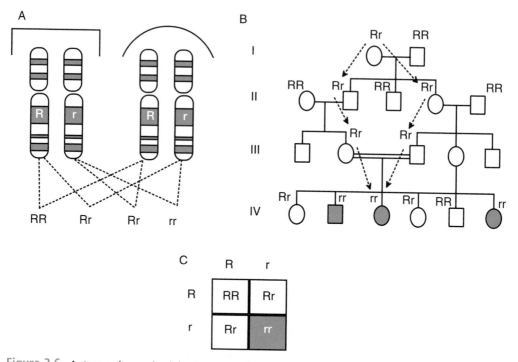

Figure 2.6. Autosomal recessive inheritance produced by segregation of normal allele R and abnormal allele r (A) at single autosomal locus (B) as predicted using a Punnett square (C).

spring can be directly visualized using the Punnett square (Fig. 2.6C).

Abnormal alleles are relatively rare in healthy populations, so the chance that two parents will share an abnormal allele is greatly enhanced if they are related. In Figure 2.6B, a typical pedigree exhibiting autosomal recessive inheritance is displayed with affected offspring deriving from parents who are first cousins. Parents who have common relatives are said to be consanguinous, and the general phenomenon of relatedness among mates is called inbreeding. As illustrated in Figure 2.6B, inbreeding provides more than one pathway for an abnormal allele r to be transmitted to a descendant. Consanguinity, symbolized by a double line in pedigrees, should alert the historian to the possibility of an autosomal recessive disorder.

Other characteristics of autosomal recessive inheritance include a horizontal pattern to the pedigree, affliction of both males and females, transmission by either males and females, and the 1/4 ratio of affected offspring to carrier parents (Fig. 2.6B, Table 2.1). Unusual presentations of autosomal recessive inheritance are summarized in Figure 2.7. In Figure 2.7A illustrates the rare circumstance where one parent may transmit both copies of a chromosome to offspring. If the chromosome bears an abnormal recessive allele, then the offspring will be homozygous abnormal and manifest the autosomal recessive phenotype (genotype rr in Fig. 2.7A). The transmission of two copies of the same chromosome from parent is called *uniparental disomy*, and it is thought to involve a trisomic zygote that corrects to two chromosomes by excluding that of one parent. In Figure 2.7A, two copies of the maternal chromosome with its abnormal allele r are retained, while the paternal chromosome with allele R has been excluded (see Chapter 10 for clinical examples of uniparental disomy).

Other unusual phenomena that fall under the rubric of autosomal recessive inheritance include compound heterozygotes and loss of

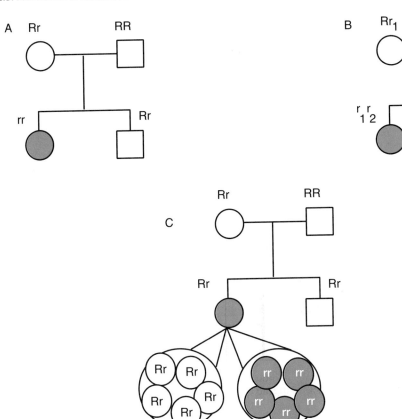

Figure 2.7. Atypical presentations of autosomal recessive inheritance.

heterozygosity. Compound heterozygotes (Fig. 2.7*B*) refer to individuals with recessive disorders that exhibit two different types of abnormal alleles. This distinction is important in understanding how the autosomal recessive disease has spread through the population (see Chapter 4). Loss of heterozygosity (Fig. 2.7*C*) refers to loss of the normal allele in certain somatic cells of an individual. Its significance was appreciated in cancer studies, where the normal allele R often has a tumor suppressor function. Loss of the normal allele through somatic mutation or chromosomal rearrangement removes constraints on growth-promoting genes in the tissue and allows it to proliferate into cancer.

Case 2B Follow-up: Review of the McKusick catalogue reveals that retinitis pig-mentosa may exhibit any of the Mendelian mechanisms of inheritance—autosomal recessive (268000), autosomal dominant (180100), and X-linked recessive (312650). The affected boy could have an X-linked recessive disease or represent a new mutation for autosomal dominant retinitis pigmentosa. His brother's visual symptoms provide the clue that two sibs may be affected, and this was confirmed by ophthalmologic examination. The likelihood of autosomal recessive inheritance is also supported by Archibald's law; this rule states that in the case of phenotypes exhibiting genetic heterogeneity (all three types of Mendelian inheritance), the most severe are likely to be autosomal recessive. The affected brothers display early onset of retinitis pigmentosa that would suggest autosomal recessive inheritance. The parental recurrence risk is now known to be 25% or 1 in 4, while that of the affected sons is low unless they marry a relative who is a carrier. Chapter 4 discusses a method for computing the unlikely chance of encountering a carrier in the general population.

■ 2.4. X-LINKED RECESSIVE INHERITANCE

Case 2C: A Man with Muscle Weakness
A 20-year-old man presents to his neurologist with weakness in his upper legs. A family history (Fig. 2.8) shows that his maternal grandfather had muscle weakness and died from heart disease; two male cousins on his mother's side have "muscular dystrophy" that developed in their late 20s. The man and his cousins wish to know their risks for having a child with muscular dystrophy.

X-linked inheritance has characteristics that reflect the different sex chromosomes in men and women. Because males have only one X chromosome and a Y chromosome that consists mostly of "junk" DNA, they are susceptible to the effects of an abnormal allele on the X chromosome. The presence of an abnormal al-

lele on the X chromosome in males, together with absence of a homologous copy on the Y chromosome, is termed *hemizygosity*. With two X chromosomes, women are less susceptible to abnormal alleles on one chromosome because they may be counterbalanced by normal alleles on the other X chromosome.

The most common form of X-linked inheritance involves recessive alleles. X-linked recessive inheritance is usually expressed in males due to their hemizygosity. Women who have one abnormal allele on their X chromosome can compensate with a normal allele on their other X chromosome; they are thus carriers of the abnormal allele but are unaffected with the disease trait (Fig. 2.9). The rule of transmission through females with affliction in males may produce an oblique pattern in the pedigree, as shown in Figure 2.9*B*.

Other characteristics of X-linked recessive inheritance include a lack of male-to-male transmission (males must transmit their Y chromosome to sons, not their X chromosome) and a 25% ratio of affected offspring from matings involving carrier women (see Table 2.1). As shown in the Punnett square (Fig. 2.9*C*), affected offspring are males, so risks can be modified according to whether male or female offspring are specified. Sons of carrier females

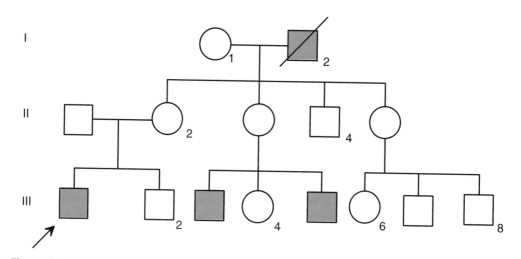

Figure 2.8. Case 3C pedigree illustrating X-linked recessive inheritance of Becker muscular dystrophy (310200).

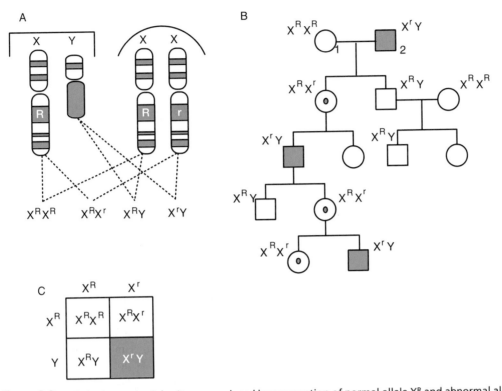

Figure 2.9. X-linked recessive inheritance produced by segregation of normal allele X^R and abnormal allele X^r (A) at a single sex chromosomal locus (B) as predicted using a Punnett square (C).

have a 50% chance to be affected; daughters of carrier females have a 50% chance to be carriers and zero chance to be affected.

Unusual presentations of X-linked inheritance are illustrated in Figure 2.10. In rare cases, a trait exhibits X-linked dominant inheritance where one abnormal allele is sufficient to cause the disease trait in heterozygous females. For many X-linked dominant diseases, the presence of the abnormal allele in hemizygous males produces a severe phenotype with lethality; the affected males often do not survive and present as spontaneous abortions (Fig. 2.10A). Examples of X-linked dominant disorders include incontinentia pigmenti (308300) with hair, teeth, and skin abnormalities, or chondrodysplasia punctata (302960) with hair, skin, and skeletal abnormalities. It is also important to realize that some X-linked recessive diseases exhibit mild disease manifestations in carrier females; the distinction between X-linked recessive and dominant is thus somewhat arbitrary and depends on the proportion of carrier females who exhibit findings and the severity of those findings.

Nonrandom X chromosome inactivation is another mechanism for producing symptoms in female carriers of X-linked diseases (Fig. 2.10B). Because two X chromosomes in females would produce a double dose of their encoded genes as compared to males, a mechanism for inactivating one of the X chromosomes in females has evolved. Female carriers of X-linked diseases are thus mosaic for cells expressing the normal X chromosome allele and those expressing the abnormal X chromosome allele. A hypothesis regarding X inactivation was formulated by Mary Lyon, (1961) who stated that the inactivation occurs at an early embryonic stage, is irreversible, and is random. Were X inactivation to occur at the 30-cell embryonic stage, then 15 cells would

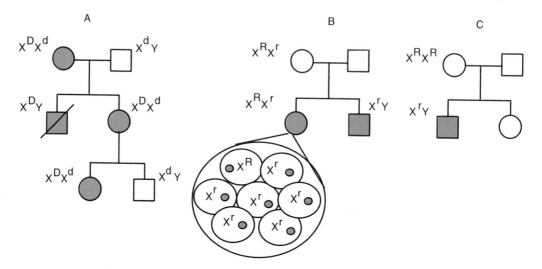

Figure 2.10. Atypical presentations of X-linked recessive inheritance.

inactivate one X chromosome and 15 the other. Every cell derived from these primordial cells will maintain this choice of inactivation, producing a 50/50 mix of cells in the average female. The exception occurs when there is bias for inactivation, such that the majority of cells inactivate a particular X chromosome. If the inactivated X chromosome happens to contain the normal allele, then the majority of tissues in that female will be deficient in the normal gene product and produce symptoms like those of an affected male. Figure 2.10*B* shows the different cells in cartoon form, with an excess of cells inactivating the X chromosome carrying the normal allele R. Such women would be likely to show partial expression of the X-linked recessive trait due to the high frequency of cells expressing the abnormal allele r.

A final exception in the rules for X-linked recessive inheritance occurs with new mutations. As with autosomal dominant inheritance, the expression of one abnormal allele in hemizygous males allows mutant individuals to have disease without inheriting it from their parent. This brings up an obvious dilemma when counseling families such as that depicted in Figure 2.10*C*. Unless additional family members provide evidence of heredity, the affected male could have inherited the X^r allele from his mother or developed it as a new mu-

tation. A simple rule for estimating the risk for mother being a carrier is to realize that mutations could occur on either of her X chromosomes or on the single X chromosome of her son. Mother thus has two of the three sites for potential mutation, and this translates to a 2/3 risk for mother to be a carrier in situations like that depicted in Figure 2.10*C*. Although the probability for new mutations actually increases with severity of an X-linked recessive disease (Haldane's law), the 2/3 carrier risk is a sufficient approximation for clinical situations.

Case 2C Follow-up: The oblique pattern of the pedigree and the affected males in Figure 2.8 clearly points to X-linked recessive inheritance. Becker dystrophy is known to be caused by milder alleles at the Duchenne muscular dystrophy locus (310200). Note that the proband's mother (II-2) is an obligate carrier as are her sisters (II-3, II-5) because they must have inherited the X chromosome with the abnormal Becker allele from their affected father. The unaffected daughters of individuals II-2 and II-5 have a 1/2 chance to be carriers and a 1/8 chance to have a child affected with Becker dystrophy. The affected males have a 1/2 chance that their daughters will be carriers, but cannot transmit the disease because their sons will not receive their X chromosome. Since Becker and Duchenne dystrophy are known to involve mutations in the dystrophin gene, DNA analysis to refine these risks or to perform prenatal diagnosis would be available (see Chapter 8).

■ 2.5. RISK CALCULATIONS FOR MENDELIAN DISORDERS

A prime ingredient in genetic counseling is the risk for genetic disease to occur in individuals and their family members. Sometimes these risks are general, such as those associated with increasing age of the prospective parent. More often the risk estimate concerns a disease that has already occurred in the family, in which case the family wants an estimate of *recurrence risk*. Couples often seek genetic counseling after having an affected child and wish to know the risk for future affected children as

well as the options for prenatal diagnosis and reproductive management. Figure 2.11 shows four sample pedigrees that illustrate the combined use of Mendelian principles, pedigree interpretation, and probabilities to calculate recurrence risks. A brief review of probabilities was presented in Chapter 1. Figure 2.12 illustrates how the methods for risk calculations apply to the pedigrees shown in Figure 2.11.

Risks When the Family History Is Normal (The Sporadic Case)

The pedigree shown in Figure 2.11A represents the most common dilemma in clinical practice: the sporadic case with a normal family history. Since the affected individual is male, it should be obvious that the three major Mendelian mechanisms could apply. The affected person could represent a new mutation for autosomal dominant or X-linked recessive disease, or the first incidence of autosomal recessive disease

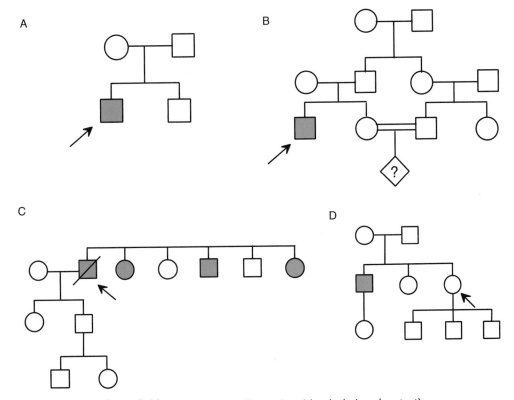

Figure 2.11. Pedigrees A–D illustrating risk calculations (see text)

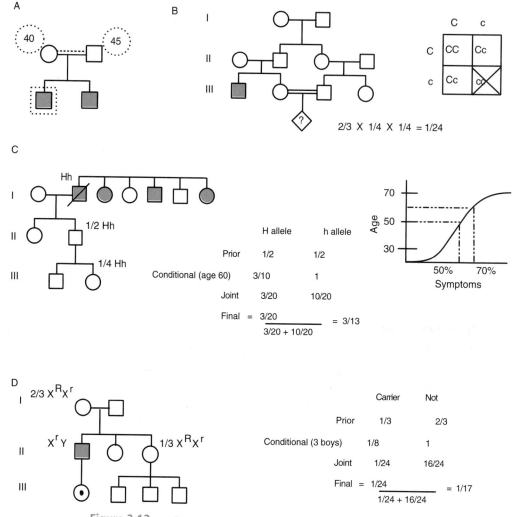

Figure 2.12. Pedigrees A–D illustrating solutions to risk calculations.

inherited from carrier parents. Other possibilities include multifactorial determination, as would be seen with many congenital anomalies (see Chapter 3), or a newly arising chromosomal disorder (see Chapter 7). The problem could also have nothing to do with genetics as many parents assume when they look back on their normal family history.

There are three ways in which a recurrence risk can be estimated in this situation with minimal family history. The first is to acquire additional information about factors that could point toward a particular mode of inheritance.

In Figure 2.12A, the pedigree is redrawn with potential factors such as consanguinity (autosomal recessive), advanced maternal age (chromosomal disease), or advanced paternal age (higher rate of new mutations consistent with an autosomal dominant trait). If none of these factors are helpful, then the disease in question may provide information if its inheritance mechanism is known. By using *Mendelian Inheritance in Man*, (1994) a first case of achondroplasia (100800—autosomal dominant implying a new mutation and low recurrence risk), cystic fibrosis (219700—autosomal recessive implying a 25% recurrence risk), or Duchenne muscular dystrophy (310200—X-linked recessive implying a 25% recurrence risk) would allow risk calculation based on a well-documented inheritance mechanism. If there were no obvious parental factors or known disease mechanisms to guide risk calculation, then a worst-case scenario could be assumed with a 25% recurrence risk. This information takes into account the possibility for autosomal or X-linked recessive disease without considering rare situations such as autosomal dominant disease with incomplete penetrance in one parent. The possibility of a 25% recurrence risk is important information for many families who have the all-or-none assumption about genetics: "It hasn't occurred in our family, therefore it can't be inherited."

Risks from Autosomal Recessive Diseases

Figure 2.11*B* shows a sample pedigree that might be encountered for an individual with an autosomal recessive disease like cystic fibrosis (219700). A consanguinous couple is expecting a child and wants to know the risk for the child to have cystic fibrosis based on the wife's affected brother (individual III-1). The steps in this risk calculation are displayed in Figure 2.12*B*. The wife's father (II-2) is an obligate carrier for cystic fibrosis (assuming correct paternity), yielding a 1/2 risk for his sister (II-3) and a $(1/2)(1/2) = 1/4$ risk for the husband (III-3) to be a carrier. These calculations recognize that primary relatives (parent-child, sibs) share 50% of their genes and thus have a 1/2 probability of sharing the abnormal allele c, as discussed in Chapter 1. The wife (III-1) has a 2/3 chance to be a carrier based on exclusion of the cc genotype that would cause her to have cystic fibrosis (see Punnett square). The risk for their prospective child to be affected (Fig. 2.12*B*) is then the joint probability of 2/3 (wife's chance to be carrier) $\times$ 1/4 (husband's chance to be carrier) $\times$ 1/4 (risk for child to be affected if both parents carriers).

Risks from Autosomal Dominant Diseases (Including Bayesian Methods)

Figure 2.11*C* illustrates a pedigree that represents a family with a neurologic disorder called Huntington chorea (143100). This disorder typically presents in middle age with unusual tremors and movements (chorea) followed by memory loss and neurodegeneration. Huntington chorea is known to exhibit autosomal dominant inheritance, so recurrence risks for relatives of affected individuals (II-1, II-2, III-1, and III-2 in Fig. 2.11*C*) are of prime importance. The risk calculations are straightforward as shown in Figure 2.12*C*, being $\times$ 1/2 for children and $1/2 \times 1/2 = 1/4$ for grandchildren of affected individuals to receive the abnormal H allele. However, a new type of risk calculation can be introduced that takes into account the *conditional* information supplied by the pedigree. This approach is called Bayesian counseling, and its elements are diagrammed in Figure 2.12*C*.

Because individual II-2 is unaffected with Huntington chorea, this conditional information affects the likelihood that he carries the abnormal H allele. The age of onset curve shown in Figure 2.12*C* indicates that 70% of 60-year-olds who were subsequently determined to have Huntington chorea exhibited symptoms by this age. The accompanying table in Figure 2.12*C* illustrates how this 30% conditional probability of having the Huntington allele without showing symptoms can affect the preexisting (*a priori*) recurrence risk for individual II-2. His 3/13 recurrence risk then impacts the risks for his children, reducing them from 1/4 to 2/26 or less than 1/5. The children are not old enough for their age to influence recurrence risk using the onset curve in Figure 2.12*C*.

Risks from X-Linked Recessive Diseases (Including Bayesian Methods)

Figure 2.11*D* provides an example of risk calculation for X-linked disorders that takes into account conditional information from the number of male offspring. Individual II-1 might have hemophilia A (306700), a disorder with chronic bleeding that often presents after circumcision in the neonatal period. The ability to manufacture factor VIII, the blood protein involved in the coagulation cascade, has allowed treatment of hemophiliacs with restoration of normal function to many. Nevertheless, risks from blood products and limitations on physical activity enforced by this disease make recurrence risks of great concern to relatives.

The first issue for risk calculation is to remember that the proband's mother (I-1) has a 2/3 chance to be a carrier provided she has no other affected relatives (Fig. 2.12D). The proband's daughter (III-1) is an obligate carrier since she must have received her father's X chromosome to be female. One sister (II-2) has no children and will have a 1/2 × 2/3 = 1/3 chance to be a carrier and a 1/12 chance that each child will have hemophilia. The other sister (III-3) has provided some conditional information by having three normal sons. The table (Fig. 2.12D) illustrates how her 1/8 chance for three normal sons if she were a carrier can be used in a Bayesian calculation to lower her carrier risk to 1/17 and her risk for the next child to have hemophilia to 1/68 (compared to 1/12 if her normal sons were not taken into account). Although rarely needed in medical genetic counseling, Bayesian probability is a useful concept that has wide application in medicine. Diagnostic decisions often use Bayesian reasoning, i.e., to render a tumor unlikely based on the degree of firmness or an X-ray shadow, even though it may not be explicitly recognized.

■ 2.6. FROM GENETIC DIAGNOSIS TO GENE ISOLATION (A PREVIEW)

In this chapter and in Chapter 1, genetic loci have been treated as theoretical entities much like Mendel's "factors" in his pioneering experiments with peas. It is important to realize that risk calculations such as those employed in Figures 2.11 and 2.12 are now being supplemented by direct DNA analysis to determine whether individuals inherit normal versus abnormal alleles. As a preview to later chapters on molecular genetics, a powerful example is given showing how Mendelian inheritance can lead to gene isolation, using two clinical examples in this chapter—achondroplasia (100800) and Huntington chorea (143100). Large families with Huntington chorea were available because of its late onset, allowing gene mapping studies that localized this gene to the tip of the short arm of chromosome 4 (Fig. 2.13). Families with achondroplasia rarely provided the multiple generations that facilitate gene mapping, but investigators soon localized the achondroplasia gene to the same region of chromosome 4. Now the extensive information on DNA in this region gleaned from studies of Huntington disease allowed the rapid selection of a candidate gene for achondroplasia—the fibroblast growth factor receptor-3 (FGFR3) gene. Because achondroplasia was known to affect the bone cartilage, genes like FGFR3 that were known to regulate connective tissue were obvious candidates. Spurred on by the correlation of location with a potential physiologic role, scrutiny of the FGFR3 DNA sequence quickly revealed mutations in individuals with achondroplasia. As shown in Figure 2.13, these mutations could be used to confirm the diagnosis in people with dwarfism and possible achondroplasia, as well as to provide prenatal diagnosis for interested families. In addition, the FGFR3 gene was added to several genes known to influence bone growth and expanded knowledge of this important subject. In vitro studies of bone growth to aid victims of trauma or osteoporosis (bone weakening that occurs with aging) thus are enhanced by knowledge of important molecules from Mendelian disorders. Figure 2.13 illustrates how medical genetics, the genome project to isolate all human genes, and knowledge of bone physiology are united in progress that will one day enhance treatment of fractures, degenerative arthritis, and growth disorders.

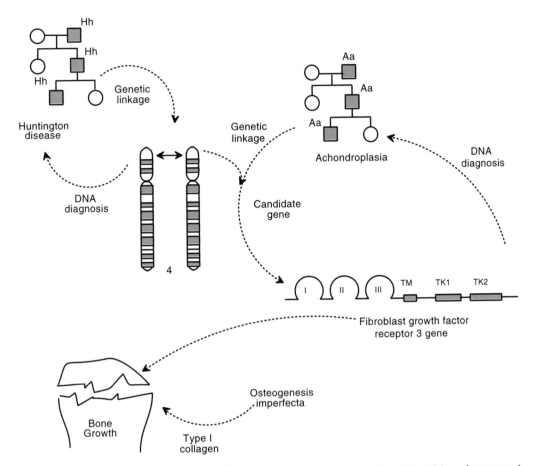

Figure 2.13. The route from Mendelian inheritance to gene characterization. Recognition of autosomal dominant inheritance of achondroplasia (left panel) allowed mapping of the responsible locus to the short arm of chromosome 4 (middle panel). Characterization of numerous genes in the 4p region had been performed because of interest in Huntington chorea, allowing election of the candidate fibroblast growth factor receptor 3 (FGFR3) locus as the achondroplasia gene through characterization of FGFR3 mutations in achondroplastic individuals. The function of specific regions in the FGFR3 gene (Ig, immunoglobulin motifs, TM, transmembrane domain, TK, tyrosine kinase domains) can then be derived by the impact of mutations in those regions. Through its association with skeletal dysplasia, the FGFR3 gene product joins others like type I collagen that are known to be important for bone growth.

PROBLEM SET 2
Mendelian Inheritance

These problems stress the principles of Mendelian inheritance, the interpretation of inheritance mechanisms from pedigrees, and the estimation of risks based on degrees of relationship and inheritance mechanisms. Mendelian principles are also explored in the more clinically oriented problem sets of Chapters 11–16.

2.1. An affected male infant born to normal parents could be an example of all the following disorders except:

   (A) an autosomal dominant disorder
   (B) an autosomal recessive disorder
   (C) a polygenic disorder
   (D) a vertically transmitted disorder
   (E) an X-linked recessive disorder

For the clinical situations, provide genetic counseling and recurrence risk information.

2.2. A couple request genetic counseling because of their family history of Norrie disease (310600; Fig. 2.14A). Norrie disease causes blindness and mental retardation. They wish to know the risk that their next child will be affected, and whether knowledge of the fetal sex would influence the recurrence risk.

2.3. A man and woman with autosomal dominant achondroplasia are planning to marry and request genetic counseling for their chances to have average-sized versus achondroplastic children. They prefer that their children have achondroplasia, but fear the homozygous lethal form of disease. The woman lost a brother to this condition (Fig. 2.14B). In addition to their recurrence risks, comment on their perspective regarding an abnormal child.

2.4. A woman with autosomal recessive sickle cell anemia has heard that the disease skips generations. She is married to her first cousin,

and wants confirmation that they have a negligible risk to have sickle cell anemia.

2.5. A woman requests genetic counseling for color blindness, questioning specifically the risks for her sons and for her daughters. Her father is color-blind, and she has heard that it is an X-linked recessive disease. Her husband has normal vision.

2.6. The pedigree shown in Figure 2.14C was taken for a family with autosomal dominant ichthyosis (146800), a disease with fishlike skin. Individual IV-4 (proband) requests genetic counseling regarding her risks for affected children.

2.7. A couple from a remote Scandinavian settlement request genetic counseling because of relatives with mental retardation. Both affected relatives are male, and they exhibit striking similarity in appearance. The couple are re-

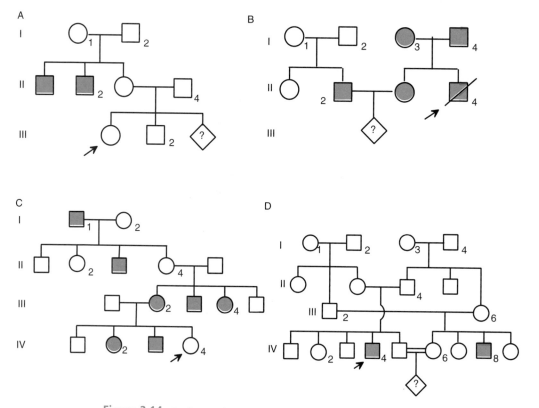

Figure 2.14. Pedigrees for problems 2.2 (A), 2.3 (B), 2.6 (C), 2.7 (D).

lated, and the two sets of potential grandparents are sibs (Fig. 2.14*D*). They recognize that definitive information may not be available, but wish to know the highest probability for mental retardation in their offspring.

2.8. A man has two sibs with small head size (microcephaly), which in severe forms (251200) may exhibit autosomal recessive inheritance. He has married his first cousin, which increases his concern about the recurrence risk for their children. The man is the fourth in his sibship, with the firstborn male affected, the second born female unaffected, and the third born female affected with microcephaly. His parents are normal, but his mother is a sib of his wife's mother who is an identical twin. He and his wife's common grandparents are normal, as are his wife's parents and his wife's brother and sister. Construct the pedigree and estimate the risk for the man's child to have microcephaly under the assumption of autosomal recessive inheritance.

2.9. A couple request genetic counseling because the wife's brother has hemophilia A (306700), an X-linked recessive disorder. The wife was the third child after a normal sister and the affected brother. Her parents are normal, as are her husband and his family. The couple have had two normal sons, and fear that their third child is due for the hemophilia gene. Construct the pedigree and estimate their recurrence risk.

2.10. A woman requests counseling because her brother, mother, and deceased grandfather all have Ehlers-Danlos syndrome type IV (130050), an autosomal dominant condition with loose connective tissue that can cause dilated blood vessels (aneurysms). The woman's maternal grandfather died from this disease, but her maternal grandmother was normal. Her mother's fraternal twin brother is unaffected, and they were the first two of four children. The woman is third born after a normal sister and her affected brother. Each of the latter individuals have two children. The woman has no symptoms of Ehlers-Danlos IV, and she has read that 90% of affected individuals will show

symptoms by her age of 35. She and her normal husband have postponed having children, but she is now considering a last chance at reproduction. Construct the pedigree and calculate both her risk for an affected child and that of her affected brother.

PROBLEM SET 2
Answers

2.10. The risk for the woman to have a child with Ehlers-Danlos syndrome type IV is 1/22, that for her affected brother 1/2.

2.9. The risk for the next child to have hemophilia A is 1/5.

2.8. The risk for microcephaly is 1/24.

2.7. Risk for mental retardation is 1/9.

2.6. The risk for ichthyosis is virtually 0.

2.5. Risk for color blindness in sons 1/2, for daughters virtually 0.

2.4. Risk for sickle cell anemia 1/8.

2.3. Risk for achondroplasia 3/4 with 1/3 of affected infants being homozygous. Less burden for achondroplasia with affected parents.

2.2. Risk for Norrie disease 1/8; 1/4 for sons, 0 for daughters

2.1. D

PROBLEM SET 2
Solutions

2.1. A sporadic case (i.e., without a family history) is by definition not an example of vertical transmission (i.e., transmission from one generation down to the next). The other listed inheritance mechanisms could all apply, as well as chromosomal disorders that can present as a de novo (new) rearrangement. The index case without a family history is a common dilemma in genetic counseling, because the lack of obvious familial transmission by no means excludes a genetic etiology.

2.2. The solution requires recognition that the grandmother (individual I-1 in Fig. 2.14*A*) is an obligate carrier because of two affected sons. Her daughter (II-3) as a 1/2 chance to be a carrier and thus a 1/8 chance for the next child to be affected. Norrie disease is X-linked recessive, so the risk is 1/4 if it is known that the baby is male, and virtually 0 if it is known that the baby is female.

2.3. Two affected parents with achondroplasia can be represented by genotypes Aa as shown in the Punnett square (Fig. 2.15*A*). Only 1 in 4 offspring will be normal (genotype aa), while 3 of 4 will have at least one A allele and present with achondroplasia. Of these achondroplastic offspring, 1 in 3 will be homozygous AA and have the lethal form of disease. The couple have a different perspective from parents without dwarfism, since the burden of a child with achondroplasia is less than the burden of accommodating an average-sized child into their modified lifestyle.

2.4. The genotype of the affected woman with sickle cell anemia must be SS, and both her parents must be AS carriers (sickle trait—Fig. 2.15*B*). Because her husband's parent is a sib to her parent, the husband's parent has a 1/2 chance to be AS and the husband has a 1/4 chance to be AS. The child will have a 1/8 chance to receive the S allele from his father and a 100%

chance to receive it from his SS mother, resulting in an overall risk of 1/8.

2.5. The woman's father is color-blind, giving her a 100% chance to receive his X chromosome with the abnormal allele (obligate carrier). She then has an overall 1/4 risk that each child will be color-blind, with a 1/2 chance for boys and a virtually 0 chance for girls to be affected.

2.6. Autosomal dominant inheritance is suggested by the pedigree because of its vertical pattern and the presence of affected males and females. The woman is unaffected, so she presumably did not receive the abnormal allele from her affected mother. She cannot transmit the disease, and the chance of a new mutation in her offspring is minimal. Although she could be an example of incomplete penetrance or germinal mosaicism, these are rare possibilities that explain the use of "virtually 0" in practice rather than "0."

2.7. The presence of consanguinity (double line in pedigree) in Figure 2.14*D* is a red flag

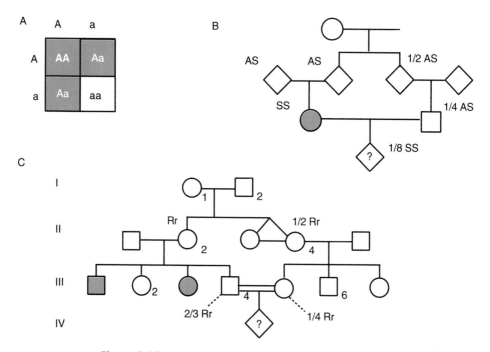

Figure 2.15. Solutions for problems 2.3 (*A*), 2.4 (*B*), 2.8 (*C*).

for autosomal recessive inheritance, and in this case one set of sibs has married another. Because each member of the couple has an affected sib, they each have a 2/3 chance to be a carrier. Given that they are carriers, there is a further 1/2 chance for each that they will transmit their abnormal allele, producing a risk of $2/3 \times 1/2 \times 2/3 \times 1/2 = 1/9$ for their prospective child to have this recessive form of mental retardation.

2.8. The pedigree in Figure 2.15C illustrates the man's two affected sibs, giving him a 2/3 risk to be a carrier for the allele causing microcephaly. His mother is an obligate carrier, so his wife's mother has a 1/2 chance to be a carrier and his wife a 1/4 chance. The chance for an affected child is thus $2/3 \times 1/4 \times 1/4 = 1/24$.

2.9. The pedigree in Figure 2.16A shows the wife's affected brother and her two normal sons, which provide conditional information to use in a Bayesian risk estimate. The table in Figure 2.16A illustrates that the condition of two normal sons lowers the woman's a priori risk to be a carrier (1/2) to 1/8, resulting in a final risk of 1/5.

2.10. The pedigree in Figure 2.16B illustrates the affected grandfather and brother of the woman, making her at 50% risk to have received the abnormal allele. The table shows how her lack of symptoms at age 35 years can be used as a condition that predicts a 10% chance to have the abnormal allele H. Her final risk to have the abnormal allele is then 1/11, and her risk to have an affected child 1/22. Her

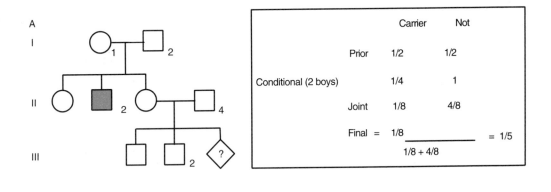

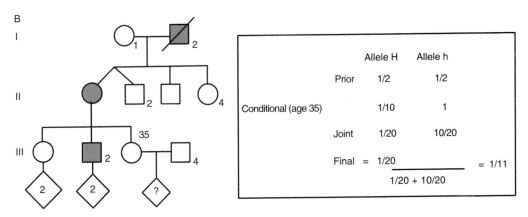

Figure 2.16. Solutions for problems 2.9 (A) and 2.10 (B).

brother is known to be affected, conferring a 1/2 risk for each of his children to be affected.

BIBLIOGRAPHY

McKusick VA. 1994. *Mendelian Inheritance in Man,* 11th ed. Baltimore: Johns Hopkins; on-line at http//:www3.ncbi.nlm.nih.gov/omim.

Lyon M. 1961. Gene action in the X chromosome of the mouse (*Mus Muscullus*). Nature 190: 372–3.

3

MULTIFACTORIAL DETERMINATION AND THE GENETICS OF COMMON DISEASES

■ LEARNING OBJECTIVES

1. Polygenic inheritance involves the interaction of alleles at several loci to produce a phenotype.
2. Multifactorial determination refers to the interaction of genes and environment to produce a phenotype.
3. Multifactorial determination may produce continuous (quantitative) phenotypes like blood pressure or, with thresholds, produce discontinuous (qualitative) phenotypes like cleft palate.
4. Knowledge of multifactorial determination plus genetic relationships allows the estimation of empiric recurrence risks.
5. Knowledge of multifactorial determination promotes the concept of heritability and introduces the use of risk factors for the prevention of common diseases.

Case 3: A Newborn with Cleft Lip and Palate

A child with cleft lip and palate (Fig. 3.1) is born to a 29-year-old mother with juvenile di-

abetes mellitus. The mother is familiar with this anomaly because her sister had cleft lip and palate. Review of the family history reveals no evidence for consanguinity or for other individuals with congenital anomalies. The mother also had a urinary tract infection in the second trimester and is concerned that antibiotics may have caused her child's anomaly.

■ 3.1. MULTIFACTORIAL TRAITS: GENES PLUS ENVIRONMENT

It is a logical step to move from single gene disorders to phenotypes that depend on the interaction of multiple alleles on several chromosomes. An example is the "tissue type" of an individual, which is a complex trait determined by *histocompatibility* and blood group antigens encoded by many different genetic loci. Because of interactions between these cell surface antigens and exposures to antigens from the environment, a person is more or less likely to develop diseases like ankylosing

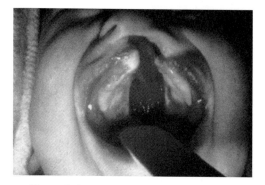

Figure 3.1. Child with cleft lip and palate.

spondylitis (arthritis of the spine), diabetes mellitus, *transfusion reaction,* transplant rejection, or a severe *hemolytic anemia* in her fetus. The interaction of multiple genes to determine a trait is called *polygenic inheritance,* and the interaction of multiple genes plus the environment is called *multifactorial determination.*

There are obviously two components to multifactorial disease: the several loci that interact to produce polygenic inheritance and the environmental factors that determine the consequences of this gene interaction. In other words, "genes propose, the environment disposes." Environment can certainly modify characteristics determined by single genes, exemplified by high rates of skin cancer in individuals with albinism (203100) and frequent sun exposure. However, environmental influence is often more evident for phenotypes gov-

erned by multiple loci. Starvation to delay growth, brain injury to depress intelligence, and stress to elevate blood pressure are examples of environmental influences on polygenic traits.

Common diseases like diabetes mellitus or schizophrenia often exhibit multifactorial determination (Table 3.1). A current emphasis of genetic medicine is the identification of genetic loci or environmental factors that are important predictors of these common diseases. These predisposing factors can then be used to identify high-risk individuals who can benefit from early treatment or prevention. Although genes are difficult to change, the modulation of environmental influences like diet, drugs, or exercise can produce dramatic health benefits.

■ 3.2. QUANTITATIVE TRAITS AND THE IDEA OF MULTIPLE GENETIC LOCI

Mendelian inheritance explains phenotypes that depend on the transmission of alleles at one genetic locus. Polygenic inheritance explains phenotypes that depend on alleles at multiple genetic loci—aggregates, in a sense, of Mendelian effects. Three types of phenotypes are associated with polygenic inheritance: multifaceted or polymorphic, continuous or quantitative, and qualitative or discrete;

TABLE 3.1. Multifactorial Disorders in the United States

Disorder or Category	Cause of Death *(rank)*	Prevalence *(% population)*	Numbers Affected *(millions)*	Hereditability (Genetic risk factors) *(high ++++ to low +)*[a]
Heart disease	1	3	7	+++ (Cholesterol uptake)
Cancer	2	5	6	+++ (Oncogenes)
Stroke	3	<1	0.6	+ (Cholesterol, blood clotting)
Accidents	4	<1	3	+ (Alcohol and drug use)
Diabetes mellitus	7–8	4	11	+++ (Insulin secretion, action)
Suicide	8–9	<1	0.1	+ (Schizophrenia, alcoholism)
Congenital anomalies[b]	9–10	5	3	+++ (Developmental genes)

[a]Approximate scale: ++++ (100% of predisposition due to genetic factors as for Mendelian disorders) to + (20% of predisposition due to genetic factors).

[b]Ranks first for neonatal causes of death.

qualitative and quantitative traits were contrasted in Figure 1.3. Figure 3.2 illustrates how the interaction of alleles at several loci might account for a multifaceted phenotype like eye color. In Figure 3.2*A*, genotype aa at a single locus blocks melanin formation and produces the pink, colorless iris of people with albinism. Albinism (203100, 203200) exhibits autosomal recessive inheritance, with genotypes AA or Aa producing sufficient melanin to produce eye color. In Figure 3.2*B*, the hypothetical loci B and C interact with locus A to produce five possible phenotypes (shades) for eye color. Polygenic inheritance has been demonstrated for many types of eye, skin, or coat color in animals, but the responsible genetic loci are rarely known. The different colors are examples of a polymorphic trait, with various color states produced by different combinations of polygenic alleles.

Another type of character associated with polygenic inheritance is continuous or quantitative, exemplified by height or blood pressure. Rather than the discontinuous traits of eye color (e.g., blue, hazel, brown), quantitative traits exhibit a range of values (e.g., weights of 68.3, 69.8, or 70 kg or the range of values for interpupillary distance illustrated in Figure 1.3). Within biologic populations, continuous traits often fall along a bell-shaped curve that depends on two factors: a mean value and the extent of variation about the mean (statistically known as the standard deviation). Figure 3.3 contrasts the discrete heights produced by alleles at the achondroplasia locus (100800) with a hypothetical curve generated by alternative genotypes at two loci. Figure 3.3*A* shows the bimodal phenotypes of average-sized (genotype aa) and little people (genotype AA), while Figure 3.3*B* illustrates the continuous range of stature that is standard in human populations. Note that the normal distribution exhibited by height in Figure 3.3*B* might be produced by five combinations of alleles at two loci for stature. In fact, the number of loci that interact with the environment to determine stature are unknown but undoubtedly large.

Note in Figure 3.3 that the mutant allele for achondroplasia truncates the continuous distribution of stature, just as the variable facets of eye color are ablated by albinism (Fig. 3.2). The gene causing achondroplasia is that for the fibroblast growth factor receptor-3 (see Section 2.6). Once identified as a locus with major effect on stature, this growth factor receptor gene becomes an interesting candidate for one of the many factors that contribute to the normal height distribution shown in Figure 3.3*B*. The discovery of such major loci is a focus of modern research on quantitative traits and multifactorial determination, illustrated by the discovery of elevated cholesterol and low-density lipoprotein (LDL) receptor mutations as predisposing factors for coronary artery disease (see Chapter 5).

Although the ability of single mutant alleles to produce qualitative phenotypes like "normal" versus "dwarfism" may be illustrated (Fig. 3.3), the ability of polygenic/multifactorial interaction to produce alternative pheno-

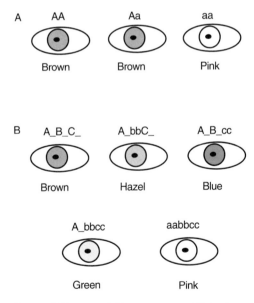

Figure 3.2. Mendelian versus multiple locus (polygenic) determination of eye color. Alleles at the locus for albinism determine whether eye color is present, and alleles at locus B or C could modify color intensity. The latter loci are theoretical, because the alleles governing eye color have not been identified.

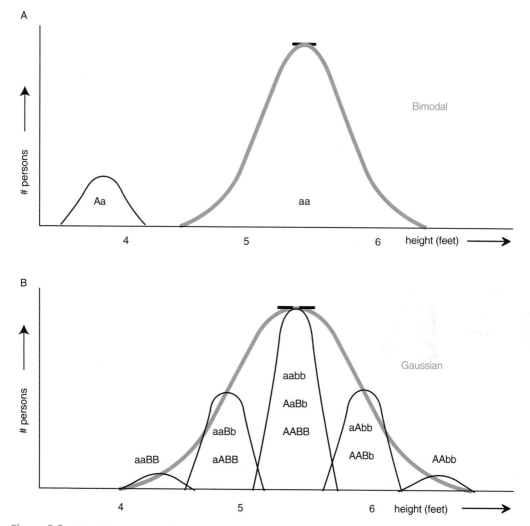

Figure 3.3. Mendelian versus polygenic determination of height. *A*, Bimodal distribution of normal and short stature (dwarfism) caused by alleles at a single locus (e.g., achondroplasia 100800). *B*, Gaussian distribution in normal population derived from alleles at two theoretical loci.

types requires the concept of threshold. Figure 3.4 shows how a threshold can operate to convert a normal distribution like that for height into a dichotomy of tall versus short. A useful analogy for the concept of genetic predisposition with threshold is that by Dr. Michael Brown of the University of Texas Southwestern Medical Center who lectures about the bruised forehead syndrome. If the statutory height of door jambs were lowered from almost 8 to 6^{1}/$_{2}$ feet, then one might see a new medical condition called the "bruised forehead

syndrome." The disorder would occur rarely in average-sized families (left distribution in Fig. 3.4), but would reach epidemic proportions in tall families (right distribution in Fig. 3.4). The threshold, literally a door jamb, converts a continuous height distribution in these families into two phenotypes: bruised (over 6^{1}/$_{2}$ feet) or normal (under 6^{1}/$_{2}$ feet). Proportionally more individuals from genetically predisposed (tall) families will have the bruised forehead phenotype (shaded area in Fig. 3.4), even though the threshold (6^{1}/$_{2}$ feet) remains the same.

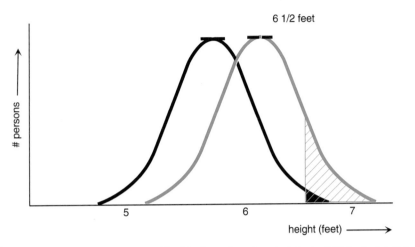

Figure 3.4. The threshold concept exemplified by lowering door height to 6½ feet. A tall family will have more alleles predisposing to tall stature, with the result that more individuals cross the threshold to present with bruised forehead syndrome.

Note that one could estimate risks for an individual to develop the bruised forehead syndrome before they crossed through a door. Such risk estimates would depend on genetic factors (e.g., parental heights) and environmental factors (e.g., nutrition). Other factors, termed *associations* could be defined such as clothes labels from stores for taller men. These labels would not be causative themselves, but would be associated with bruised forehead syndrome through the behaviors of tall individuals. Analogous research for associations, identified as genetic or environmental factors, is one avenue for defining risk factors in multifactorial diseases.

■ 3.3. SETTING THE THRESHOLD FOR MULTIFACTORIAL DISEASE: HEREDITY AND ENVIRONMENT

The use of thresholds to convert a continuous distribution into a bimodal or discontinuous phenotype can be used to explain the inheritance of congenital anomalies. Recurrence risks for congenital anomalies like cleft palate can be estimated from surveys that tabulate how often a parent with cleft palate has an affected child. These *empiric risks* can be explained by postulating a threshold level that separates individuals with and without anomalies. In the case of cleft palate, a continuous distribution for individual liability is transformed into a yes/no decision for clefting as shown in Figure 3.5.

The influence of heredity on the incidence of cleft palate is readily appreciated from the data in Table 3.2. Figure 3.5 illustrates how affected relatives can increase the liability for cleft palate in the presence of a fixed threshold. Assume that three loci X, Y, and Z are involved in the polygenic inheritance of cleft palate and that abnormal alleles x, y, and z must occur at each locus to produce cleft palate. If the abnormal alleles each occur in 10% of the population, then the general frequency of cleft palate would be 1 in 1000 (people with genotype x-/y-/z- = 0.1^3). In Figure 3.5A, this 1/1000 frequency is represented by the shaded region to the right of the cleft palate threshold (T1).

In Figure 3.5B, children (first-degree relatives) of individuals with cleft palate are depicted. With the same threshold, genotype a-/b-/c- is again required to produce cleft palate, but its frequency increases to 1 in 8 ($1/2^3$) because each abnormal allele has a 1/2 chance to be transmitted from the a-/b-/c- parent. By selecting first degree relatives of indi-

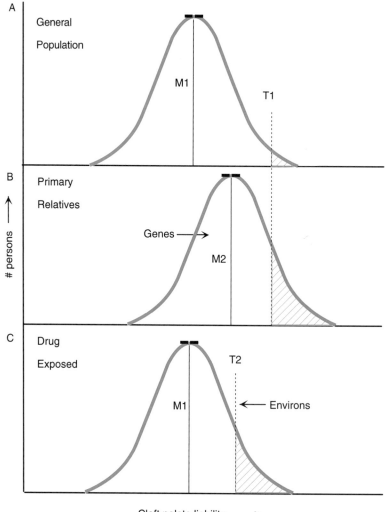

Figure 3.5. Genetics or environment can increase the likelihood for cleft palate. *A*, distribution of predisposition towards cleft palate in the general population; *B*, distribution in primary relatives of people with cleft palate as illustration genetic factors; *C*, distribution in offspring of mothers taking hydantoin as illustration of in utero environmental factor.

viduals with cleft palate, the distribution for cleft palate liability has shifted to the right, producing a much higher frequency of cleft palate (shaded area) in offspring of these individuals. The actual risk for offspring of individuals with cleft palate is 3–4%, representing a 30/40-fold increase over the incidence in the general population (Table 3.2). Figure 3.5*B* illustrates the role of polygenic inheritance in increasing cleft palate liability when environ-

mental factors (e.g., the threshold) remain the same.

Figure 3.5*C* illustrates the influence of environment in the multifactorial determination of cleft palate. Environmental factors are clearly demonstrated by studies of *monozygotic twins* who are genetically identical. For congenital anomalies like cleft palate, only 40% of identical twin pairs will share (be concordant for) the anomaly. The 60% of monozygotic twin pairs

■ TABLE 3.2. Empiric Recurrence Risks for Selected Congenital Anomalies

Disease	Identical Twins (%)	First-Degree Relatives (%)	Second-Degree Relatives (%)	Third-Degree Relatives (%)	General Population (%)
Pyloric stenosis	55–60	7.5	2.0	0.4	0.3
Cleft lip/palate	38–40	3–4[a]	0.7–0.8	0.3	0.1
Congenital heart disease	35–50	3–4	0.7	0.2	0.4–0.8
Club foot	30–32	2.5	0.5	0.2	0.1
Congenital hip dislocation	33	5	0.6	0.4	0.2

[a]If unilateral, but 7–8% if bilateral (more severe).

who are discordant for cleft palate must experience differences in the uterine environment, most likely due to differences in vascular supply. Figure 3.5*C* presents a hypothetical illustration of these environmental effects, shown as an alteration in the threshold. If a "lower" threshold (T2) for cleft palate is caused by altered uterine vascular supply, then the same distribution for cleft palate liability will result in more individuals with cleft palate.

Another example of altered threshold for cleft palate is produced by exposure to the drug Dilantin (phenytoin), which must be taken by some epileptic mothers to prevent convulsions during pregnancy. Offspring of mothers taking phenytoin during the first trimester of pregnancy have a pattern of anomalies called the fetal hydantoin syndrome that includes cleft palate. Adrenal corticosteroids have also been implicated in cleft palate by Fraser (1976), who used a mouse model to reveal factors like palatal width or tongue size that modify the threshold. Although knowledge of particular alleles or environmental factors that influence the thresholds for congenital anomalies may remain unknown, the multifactorial determination/threshold model rationalizes the empiric recurrence risks that have been derived for many congenital anomalies (see Table 3.2).

Case 3 Follow-up: The three- to five-fold increase of congenital anomalies in infants of diabetic mothers prompted consideration of diabetes as a factor in lowering the threshold for cleft palate in the infant pictured in Fig.

3.1. Infants of diabetic mothers may exhibit growth delay in the first trimester of pregnancy when the maternal diabetes is out of control. This early growth delay with its higher risk for congenital anomalies contrasts with the later growth increase precipitated by excess fetal insulin secretion. Poor diabetic control in the third trimester often produces a large, plethoric baby with alterations in blood glucose or calcium.

■ 3.4. GENETIC RELATIONSHIPS

As demonstrated in Figure 3.5*B*, the estimation of recurrence risks for multifactorial disorders is very dependent on genetic relationships. Because one-half of a parent's genetic material is transmitted to each offspring, the proximity to affected individuals will have a large effect on liability to multifactorial disease. In Figure 3.6, degrees of relationship are illustrated by reference to an affected individual or proband. Identical twins (individual III-2 in Fig. 3.6A) will have identical genes; they have a probability of 1 to share an abnormal allele. Children, parents, and siblings are first-degree or primary relatives with one-half of their genes in common. Grandparents, grandchildren, aunts, and uncles have one quarter of their genes in common with a propositus and are second-degree or secondary relatives. Great-grandparents, great-aunts or uncles, cousins, nephews and nieces have one eighth of their genes in common and are tertiary or third-degree rela-

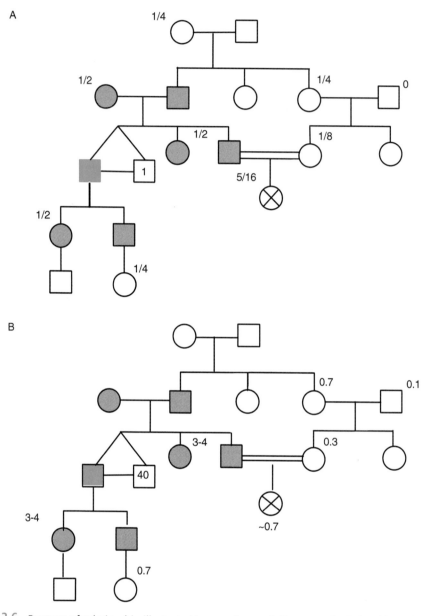

Figure 3.6. Degrees of relationship illustrated in a pedigree. *A*, Degrees of relationship and probabilities of sharing an abnormal allele r with the propositus; *B*, degrees of relationship and empiric recurrence risks for a disorder affecting the proband.

tives. The proportion of genes in common is also known as the *coefficient of relationship.* Rather than memorizing specific values, the coefficient of relationship can always be derived from the pedigree by including a factor of one-half for every generation between two individuals. An exception to the rule occurs with inbreeding or consanguinity, because ancestors are connected to offspring by more than one hereditary path (e.g., individual IV-3 in Fig. 3.6*A*).

The importance of relationship in genetic risk calculations can be illustrated by assuming the proband has a rare allele designated r. Examining Figure 3.6A once more, the chance is 1/2 that each primary relative has allele r and 1/4 for each secondary relative. These numbers ignore the possibility of multiple origins for allele r since it is rare and there is no inbreeding in this pedigree. If the propositus has an identical twin separated at birth, there would be a 100% chance that the twin has allele r. The chance would be 1/2 for a fraternal twin, 1/2 for a sibling, and 1/8 for a cousin.

If r were an allele causing severe disease in later life, like Huntington chorea, then these chances for allele sharing would have important implications for retirement and life insurance planning. Reasoning in the opposite direction, one might also use the sharing of allele r to determine the probability of relationship. This approach becomes powerful when there are many alleles at a locus (i.e., r1–r10) and is used in forensic medicine and paternity testing (see Chapter 8).

■ 3.5. CALCULATING RECURRENCE RISKS USING THE MULTIFACTORIAL DETERMINATION/ THRESHOLD MODEL

For most multifactorial disorders, empiric risk tables have been constructed from surveys of families with affected individuals. Tables 3.2 and 3.3 are examples of recurrence risks based on population studies. Using these tables, it is possible to estimate risks for individuals based on their family history. In Figure 3.6B, the degree of relationship shown in Figure 3.6A is

used to estimate recurrence risks for cleft palate in each individual. It should be remembered that risks based on family history assume a constant threshold for the general population as illustrated in Figure 3.5A and 3.5B. In certain families or in certain individuals with different environmental or pharmacologic exposures, changes in threshold (as in Fig. 3.5C) may change recurrence risks. Alertness for peculiarities of inheritance or environment is always necessary when counseling for multifactorial disorders.

Pyloric stenosis (narrowing of the lower stomach valve) was the first congenital anomaly to be related to a multifactorial determination/threshold model. This anomaly is one of the most common requiring surgical intervention during childhood and has an overall incidence of about three per thousand in the general population (see Chapter 13). It should be realized that improved operative techniques were required before the genetics of pyloric stenosis could even be studied, because 80% of infants died from medical management alone. By collecting data on 174 males and 48 females who survived operation for pyloric stenosis, a geneticist named Cedric Carter showed a dramatic increased frequency of the anomaly in primary relatives of these individuals (Fig. 3.7; see Fraser, 1976). Note that relatives of affected females have a greater increase in liability for pyloric stenosis than do relatives of affected males (Fig. 3.7). Carter reasoned that this was because females, being the atypically affected sex, must have genotypes with greater numbers of deleterious alleles before they cross the threshold and exhibit

■ **TABLE 3.3.** Empiric Recurrence Risks for Selected Multifactorial Diseases

Disease	Identical Twins (%)	First-Degree Relatives (%)	Second-Degree Relatives (%)	General Population (%)
Type I diabetes mellitus	30–50	4–6	2–3	0.2
Type II diabetes mellitus	90	10–15	3–5	2–5
Coronary artery disease	39–44	14–25		
Schizophrenia	6–86	3–18	2–4	0.5
Autism	92	4.5	0.1	0.04

Source: Data from Motulsky and Brunzell (1992); Rotter et al. (1992).

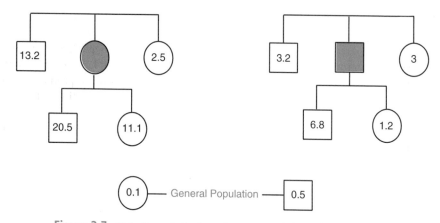

Figure 3.7. Risks for pyloric stenosis among relatives of an index case.

the abnormal phenotype. In other words, affected females must have a greater genetic predisposition for the anomaly that is then passed on to offspring. The shift in distributions for pyloric stenosis liability would be similar to that diagrammed in Figure 3.4 for bruised forehead syndrome, with females shifted toward lower liability. Females who sustain bruised foreheads will be much more atypical for height (over 6½ feet) than are affected males, and their hereditary contribution to stature in offspring is likely to be greater. For pyloric stenosis of course, as with most congenital anomalies, there is no convenient measure of liability that is analogous to stature in the bruised forehead syndrome.

Pyloric stenosis is representative of several modifications to recurrence risk that are necessary when dealing with multifactorial determination. Table 3.4 lists these modifications, which include the number of affected relatives, the sex of affected relatives, and the severity of

disease. For malformations like cleft palate, severity relates to the extent of malformation (i.e., does clefting involve the entire palate? Is it on one or both sides?). For disorders like diabetes mellitus, severity often relates to the age of onset. Juvenile-onset diabetes mellitus (type I diabetes) usually requires exogenous insulin therapy, while adult-onset diabetes mellitus (type II diabetes) often does not. As with female sex for pyloric stenosis, severe or early-onset disease in relatives indicates a higher genetic predisposition with higher risks for family members to be affected. Based on the numbers in Tables 3.2–3.4, risks for individuals with the indicated multifactorial disorders can be estimated using knowledge about family history and disease severity.

Case 3 Follow-up: A more detailed gestational and family history was taken during evaluation of the child in Figure 3.1. The mother's diabetes had been difficult to con-

■**TABLE 3.4.** Factors That Modify Risk in Multifactorial Determination

Relationship or Characteristic	Increased Risk *(fold)*	Usual Risk *(%)*
General population	1	0.1
First degree relative affected	30–50	3–5
Second degree relative affected	5–7	0.5–0.7
Third degree relative affected	2–3	0.2–0.3
Two first degree relatives affected	60–100	6–10
Severe disease	2–3	
Atypical sex affected	3–5	

trol during the first trimester of pregnancy, and her glucose levels were often elevated. The fetus had early growth delay with subsequent improvement and a normal birth weight. The family history revealed no other relatives with congenital anomalies except for mother's sister with cleft lip/palate. Based on affected second-degree and first-degree relatives, the multifactorial recurrence risk for cleft lip/palate in the next pregnancy would be 4–5%. However, the presence of maternal diabetes raised another possibility for the cause of cleft palate. The mother's father had adult-onset diabetes mellitus and one of her three brothers had juvenile diabetes mellitus.

■ 3.6. THE MEASUREMENT OF GENETIC PREDISPOSITION (HERITABILITY): TWIN STUDIES

It should now be appreciated that diseases can be placed on a continuum from genetic to environmental cause, with Mendelian disorders on the genetic extreme and toxic or infectious disorders on the other. Genetics is almost always a part of the story for a particular disease, but it is rarely the whole story. When family studies reveal the obvious patterns of Mendelian inheritance, then genetic causation is secure and environment is relegated to a role in phenotype expression. When Mendelian patterns are not evident, then the extent of hereditary influence must be evaluated by other means. The extent of hereditary influence on a disease or phenotype is called *heritability,* and considerable effort in the field of quantitative genetics has been devoted to its measurement.

The larger the heritability, the greater the role of genes in determining phenotypic variation. Mendelian disorders presenting early in pregnancy will thus have a heritability of 1, while those presenting later in life may have heritabilities less than 1 due to environmental modification. For phenotypes without Mendelian patterns of inheritance, the heritability measures the degree of genetic influence on multifactorial determination. Heritabilities of 0.7–0.8 have been estimated for disorders like

schizophrenia or asthma, 0.6–0.7 for cleft lip/palate or coronary artery disease, and 0.3–0.4 for peptic ulcer or congenital heart defects. Infectious diseases will have low heritability, but epidemics can certainly produce clusters in families that must be distinguished from genetic factors. Even in infectious diseases, host immune responses may bring genetics into the story.

Table 3.5 lists some methods for determining heritability, drawn from the reference of King et al. (1992), which summarizes heritability studies for many common diseases. Twin studies are the most powerful, because *identical twins* raised together, identical twins raised apart, and *fraternal twins* provide cohorts that contrast genetic and environmental influences on phenotype. Twins have an incidence of about 1% in the population and occur by several mechanisms. Identical twins result from early division and separation of the zygote, producing two embryos from the same genetic material. Fraternal twins result from the fertilization of two ova with two sperm, producing two individual embryos. Most fraternal twins derive from the same father (50% of genes in common), but they occasionally

■ TABLE 3.5. Methods for Determining Heritability of Common Diseases

Method	Example
Familial aggregation	Higher incidence in twins, relatives of affected patients
Ethnic differences	Higher incidence in certain ethnic groups
Twin studies	Higher incidence in monozygotic versus dizygotic twins
Adoption studies	Higher incidence in biologic versus adoptive parents
Allele association	Higher incidence of HLA alleles in diabetes mellitus
Presence in Mendelian disorders	Mendelian disorders with diabetes mellitus as one component

arise from different fathers (25% of genes in common). Fraternal twins have separate amnions and placentas, although these may fuse together and be difficult to distinguish. Identical twins may have fused or separate placentas depending upon the embryonic timing of separation, and the demonstration of *monochorionic twins* (single placental membrane) is often taken as evidence for monozygosity. A problem with the older literature on twin studies is uncertainty in methods for distinguishing *monozygous* from *dizygous* twins. *DNA fingerprinting* (see Chapter 8) now allows definitive determination of twin status as opposed to methods based on facial appearance, placental examination, or blood type sharing. The frequency of monozygotic twins is similar in all populations and is about 1 in 260 live births. The frequency of dizygotic twins varies among populations and is about 1 in 87 live births in North America.

Twins are *concordant* when they share a particular trait, *discordant* when they do not. Table 3.3 illustrates that concordance rates in identical twins have a strong correlation with heritability, and there are several formulas relating the two measures. Often the concordance in identical twins is weighed against the concordance in *dizygotic twins* (only 50% related) to produce an estimate of heritability. Although very powerful, twin studies are susceptible to bias. The best studies of heritability ascertain all patients and relatives with a disease, then evaluate concordance as a function of relationship. Studies that focus only on twins with the disease may exaggerate the number of concordant pairs because these are more striking, or because identical twins tend to volunteer together more often than do fraternal twins.

Other methods for evaluating heritability include ethnic differences and familial aggregation of diseases (Table 3.5). These are weaker methods than twin studies because environmental factors may differ so greatly among ethnic groups and increasingly mobile families. Adoption studies are useful, because adoptive parents are matched with offspring

environmentally, while their biologic parents are matched genetically.

The most powerful method for discovering evidence for heritability is exemplified by the discovery of hypercholesterolemia as a factor in coronary artery disease through study of individuals with early-onset heart attacks. Within each multifactorial disease category, there are usually rare families or syndromes that exhibit Mendelian inheritance, providing a vehicle for gene identification. In this context, Mendelian diseases may produce more severe phenotypes that are masked within the extremes of a polygenic distribution. Chapter 5 discusses the approach for elucidating genetic and environmental risk factors for multifactorial diseases.

PROBLEM SET 3
Multifactorial Determination

Tables 3.2–3.4 summarize risks for an individual to be affected with a disease according to its presence in a particular relative or population group. Refer to these tables when answering the questions.

Provide the one best answer to the following questions:

3.1. A father has a child with a heart defect and learns that his mother had a heart defect. He has two normal children. What is the risk for his next child to have a congenital heart defect?

(A)	35–50%	(D)	0.7%
(B)	6–8%	(E)	0.2%
(C)	3–5%		

3.2. A mother with unilateral cleft lip/palate has a child with unilateral cleft lip/palate. Her risk for the next child to be affected with unilateral cleft lip/palate is:

(A)	38–40%	(D)	3–4%
(B)	10–12%	(E)	0.1%
(C)	6–10%		

3.3. Males affected with pyloric stenosis are five-fold more common than affected females. Based on this knowledge, the recurrence risk for offspring of a father who had pyloric stenosis would be:

(A) 55–60%
(B) > 7.5%
(C) 7.5%
(D) < 7.5%
(E) 0.4%

3.4. A mother who had pyloric stenosis during infancy requests counseling regarding the chance that her newborn son has the condition. The son is feeding poorly in the nursery, but does not yet have obvious vomiting. Consult the data in Figure 3.7 for sex-specific recurrence risks in addition to that in Tables 3.2 and 3.3.

(A) 20.5%
(B) 13.2%
(C) 11.1%
(D) 6.8%
(E) 2.5%

3.5. An adopted individual, age 46, discovers an identical twin who died of coronary artery disease in the past year. Although the individual has no symptoms of coronary artery disease, what is his or her risk to develop the disorder?

(A) higher than 39–44%
(B) 39–44%
(C) lower than 39–44%, but higher than 30%
(D) 14–25%
(E) lower than 14–15%

Many of the more common birth defects like cleft palate or congenital heart disease exhibit multifactorial determination. Although specific empiric risks can be specified as in Tables 3.2 and 3.3, general risks can be borne in mind relative to an affected person: identical twin, 20–30%; first-degree relative, 3–4%; two first-degree relatives, 5–8%; three first-degree relatives, 9–12%; second-degree relatives, 0.7–2%; third-degree relatives and general population, less than 0.5%. By reference to the person with a birth defect, match the relatives below with their proportion of genes in common and their concordance or recurrence risk:

(A) 100% genes in common, 20–30% concordance risk
(B) 50% genes in common, 3–4% concordance risk
(C) 50% genes in common, 3–4% recurrence risk

(D) 25% genes in common, 2% recurrence risk
(E) 12.5% genes in common, < 0.5% recurrence risk

3.6. Twin brother whose twin sister has cleft palate by ultrasound

3.7. Unborn sibling of a child with congenital heart defect

3.8. Grandchild of a person with spina bifida

PROBLEM SET 3
Answers

	3.6. B	**3.3. D**
3.8. D	**3.5. B**	**3.2. C**
3.7. C	**3.4. A**	**3.1. C**

PROBLEM SET 3
Solutions

3.1. Congenital heart defects fit the model of multifactorial determination, allowing the tabulation of empiric risks from studies of affected families. The next child to the father will have a sibling (primary relative) with congenital heart disease, giving a recurrence risk of 3–4%. The paternal grandmother also had a heart defect, resulting in an additional 0.7% risk because a second-degree relative is affected. The 3–4 plus 0.7% risk gives a final risk of approximately 4–5% (answer C). Note the difference between the empiric risks used for multifactorial determination and those if autosomal dominant inheritance of heart defects were involved: In the latter case, the father would exemplify incomplete penetrance and have a 50% recurrence risk.

3.2. The mother's next child will have two primary relatives with unilateral cleft lip/palate—the mother and sibling. Table 3.4 indicates that the risk for a multifactorially determined congenital anomaly increases 60–100-fold over that in the general population when two primary relatives are affected. Table 3.2 lists the general population incidence of cleft palate as 0.1%, yielding a 6–10% risk for individuals with two primary relatives affected (answer C).

3.3. Recurrence risks for multifactorial diseases are referred to as empirical because they are based on family history and population data. In Table 3.2, a 7.5% risk for pyloric stenosis is listed when there is an affected primary relative. Risks also vary according to the sex of affected individuals, because females may predominate in disorders such as neural tube defects and males may predominate in disorders such as pyloric stenosis. Since males are the typically affected sex with pyloric stenosis, a lower number of predisposing alleles are required to produce the disorder in males (lower threshold). The lower number of alleles in turn predicts a lower recurrence risk for primary relatives (i.e., < 7.5%, answer D).

3.4. Females have a lower incidence of pyloric stenosis, indicating a higher threshold for pyloric stenosis. Affected females will have a higher number of predisposing alleles, conferring a higher recurrence risk than for affected males as shown in Figure 3.7. Since the woman's child is male, he has a 20.5% chance to develop pyloric stenosis (answer A). This high risk would encourage the managing physicians to visualize the pylorus using ultrasound so that the need for surgery could be determined.

3.5. The concordance rate for the monozygous twin of an affected individual to develop coronary artery disease is listed as 39–44% in Table 3.3 (answer B). This risk is average, which is about 39% for males (the more commonly affected sex) and 39% for females. The actual risk for the individual would depend on his or her sex.

3.6–3.8. The twins are different sexes and must be dizygous, with 50% of their genes in common like siblings. When twins share an anomaly, they are concordant (answer 3.6-B). Siblings also share 50% of their genes, and the probability for recurrence of an anomaly in a subsequent sibling is called a recurrence risk (answer 3.7-C). The degree of relationship depends on genetic distance, with first-degree (primary) relatives such as siblings, parents, and children sharing one-half or 50% of their genes. Second-degree (secondary) relatives (grandparent-grandchild, uncle / aunt-niece / nephew) share one-fourth of their genes (answer 3.8-D). Third-degree relatives (first cousins) share one-eighth of their genes such that the recurrence risk for a multifactorial disorder in a third-degree relative approaches the background risk (i.e., incidence in the general population).

BIBLIOGRAPHY

Emery AH, Rimoin DL. 1990. *Principles and Practice of Medical Genetics,* 2nd ed. Edinburgh: Churchill Livingstone.

Fraser FC. 1976. The multifactorial disease concept—uses and misuses. *Teratology* 6:225–270.

King RA, Rotter JI, Motulsky AG, eds. 1992. *The Genetic Basis of Common Diseases.* New York: Oxford University Press.

Motulsky AG, Brunzell JD. 1992. The genetics of coronary atherosclerosis. In: King RA, Rotter JI, Motulsky AG, eds. *The Genetic Basis of Common Diseases.* New York: Oxford University Press, pp. 150–169.

Rotter JI, Vadheim CM, Rimoin DL. 1992. Diabetes mellitus. In: King RA, Rotter JI, Motulsky AG, eds. *The Genetic Basis of Common Diseases.* New York: Oxford University, pp. 413–81.

4

POPULATION GENETICS

■ LEARNING OBJECTIVES

1. Population genetics examines genetic variation among groups of individuals. Its most clinically relevant principle is the Hardy-Weinberg law, which allows the calculation of allele and genotype frequencies within populations.
2. Human genetic variation is ubiquitous and massive, explaining individual differences and genetic diseases.
3. Allele frequencies often differ among ethnic groups, with changes related to selection, founder effects, or genetic drift. These differences have important implications for genetic screening and prenatal diagnosis.
4. Human genetic variation is necessary for adaptation and evolution, which provides an important perspective on inherited disease.

Case 4: *An Affected Relative*

An engaged couple presents for counseling because the woman's brother has cystic fibrosis (219700). She has two normal siblings, and her fiancee's family history is unremarkable. The couple wishes to know their risk for having a child with cystic fibrosis and whether genetic tests are available to better define their risks.

■ 4.1. POPULATION GENETICS AND HUMAN VARIATION

Population genetics is concerned with the nature and mechanism of genetic variation among groups of individuals. Across relatively short time frames like those of recorded human history, population genetics is mostly a study of ethnic differences and group migrations. Across longer time frames like those of vertebrate evolution, population genetics explains changes in allele frequencies that underlie adaptation and natural selection. At the clinical level, population genetics is used to calculate allele frequencies relevant to genetic counseling or to the chance for atypical drug responses. It also provides perspective on the extensive variation among human beings that is a key to anticipatory medical care and screening programs.

The remarkable degree of genetic variation among humans, though evident from protein structure, has become dramatically evident at the DNA level. DNA sequence variation occurs once every 200 to 500 nucleotides in a average stretch of DNA, although noncoding regions are much more variable than those central to gene function. This variation is essential for adaptation, and the chance voyage

59

from amoeba to man would never have occurred if new mutations and polymorphisms were not extensive. Genes and genomes are wired for change, and genetic disease is as inevitable for humans as it is for the simplest algae. This chapter examines the nature of genetic variation in human populations, and emphasizes the relevance of human variation to health care.

■ 4.2. MUTATION: THE CAUSE OF POLYMORPHISM AND DISEASE

Mutations are changes in the structure or arrangement of genes. Mutations alter DNA or chromosomal structure of their cell of origin and are transmitted to all daughter cells by

DNA replication. There are several categories of mutation as defined by their distribution within the organism and by their molecular mechanism. Although classical population genetics concerns the distribution of mutations within populations, it is important to realize that mutations begin within one gene or chromosomal region, raising issues about the spread of mutations within the cellular genome and among other cells in the organism.

Mutations may be detected at the DNA level as extra, deleted, or substituted nucleotides; at the RNA or protein level as altered RNA sizes or deficient enzyme activity, and at the chromosomal level as larger deletions, duplications, or rearrangements (translocations) (Fig. 4.1). Causes of mutations include mutagenic chemicals that bind or react with DNA, physical

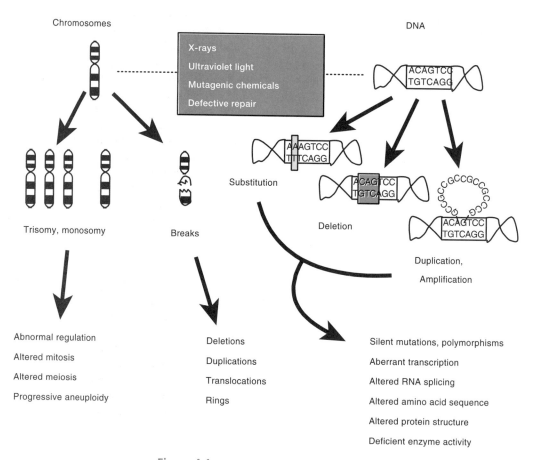

Figure 4.1. Types and causes of mutations.

agents such as X rays or ultraviolet light that damage DNA by collision, or metabolic alterations such as folic acid deficiency that alter the regulation of DNA synthesis. These forces are counterbalanced by processes of DNA repair that fill in deleted regions or nicks in the DNA strands, and by cellular metabolites that inhibit oxidation or absorb physical agents. The result of this genetic yin and yang is somewhat unexpected in that mutations are highly selective: Some genes and some gene or chromosomal regions have particularly high rates of mutation and are called *hot spots*. It is also clear that certain DNA sequences favor the occurrence of mutations, so that endogenous gene structure as well as damage from exogenous agents may predispose to mutations. Molecular mechanisms for errors in DNA replication and repair are reviewed in Chapter 6.

Mutations can also be categorized as germline mutations or somatic mutations. Early in embryogenesis, complex organisms separate their reproductive cells (*germ-line* cells) from other cells in the body or soma (*somatic* cells). In humans, this separation is accomplished by differentiation of the *primordial germ cells* from the yolk sac. If a mutation occurs in one of the somatic cells, then an embryo with *somatic mosaicism* is produced that is a mixture of normal and mutant cells. If the mutation arises in a primordial germ cell during germ cell differentiation, then an embryo with *germline mosaicism* is produced. After progressing through the stages of birth and puberty, individuals with germinal mosaicism will produce a mixture of normal and mutant gametes with the chance for normal or mutant offspring. The consequences of somatic and germ-line mutations for pedigrees or phenotypes are discussed in Chapters 7 and 10.

Mutations that severely impair function may cause death of the organism (*lethal* mutations) or prevent its reproduction (*genetic lethality*). Those that are compatible with reproduction can be transmitted from the mutated or founding individual to others in the population. Intuitively, a relationship between disease severity and mutation rate can be predicted as formulated by Haldane with regard to X-linked recessive disorders (see Chapter 2). The more severe the genetic disease, the higher the proportion of cases due to new mutation. As a result of this prediction, severe and lethal cases of osteogenesis imperfecta (166200) were thought to be autosomal recessive because no cases of parental transmission were observed and occasional cases of affected siblings were described. Molecular analyses have now demonstrated that such cases are due to autosomal dominant inheritance with germline mosaicism in one parent. Mutations are thought to arise during the differentiation of primordial germ cells in the 8–10-week fetus, producing a mixture of normal and mutant gametes that can yield affected siblings from normal parents.

At the other extreme from lethal mutations are *neutral* mutations that have no impact on form or function. Examples include *silent* mutations (nucleotide substitutions) that do not alter the protein reading frame or amino acid sequence. If neutral mutations reach a frequency of 1% in the population by mechanisms to be discussed below, they are called *polymorphisms*. As noted in Chapter 1, polymorphic traits and polymorphic sequence variations are ubiquitous in human populations due to the abundance of benign or neutral mutations.

Mutation rates can be estimated for certain genetic loci and are expressed as the number of mutations per million gametes per generation. In bacteria and viruses, the rate of point mutations depends greatly on the locus considered, ranging from 0.001 to 10. Higher rates in flies (0.1–10) and mice (10–20) approach the mutation rates estimated for certain genetic diseases of man. Mutation rates for the dominant conditions such as achondroplasia (10–50) or neurofibromatosis (100–250) are comparable to those of X-linked recessive conditions like Duchenne muscular dystrophy (50–100). Rates for chromosomal rearrangements are higher at 200–350 new mutations per million gametes per generation.

While human mutation rates of 1–100 per million gametes per locus per generation may seem low, these rates become more significant when multiplied by the estimated 100,000 genes in each cellular genome. The implication of one mutation per individual per generation seems incompatible with species survival and has been called the *genetic load*. The paradoxical success of humans and other species with large, high-maintenance genomes must be explained by the fact that most mutations are harmless and lead to polymorphisms. Although the copious genesis of polymorphisms may be beneficial for adaptation and evolution, their heritage of genetic variation poses medical challenges for patients when they are exposed to novel antigens or drugs.

■ 4.3. HUMAN POLYMORPHISMS: THE ABO AND RH BLOOD GROUPS

The ABO and Rh blood groups are examples of human polymorphisms with significant medical consequences. The ABO locus is on chromosome 9 and encodes a carbohydrate-transferring enzyme that modifies a membrane protein. As shown in Figure 4.2, individuals with the O version of this transferase do not

modify the H membrane protein, which then can be detected as the "O" antigen. If alleles A or B are present at the ABO locus, then their encoded transferases place a galactosamine or galactose residue on the membrane protein, producing respective A or B antigens. Because the H membrane protein is abundant in red blood cells, its carbohydrate status is very important for blood transfusions.

The phenomenon of immune tolerance explains why antigens present during early fetal life become recognized as "self" (Benjamini et al., 1996). Individuals with A antigen do not acquire tolerance for B antigen, and produce serum antibodies to type B membrane proteins if challenged after birth. Infusion of type B red blood cells produces antigen-antibody complexes in such individuals, causing fever and damage to internal organs known as a transfusion reaction. Figure 4.2 illustrates the transfusion incompatibilities that result from different ABO blood types. Note that type O individuals are "universal donors" because their red blood cells (washed free of serum antibodies) will not provoke reactions in type A, B, or AB individuals. Type AB individuals are universal recipients because they acquire tolerance to both A and B antigens.

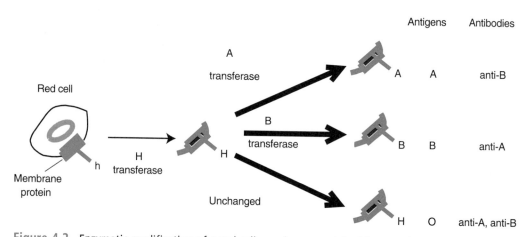

Figure 4.2. Enzymatic modification of a red cell membrane protein (h) to produce alternative membrane antigens A, B, and O. Individuals producing an antigen on their red blood cells (e.g., A antigen) develop tolerance to that antigen in fetal life, but can produce antibodies to other antigens (e.g., B antigen) if sensitized by maternal blood or later exposures (e.g., foods, infections).

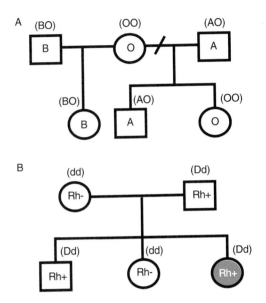

Figure 4.3. Mendelian segregation of alternative alleles to determine genotypes and blood types of offspring. *A*, ABO blood group alleles; *B*, Rh blood group alleles with sensitization of an Rh– mother by an Rh+ male offspring and later Rh disease (filled symbol) in a subsequent female offspring.

The genetics of transfusion reactions due to variation at the ABO blood group is shown in Figure 4.3*A*. Because the ABO locus occurs on an autosome, each individual has two ABO alleles. The pedigree illustrates a union between a type O woman and type A man; the blood types imply a homozygous OO genotype for the woman with possible AA or AO genotypes for the man. The woman also has a type B child that must be the product of another union, since the father has to be type B or AB. This family illustrates the use of genetic polymorphisms for *paternity testing*. Note also that children who inherit A or B alleles from their father can produce antibodies to these antigens during pregnancy if present in their mother.

During gestation, sufficient fetal blood enters the maternal circulation to provoke a maternal antibody response. A strong maternal response usually requires that the mother has been sensitized previously, perhaps from intestinal bacteria that carry antigens similar to those of the human ABO system. Once the sensitized mother is exposed to fetal antigens, her responding antibodies cross the placenta and complex with fetal red cells. Fetal cells coated with maternal antibodies are then destroyed by the fetal immune system, producing a low red blood cell count (anemia) and excess bilirubin (jaundice) due to hemoglobin degradation. Although infants with ABO blood group incompatibility are usually mildly affected, maternofetal incompatibility because of other red cell antigens can be lethal.

The Rh blood group, named for its discovery using Rhesus monkeys, consists of a major locus encoding a D antigen and a minor locus encoding C and E antigens. For practical purposes, alleles at the D locus determine medical problems. Women who are dd homozygotes do not produce D antigen and are called Rh negative (Rh–), while those with Dd or DD genotypes produce D antigen on their red blood cells and are Rh positive (Rh+). Rh disease occurs when an Rh– woman marries an Rh+ man, giving them the possibility of conceiving an Rh+ fetus. Figure 4.3*B* illustrates that a man with DD genotype has a 100% chance to produce a Dd (Rh+) fetus, while a man of genotype Dd has a 50% chance. If the Rh– (genotype dd) mother has been previously sensitized by a transfusion of Rh+ blood or by a gestation with an Rh+ child, she will produce antibodies to her Rh+ (genotype Dd) fetus. The resulting anemia and jaundice may be so severe that they lead to fetal death if an in utero transfusion is not performed.

Because of Rh disease, all blood donations are typed as Rh+ or Rh– with the latter used for Rh– women. Rh– women can also be given Rhogam after an emergent Rh+ transfusion or as a precaution during pregnancy. Rhogam is an immune globulin that binds to the D antigen on red cells and blocks it from eliciting an immune response. For public health reasons, it would be helpful to know the proportion of Rh– women or of ABO blood types in a population in order to plan for pregnancy management and blood banking. Such predictions are possible using the Hardy-Weinberg law.

■ 4.4. POPULATION FREQUENCIES OF POLYMORPHISMS: THE HARDY-WEINBERG EQUILIBRIUM

Hardy and Weinberg independently demonstrated that Mendelian segregation of alleles predicted a relationship among allele and genotype frequencies in a population. Suppose it is known that the alternative alleles C and c at a single diploid locus have frequencies of p and q in a population, for example, p = 0.9 (90% of alleles) and q = 0.1 (10% of alleles). This example assumes that every allele at the diploid locus is either C or c, meaning that p + q = 1. The frequencies of genotypes in this population can be determined from the allele frequencies by using the familiar Punnett square (Fig. 4.4A). The chance for the maternal

egg to contain allele C or c is given by frequency p or q, respectively, as is the chance for the paternal sperm to contain allele C or c. As shown by the Punnett square, the chance that two C gametes fertilize is p², that C and c gametes fertilize is pq taken twice (possibilities of C ovum with c sperm and vice versa), and that two c gametes fertilize is q². The *Hardy-Weinberg law* states that under certain assumptions, populations with allele frequencies of p and q have corresponding genotype frequencies of p², 2pq, and q². The implications for a population of 100 people is shown in the right portion of Figure 4.4A.

The Hardy-Weinberg law relies on several assumptions that can be deduced by conceptual experiments. If individuals with cc genotypes only married each other, then the fre-

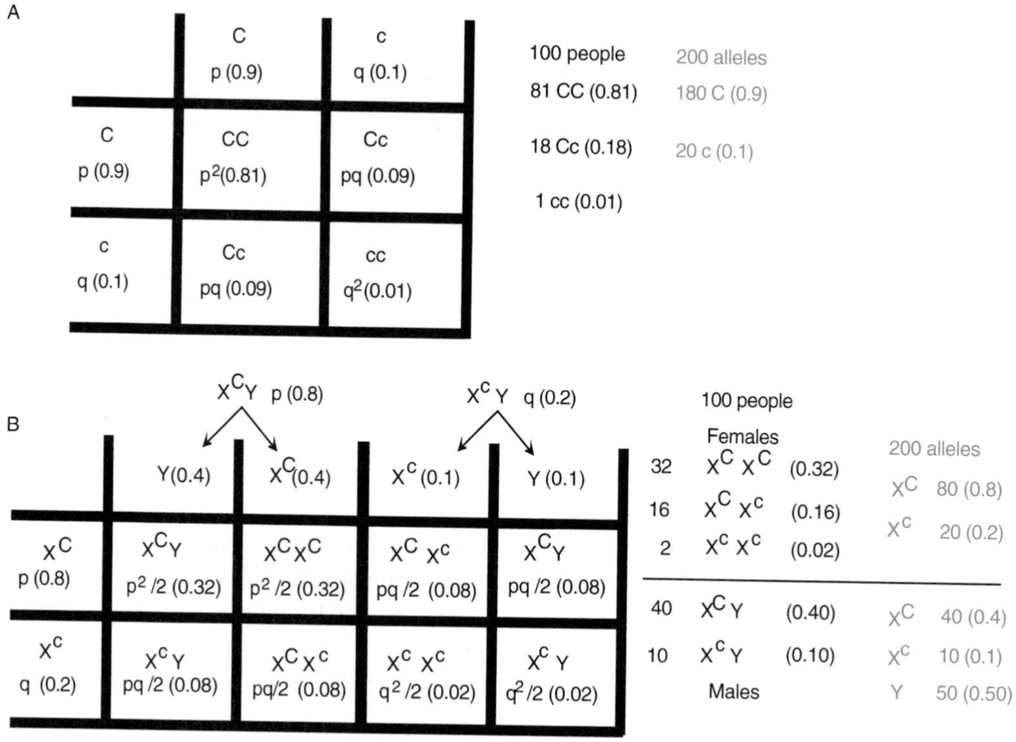

Figure 4.4. The Hardy-Weinberg equilibrium, illustrated for an autosomal locus with alleles C and c (*A*) and an X-linked recessive locus with alleles X^c and X^c. The Punnett squares illustrate how matings among individuals with particular alleles in one generation can generate comparable allele and genotype frequencies in the next generation. To the right, these allele and genotype frequencies are related to proportions of individuals in the population.

quency of allele c would increase in the population. The tendency for individuals of particular genotypes to breed is called *assortative mating,* and its occurrence will negate the relationship between allele and genotype frequencies predicted by the Hardy-Weinberg law. Another exception would occur if individuals with genotype cc had three times as many children as individuals with allele CC; the frequency of allele c would again increase. Equal reproductive success among individuals with genotypes CC, Cc, or cc is necessary for validity of the Hardy-Weinberg law. Reproductive success of a genotype is termed *fitness,* and changes in genotype frequency due to reproductive advantage or disadvantage is termed *selection.*

When the measured genotype frequencies in a population observe the expected relationship with allele frequencies, then the population is said to be in Hardy-Weinberg equilibrium. Actual populations frequently show deviations from the Hardy-Weinberg equilibrium, and these deviations can provide insights

about factors such as assortative mating or selection in the population under study.

The Hardy-Weinberg law also can be applied to loci on the X chromosome, since the allele frequencies are manifest in males. In Figure 4.4B, the alternative X chromosome alleles X^C and X^c are illustrated together with their counterpart Y chromosome allele present in males. Since few Y chromosome alleles function, the frequencies of X^C and X^c alleles are equal to the proportions of $X^C Y$ and $X^c Y$ genotypes in males. If the X^C allele prevented color blindness, then the proportions of normal to color-blind males would reflect the frequencies of X^C and X^c alleles. Figure 4.4B illustrates how the Punnett square can be used to convert X^C / X^c allele frequencies to genotype frequencies in males and females according to the Hardy-Weinberg law.

In Figure 4.5, a similar illustration of the Hardy-Weinberg law is provided for the ABO blood group locus, a single locus with three alleles. If O, A, and B alleles occur at frequencies p, q, and r in the population, then the ho-

	O p (0.7)	A q (0.2)	B r (0.1)
O p (0.7)	OO p^2(0.49)	AO pq (0.14)	BO pr (0.07)
A q (0.2)	AO pq (0.14)	AA q^2(0.04)	AB qr (0.02)
B r (0.1)	BO pr (0.07)	AB qr (0.02)	BB r^2(0.01)

100 people   =   200 alleles

49 type O (OO)   140 O

32 type A (OA) 36   40 A
        (AA)   9

15 type B (OB) 12   20 B
        (BB)   1

4 type AB (AB)

Figure 4.5. Implications of the Hardy-Weinberg law for A, B, and O alleles at the ABO blood group locus. The Punnett square illustrates the relationship of allele and genotype frequencies (left), with corresponding proportions of genotypes and blood types in a population (right).

mozygous genotypes OO, AA, and BB will occur at frequencies of p^2, q^2, and r^2. The heterozygous genotypes AO, BO, and AB will occur at frequencies of 2pq, 2qr, and 2pr, respectively. Figure 4.5 demonstrates that frequencies of 0.7, 0.2, and 0.1 for the O, A, and B alleles convert to frequencies of 0.49 (OO), 0.04 (AA), and 0.01 (BB) for the corresponding homozygous genotypes. When heterozygous AO (.28), BO (.14), and AB (.04) genotype frequencies are included, then the population frequencies for blood types O (49%), A (32%), B (15%), and AB (4%) can be calculated (Fig. 4.5). In Table 4.1, actual frequencies for these blood groups are shown in various segments of the American population. The example allele frequencies in Figure 4.5 correlate best with the actual blood type (genotype) frequencies of African-Americans. If it were assumed that their higher proportions of blood group B were discrepant from the frequency of allele B, then a selective advantage or assortative mating favoring this allele could be postulated. Problem Set 4 gives examples of such analyses.

The hypothetical genotype frequencies shown in Figure 4.5 can be used to illustrate the concept of *heterozygosity*, an important measure of allelic variation at a genetic locus. For any given allele, the frequency of homozygous individuals is relatively simple to calculate as the square of allele frequency. For the ABO blood group locus, homozygous individuals with genotypes OO, AA, or BB total 0.49 + 0.04 + 0.01 = .54 or 54% of individuals. Heterozygotes must constitute the remaining 46% of the population, providing a quantitative estimate of heterozygosity for the ABO locus.

The heterozygosity of a locus is important in providing genetic testing or designing genetic linkage studies. When heterozygosity is high, genetic testing is more difficult, because the assay of many different alleles is required. High heterozygosity increases the value of a locus for genetic linkage studies, because the possibility of distinguishing parental alleles is increased. These aspects of heterozygosity are revisited when discussing molecular genetics (Chapter 8). An average heterozygosity for an organism can also be calculated if genotype frequencies at multiple independent loci are known. As discussed in Section 4.7, a higher proportion of heterozygous loci (higher genetic diversity) is associated with increased fitness of populations.

Case 4 Follow-up: Because cystic fibrosis is inherited as an autosomal recessive trait, the woman whose brother has cystic fibrosis has a 2/3 chance to be a carrier. The chance that her unrelated fiancee is a carrier can be estimated by assuming that the cystic fibrosis locus is under Hardy-Weinberg equilibrium. If the normal cystic fibrosis allele is represented by C and the abnormal allele by c, then affected individuals (genotype cc) can be counted in the population (see Fig. 4.3). The usual prevalence in Caucasian populations is 1 in 2500 persons, which therefore equals q^2. The chance for the fiancee to be a carrier is equal to the frequency of carriers in the population, = 2pq. Since q must equal the square root of 1/2500 = 1/50, 2pq = 1/25. The couple's risk to have a child with cystic fibrosis is therefore 2/3 (woman to be a carrier) X 1/25 (fiancee to be a carrier) X 1/4 (chance for affected child

■TABLE 4.1. Frequencies of ABO Blood Groups in Americans

Blood Group	Caucasian (%)	African (%)	Indian (%)	Asian (%)
O	45	49	79	40
A	4	27	16	28
B	11	20	4	27
AB	4	4	1	5

Source: Benjamini et al. (1996), p. 364.

given that both are carriers) = 1/150. When counseled that a carrier test could modify their odds for an affected child, the couple opted for testing.

■ 4.5. POPULATION DIFFERENCES IN ALLELE FREQUENCIES: EXAMPLES AND MECHANISMS

The most important aspect of population genetics for medical practitioners concerns the differences in allele frequencies among ethnic groups. Ethnic differences are important when considering a differential diagnosis, when providing prenatal counseling and testing, or when designing genetic screening protocols. The reasons for ethnic differences concern the different origins and environments of human populations. Geography and genealogy produce changes in allele frequencies by five major mechanisms that are diagrammed in Figure 4.6. Two of the mechanisms for increased frequency are dependent on changes in population size (A, B), while the others (C–E) maintain a relatively constant population size. Although these mechanisms can be demonstrated mathematically by calculating their effects on the Hardy-Weinberg equilibrium, they are presented conceptually here for the purposes of clinical correlation.

Founder Effect

Figure 4.6A illustrates the phenomenon known as *founder effect*. When a new allele (M in Fig. 4.6) arises by mutation in a population, it may increase in frequency if it happens to occur in a reproductively prolific family. These "founders" leave behind a disproportionately large number of offspring, whose success increases the proportion of M alleles in the remainder of the population. Founder effects are most dramatic when the initial population is small or when a small population migrates to colonize a new region. A classic example of a founder effect concerns an American family with an X-linked recessive disorder called

nephrogenic diabetes insipidus (304800). In this disorder, the kidneys do not respond to antidiuretic (water-conserving) hormone that is made by the posterior pituitary gland in response to increased blood sodium (i.e., when the individual becomes dehydrated). New England individuals with this mutation could be traced to ancestors who arrived on the ship Hopewell. Because of this ancestral seeding, there is a disproportionately high incidence of diabetes insipidus in the descendants of Hopewell passengers.

Genetic Drift

A second mechanism for changes in allele frequencies is *genetic drift* (Fig. 4.6B). According to Mendelian inheritance, the mutant allele M would initially occur in heterozygotes with a normal allele m, and the random chance of fertilization would determine which allele is transmitted to offspring. If M were transmitted more frequently, just as four coin flips may occasionally yield four heads, then more offspring with M than m alleles would be conceived. Chance favoring one allele over another is particularly important when populations reach low levels—for example, after epidemics, wars, or famines. In biology, the contraction of a population prior to reexpansion is called a *bottleneck,* and genetic drift can have a potent effect on allele frequencies during bottlenecks.

Although the scientific approach to human history is too recent to reveal obvious examples of genetic drift, experiments in short-lived organisms like the fruit fly have demonstrated its operation. A common experimental design is to divide a genetically equilibrated population into small groups, then to evaluate allele frequencies among these groups as they produce larger populations. Despite controls to maintain constant environments, the groups will evolve quite different allele frequencies due to random favoring of certain alleles.

A human example of genetic drift might involve the division of a genetically homogenous and interbreeding population among

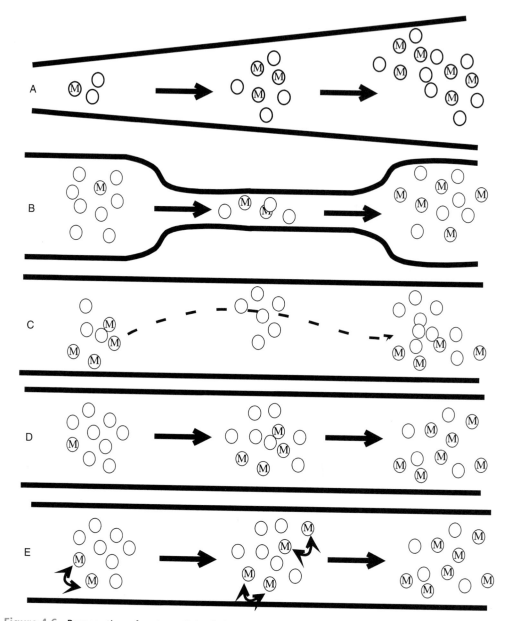

Figure 4.6. Propagation of mutant alleles (M) in populations of changing (*A,B*) or constant (*C–E*) size. *A*, Founder effect with higher frequencies of allele M in descendents reflecting its presence in a few ancestors; *B*, genetic drift showing a chance increase in allele frequency due to sampling error during a time of low population (bottleneck); *C*, gene flow showing increase in allele frequency due to migration and intermarriage; *E*, assortative (preferential) mating between individuals with mutant alleles leads to increased allele frequency; *D*, positive selection for allele M due to better fitness (more offspring) with its corresponding phenotype. Positive selection in heterozygotes may compensate for the decreased fitness (negative selection) of affected homozygotes.

small valleys within a mountain range. Prior to the development of modern roads and transportation, each valley might harbor a small and relatively isolated human population. A disproportionately high incidence of Rendu-Weber-Osler disease (187300) has been documented in the Haut-Jura region of France, with 120 affected individuals living in a 100mi^2 area. Rendu-Weber-Olser disease causes blood vessel dilations (telangiectasias) that produce red areas like birthmarks on the skin. Because this autosomal dominant disease is compatible with long survival, random proliferation from a few affected individuals may have increased its frequency in this relatively isolated population. Note that it is difficult to distinguish genetic drift from a founder effect without studies of surrounding areas to exclude the migration of founders.

Migration and Gene Flow

On a larger scale, migration and intermixing of populations may change allele frequencies according to differences within each population. Changes due to migration are called *gene flow,* because the changes in allele frequency can be related to the migration of a distinct population into other geographic areas (Fig. 4.6C). Although the impact of the migrating (invading) population are accentuated by decimation of the existing population, effects of gene flow do not depend on a small population size. A commonly cited example of gene flow concerns the differences in frequency of ABO blood group B alleles. Group B has its highest frequency in Asia (see Table 4.1), with a gradual decrease in frequency across Europe that corresponds to the routes of conquerors like Genghis Khan. High frequencies of α-1-antitrypsin mutations in Scandinavia also exhibit a gradient across northern Europe that corresponds to the routes of Viking conquests. A compelling argument for gene flow is provided by data (e.g., Cavalli-Sforza et al., 1993) showing that genetic differences today can be explained by migrations during Paleolithic times when small

population sizes accentuated the role of genetic drift. As higher resolution DNA analyses were employed to demonstrate genetic differences, a correspondence between gene flow and language acquisition has become evident.

Nonrandom Mating

Although unbiased or random mating is a basic assumption for the Hardy-Weinberg law, selection of mates is far from random in many biologic species including humans. Attributes such as strength, health, youth, and intelligence are often desired in mates, particularly among organisms that form attachments extending beyond the act of fertilization. When mates join together because of shared phenotypic characters and their corresponding genotypes, the mating is called *assortative*. In Figure 4.6E, matings between individuals with M alleles are favored compared to matings between other individuals. This *assortative mating* is positive toward the M allele and negative toward other alleles at the locus. Both positive and negative assortative matings occur in human and animal populations.

One example of assortative mating is the beneficial trend for patient or parent support groups in the area of chronic disease. Affected individuals or family members not only share medical and psychosocial information about the disease, but are brought together through meetings and volunteer activities. The common result is illustrated by the frequency of matings between people with achondroplasia (100800) that occurs through the valuable activities of the Little People of America (LPA). The LPA is not only a boon to self-image, medical care, and longevity for people with short stature, it also catalyzes matings between achondroplasts that are much more common than would be expected from the 1 in 25,000 prevalence of the disorder.

Other phenotypes selected for assortative mating include height, intelligence, and ethnic background. Assortative mating for similar ethnicity tends to conserve ethnic differences in gene frequencies, acting like geographic isolation in preventing gene flow. Mating between relatives (inbreeding) can be viewed as an extreme of assortative mating, where the circumstance of family gatherings and the sharing of familial characteristics promotes the sharing of rare alleles through common descent. The disadvantages of such matings are manifested by the risks for homozygosity of rare recessive alleles. Inbreeding produces a decrease in heterozygosity for polymorphic Mendelian loci, leading to increased frequencies of rare alleles and producing autosomal recessive diseases. Matings outside of the family and ethnic background increase heterozygosity and tend to counteract the effects of rare recessive alleles. A positive effect for outbreeding is clearly documented in plants, where it is called heterosis or hybrid vigor.

Selection

Long-term changes in allele frequencies can occur because certain alleles benefit the survival and reproduction of their host individuals (Fig. 4.6D). This effect is called *selection,* and it is related to the reproductive success or fitness of the individual. Selection is thought to account for the high frequencies of sickle cell hemoglobin alleles (141900) in Africans and of cystic fibrosis alleles (219700) in Caucasians. In Africa, the frequency of the sickle cell alleles parallels the number of cases of a parasitic disease called malaria. One stage of the malaria parasite involves reproduction in human blood cells, with release of offspring and destruction of red cells. The reproductive cycles produce fever and anemia in the human host, leading to severe and sometimes fatal disease. Because of the parallel between the frequencies of sickle hemoglobin alleles and malarial infection, it is thought that individuals with sickle cell trait (one sickle hemoglobin allele) are more resistant to malaria. Over time, this resistance would favor the reproduction of individuals with sickle cell trait over those with normal hemoglobin and produce higher frequencies of the sickle cell allele. These higher frequencies are maintained in Americans of African descent because of gene flow, continued malarial infection in the Southern states, and assortative mating (positive among African-Americans, negative among African-Americans and Caucasians because of sociopolitical factors and former miscegenation laws).

Cystic fibrosis (219700) is a disorder of chloride transport that is caused by mutations in the cystic fibrosis transmembrane regulator (CFTR). The CFTR forms a pore in the membranes of lung and gut cells that mediates chloride transport; the CFTR also responds to cellular energy status revealed by the concentrations of adenosine triphosphate (ATP) and cyclic adenosine monophosphate (AMP). It is now recognized that the cholera bacterium (*Vibrio cholerae*) can increase cyclic AMP levels, stimulate the CFTR, increase chloride ion secretion into the gut, and cause severe diarrhea. Cholera has been an epidemic disease in temperate climates like Europe, and it was postulated that the relatively high frequency of cystic fibrosis in Caucasians arose because heterozygotes have increased cholera resistance.

Heterozygote advantage toward cholera infection has now been demonstrated in a mouse model of cystic fibrosis (Gabriel et al., 1994). Mice lacking a functional CFTR (homozygous abnormal) exhibited no increase of intestinal chloride after exposure to cholera toxin, and heterozygotes exhibited only half the increase in intestinal chloride secretion as compared to homozygous normal mice. Acting over long periods, better survival of CFTR heterozygotes would increase the frequency of mutant CFTR alleles in the Caucasian population. Gene flow through immigration, assortative mating, and continued exposure to cholera could explain the remarkably high frequency of cystic fibrosis in Caucasian Americans. As emphasized in Section 4.6, increased fitness of heterozygotes (heterozygote advantage) can more than compensate for negative fitness of affected homozygotes because heterozygotes are much more numerous ($2pq > q^2$) for most recessive disorders.

■ 4.6. CONSEQUENCES OF POPULATION VARIABILITY FOR NEONATAL, CARRIER, AND PRENATAL SCREENING

In addition to its implications for general medicine, exemplified by tranfusion reactions and drug responses, population genetics is important in prenatal diagnosis and genetic screening. The high degree of human polymorphism, coupled with the factors outlined in Figure 4.6, means that the frequency of many genetic diseases depends on ethnic background. Table 4.2 summarizes some well-known examples of allele frequency differences among different ethnic groups. Diseases like sickle cell anemia (141900), α- or β-thalassemias (273500), α-1-antitrypsin deficiency (107400), Tay-Sachs (272800), and cystic fibrosis (219700) have frequencies in certain ethnic groups that mandate the consideration of genetic risks. As illustrated in Table 4.2, sickle cell anemia would be considered in African-Americans, cystic fibrosis in Caucasian Americans, α-1-antitrypsin deficiency in Caucasians of Scandinavian origin, and Tay-Sachs disease in Ashkenazi Jews.

Two approaches are relevant to individuals with higher genetic risk based on ethnic background. The first is a family history to identify potential relatives affected with the disease in question. Once the ethnic background is documented, specific questions targeting high-risk diseases are often more successful than general questions. Relatives with Tay-Sachs disease are more likely to be found in Jewish than in African-American families, and mentioning the disorder by name may prompt the family to remember or uncover such individuals. If an affected relative is found, risks for shared alleles often eclipse those for the ethnic group at large, reaching 1 for identical twins, 1/2 for siblings or parents, 1/4 for grandparents, etc.

The second approach that derives from higher gene frequencies in selected ethnic groups involves testing of the entire population. Strategies for testing every individual in a population without regard to family history or symptoms are called screening strategies or, in the context of genetic diseases, *genetic screening*. Genetic screening may be performed on newborns or adults at risk for disease or on adults at risk to transmit the disease. The types and ethical implications of genetic screening are discussed in Chapter 12. Here, the effects of disease frequency and screening accuracy are considered.

■ **TABLE 4.2.** Incidence, Gene Frequency, and Ethnic Predilection of Selected Genetic Diseases

Disease	Ethnic Group (%)	Heterozygote Frequency (%)	Homozygote Frequency (%)
α-1-Antitrypsin deficiency	Scandinavian	1/20	1/2000
African-Americans	1/125	1/100,000	
Cystic fibrosis	Caucasian Americans	1/50	1/2500
African-Americans	< 1/200	1/40,000	
Neurofibromatosis	All groups	1/3000	1/2.25 million
Tay-Sachs	Jewish Americans	1/30	1/3900
Caucasian Americans	1/170	1/112,000	
Sickle cell anemia	African-Americans	1/12	1/1875
Caucasian Americans	< 1/70	<1/20,000	
α-Thalassemia	Selected Chinese regions	1/20	1/2400
African-Americans	1/250	1/50,000	
β-Thalassemia	Sardinians	1/35	1/3000
Caucasian Americans	< 1/350	1/30,000	

Source: McKusick (1994).

As outlined previously, the frequency of affected individuals in a population (q^2) allows the frequency of carriers ($2pq$) to be estimated by assuming Hardy-Weinberg equilibrium. If a homogenous Caucasian population with 300,000 annual births is considered (similar to that of Texas), the cystic fibrosis allele frequency (q) will be about 1/50 (1 in 2500 incidence). There will be 120 affected infants (300,000 × q^2) and 12,000 carrier mothers (300,000 × $2pq$) of these infants. One screening strategy might target the mothers, since the first prenatal visit offers a convenient opportunity for genetic counseling and the collection of blood samples for DNA testing. If 70% of carrier mothers could be detected (as was true when the cystic fibrosis gene was first isolated), then 8400 would be identified and 2600 missed. Among the 8400 husbands of the detected carriers, $2pq$ or 336 should be carriers and 70% (235) would be detected. If all 235 carrier couples selected prenatal diagnosis, then 1/4 of their fetuses or ~59 affected fetuses would be detected. Even assuming full compliance, screening a population of 300,000 pregnant women and 8400 husbands would lead to detection of only 59 or less than half of the affected fetuses.

Several problems attend this method of carrier screening besides the obvious ones of women undergoing no prenatal care or couples refusing male screening or prenatal diagnosis. There may be financial coercion to act on the screening results if affected children are excluded from insurance coverage when couples choose to proceed with affected pregnancies. Carriers may encounter prejudice from society or relatives and suffer loss of self-image. False negatives are a problem because the 70% detection rate would falsely reassure 30% of carriers and 50% of the 480 couples at 1/4 risk for an affected fetus. This concern led an expert panel from the American Society of Human Genetics to recommend against heterozygote screening until a detection rate of greater than 90% was achieved for the cystic fibrosis gene test. This sensitivity has now been achieved, but carrier screening has proceeded only in small pilot programs because of the foregoing concerns. Use of the Hardy-Weinberg law in devising screening strategies should be apparent from this example. Methods to compare the reliability of screening tests are discussed in Chapter 5, and additional ethical concerns are addressed in Chapters 12 and 16.

Case 4 Follow-up: Because the wife had a sibling with cystic fibrosis, this couple would qualify for heterozygote screening to modify their 1/150 a priori chance to have a child with cystic fibrosis. First, the affected sibling would be tested to see if one or both mutant alleles were detected by the DNA test. If both were detected, then testing of the wife to determine her carrier status would be 100% sensitive, and prenatal diagnosis could be performed regardless of the husband's carrier status. If one mutant allele were detected in the affected sibling, then a negative test on the wife would reduce her carrier risk to 1/3 and require testing on the husband. Negative testing of her husband would give him a carrier risk of 1/25 × (1-the detection rate), or 1/25 × 1/3 = 1/75 if the detection rate were 67%. Their risk for an affected fetus would be lowered to 1/3 × 1/75 × 1/4 = 1/900, still higher than that for the general Caucasian population (1/2500). If this couple had no relative with cystic fibrosis, their chance to be carriers after negative screening at 67% detection rate would be 1/3 × $2pq$ = 1/75, and their chance to have an affected fetus would be lowered from the population incidence (1/2500) to 1/21,500. Individual couples might select this option, but population screening with a 67% detection rate would mean that 1 in 9 couples at 1/4 risk were falsely reassured.

■ 4.7. EVOLUTION AS CHANGES IN GENE FREQUENCIES IN RESPONSE TO ENVIRONMENT

Among the mechanisms for changing allele frequencies in populations that were diagrammed in Figure 4.6, selection was highlighted in Darwin's classic treatise on the origin of species published in 1859. Selection was actually the second thesis of Darwin's theory, the first being that all organisms originated by descent from common ancestors (Futuyma, 1986). These genetic ingredients of Darwinian theory were given substance by the rediscovery of Mendelian inheritance as applied to populations. Over the first half of the twentieth century, genetic mechanisms were integrated with fossil evidence to produce a neo-Darwinian or modern synthesis. Although there is still debate about the extent to which gene frequency changes (microevolution) are responsible for the development of complex anatomic structures like the vertebrate eye (macroevolution), the forging of evolutionary processes from genetic changes in response to environment is generally accepted. An important lesson for clinical genetics is to recognize genetic disease as the heritage of diversity that was required for humans to emerge as sentient and communicative vertebrates. A corollary is that useful gene sequences and their corresponding phenotypes are preserved as islands in this sea of evolutionary change.

The recognition of genetic diversity as an essential for evolution provides answers for questions concerning the reasons for genetic disease. It is often difficult for couples to understand how and why a particular genetic mutation should have inflicted tragic consequences on their child. The drive for diversity that makes each individual the carrier for an estimated 5–10 mutant alleles can be invoked to rationalize autosomal recessive diseases, and the universal need for mutations can be cited for new cases of autosomal dominant or X-linked disease. Although this abstract evolutionary perspective may seem scant comfort in the face of severe genetic anomalies, it does counter the guilt and blame that may accompany the transmission of abnormal alleles.

The corollary of gene preservation during evolution has a practical implication that is expanded upon in Chapter 8 concerning molecular genetics. Although each protein exhibits a different rate of evolutionary change, its number of amino acid changes over time is approximately linear. Linear rates of change in protein or DNA structure over evolutionary time has been likened to the regular ticks of a second hand and is called a *molecular clock*. The different timing of changes among different genes or among different segments of the same gene reflect their necessity for organismal function. Proteins like cytochrome c or globin have slower clocks because these proteins are so critical for electron transport or red blood cell oxygenation, respectively. Evolutionary comparisons of gene or protein sequences thus serve two purposes: they can define ancestral relationships among organisms and define genes or regions of genes that have important functions. As discussed in Chapters 8 and 9, functional preservation of genes between organisms as diverse as flies and humans is quite striking, and this conservation provides a tool for discovering human genes based on their similarity to those in simpler organisms.

The twin themes of diversity and functional conservation in evolution may seem contradictory unless a more holistic view of genome and organism is maintained. Whole organism characteristics like growth and development, energy and appetite, reproduction and aging, are composites of many cell and organ functions. Cellular functions in turn reflect the kaleidoscope of enzymes, proteins, and metabolites produced by the genes selected for expression in each differentiated cellular genome. These gene/cell/organ interactions are channeled into a physiology and physiognomy that is characteristic of the organism, producing a steady state known as *homeostasis* (Scriver, 1984). Homeostasis melds diverse genes and proteins into a standard human character that is counted upon equally by anesthetists and astute politicians.

In the metabolic/physiologic sense, homeostasis embodies Bernard's "internal milieu" where standard values of temperature, heart rate, or metabolites are maintained regardless of protein differences or environmental extremes. Just as a buffer resists changes in pH, homeostasis resists disturbance in the internal milieu: a 10° rise in environmental temperature or a fluid intake of 1 L does not produce the corresponding changes in body temperature or volume. Homeostatic mechanisms like sweating and water excretion will compensate until a threshold is reached where the buffering mechanisms fail. Dysfunction and its extreme, called disease, occur when homeostasis is overwhelmed. Balance may be shifted by extrinsic factors (e.g., environmental extremes) or intrinsic factors (e.g., genetic mutations) as described in Chapter 3 on multifactorial determination. The increasing impact of genetic factors in certain medical realms such as infant mortality reflects the persistence of genetic mutation despite improved control of environmental agents.

If homeostasis is viewed as a buffering state made possible by networks of gene products, then genetic variation can be seen to have value for the individual organism as well as for populations that must evolve by adapting to changing environments. Genetic variation produces differences between alleles at more loci, increasing average heterozygosity and providing broader ranges of activity for many enzymes and proteins. This in turn allows greater versatility for inactivating toxins or withstanding environmental extremes. The greater buffering capacity provided by genetic variation and heterozygosity is a strong selective advantage for the organism as a whole that overcomes the disadvantage to rare, homozygous individuals. Genetic diversity is thus a boon to individuals and populations that is promoted by outbreeding and reduced by inbreeding or geographic isolation. Maximal genetic diversity favors individual homeostasis and resistance to injury, improving adaptation for groups of individuals.

■ 4.8. SOCIOLOGICAL IMPACT ON GENE FREQUENCIES: FALLACIES UNDERLYING REPRODUCTIVE SANCTIONS

The political policies of nations, transformed into laws for their populations, can impact al-

lele frequencies through the mechanisms illustrated in Figure 4.6. Medical care is one expression of national law, and practice decisions or public health policies that selectively impact one part of the population can influence allele frequencies. Some effects on allele frequencies are easy to predict (e.g., the effect of immigration laws on gene flow) while others are more complex and have led to tragic fallacies.

Fallacies Concerning Affected Individuals

A classic fallacy, or group of fallacies, was the misguided attempt to sterilize individuals with mental deficiency under the aegis of eugenics (Gould, 1981; Larson, 1995). It is ironic that many of the estimated 20,000 U.S. sterilizations targeted individuals who were already infertile like those with Down syndrome. Others had mental disability due to environmental or multifactorial determination, so that sterilization on the assumption of high transmission risk was misinformed. Even for the few that were reproductively capable and had mental disability due to Mendelian inheritance, application of the Hardy-Weinberg law would have demonstrated the inefficiency of sterilizing homozygotes.

In Figure 4.7A, the effect of reproductive sanctions on homozygotes affected with a disorder having the frequency of cystic fibrosis is illustrated. For 2500 individuals with an autosomal recessive disease like cystic fibrosis, normal homozygotes (p^2 = 2401 people) and heterozygotes ($2pq$ = 98 people) will far outnumber affected homozygotes (q^2 = 1 person). Prohibiting the reproduction of the single affected person, whether by prenatal termination, postnatal withdrawal of medical care, or adult sterilization, will minimally affect disease frequency in the next generation. Assuming no heterozygote selection, no assortative mating, and 1 child per individual, the 98 heterozygotes will contribute on average 49 mutant alleles to the next generation compared to 1 mutant allele by the single homozygote. The major reservoir of abnormal alleles is in het-

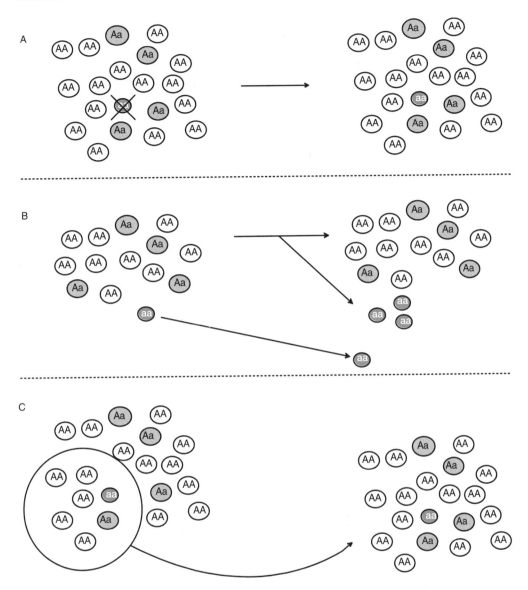

Figure 4.7. Three eugenic fallacies. *A*, Sterilization or removal of individuals with autosomal recessive disorders will have minimal effects on population incidence of disease because heterozygous carriers will produce equal numbers of affected individuals in the next generation. *B*, Each individual carries at least five mutant alleles that can yield affected offspring in the next generation if they match up with mutant alleles in their spouse. Prohibitions on the reproduction of people with genetic diseases will not impact the frequency of carrier matings or of new mutations. *C*, Selection of a subset of a population to propagate new offspring (stirpiculture) will not change allele frequencies in offspring unless there is screening for carriers and for new mutations. Selection of "superior" individuals based on limited characteristics (strength, beauty, intelligence) will ignore heterozygosity for recessive diseases that exact their toll in offspring.

erozygotes, so removing affected homozygotes from the gene pool will have minimal effects on allele frequencies (Fig. 4.7A). One would have to screen for heterozygotes (Table 4.2) and enforce reproductive sanctions on phenotypically normal individuals before any impact on the frequency of abnormal alleles was realized.

Fallacies Concerning "Genetically Defective" Individuals

Although reproductive sanctions make little sense for homozygotes with recessive disorders, the larger goal of the eugenics movement was to discourage any individual with "defective" genes from reproducing so as to improve the gene pool of the next generation. Figure 4.7B illustrates the misguided assumptions of this strategy by evaluating a single Mendelian locus, although the fallacy applies to multifactorial and chromosomal disorders with even greater force. Many individuals have higher risks for transmitting disease despite being phenotypically normal. Heterozygous carriers of alleles that can cause recessive disease (Aa genotypes in Fig. 4.7B), chromosomal translocation carriers, older fathers, older mothers, individuals with germ-line mosaicism, individuals with multiple mutant alleles below the threshold for multifactorial disease, and so forth, will have higher risks for genetic disease in offspring. Reproductive sanctions targeting those with overt genetic disease thus misses the huge load of predisposition and sporadic disease that accounts for a 3–5% risk in every pregnancy.

Higher rates of transmission are possible from the estimated 1% of individuals affected with Mendelian disorders, although the negligible impact of affected homozygotes with recessive disease was demonstrated in Figure 4.7A. People with autosomal dominant disorders would have a 50% recurrence risk, and fertile males with X-linked recessive disorders have a 100% chance to transmit abnormal alleles to their daughters. Perspective on Mendelian diseases requires the reminder that at

least 4000 Mendelian disorders are known, with an average prevalence no greater than 1 in 40,000 each (= q^2, range between 1/3000 and 1/100,000 or less). Carrier frequencies (2pq) averaging $2 \times 1/200 = 1/100$ for each of 4000 diseases imply that each individual is heterozygous for about 40 disease-associated loci. When only recessive rather than manifesting (dominant) diseases are involved, estimates suggest 5–6 heterozygous loci per individual. Regardless of the exact number, sanctions against all predisposed or heterozygous individuals would eliminate reproduction altogether. Figure 4.7B illustrates that the elimination of genetic risk makes sense only at the level of individual options and choices; elimination of genetic disease from the population represents a contradiction.

Fallacies Concerning "Genetically Superior" Individuals

American religious groups of the early 1800s conducted several interesting experiments in the social manipulation of reproduction. Groups like the Shakers frowned on reproduction because of religious reasons and produced valuable furniture but few descendants. Other groups like the Mormons relaxed social restrictions like monogamy and thrived. The Oneida colony of New York tried a different approach that serves to debunk another fallacy of the eugenics movement. They instituted a technique called stirpiculture, in which a few prized individuals are given the privilege of reproduction for the entire population (Stevenson, 1993). The Oneida colony selected a small group of men and women with desirable mental and physical features (including the male leaders of course) to engage in reproduction; other young men were taught restraint from orgasm as a birth control measure. Children of the select reproductive group were raised communally, and the strategy did produce an enduring colony for several generations. While descendants of the Oneida colony persist, there are few modern claims for superiority except perhaps in the craft of silverware.

In Figure 4.7*C*, the fallacy of selecting a phenotypically superior group within the population as a seed for reproduction is diagrammed. Unless methods for carrier testing are developed that can screen every human locus, individuals in the reproductively privileged group will have the same 5–40 mutant alleles as those from the population at large. Breeding for a few desirable characteristics is possible, as illustrated by dogs and racehorses, but overall improvement of the population is doomed to failure by the subclinical diversity of mutant alleles. In fact, the selection of a few individuals for breeding brings forward the hazards of inbreeding, illustrated by the fragile health of many canine and racehorse breeds. Although the Oneida experience was an eccentric curiosity, fallacies like racial hygiene and super-races have had terrible consequences (e.g., Muller-Hill, 1988).

Segments of populations, whether they are perceived as superior individuals or as identifiable ethnic groups, have significant carrier rates that can result in genetic disease. Ethnic groups have different carrier frequencies for particular genetic diseases, but their overall genetic load (number of alleles with potential adverse consequences) is similar. While differences in gene frequencies among races are inevitable because of founder effects, genetic drift, and differences in environment that influence selection, the differences are trivial compared to the inexhaustible well of genetic diversity shared by all human and biological populations. Ethnic differences are important for guiding medical care, but the lessons of genetics and evolution argue strongly for equal opportunity of reproduction rather than for geopolitical restrictions. The central issue for humanity is to balance population with environmental resources, not to engineer the population according to prejudice and fallacious genetic reasoning (Neel, 1995).

PROBLEM SET 4
Population Genetics

Select the single most appropriate answer for the following questions. For allele frequency calculations, round off fractions such as 7/8 or 15/16 to 1.

4.1. A woman has a brother with sickle cell anemia. She marries an unrelated man with a normal family history. Given a 1/16 frequency for the sickle globin allele, what is their risk to have an affected child (equate 15/16 to 1)?

  (A) 1/4   (D) 1/24
  (B) 1/6   (E) 1/48
  (C) 1/8

4.2. A population has a 1/3000 frequency of individuals with cystic fibrosis. If all affected individuals were sterilized, the frequency of those affected in the next generation would be:

  (A) Reduced by 2/3
  (B) Reduced by 1/2
  (C) Reduced by 1/3
  (D) Reduced to O
  (E) Approximately the same

4.3. In a population in which random mating occurs, 50% of the people are heterozygotes for a mutant allele. In the following generation, the frequency of heterozygotes will be:

  (A) 100%   (D) 25%
  (B) 75%   (E) 0%
  (C) 50%

4.4. Of the following assumptions that must be valid for a population to be in Hardy-Weinberg equilibrium, which is the least likely to hold for modern Americans?

  (A) No positive or negative selection
  (B) No assortative mating
  (C) Low rates of mutation
  (D) Large populations to dilute the effect of genetic drift
  (E) No migrations to alter frequencies by gene flow

Match the following questions with one or more correct answers.

4.5–4.7. Match the following definitions with the terms below:

  (A) Gradual diffusion of genes between populations
  (B) Produces identical alleles in relatives
  (C) Mutation to produce multiple alleles at a locus
  (D) Random fluctuation of genes in small populations

(E) Identical alleles in descendants of a small group

4.5. Founder effect

4.6. Genetic drift

4.7. Gene flow

4.8–4.10. Match each of the ethnic groups listed below with the genetic disorder commonly associated with it.
(A) Cystic fibrosis
(B) α-Thalassemia
(C) Tay-Sachs disease
(D) α-1-Antitrypsin deficiency
(E) Glucose-6-phosphate dehydrogenase deficiency

4.8. African-Americans

4.9. Chinese Americans

4.10. Jewish Americans

PROBLEM SET 4
Answers

		4.4. E
4.10. C	4.7. A	4.3. C
4.9. B	4.6. D	4.2. E
4.8. E	4.5. E	4.1. E

PROBLEM SET 4
Solutions

4.1. The pedigree in Figure 4.8*A* illustrates the woman and her brother with sickle cell anemia (genotype SS). The woman has a 2/3 chance to have sickle cell trait (genotype AS), while her husband has a chance of $2pq = 1/8$, where p is the frequency of allele A (15/16 or ~ 1) and q is the frequency of allele S (1/16). The chance for an affected fetus is the chance for the wife to be sickle trait (2/3) X the chance for the husband (1/8) X the chance that they will have an affected fetus if both are carriers (1/4) = 1/48 (answer E).

4.2. In a population at Hardy-Weinberg equilibrium, the ratio of heterozygous carriers to homozygous affected individuals with an autosomal disease is $2pq/q^2$. The highest values for q will be about 1/60 for recessive diseases like

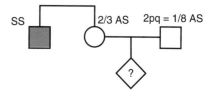

Figure 4.8. Solution for question 4.1

Tay-Sachs in Ashkenazi Jewish populations, meaning that the ratio of carriers to affected individuals is at least 120 to 1. For the usual recessive disorder with a frequency of 1/100,000 or so, the ratio is over 300 to 1. If they survive to reproduce, rare affected homozygotes marry normal heterozygotes and produce carrier but not affected offspring. Heterozygous couples, on the other hand, produce an equivalent number of affected homozygotes in the next generation (q^2), negating any restrictions directed at affected homozygotes (answer E).

4.3. The Hardy-Weinberg law predicts that the frequency of normal homozygotes (p^2), heterozygotes ($2pq$), and affected homozygotes (q^2) remains the same in subsequent generations if the population is at equilibrium (answer C). Random mating is one of the prerequisites for the population to be at Hardy-Weinberg equilibrium.

4.4. Assortative mating with preferences for like ethnicity or social class is common in the United States. With modern transportation and communication, isolated and inbred populations that exhibit chance increases in low frequency alleles are rare. Migration within and immigration from without are very common, producing changes in gene frequency by gene flow (answer E).

4.5–4.7. Genetic drift refers to the random fluctuations seen in gene frequencies over time (answer D). These fluctuations are more significant in small populations with few alleles. Gene flow, on the other hand, is the slow diffusion of genes from one population to another through migration and intermarriage (answer

A). A founder effect describes the propagation of mutant alleles to descendants from one or a few ancesters (answer E). It follows that the descendants will have similar mutant alleles because they derive from the ancestral founder(s). Multiple alleles at a locus are referred to as polymorphism if one of the less common alleles has a population frequency of 1%.

4.8–4.10. Different ethnic groups may develop different frequencies of certain alleles because of unique alleles in their ancestors (founder effect), chance fluctuations in allele frequencies during periods of small population size (genetic drift), and living in different environments (selection). Once present, these differences in allele frequencies may be perpetuated by assortative mating or migrations, so that immigrant groups like African Americans retain their ancestral predisposition to sickle cell anemia. Genetic counseling regarding carrier testing or prenatal diagnosis must therefore take into account the ethnic background, since African-Americans have higher frequencies of glucose-6-phosphate dehydrogenase deficiency alleles, Ashkenazi Jews of Tay-Sachs alleles (answer C), Greeks and other Mediterranean peoples of β-thalassemia alleles, orientals of α-thalassemia alleles (answer B), Scandinavians of α-1-antitrypsin deficiency alleles, and Caucasians of cystic fibrosis alleles.

BIBLIOGRAPHY

General Texts and References

Benjamini E, Sunshine G, Leskowitz S. 1996. *Immunology: A Short Course,* 3rd ed. New York: Wiley-Liss, Inc.

Cavalli-Sforza LL, Menozzi P, Piazza A. 1993. Demic expansions and human evolution. *Science* 259:639–646.

Futuyma DJ. 1986. *Evolutionary Biology,* 2nd ed. Sunderland, MA: Sinauer.

Gould SJ. 1981. *The Mismeasure of Man.* New York: WW Norton.

Hartl DL. 1980. *Principles of Population Genetics.* Sunderland, MA: Sinauer.

Larson EJ. 1995. *Sex, Race, and Science. Eugenics in the Deep South.* Baltimore: Johns Hopkins.

McKusick VA. 1994. *Mendelian Inheritance in Man,* 11th ed. Baltimore: Johns Hopkins; online at http://www3.ncbi.nlm.nih.gov/omim.

Muller-Hill B. 1988. *Murderous Science. Elimination by Scientific Selection of Jews, Gypsies, and Others in Germany, 1933–1945.* Oxford University: Oxford.

Nei M. 1987. *Molecular Evolutionary Genetics.* New York: Columbia, p. 49.

Specific References

Gabriel SE, Brigman KN, Koller BH, Boucher RC, Stutts MJ. 1994. Cystic fibrosis heterozygote resistance to cholera toxin in the cystic fibrosis mouse model. *Science* 266:107–109.

Harris H. 1966. Enzyme polymorphisms in man. *Proc Roy Soc Lond* B164:298–310.

Jacobs PA, Funkhouser J, Matsuura J. 1981. Mutations of human chromosomes. In Hook EB, Porter IH, eds. *Population and Biological Aspects of Human Mutation.* New York: Academic Press, pp. 133–145.

Morton NE. 1981. Mutation rates for human autosomal recessives. In Hook EB, Porter IH, eds. *Population and Biological Aspects of Human Mutation.* New York: Academic Press, pp. 65–89.

Neel JV. 1995. The neglected genetic issue: The how and why of curbing population growth. *Am J Hum Genet* 56:538–542.

Scriver CR. 1984. An evolutionary view of disease in man. *Proc R Soc Lond B*220:273–298.

Stevenson RE. 1993. Stirpiculture. *Proc Greenwood Genet Center* 12:3–6.

5

MEASURING GENETIC PREDISPOSITION: COMMON DISEASES, PHARMACOGENETICS, AND ECOGENETICS

■ LEARNING OBJECTIVES

1. Individual genetic variation in the form of polymorphic alleles and proteins explains differences in susceptibility to common diseases, drug side effects, and environmental injuries.
2. Mendelian diseases may produce extremes within a phenotypic spectrum, highlighting biomarkers like serum cholesterol that can be used as risk factors in the general population.
3. The value of risk factors for population screening can be quantified in terms of sensitivity, specificity, and positive predictive value.
4. Biomarkers and family history can be combined to estimate disease risk using the principles of Bayesian counseling.
5. Enzyme polymorphisms affecting drug metabolism can produce devastating side effects in genetic predisposed individuals.

6. Enzyme polymorphisms affecting metabolism of environmental agents place some individuals at high risk for toxicity or cancer.

*Case 5. **Death During Surgery***
An 8-week-old child is brought to the emergency room because of projectile vomiting and sleepiness. The initial electrolytes reveal an elevated chloride and an alkaline pH that is typical of hypochloremic alkalosis. There are increased peristaltic waves visible over the child's abdomen, and an olivelike mass is palpated that suggests the diagnosis of pyloric stenosis. A family history reveals that the child's mother had stomach surgery when she was an infant, and that the mother and father are first cousins. A successful operation for pyloric stenosis is performed, but the child has difficulty breathing after extubation. A code is called for emergency resuscitation.

81

■ 5.1. MEASUREMENT OF GENETIC PREDISPOSITION: RISK FACTORS FOR COMMON DISEASES

The two aspects of multifactorial determination, genetics and environment, provide complementary strategies for preventive management. Both aspects of prevention require the definition of risk factors that influence the likelihood that a particular individual will develop a disease or a complication of that disease. Risk factors may consist of *biomarkers* like serum cholesterol or enzyme levels, or they may be lifestyle components like obesity or cigarette smoking. Once risk factors are defined, they can be used to formulate a clinical pathway for preventive management. An approach to defining risk factors for common diseases is illustrated with coronary artery disease and diabetes mellitus. The discussions are adapted from two useful texts on the genetics of common diseases (King et al., 1992; Emery and Rimoin, 1990).

Coronary Artery Disease

A familial predisposition to heart attacks was recognized in the nineteenth century. The cause of myocardial infarction is atherosclerosis or "hardening of the arteries." When atherosclerosis occurs in arteries supplying the heart muscle (coronary arteries), the resulting atherosclerotic plug or plaque can gradually occlude blood flow, causing heart muscle damage (myocardial infarction). Contents of the atherosclerotic plaque include lipids like cholesterol, blood clotting components like fibrin, and blood cells like macrophages and lymphocytes. Although plaque evolution is a complex and much-investigated topic, its lipid and fibrin contents correlate with some of the risk factors revealed by genetic and population studies.

Coronary artery disease is a common disorder, accounting for at least 25% of all deaths in the United States. Population studies have been instrumental in defining risk factors, because countries like Japan have a sixfold lower incidence of the disorder. Genetic involvement is suggested by the threefold higher rate in men, although women catch up after menopause (Fig. 5.1A). Familial tendencies include the fivefold higher mortality rates of males who have first-degree relatives that died of premature heart disease (heart attack prior to age 55). Female first-degree relatives also have a higher mortality risk (2.5-fold) if a male relative has premature heart disease. An example of twin studies is the Scandinavian data showing a 39–66% monozygous concordance rate and a 25–26% dizygous concordance rate for heart attacks in males, with 44% and 14% respective rates in females (Fig. 5.1A).

The genetic predisposition to heart attacks suggested by familial aggregation has been dissected by several techniques. Prominent among these was the study of families with numerous members having extreme (premature) coronary artery disease; these studies led to the recognition of autosomal dominant hypercholesterolemia (143890) that derives from mutations in the low density lipoprotein receptor (Goldstein et al., 1973; 1995). People with hypercholesterolemia are at the high extreme of the serum cholesterol distribution for the normal population (Fig. 5.1B, upper panel), and affected families exhibit a biphasic distribution that reflects heterozygous or normal status (Fig. 5.1B, lower panel). Study of hypercholesterolemia families revealed three distributions of cholesterol (Fig. 5.1C): very high levels for homozygous abnormal individuals, high levels for heterozygotes, and a normal range for individuals who were homozygous normal. Individuals with homozygous or heterozygous hypercholesterolemia exhibit an extreme phenotype that illustrates a gene of major effect in the multifactorial determination of coronary artery disease. Other Mendelian disorders are associated with heart attacks as shown in Table 5.1.

The dramatic success in defining the cause of hypercholesterolemia stimulated investigations into other serum lipids that might reflect a predisposition to heart attacks. Many lipid factors have been found, including triglycerides and a glycoprotein named Lp(a). Added to these risk factors are families who have ele-

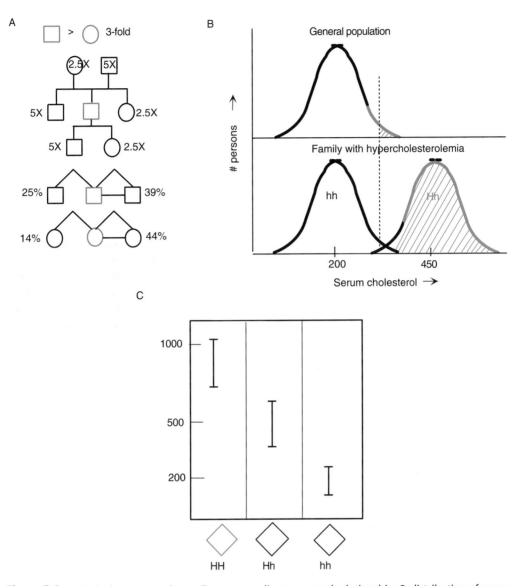

Figure 5.1. A, Risks for coronary heart disease according to sex and relationship; *B*, distribution of serum cholesterol in the normal population (upper panel) and in a family with hypercholesterolemia (lower panel); *C*, serum cholesterol levels in hypercholesterolemia homozygotes (HH), heterozygotes (Hh), and unaffected individuals (hh) in the same family. Data taken from Motulsky and Brunzell (1992); Goldstein et al. (1995).

vated numbers of heart attacks in the face of normal serum lipids and cholesterol. Carriers of an autosomal recessive metabolic disorder called homocystinuria (236200), associated with increased clotting tendencies, may have an increased risk for coronary thromboses. Di-

abetes mellitus (see following paragraphs), obesity, and hypertension all are multifactorial diseases with genetic predisposition that increase the risk for coronary artery disease. Figure 5.2 illustrates the complex interaction of genetic and environmental risk factors in pro-

■ **TABLE 5.1.** Mendelian Disorders Associated with Diabetes or Coronary Artery Disease

Inherited Disorder	Findings
Diseases causing coronary artery disease	
Hypercholesterolemia (143890)	Corneal deposits (arcus senilis), fatty deposits (xanthomas)
Cholesterol ester storage disease (278000)	Stored lipid causing large liver and spleen
Homocystinuria (236200)	Tall and thin body build (Marfanoid habitus, lens dislocation, blood clots)
Lipoprotein lipase deficiency (238600)	Hypertriglyceridemia
Diseases causing diabetes mellitus	
Multiple endocrine neoplasia type I (131100)	Pituitary, parathyroid, and pancreatic tumors; peptic ulcers
Myotonic dystrophy (160900)	Cataracts, myotonia, myopathic facies
Bardet-Biedl syndrome (209900)	Obesity, hypogonadism, polydactyly
Donahue syndrome (leprechaunism; 246200)	Dwarfism, lipodystrophy, large hands and feet, large genitalia

Note: The mode of inheritance is indicated by the starting digit of the McKusick number in parentheses (1, autosomal dominant; 2, autosomal recessive).

moting the progression from a normal vascular system to plaques to myocardial infarction. It is obvious that the dramatic event of myocardial infarction is far removed from the genetic endowment within a newborn child. Yet each individual's genome contains a unique combination of alleles that may make them vulnerable for a severe disease later in life. Even environmental risk factors for coronary heart disease—factors like obesity, smoking, or stress—depend somewhat on individual genes that predispose to aggressive personalities and/or addictive behaviors (Fig. 5.2).

Diabetes Mellitus

Diabetes mellitus is a disorder of glucose metabolism that is caused by defective insulin action. Two major types have been recognized: early onset (juvenile or type I) and later onset (adult-onset or type II) diabetes mellitus. Type I juvenile diabetics usually require insulin therapy, whereas type II adult-onset diabetes often can be treated by dietary modification and oral glucose-lowering medications. Although there is clearly a genetic predisposition to diabetes mellitus, it has been described as a geneticist's nightmare because of its common occurrence (2–5% of adults), variable presentation (up to 11% of adults have altered glucose uptake as measured by their tolerance of oral glucose), and difficulty in diagnosis (type I may be confused with type II, and normal women may manifest diabetes during pregnancy). The data shown in Figure 5.3 have broad ranges, reflecting different recurrence risks in different populations (King et al., 1992; Emery and Rimoin, 1990).

Evidence for familial clustering of diabetes mellitus is shown in Figure 5.3. The incidence of type II (adult-onset) is at least 20 times that of type I, although the juvenile can be viewed as a more extreme and severe phenotype with greater impact on lifespan. As a result, concordance rates for monozygous twins can approach 100% if they are followed to old age when the type II abnormality becomes common. Overall, the risk for a dizygous twin is about that of the risk for a sibling: 3–30% depending on the duration and sensitivity of diabetes testing. In certain populations such as the Pima Indians, diabetes acts almost like an autosomal dominant trait. Primary relatives of affected individuals exhibit the expected 50% chance to be affected, and monozygous twins are almost 100% concordant. These twin and family studies suggesting genetic predisposition to diabetes are supported by the presence of numerous Mendelian disorders that have an increased risk for diabetes (Table 5.1).

Dissection of this familial aggregation for diabetes has revealed a major influence of

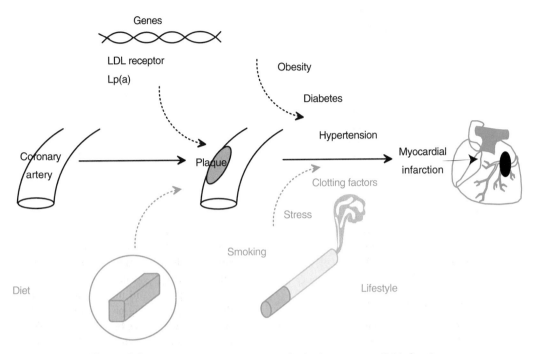

Figure 5.2. Pathway from atherogenic diathesis to myocardial infarction.

genes regulating the immune system. A preliminary clue was the finding that several autoimmune disorders—diseases where the body's immune system attacks its own organs—exhibit increased incidence in individuals with diabetes mellitus. This association applies to autoimmune diseases like myasthenia gravis (muscles), Hashimoto's thyroiditis (thyroid), pernicious anemia (stomach), and certain forms of Addison's disease (adrenal gland). Because many autoimmune diseases exhibit an association with particular HLA antigens, extensive research on diabetes mellitus identified several alleles in the HLA region on chromosome 6 that are associated with the diabetic phenotype. Several are diagrammed in Figure

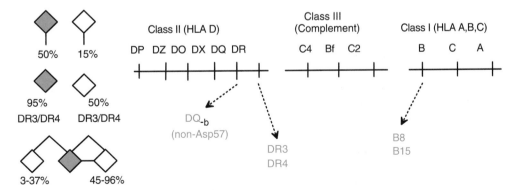

Figure 5.3. Familial risks in diabetes mellitus (left panel); illustration of the HLA locus (right panel). From Rotter JI et al. (1992).

5.3, including the DR3/DR4 alleles that occur in 95% of type I diabetics and 50% of the general population. Also striking is the single amino acid difference in the DQ-β surface protein: People with an aspartic acid residue at this locus have a 10–20-fold lower risk for diabetes. Molecular testing for this DQ-β polymorphism can thus refine risks in families. For example, the 4–6% risk conferred on a child by a parent with diabetes could be lowered if the parent had a predisposing DQ-β allele but did not give it to his child. Conversely, transmission of the high-risk DQ-β allele would place the child at the upper range of risk to develop diabetes mellitus.

The dissection of familial risk to reveal specific HLA surface molecules that predispose to diabetes is thus similar to the elucidation of autosomal dominant hypercholesterolemia as a locus of major effect in the development of coronary artery disease. As with the attention to lipid factors catalyzed by hypercholesterolemia, the HLA association with diabetes has focused attention on autoimmunity to the pancreatic insulin-producing cells in the early stages of diabetes. Population studies have shown that 30–40% of juvenile diabetics have antibodies to islet cells compared to 5–8% of adult-onset diabetics. Because of this role of HLA-influenced autoimmunity, investigators have considered the possibility of administering inhibitors of the immune system to patients with high susceptibility HLA types (DR3 or DR4) in an attempt to prevent the onset of juvenile diabetes. The elucidation of risk factors, whether in the form of cholesterol or glucose-elevating genes, thus leads directly to the possibilities for screening and prevention.

■ 5.2. ASSESSMENT OF RISK FACTORS: POSITIVE PREDICTIVE VALUE

Although the many genetic loci involved in predisposition to coronary artery disease or diabetes mellitus defy simple genetic testing, high serum cholesterol or poor glucose tolerance can identify susceptible individuals before symptoms begin. The recognition of predisposition may confer advantages through drug therapy or lifestyle modification, but it also may initiate problems with anxiety or insurability. It is therefore necessary that health professionals have an approach for evaluating predictive testing.

Disease status

	Affected	Unaffected
Test result positive (+)	a True positive	b False positive
Test result negative (−)	c False negative	d True negative

Sensitivity (What % of affecteds are truly positive) $= \dfrac{\text{\# true positives}}{\text{\# affecteds tested}} = \dfrac{a}{(a + c)}$

Specificity (What % of unaffecteds are truly negative) $= \dfrac{\text{\# true negatives}}{\text{\# unaffecteds tested}} = \dfrac{d}{(b + d)}$

Positive predictive value (What % of positive tests are truly affected) $= \dfrac{\text{\# true positives}}{\text{\# positive tests}} = \dfrac{a}{(a + b)}$

Negative predictive value (What % of negative tests are truly unaffected) $= \dfrac{\text{\# true negatives}}{\text{\# negative tests}} = \dfrac{d}{(c + d)}$

Figure 5.4. Assessment of diagnostic tests or risk factors.

The diagram in Figure 5.4 separates individuals into four categories according to the presence or absence of a characteristic (i.e., affected or unaffected with a disease) and a positive or negative test result for that characteristic. In order to use the diagram, it is necessary to have test data on a population where the number of individuals with or without the characteristic are independently known. The quadrants in Figure 5.4 then reflect true positives (a, affected individuals who test positive), false positives (b, unaffected individuals who test positive), true negatives (d, unaffected individuals who test negative) and false negatives (c, affected individuals who test negative). These four values allow the calculation of key information regarding the laboratory test or risk factor as listed beneath the diagram in Figure 5.4.

The importance of testing parameters can be illustrated by considering the impact of acquired immunodeficiency syndrome (AIDS)

testing during routine blood donation. Individual donors would insist on a high positive predictive value, because unaffected people with a positive test (quadrant b in Fig. 5.4) would be devastated. Blood banks, on the other hand, would be most concerned about a high negative predictive value because affected people with a negative test (quadrant c in Fig. 5.4) would contaminate the blood supply. Public health officials would focus on the sensitivity of testing, because they would want to identify all affected individuals in order to minimize transmission (a/a + c in Fig. 5.4). Advocates for personal liberties would focus on the specificity of testing (d/b + d in Fig. 5.4), because they would be concerned about false positive tests that subjected individuals to social and insurance discrimination.

In Figure 5.5, these principles for evaluating tests and risk factors are applied to a multifactorial disease. In Figure 5.5A, the impact of

A

	50 affected	950 unaffected
Affected relative	10	90
None	40	860

Sensitivity = 10/50 = 20%

Specificity = 860/950 = 91%

Positive predictive value = 10/100 = 10%

Negative predictive value = 940/988 = 95%

B

	500 affected	500 unaffected
Affected relative	100	50
None	400	450

Sensitivity = 100/500 = 20%

Specificity = 450/500 = 90%

Positive predictive value = 100/150 = 67%

Negative predictive value = 450/850 = 53%

C

	50 affected	950 unaffected
DR3/DR4 +	48	475
DR3/DR4 -	2	475

Sensitivity = 48/50 = 96%

Specificity = 475/950 = 50%

Positive predictive value = 48/475 = 10%

Negative predictive value = 475/477 = 99%

D

	50 affected	950 unaffected
Diabetes allele +	50	1
Diabetes allele -	0	949

Sensitivity = 50/50 = 100%

Specificity = 949/950 = 100%

Positive predictive value = 50/51 = 99%

Negative predictive value = 949/949 = 100%

Figure 5.5. Assessment of risks for diabetes mellitus based on population and testing data. *A*, Implication of affected primary relative in general population; *B*, implication of primary relative in study group of 500 diabetics and 500 controls; *C*, implication of testing for DR3/DR4 HLA alleles; *D*, implications of testing using a hypothetical "diabetes allele" that is always present in affected individuals.

an affected primary relative on the risk to de-velop diabetes mellitus is examined. The data imply a 5% prevalence of diabetes in a popula-tion of 1000 offspring, with affected primary relatives documented in 10 of 50 affected off-spring and 90 of 950 unaffected offspring. The sensitivity of the test or risk factor (affected primary relative) in determining the diabetic status of offspring is $a/(a + c) = 10/50 = 20\%$, the specificity $d/(b + d) = 860/950 = 91\%$, and the positive predictive value $a/(a + b) = 10/100 = 10\%$. The positive predictive value gives the proportion of individuals with a primary rela-tive who will develop diabetes (type I or type II unspecified). Although the 10% positive predictive value is useful as a risk factor, it might be less useful for population screening unless there were good benefits for presympto-matic diagnosis: Note that 100 individuals would have to be screened for every 10 that would develop diabetes. The specificity of 91% indicates that about 9% of the population would be falsely suspected of having diabetes based on the presence of an affected primary relative. The high false positive rate would mitigate against screening unless the benefits of early diagnosis outweighed the potential in-juries to peace of mind and insurability.

In panel B of Figure 5.5, the incidence of di-abetes mellitus is raised to an unrealistic 50%, meaning that 500 of the 1000 offspring will be affected. Note that the positive predictive value of having an affected primary relative is now a respectable 67% despite the same low sensitivity of 20%. Two in every three individ-uals positive for the risk factor (affected pri-mary relative) will develop diabetes. This ex-ample demonstrates that the positive predictive value of a test increases in proportion to the prevalence of disease.

Panels C and D of Figure 5.5 emphasize the effect of test specificity on the positive predic-tive value. Although a positive test for the diabetes-associated HLA-DR3 or DR4 haplo-types has a high sensitivity (96%), the occur-rence of these antigens in 50% of the popula-tion produces a low specificity (50%) and a low positive predictive value (10%—Fig.

5.5C). If there were a more specific test, exem-plified by a hypothetical allele with major ef-fect on diabetes analogous to the LDL receptor in coronary artery disease, then a specificity of almost 100% could be expected from DNA testing for that allele (Fig. 5.5D). Note that this high specificity elevates the positive predictive value to 99% despite a similar sensitivity (100%—Fig. 5.5D). The example in Figure 5.5D is hypothetical, but one can envision de-finitive tests for alleles predisposing to dia-betes in populations where the disorder virtu-ally exhibits Mendelian inheritance (e.g., the Pima Indians).

■ 5.3. COMBINED RISK FACTORS AS THE GUIDE TO PREVENTION

For most genetic diseases, early detection af-fords possibilities for therapy or for avoiding complications. Mendelian diseases such as sickle cell anemia (141900) may be amelio-rated by routine blood transfusions, and multi-factorial disorders like diabetes may be ame-liorated by rigid control of blood glucose to prevent hyperglycemia and blindness. Early diagnosis also allows genetic counseling be-fore additional children are conceived, provid-ing couples with reproductive options. For Mendelian diseases like sickle cell anemia, testing for abnormal alleles often provides an early and inexorable diagnosis. For multifacto-rial diseases like diabetes or coronary artery disease, the probability for disease must be es-timated so that full-blown and catastrophic symptoms can be avoided. Because of the many factors involved in multifactorial deter-mination, methods for combining probabilities from several risk factors must be employed.

Chapter 2 presented Bayesian methods for modifying probabilities according to condi-tional information. Although there is no ade-quate substitute for population studies (em-piric risks) in the assignment of risk categories, the Bayesian approach provides an approximate method for combining risk factors to obtain a fi-nal probability for disease. This approach is useful to consider because it quantifies the procedure that every health professional uses in medical decision making (see Goldman, 1994).

Assume that an individual has a genetic risk factor for coronary artery disease in the form of an affected brother. From empiric data, his risk for developing coronary artery disease is 20% or 1/5. To further refine this genetic risk, a serum cholesterol test is obtained with the sensitivity and specificity for coronary artery disease shown in Figure 5.6A. It can be assumed that individuals with autosomal dominant hypercholesterolemia have been excluded from the population used for these calculations. If the individual has a positive test (defined here as cholesterol above 280 mg per dl), then the conditional probability for developing coronary artery disease is the true positive rate (sensitivity) = .75 and the conditional probability for not developing coronary artery disease is the false positive rate (b/b + d in Fig. 5.4 or 1 − specificity) = 1 − .9 = 0.1. The chance that the positive test predicts coronary artery disease is thus .75/(.75 + .1) = .75/.85 = 15/17. Calculation of joint and final probabilities as displayed in Figure 5.6B reveals that the condition of a positive serum cholesterol result increases the final probability of coronary artery disease from 20% to 15/23 or about 65%. Were the man to have a negative serum cholesterol result, his risk would be lowered 5/77 or about 6.5%. The use of serum cholesterol testing plus the family history yields a more accurate probability for developing coronary artery disease that has important implications for preventive management. The choice between relatively benign measures such as stress testing (monitoring the electrocardiogram while exercising) versus coronary angiography (injection of dye to visualize arterial diameter) depends on the magnitude of risk for myocardial infarction.

In practice, risk factors may not be quantified sufficiently to calculate exact probabilities for disease. Often a qualitative approach to both risk estimation and medical decision-making is used, based on the intuition that two risk factors like a positive family history and a high serum cholesterol are of greater concern than one. Nevertheless, it is important to appreciate the process by which diagnostic testing can be integrated with genetic risk information to estimate disease probabilities. The magnitude of risk together with the burden of disease will guide genetic counseling and preventive management strategies.

Once risk factors have been defined, the focus shifts to disease prevention and management. As an introduction to the clinical examples in Part III, it is useful to review the difference between primary, secondary, or tertiary preventive measures. Consider the production of hearing loss by noise. Primary prevention would involve eliminating the onset of the disorder, as in the removal of an individual from a noisy workplace. Secondary prevention concerns the avoidance of complications from

A

	20 affected	105 unaffected
Cholesterol >280	a (15)	b (10)
Cholesterol <280	c (5)	d (95)

Sensitivity = 15/20 = 75%

Specificity = 95/105 = 90%

Positive predictive value = 15/25 = 60%

Negative predictive value = 95/100 = 95%

Number affected in population = 20/125 = 16%

B

	Affected	Not
Prior (affected relative) =	1/5	4/5
Conditional (cholesterol >280) (= chance false positive/total) = 0.75/0.85 =	15/17	2/17
Joint =	15/85	8/85

$$\text{Final} = \frac{15/85}{15/85 + 8/85} = 15/23$$

Figure 5.6. The use of elevated serum cholesterol as a risk factor for coronary artery disease. A, Test results in a hypothetical population with cholesterol above or below 280 mg per dl; B, modification of risk from an affected sibling using conditional probabilities from cholesterol testing by Bayesian analysis.

the problem, as in detecting hearing loss early so that a child does not have speech delay. Tertiary prevention involves the amelioration of complications once they are detected, such as the use of hearing aids and speech therapy to improve language acquisition in a deaf child (Marge, 1984). For coronary artery disease, primary prevention would eliminate any coronary artery blockage, secondary prevention would minimize heart muscle damage after coronary artery blockage is detected (e.g., with fibrinolytic drugs), tertiary prevention would minimize the adverse consequences of heart muscle damage (e.g., cardiac stimulants, pacemakers, etc.).

In the context of genetic diseases, primary prevention would prevent the disease phenotype in individuals harboring the abnormal genotype. This could be accomplished by gene or enzyme replacement therapy or by dietary restriction in metabolic diseases such as phenylketonuria (261600). Gene therapy provides the greatest hope for primary prevention of genetic disease (see Chapter 10). Genetic counseling or prenatal diagnosis may prevent the birth of affected individuals, but these strategies are no more examples of primary prevention than would be the execution of predisposed individuals before they develop coronary artery disease. Genetic counseling is essential for informed reproduction, but the lack of primary prevention often makes reproductive decisions difficult. The eugenics movement confused these issues and mistakenly endorsed reproductive controls as preventive measures for society (see Section 1.10).

In contrast to primary prevention by future advances in gene therapy, secondary and tertiary prevention are available strategies for the majority of genetic disorders. The ounce of prevention lies in forestalling complications or ameliorating their consequences; the pound of cure lies in improved outcome for the patient because of fewer disabilities. In the case of multifactorial diseases, risk factors guide preventive management by dictating the probability for disease and the aggressiveness of intervention. As cost-effectiveness becomes paramount in the revolution toward managed

care, the interpretation of genetic mechanisms and of genetic testing assumes importance in all areas of medicine.

■ 5.4. PHARMACOGENETICS: VARIABLE DRUG RESPONSE DUE TO GENETIC POLYMORPHISM AND ETHNIC DIFFERENCES

From the examples of common diseases, it is clear that each human being has a genetic individuality that confers specific advantages and frailties. These genetic predispositions may also influence the way an individual responds to drugs (*pharmacogenetics*) or to environmental agents (*ecogenetics*). Genetic analysis may thus assess individual risk for drug reactions or environmental injury, and this is an important new area for clinical genetics.

The frequency of human polymorphism, the advantages of heterozygosity, and the various mechanisms for changing population frequencies that were discussed in Chapter 4 are relevant to individual differences in drug response. One might expect an adverse drug reaction like succinylcholine apnea (lack of recovery from anesthesia with succinylcholine) to disappear from the population because of its severe consequences. However, the high frequency of heterozygotes for enzyme variants that cause most drug reactions, the normal health of carriers, and the slow changes in allele frequency due to negative selection on homozygotes have maintained a low but constant frequency of these diseases. Table 5.2 lists several abnormal drug responses that are mediated through polymorphic alleles that exhibit variability among ethnic groups. These examples of variable drug response should provide an unforgettable lesson on the importance of genetic variation for medical practice.

Glucose-6-Phosphate Dehydrogenase Deficiency (G6PD)

G6PD is an enzyme that generates reduced nicotinamide adenine dinucleotide phosphate (NADPH), a substance that is critical for main-

■**TABLE 5.2.** Selected Loci Producing Altered Drug Responses in Humans

Locus/Enzyme	Alleles (frequency in population)	Consequences
Glucose-6-phosphate deficiency (G6PD; 305900)	G6PD alleles > 400 known (up to 2/3)	Hemolytic anemia, neontal jaundice, fatal hemolytic crisis
Succinyl choline apnea (butyrylcholinesterase deficiency; 177400)	K (1/10) A (1/60) S (1/330) J (1/3600)	Paralysis after succinylcholine anesthesia, cocaine intoxication
Debrisoquine oxidase (Cytochrome P450—CYP2D6; 124030)	CYP2D6 alleles (up to 1/5)	Poor metabolism of drugs including antihypertensives, beta-blockers, antidepressants
Malignant hyperthermia (Ryanodine receptor—RYR1; 145600; 180901)	RYR1 alleles (?1/100) Other loci (?)	Hyperthermia, tachycardia, muscle rigidity

taining the stability of cellular glutathione and catalase. Red blood cells are particularly dependent on G6PD and its reducing functions, because their limited protein repertoire includes no other sources for NADPH. The recognition of individuals who were susceptible to sudden destruction of red blood cells (hemolysis) after exposure to certain drugs led to the documentation of polymorphism at the G6PD locus on the X chromosome. Investigation of G6PD enzyme activity and of G6PD gene structure has demonstrated more than 400 mutant alleles at this locus that result in deficient G6PD activity (305900). The phenotype of G6PD deficiency exhibits X-linked inheritance, with the majority of affected males living normal lives. The mild phenotype of most males with G6PD deficiency plus the suspected resistance of carrier females and affected males to malaria accounts for its status as the most common enzyme defect in humans. More than 400 million people have G6PD deficiency worldwide (Luzzatto and Mehta, 1995).

Individuals with G6PD deficiency are susceptible to both dietary and pharmacologic insults. The onset of pallor, pink urine due to hemoglobin excretion, and severe anemia after ingestion of broad (fava) beans has been recognized for centuries. When the same individuals reacted to both fava beans and primaquine (an

antimalarial drug), an enzyme defect was suspected and proved to be G6PD deficiency. The demonstration of X-linked recessive inheritance led to mapping of the G6PD locus to the long arm of the X chromosome, and the responsible gene has been thoroughly characterized at the molecular level.

The frequency of G6PD deficient alleles correlates strongly with the incidence of malaria except in regions like the southern United States where malaria was recently eradicated. Frequencies as high as 0.65 for G6PD alleles (in Kurdish Jews) mandate caution when using provocative drugs like antimalarials, sulfa or furantoin antibiotics, and a variety of dye preparations. Recall from Figure 4.4*B* that the frequency of mutant alleles (q) equals the proportion of hemizygous mutant males. Most affected males will not be symptomatic. A selective advantage for G6PD deficient alleles in malarial areas has been supported by in vitro studies showing decreased survival of the parasite in red blood cells from carrier females or affected males. Also consistent with selection as the mechanism for high G6PD frequencies are the many different G6PD alleles demonstrated at the molecular level (Luzzatto and Mehta, 1995). Recall of the discussion in Chapter 4 indicates that increasing frequency of one mutant allele would be expected in populations affected by founder effect, genetic drift, gene flow, or assortative mating. Only selection would promote the ascendancy of multiple mutant alleles, each arising independently in a malaria-infested region.

Succinylcholine Apnea

The medical importance of the autonomic nervous system led to the discovery of plasma cholinesterases that metabolize parasympathetic mediators such as acetylcholine. A particular form of plasma cholinesterase was first called pseudocholinesterase, then butyrylcholinesterase (177400). The clinical relevance of this enzyme became apparent when prolonged paralysis and absent breathing (apnea) were observed after routine anesthesia. The responsible anesthetic agent, succinylcholine, is a powerful muscle relaxant used at the beginning of anesthesia to facilitate intubation and artificial ventilation. Once surgery was completed, some patients failed to recover from anesthesia, remaining paralyzed and ventilator-dependent for many hours. Many patients died from hasty and inappropriate resuscitative measures when this prolonged recovery was not anticipated.

The cause in many cases of succinylcholine apnea was shown to be deficiency of butyrylcholinesterase in plasma. The locus for this enzyme is autosomal and has been mapped to chromosome 3. Molecular characterization of the gene has defined several mutant alleles with varying degrees of enzyme deficiency. Table 5.2 shows that allele frequencies range from about 1/10 for milder variants to 1/360 for severe variants, predicting an incidence of homozygotes between 1 in 100 to 1 in 150,000 people. Those few surveys employing DNA analysis have shown considerable differences among ethnic groups, exemplified by the A allele with frequencies of 1/50 in Caucasians, 1/200 in African-Americans, and 1/5000 in Asians. Anticipation of the problem allows screening of individuals for enzyme deficiency and provision of appropriate resuscitation and recovery methods. Unfortunately, cocaine is another cholinergic drug that is metabolized by

butyrylcholinesterase, and lethal reactions to nasal cocaine sprays administered for the control of bleeding have been described. Equally unsettling is the effect of this polymorphic locus on cocaine drug abuse, with the possibility that fatal reactions to seemingly normal doses might represent a pharmacogenetic disease (Kalow and Grant, 1995).

Case 5 Follow-up: The child failed to respond to emergency resuscitation, partly because of rushed and overreactive therapy. Succinylcholine apnea due to butyrylcholinesterase deficiency (homozygous abnormal alleles) was suspected and confirmed by autopsy studies. Blood butyrylcholinesterase assays were then performed on the child's three siblings, identifying one with similar butyrylcholinesterase deficiency. Autosomal recessive inheritance of this enzyme deficiency was explained to the parents, along with their increased risk for children with recessive diseases because of consanguinity. Once the predisposition to succinylcholine apnea was identified in the sibling, appropriate anesthetic and postoperative precautions could be instituted.

Debrisoquine Oxidase and Cytochrome P450 Polymorphism

The cytochrome P450 superfamily includes a large group of related proteins that comprise the body's main defense against toxic agents. Most active in liver, the P450 enzymes provide a diverse range of substrate activity that allow most environmental chemicals to be metabolized by one or more of these enzymes. It was therefore surprising among the many P450 enzymes to discover a CYP2D6 locus at which genetic variation affected the metabolism of several key drugs. The initial observation occurred when an investigator developed severe hypotension (low blood pressure) while testing an antihypertensive drug called debrisoquine. This extreme effect was due to slow metabolism of the debrisoquine, and the people exhibiting this phenotype were called "poor metabolizers." Now it is known that the poor metabolizer phenotype exhibits autosomal recessive inheritance, with the causative CYP2D6 locus on chromosome 22. Numerous CYP2D6 mutant alleles have been characterized, with frequencies ranging from 1/100 up to 1/3 (Table 5.2). The corresponding homozygote frequencies of 1 in 10,000 to 1 in 10 emphasize that a sizable fraction of the population may metabolize CYP2D6 substrates differently. These substrates include drugs such as propranolol, a beta-blocker that slows the heart rate, amitryptyline, a tricyclic antidepressant, and even cough suppressants such as dextromethorpan. Awareness of this genetic variation is obviously important for several medical specialties, particularly in cardiology or psychiatry where poor metabolism may lead to drug side effects (e.g., tremors with antidepressants) that mimic the indications for treatment.

Malignant Hyperthermia

Although this disorder probably began with the first use of chloroform or ether anesthesia, the familial pattern of malignant hyperthermia was not recognized until 1960 (Kalow and Grant, 1995). The hyperthermic crisis consists of severe muscle spasm, with arching of the back to the degree that the head and heels touch the table. Temperature rises as great as $2°$ per hour may occur, and there is muscle breakdown with release of potassium and clogging of renal excretion. A high serum potassium may cause cardiac arrhythmias and congestive heart failure that is exacerbated by kidney failure. Untreated crises can be fatal 80% of the time, but modern management has reduced this to 10%. Many cases exhibit autosomal dominant inheritance, and a specific gene for the ryanodine receptor has been located on chromosome 19. Some cases do not involve the ryanodine receptor, and multifactorial determination with the ryanodine receptor as a locus of major effect is likely.

Malignant hyperthermia is observed in about 1 in 15,000 operations on children and about 1 in 100,000 on adults. The maximum

frequency for ryanodine receptor mutant alleles is therefore about 1 in 120. The ryanodine receptor locus was discovered in pigs, where a hyperthermia crisis occurs during stresses like transport, fighting, or mating. Poor quality of pork after such crises led to the discovery of the ryanodine receptor, which requires homozygous mutation to produce hyperthermic crisis. However, provocative stimulation with anesthetics such as halothane can produce the crisis in heterozygous pigs, making the distinction between autosomal dominant or recessive inheritance one that depends on environment conditions. Few humans have the same mutant allele delineated in pigs, and the broader range of ryanodine receptor mutations may account for dominant inheritance in humans. From the population perspective, mutant ryanodine receptors were traced to a founder pig in England, whose progeny were favored by breeders because they had a lean and muscled phenotype. This meaty phenotype also occurs in heterozygotes, allowing continued selective breeding based on heterozygote advantage in the marketplace. As emphasized previously, crises occurring in homozygotes will be infrequent compared to the favored meaty phenotype with $2pq/q^2 = 2p/q$ from the Hardy-Weinberg equation (Chapter 4) giving the ratio of good meat over bad.

■ 5.5. ECOGENETICS

The idea that individual mutations can alter drug metabolism and produce dangerous side effects has more general application to all chemical and physical agents in the environment, a field known as ecogenetics. Three major categories of environmental exposures are summarized in Table 5.3, including dietary, radiation, and chemical agents. If certain genetic polymorphisms can be identified as biomarkers that predict higher or lower risk for environmentally caused diseases, then such markers would have important implications for prevention and public health.

■TABLE 5.3. Ecogenetic Loci That Modify Responses to Environmental Agents

Type of Agent	Disorder	Consequences
Dietary lactose	Lactose intolerance (150220)	Lactase deficiency, severe diarrhea
Dietary folic acid	Coronary artery disease	Increased blood homocysteine due to MTHFR (236250) polymorphism and folate deficiency
	Neural tube defects	Folate deficiency,?increased susceptibility with MTHFR or folate receptor polymorphisms
Dietary iron	Hemochromatosis (235200)	Increased iron storage, heart and liver failure
Inhaled tobacco smoke	Lung cancer	Aryl hydrocarbon hydroxylase inducibility (108340); low levels of enzyme may protect against cancer by limiting levels of toxic metabolites
Ultraviolet light	Albinism (203100)	Lack of melanin, skin cancers
	Xeroderma pigmentosum (278700)	Defective DNA repair, skin cancers

Note: MTHFR, methylene tetrahydrofolate reductase

Dietary Ecogenetics

Variation in susceptibility to coronary artery disease because of dietary fat has already been related to genetic mutations like that for hypercholesterolemia. Of recent interest has been another risk factor for coronary artery disease relating to elevated blood levels of the amino acid homocysteine. Although two inborn errors of metabolism called homocystinuria (236200) and methylene tetrahydrofolate reductase (MTHFR, 236250) could cause elevated homocysteine levels, a more common cause is polymorphism of the MTHFR enzyme. The polymorphic allele encodes a more thermolabile enzyme that combines with low dietary intake of folic acid to produce elevated homocysteine levels and higher risk for coronary artery disease. Some studies have found between 17% and 28% of individuals with coronary artery disease to be homozygous for this common MTHFR polymorphism. An estimated 50% of female and 9% of male deaths from coronary artery disease could be prevented (~50,000 annual deaths in the U.S.) could be prevented by fortification of flour and cereal products with folic acid, with resulting

decrease in homocysteine levels (Motulsky, 1996).

Another potential effect of the MTHFR polymorphism that is not yet demonstrated may concern the preventive effects of folic acid supplementation on birth defects. In some populations, folic acid supplementation before conception and during pregnancy can lower the risk for defects of the neural tube or heart by as much as 50%. Polymorphisms affecting folate absorption or metabolism may thus influence the risk for certain birth defects, and the identification of such individuals would allow prevention through preconceptional supplementation of folic acid.

Other diseases related to genetic differences in the handling of dietary agents (Table 5.3) include lactose intolerance due to lactase deficiency (150220), iron toxicity due to hemochromatosis (235200), and hemolysis from fava beans due to glucose-6-phosphate dehydrogenase deficiency that was mentioned previously.

Chemical Ecogenetics

The cytochome P450 family of proteins is an important metabolic shield from toxic chemicals found in the environment. Genetic variants (polymorphisms) in these proteins have the potential to confer greater or lesser risk for toxicity to cells, including the risk of mutations caused by chromosomal or DNA damage. The cytochrome P450 protein 1A1 contributes to an enzyme activity called aryl hydrocarbon hydroxylase (AHH) that exhibits genetic variation (Nebert et al., 1996). Individuals with increased activity of AHH enzyme, correlating with specific nucleotide changes in the AHH gene CYP1A1, are at higher risk to develop lung and breast cancer (Table 5.3). Although CYP1A1 gene variation and cancer risk are not sufficiently correlated for routine clinical use, the AHH and related polymorphisms are being studied as a way to identify individuals at high risk for environment carcinogenesis. Knowledge of high-risk status would allow cancer prevention by modifications of habitual (i.e., tobacco use) or occupational exposures (Nebert et al., 1996).

Physical Ecogenetics

Ultraviolet radiation through sunlight is a leading cause of skin cancer in all individuals, but particularly in those with genetic predisposition to fair skin (Fig. 5.3). The group of genetic diseases that interfere with melanin pigment production (e.g., albinism, 203100) remove an important absorber of ultraviolet light and cause marked susceptibility to skin cancer. Fair skin is a visible sign of polygenic predisposition to skin cancer, heightened in extreme Mendelian phenotypes like albinism. Other factors predisposing to skin damage from sunlight are defects in the DNA repair machinery that occur in diseases such as xeroderma pigmentosum (278700). Several different genetic loci encoding DNA repair proteins can be mutated to produce this disease, and all have extremely high rates of skin cancer with death in the teenage years. By analogy to the MTHFR and AHH polymorphisms mentioned above, it is likely that polymorphisms affecting DNA repair enzymes will one day be useful as predictors of cancer risk.

PROBLEM SET 5
Ecogenetics, Multifactorial Determination, and Risk Factors

5.1. Comment on genetic and/or environmental risk factors that could refine an adoptive man's risk for coronary artery disease.

5.2. A man learns that his fraternal twin has developed type I diabetes mellitus at age 17. He has HLA testing and finds that his DR haplotypes are different from his twin's, and that he does not have the DR3 or DR4 alelle. His risk to develop type I diabetes is

(A) 90% (D) 4–6%
(B) 30–50% (E) < 4–6%
(C) 10–15%

5.3. As exemplified by HLA DQβ haplotypes in type I diabetes mellitus, the use of an individual's HLA status to refine recurrence risks requires

(A) genetic linkage of a disease allele with an HLA allele.
(B) concurrent segregation of a disease allele and a particular HLA allele in the family.
(C) cotransmission of the disease phenotype and a particular HLA allele in an individual family.
(D) higher frequency of a particular HLA allele in affected individuals from many families.
(E) location of a disease allele (allele of major effect) near the HLA locus on chromosome 6.

A population study defines 20 of 125 individuals who have overt coronary artery disease, among whom 15 had serum cholesterol values above 280 mg per dl. Ten individuals in the normal population had a value over 280. Match the following percentages with the probabilities below, and provide the appropriate term for that probability (e.g., positive predictive value):

(A) 95% (D) 60%
(B) 90% (E) 16%
(C) 75%

5.4. Chance for untested individual in the population to be affected

5.5. Chance that individual with cholesterol > 280 is affected

5.6. Chance that an unaffected individual will have normal cholesterol

5.7. Chance that individual with normal cholesterol is unaffected

5.8. A man loses a child because of failure to recover from anesthesia. A diagnosis of succinylcholine apnea is made, and the man and his wife test positive as carriers for the A mutant allele (see Table 5.2). Later, the man remarries and has a second family. What are the risks that his new children will be AA homozygotes?

(A) 1/30   (D) 1/480
(B) 1/60   (E) 1/540
(C) 1/240

PROBLEM SET 5
Answers

5.8. C
5.7. A (negative predictive value)
5.6. B (specificity)
5.5. D (positive predictive value)
5.4. E (disease prevalence)
5.3. D
5.2. E
5.1. Male sex, other affected relatives, obesity, serum cholesterol levels, stressful personality, hypertension, coexisting disorders (diabetes, homocystinuria).

PROBLEM SET 5
Solutions

5.1. The presence or absence of affected relatives provides insight into the genetic component of multifactorial disease. For congenital anomalies like cleft lip/palate, the environmental components manifest during pregnancy and consist of maternal illnesses or drug exposures, in utero positioning or blood supply. For later onset multifactorial disorders like coronary artery disease, it is often possible to define both genetic and environmental components that serve as risk factors to estimate the degree of predisposition. Male sex, affected relatives, obesity, high fat diets, high serum cholesterol levels, hypertension, diabetes, and

cigarette smoking are risk factors for coronary artery disease. Low age of onset (extreme severity) increases the probability for genetic factors such as mutations in the LDL receptor (hypercholesterolemia). Note the interweaving of genetic and environmental factors in coronary artery disease, since many of the risk factors (e.g., obesity, hypertension, diabetes mellitus) also have a genetic predisposition.

5.2. The male dizygous twin is equivalent to a sibling who would confer a 4–6% recurrence risk for juvenile diabetes type I. The use of histocompatibility locus antigen (HLA) testing allows refinement of that risk, since the man did not inherit either the DR3 or DR4 alleles that are likely to be present in his brother. The man's risk can thus be lowered to less than 4–6% (answer E).

5.3. Individuals affected with autoimmune disorders such as juvenile diabetes mellitus, ankylosing spondylitis, or rheumatoid arthritis often have increased frequencies of particular HLA alleles, a phenomenon termed allele association or linkage disequilibrium. Allele associations are revealed by HLA typing of multiple individuals with a particular disease (correct answer D). Usually, the association involves unknown factors in the immune response rather than location of a disease allele near to the HLA locus on chromosome 6. This is particularly true for multifactorial disorders that have multiple contributing alleles, even though one or more may have major impact on the phenotype. The Mendelian disorders congenital adrenal hyperplasia (201910) and hemochromatosis (235200) exemplify genetic linkage with the HLA locus; these loci reside near the HLA locus on chromosome 6 such that families may exhibit cotransmission of particular HLA alleles with disease alleles (as incorrectly suggested by answers A, B, C, and E). In the case of genetic linkage, the cotransmitted allele varies according to the phase of HLA and disease alleles in a parent. In the case of allele association, the same HLA allele always has a higher frequency in affected individuals, regardless of family context.

5.4–5.7. The data set is that used to construct the table in Figure 5.6*A* as discussed in the text. Of 125 individuals, 20 (16%) had symptoms that rendered them affected with coronary artery disease (answer 5.4-E: disease prevalence). The affected and unaffected individuals in this population are tabulated according to elevated or normal cholesterol testing in Figure 5.6*A*; in this case a serum cholesterol level above 280 mg per dl is the criterion for abnormality. The chance that a person with high cholesterol is affected = a/(a+b) = 15/25 = 60% (positive predictive value, answer 5.5-D); that for an unaffected person to have normal cholesterol d/(b+d) = 95/105 = 90% (test specificity, answer 5.6-B); that for a person with normal cholesterol to be unaffected is d/(c+d) = 95/100 = 95% (negative predictive value or answer 5.7-A). Not requested is the chance that an affected person will be recognized by an elevated cholesterol level = a/(a+c) = 15/20 = 75% (test sensitivity). Note that increasing the frequency of coronary artery disease in the population would increase this relatively low positive predictive value, given the same sensitivity for cholesterol screening.

5.8. The man and his first wife are carriers (genotype AU, where U is the normal butyryl-cholinesterase allele and A is the mutant allele—see Table 5.2). The second wife has a chance of 2pq to be a carrier where p is the frequency of allele U (59/60) and q the frequency of allele A (1/60). The chance that each of their children has genotype AA with susceptibility to succinylcholine apnea is 1/60 X 1/4 = 1/240 (answer C).

BIBLIOGRAPHY

Emery AH, Rimoin DL. 1990. *Principles and Practice of Medical Genetics,* 2nd ed. Edinburgh: Churchill Livingstone.

Goldman L. 1994. Quantitative aspects of clinical reasoning. In Isselbacher KJ, Braunwald E, Wilson JD, Martin JB, Fauci AS, Kasper DL, eds. *Harrison's Principles of Internal Medicine,* 13th ed. New York: McGraw-Hill, pp. 43–48.

Goldstein HL, Hazzard WR, Schrott HG, Bierman EL, Motulsky AG. 1973. Hyperlipidemia in coronary heart disease. II. Genetic analysis of lipid levels in 176 families and delineation of a new inherited disorder. *J Clin Invest* 81: 1653–1660.

Goldstein JL, Hobbs HH, Brown MS. 1995. Familial hypercholesteromia. In Scriver CR, Beaudet AL, Sly WS, Valle D, eds. *The Metabolic and Molecular Bases of Inherited Disease,* 7th ed. New York: McGraw-Hill, pp. 1981–2030.

Kalow W, Grant DM. 1995. Pharmacogenetics. In Scriver CR, Beaudet AL, Sly WS, Valle D, eds. *The Metabolic and Molecular Bases of Inherited Disease.* New York: McGraw-Hill, pp. 293–326.

King RA, Rotter JI, Motulsky AG, eds. 1992. *The Genetic Basis of Common Diseases.* New York: Oxford University Press.

Luzzatto L, Mehta A. 1995. Glucose 6-phosphate dehydrogenase deficiency. In Scriver CR, Beaudet AL, Sly WS, Valle D, eds. *The Metabolic and Molecular Bases of Inherited Disease.* New York: McGraw-Hill, pp. 3367–3398.

Marge M. 1984. The prevention of communication disorders. *American Speech-Language-Hearing Association,* 26:29–33.

Motulsky AG. 1996. Nutritional ecogenetics: Homocysteine-related arteriosclerotic vascular disease, neural tube defects, and folic acid. *Am J Hum Genet* 58:17–20.

Motulsky AG, Brunzell, JD. 1992. The genetics of coronary atherosclerosis. In King RA, Rotter JI, Motulsky AG, eds. *The Genetic Basis of Common Diseases.* New York: Oxford University, pp. 150–169.

Nebert DW, McKinnon RA, Puga A. 1996. Human drug-metabolizing enzyme polymorphisms: effects on risk of toxicity and cancer. *DNA Cell Biol* 15:273–280.

Rotter JI, Vadheim CM, Rimoin DL. 1992. Diabetes mellitus. In King RA, Rotter JI, Motulsky AG, eds. *The Genetic Basis of Common Diseases.* New York: Oxford University, pp. 150–169.

Part II

LABORATORY GENETICS, NEW DEVELOPMENTS

6

FROM GENE TO TRAIT: LEVELS OF GENETIC INFORMATION

■ LEARNING OBJECTIVES

1. The pathway from genotype to phenotype involves molecular levels of gene, mRNA, protein, cytoplasmic organization, intercellular communication, and physiologic function.
2. The DNA double helix structure allows DNA hybridization studies that measure the presence and/or dosage of complementary DNA strands.
3. Gene (DNA segments) occur in single or multiple copies per genome.
4. Nucleotide sequences in genes are replicated during cell division and expressed as RNA or protein to control cell functions.
5. Regulation of gene expression occurs at the levels of chromatin structure, DNA transcription, mRNA translocation, and protein activity.
6. Cytoplasmic, cytoskeletal, organellar, and extracellular matrix proteins form an interconnected network that responds to internal and external signals.
7. Hormones and other regulatory molecules produce alterations in gene expression through the universal process of signal transduction.

8. Genetic anemias provide examples of how mutation can alter various levels of hierarchical function to produce genetic disease.

Case 6: ***Seeking a Gene Screen***
A couple requests genetic counseling because they have two sons with severe mental disability. They wish to have a gene screen performed that will provide a laboratory diagnosis and allow prenatal diagnosis during their next pregnancy.

■ 6.1. INTRODUCTION

Beneath the surface phenotype of human beings are communities of organs, tissues, cells, organelles, and organized cytoplasm that make up an internal milieu. The cell is the primary unit for this milieu, sending or receiving signals and performing functions according to its genetic program. Genetic instructions are sent from the center of each cell in the form of a universal *genetic code*. The genetic code is rather simple, involving a linear sequence of *nucleotides* assembled as DNA, but its complex decoding by cells involves RNA, protein, and small molecule intermediates. Cells usually have identical coding material in the form of a complete set of genes known as the *genome;* they acquire different shapes and functions by reading select portions of the genomic code. Cell differentiation produces more than 200 cell types in humans, all interacting to produce a characteristic human anatomy and physiology.

The pathway from genes, cells, and organs to the regulated internal milieu known as life is diverse and multifaceted. Despite considerable redundancy and abilities for repair, the pathways from genes to function are susceptible to internal failings that manifest as predisposition or disease. The pathways of genetic information, extending from the DNA nucleotide to cellular function, are reviewed in this chapter as a basis for understanding genetic disease. These steps provide opportunities for laboratory analysis, which in turn has the potential for objective, presymptomatic, and/or prenatal diagnosis.

Methods for DNA, protein, and cell analysis (histology) are so universal in medicine that they receive treatment in many undergraduate courses and allied disciplines. Blood banking, transplantation, immunology, medical biochemistry, developmental and cancer biology all use techniques for cell and protein analysis that transcend the genetic domain. Each field provides examples of the genetic hierarchy wherein regulatory changes at the gene and protein level determine the identity, interaction, and differential function of cells. This chapter presents a brief overview of gene structure and regulation, emphasizing how steps in gene expression relate to strategies for the laboratory diagnosis of genetic disease. More detailed treatment of DNA structure and expression can be accessed on the companion website at http://www.wiley.com/wilson/.

Despite the remarkable simplicity of the genetic code and its provision of a unifying approach to disease, the diverse pathways from gene to trait can be extremely complex. One difficulty concerns the multiple levels that separate gene structure from organ function, while another concerns the remarkable miniaturization that underlies the molecular basis of life (Table 6.1). Molecular medicine is an abstract science, visualized indirectly by using amplifying chemical reactions, microscopy, or crystallography. It is like the nested Russian eggs on a much smaller scale, each shell opening to a new layer of complexity that proceeds from the microscopic cell to the Angstrom scale of atomic structure. The most dramatic example of this scale reduction is that of DNA structure. Each genomic length of mammalian DNA is about 1 m, yet it must be compacted into a cell nucleus with an average diameter of 10 μm. Despite these complexities of hierarchical levels and progressive miniaturization, their clear understanding is essential if health professionals are to explain genetic diseases to families. Although the steps of genetic regulation are many and complex, they provide a powerful and unifying approach to all diseases that are influenced by genes (Table 6.2).

▉ TABLE 6.1. Elements of the Genetic Hierarchy

Element	Size[a]
Atoms, covalent bond	1.5 Å
Hydrogen bond	3 Å
Sugars, amino acids, nucleotides, base pairs (bp)	0.3–.5 nm
DNA helix (width)	2 nm
DNA helical turn (10 bp)	3.4 nm
Nucleosome (146 bp)	11 nm
Chromatin fiber (width)	30 nm
Looped domain (10^5 bp)	300 nm
Chromosome band	1 μm
Chromosome (2×10^8 bp)	10 μm
Human genome (3×10^9 bp) (1 m length)	10 μm
Globular proteins	2–10 nm
Fibrillar protein (e.g., collagen)	30–100 nm
Ribosomes	30 nm
Mitochondrion	0.5–1 μm
Eucaryotic nucleus	10 μm
Procaryotic cell	1–10 μm
Eucaryotic cell	10–100 μm

[a]Recall that 1 nanometer (nm) = 10 Angstrom (Å)units and 10^{-9} meters.

■ **TABLE. 6.2.** Levels of Gene Regulation Illustrated by Human Genetic Disease

Regulatory Level	Gene Action	Disease Examples
Chromatin structure	Chromatin condensation	Roberts syndrome (268300)—cleft palate and absent limbs
Gene organization (DNA rearrangements within repetitive DNAs)	Unequal crossing over at *Alu* repeats to cause gene deletions	Hypercholesterolemia (143890)— lipid plaques and heart attacks
	Unequal crossing over to alter numbers of DNA repeats	Fragile X syndrome (309550) Color blindness (303700)
Gene organization (DNA duplications)	Duplication of a 22 kD protein component of peripheral myelin	Charcot-Marie-Tooth disease (118220)—decreased innervation of the limbs with foot drop
DNA replication and repair	Deficiencies of DNA repair enzymes or DNA transcription factors	Cockayne syndrome (216400)— accelerated aging; diabetes and heart attacks in the second decade.
RNA transcription	Deficiencies of transcription factors	Rubinstein-Taybi syndrome (268600)—mental and growth deficiency, broad thumbs and toes
RNA splicing, stability	Mutations in splice sites	Type I collagen mutations causing osteogenesis imperfecta (166200)—multiple bone fractures, deafness
Protein structure	Alterations of structural proteins	Marfan syndrome (154700) with altered fibrillin
Protein structure	Defective protein processing	Hyperproinsulinemia (176730) caused by defective processing of insulin to remove the C peptide
Organellar function	Altered protein secretion by the Golgi-ER-lysosome (GERL) apparatus	α-1-antitrypsin deficiency (107400)— Z allele causes defective protein secretion and liver disease
Organellar function	Defective lysosomal enzyme uptake	Inclusion cell disease (252500)— storage of lysosomal substrates
Organellar function	Defective uptake of mitochondrial enzymes	Ornithine transcarbamylase deficiency (321250)—defective uptake of the enzyme into mitochondria
Organellar function	Defective uptake of peroxisomal proteins	Zellweger syndrome (214400)— severe neurologic dysfunction
Surface molecules, receptors	Defective cellular uptake	Hypercholesterolemia (143890) with defective uptake of low density lipoprotein due to receptor deficiency
Extracellular matrix	Alterations of matrix proteins	Ehlers-Danlos syndrome type IV (130050)—defective type III collagen produces severe joint laxity
Extracellular matrix	Alterations of cell adhesion proteins	MASA syndrome (307000)— deficiency of L1CAM cell adhesion molecule

Case 6 Follow-up: The counselor must apprise the parents of various levels of genetic information and explain that brain function is dependent on many different cell types and genes. A specific diagnosis regarding the cause for developmental delay in these boys must be found in order to address the family's concerns. Diagnostic testing may involve multiple levels of the genetic hierarchy, from radiologic imaging (e.g., head magnetic resonance imaging (MRI) scan), tissue studies (white blood cell staining), karyotyping, protein assays, or DNA analysis. Although the affliction of two siblings does suggest an inherited disorder, a specific diagnosis must be entertained before specific gene (DNA) testing can be considered. More than 100,000 genes are thought to be present in the human genome, many of which have yet to be discovered. The parents must understand that no screen for gene mutations is available in the way that a routine karyotype can screen for more than 100 different chromosomal abnormalities.

Because the disease involves brain function, it is likely that a gene is involved that disrupts central nervous system development or function. Unfortunately, more than 1000 human genetic diseases affect the brain and cause mental retardation. The two affected males suggest the operation of autosomal or X-linked recessive inheritance, but a specific diagnosis requires either the recognition of a characteristic phenotype (nonspecific in this case) or the documentation of an abnormal laboratory test. This laboratory test could involve DNA, RNA, protein, or cellular levels of the genetic hierarchy, and the route from gene to phenotype must be appreciated in order to convey this requirement to the family.

■ 6.2. GENE STRUCTURE

The fundamental unit of DNA structure is the *nucleotide,* containing a deoxyribose sugar and a purine or pyrimidine base. Two strands of connected nucleotides run in opposite directions to comprise the DNA double helix. The synthesis of DNA copies (DNA replication) or of RNA copies (RNA transcription) from one strand is directional, proceeding from the 5'-triphosphate end to the 3'-hydroxyl end (*5 to 3 prime* direction). The DNA strand used for RNA transcription in the cell is often called the *sense strand,* while its base-paired complement is called the *antisense strand.* Information is stored in the cell nucleus as a sequence of nucleotides in DNA (*DNA sequence*), transferred to the cytoplasm as complementary *messenger RNA* (*mRNA*), and translated into proteins that mediate most cellular functions.

The DNA duplex can be separated into complementary strands at appropriate temperatures, then annealed or hybridized to reform the stable helix. This tendency for complementary strands to reanneal is exploited in the laboratory as a technique called *DNA hybridization.* By manipulating conditions of temperature, salt concentration, DNA strand length, and concentration, selective hybridization of particular DNA duplexes can be obtained. In most medical applications, one strand of DNA is labeled with fluorescence or radioactivity and called a *DNA probe.* Excess, labeled DNA strand (DNA probe) competes against endogenous DNA strands in a tissue sample or solid support to produce a DNA hybrid; the amount of DNA hybrid is then quantified by the amount of radioactivity or fluorescence that remains in the sample after extensive washing.

Higher Levels of DNA Structure—Loops, Chromatin, and Chromosomes

Linear duplex DNA is greatly compacted in the cell through binding of proteins and extensive coiling (supercoiling). The degree of secondary and tertiary coiling produces a chromosome that is much wider and shorter than its constituent DNA molecule. The coiled 10^8 bp of DNA that comprises an average human chromosome is visible in the light microscope, while the 30,000–40,000 bp (*30–40 kilobases or kb*) of DNA that comprises an average human gene can only be visualized in the electron microscope after special laboratory manipulations (Fig. 6.1). DNA regions are differentiated by nucleotide sequencing, and the linear DNA duplex that comprises each gene is often diagrammed as a single line. Regions of the gene that contain particular DNA sequences of interest may be represented by boxes along the line, including the *exons* (transcribed regions) or the intervening sequences (*introns*) that separate them. It is important to realize that the lines and boxes represent a continuous stretch of duplex DNA, identical in structure but distinguished by particular DNA sequences (Fig. 6.1). Because most genes are autosomal, it is also important to realize that diploid cells (most somatic cells) have two copies of the gene in question even if only one is diagrammed.

In complex organisms, the great majority of DNA is complexed with a regular set of histone proteins to produce a unit called the nu-

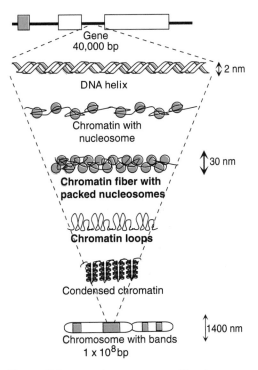

Figure 6.1. Steps in DNA supercoiling between the 2 nm double helix and a 1400 nm chromosome.

cleosome. Additional folding produces loops, chromatin fibers, and chromosomes (Fig. 6.1). Some areas of chromosomal DNA lack nucleosomes, and these are often areas that contain DNA-binding proteins associated with high levels of gene expression. Variable amounts of chromatin condensation produce dense chromosomal regions called *heterochromatin* and the chromosome bands that are visible after incubation with certain dyes. Because there are 10–20 bands per chromosome at routine resolution, each *chromosome band* contains sufficient DNA to encode at least 20 genes (Fig. 6.1, Table 6.1).

Differences in Gene Populations Revealed by DNA Hybridization Studies

If animal genomes were large aggregates of the same type of DNA, then experiments analyzing the melting and reannealing of this DNA should yield a relatively uniform hybridization curve (*A* in Fig. 6.2). The actual experiment revealed a surprising and revolutionary genetic discovery (*B* in Fig. 6.2). Although 70% of the DNA exhibited a slow and uniform reannealing curve, about 30% was unexpectedly rapid and heterogenous. The rapidly reannealing fraction was due to the presence of *repetitive DNA* in complex organisms—DNA sequences that occurred hundreds or thousands of times per cellular genome. Human DNA is thus composed of *unique DNA sequences* having one copy per haploid genome (two per diploid genome for autosomal loci) and of *repeated DNA sequences* with several to millions of copies per genome. The lower part of Figure 6.2 shows some representative DNAs with their approximate location on the reannealing curve. Single copy genes such as that for neurofibromatosis (162600) reanneal slowly with the bulk of the genomic DNA, while multiple copy, repetitive DNAs reanneal at faster rates that depend on their number of copies.

Of many groups or *families* of repetitive DNA, satellite DNAs are the most abundant and comprise 3–5% of many animal genomes. Histone protein and ribosomal RNA genes,

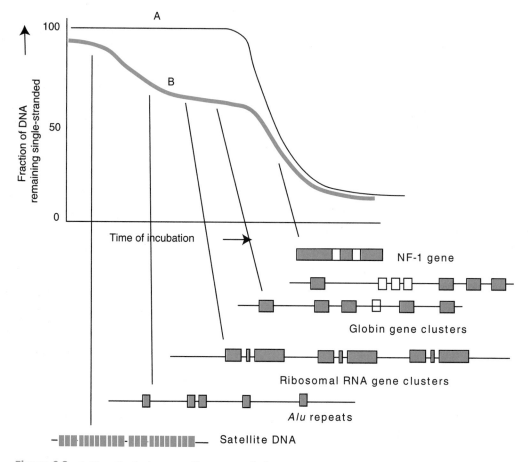

Figure 6.2. *A,* Hypothetical reannealing curve of a homogenous population of DNA segments. *B,* actual reannealing curve of DNA from humans or other mammals showing two phases representing repetitive and single copy DNA. The positions within the hybridization curve of DNA segments from single copy (e.g., neurofibromatosis-1 or NF-1 gene), low repetitive (e.g., globin gene family with 10–20 genes of similar sequence), or highly repetitive genes are shown.

with 100–1000 copies per genome, also fall into the repetitive DNA category and are confined to a few chromosomal regions. At the other extreme are globin or actin genes that comprise a small gene family with 10–20 members per genome. These genes are similar throughout their coding and noncoding portions, suggesting that they derived from a common ancestral gene by the process of gene duplication. Genes may also contain small regions or *motifs* that serve as a family crest to imply related structure and functions. An example is the homeobox motif, a 180-bp unit that allows its transcribed protein to bind

DNA. More than 300 homeotic genes that contain this motif are present in humans, comprising a gene family with important functions in embryonic and cellular differentiation.

■ 6.3. GENE REPLICATION AND EXPRESSION

Because each mistake in replication is a potential mutation that can be costly to the cell and organism, special mechanisms have evolved for DNA copying (DNA replication) and DNA editing (DNA repair). Similar DNA-binding proteins and enzymes are involved in these processes, and an entire group of genetic diseases involves defects in DNA repair. Because breaks in the DNA duplex are like broken links in the chromosomal chain, it is not surprising that patients with abnormal DNA repair may exhibit higher numbers of fragmented or nicked chromosomes (chromosome breakage).

The mechanisms for DNA replication, repair, and recombination all begin with a primer or template that guides new strand synthesis through base pairing. Except for RNA priming during DNA replication, many steps in DNA replication, repair, recombination, and even transcription are similar. There are DNA-binding proteins (DNA helicases for replication, transcription factors for RNA transcription), endonucleases that remove nucleotides in DNA to produce nicks or gaps, and topoisomerases that make nicks to relieve the strain of helical coiling that accompanies DNA synthesis. A general knowledge of these processes is relevant to clinical genetics in several ways. First, many genetic diseases and genetically predisposed cancers involve defective DNA repair or abnormal transcription factors. Second, the process of DNA recombination is fundamental to concepts such as allele segregation, Mendelian inheritance, and linkage analysis. Third, this natural array of DNA-binding proteins and DNA-modifying enzymes has been harnessed in the laboratory for use in gene cloning, protein farming, and gene therapy experiments.

Gene Expression and the Genetic Code

Certain regions of DNA specify genetic information in the form of a code (Table 6.3). The DNA sequence is first transcribed into messenger RNA (mRNA), then read as 3-bp codons that direct the insertion of specific amino acids. As with DNA replication, base pairing directs the transcription of RNA from the DNA sense strand and the selection of transfer RNA (tRNA) molecules containing the appropriate amino acids. Each variety of tRNA molecule combines a unique 3-bp anticodon with a par-

ticular amino acid, allowing translation of the base pair sequence of mRNA into the amino acid sequence of protein (Table 6.3). The flow of genetic information is from cell nucleus to cytoplasm, using RNA messages to direct protein synthesis by the cytoplasmic ribosomes. The genetic code predicts colinearity of the 5′ to 3′ nucleotide sequence of a DNA sense strand with the amino- to carboxy-terminus amino acid sequence of its product protein.

The actual regions of cellular DNA that serve as templates for RNA and protein are highly selected by means of initiation and termination mechanisms (Fig. 6.3). There are *promoter elements* that bind transcription factors and RNA polymerase enzyme to begin RNA synthesis at the appropriate 5′-end of the gene. The initial RNA transcript is chemically modified with a 5′-methylguanosine and a 3-polyadenylate tail; it is also processed to remove intervening sequences (introns) from the regions that encode protein synthesis (exons). There are punctuation signals in the genetic code that set the frame of translation; otherwise, a given DNA sequence could yield three different amino acid sequences depending on which nucleotide was chosen to initiate the first codon. Punctuation signals include the AUG codon for methionine that is used to initiate protein synthesis and three stop codons (UAA, UAG, and UGA) that signal termination of the protein chain. Most mRNAs also contain untranslated regions (UTRs) upstream (5′) and downstream (3′) of the exons. These constraints on transcription and translation mean that only about 1% of the DNA sequences in most cells reaches the cytoplasm as mature mRNA, and even less is actually translated into the amino acid sequence of cellular protein.

The transfer of genetic information to the cytoplasm follows a characteristic path from DNA to RNA to protein that has been called the *central dogma*. The molecular characteristics of this pathway define expected causes for genetic disease and provide certain strategies for investigation. Single gene disorders can be approached with the goal of defining changes in

■TABLE 6.3. The Genetic Code

1	2-U		2-C		2-A		2-G		3
U	UUU	Phe (F)	UCU	Ser (S)	UAU	Tyr (Y)	UGU	Cys (C)	U
	UUC	Phe (E)	UCC	Ser (S)	UAC	Tyr (Y)	UGC	Cys (C)	C
	UUA	Leu (L)	UCA	Ser (S)	UAA	Stop	UGA	Stop	A
	UUG	Leu (L)	UCG	Ser (S)	UAG	Stop	UGG	Trp (W)	G
C	CUU	Leu (L)	CCU	Pro (P)	CAU	His (H)	CGU	Arg (R)	U
	CUC	Leu (L)	CCC	Pro (P)	CAC	His (H)	CGC	Arg (R)	C
	CUA	Leu (L)	CCA	Pro (P)	CAA	Gln (Q)	CGA	Arg (R)	A
	CUG	Leu (L)	CCG	Pro (P)	CAG	Gln (Q)	CGG	Arg (R)	G
A	AUU	Ile (I)	ACU	Thr (T)	AAU	Asn (N)	AGU	Ser (S)	U
	AUC	Ile (I)	ACC	Thr (T)	AAC	Asn (N)	AGC	Ser (S)	C
	AUA	Ile (I)	ACA	Thr (T)	AAA	Lys (L)	AGA	Arg (R)	A
	AUG	Met (M)	ACG	Thr (T)	AAG	Lys (L)	AGG	Arg (R)	G
G	GUU	Val (V)	GCU	Ala (A)	GAU	Asp (D)	GGU	Gly (G)	U
	GUC	Val (V)	GCC	Ala (A)	GAC	Asp (D)	GGC	Gly (G)	C
	GUA	Val (V)	GCA	Ala (A)	GAA	Glu (E)	GGA	Gly (G)	A
	GUG	Val (V)	GCG	Ala (A)	GAG	Glu (E)	GGG	Gly (G)	G

DNA sequence that alter the amount or amino acid sequence of its product protein. Genes can therefore be recognized in groups of random DNA sequences by their lack of stop codons (*open reading frames*) or by their complementarity to cellular mRNA as assessed by nucleic acid hybridization. As shown in Figure 6.3, synthetic DNA strands composed only of thymidine (oligo-dT) can be synthesized and used to purify HnRNA and mRNA with polyadenylate tails (polyA RNA). When a single mRNA can be purified, as was possible for globin mRNA from reticulocytes, the oligo-dT molecules hybridize with the polyA tails of RNA and prime synthesis of a DNA copy (complementary DNA or cDNA). The cDNA is a gene copy (without introns) that can be cloned for DNA sequencing of the gene or for bulk manufacture of protein products. Techniques for isolating and characterizing genes and their mutant alleles are presented in Chapter 8.

The central dogma allows understanding of the molecular varieties of mutation that can lead to genetic disease (Fig. 6.4). Single nucleotide changes are collectively known as *point mutations*. When a point mutation occurs outside of functional DNA regions, or when it does not change the amino acid sequence of encoded protein (*silent mutation*), it has no medical significance and is a *DNA polymorphism* (Fig. 6.4B). If it affects a promoter element or one of the transcription factors guiding RNA polymerase, the point mutation increases or decreases amounts of mRNA transcript and of its corresponding protein (Fig. 6.4H). Decreased amounts of protein can also be produced by mutations that remove or add splice junctions, because improperly processed mRNAs are often degraded before they can be translated (Fig. 6.4G). Finally, single nucleotide changes can alter the codon and produce amino acid substitutions (*missense mutations,* Fig. 6.4C). More dramatic changes in amino acid sequence can be produced by mutations that insert or delete one or more nucleotides from a DNA sense strand, causing *chain terminating* mutations through production of a stop codon (Fig. 6.4D) or *nonsense mutations* (Fig. 6.4E) through shifts in the reading frame.

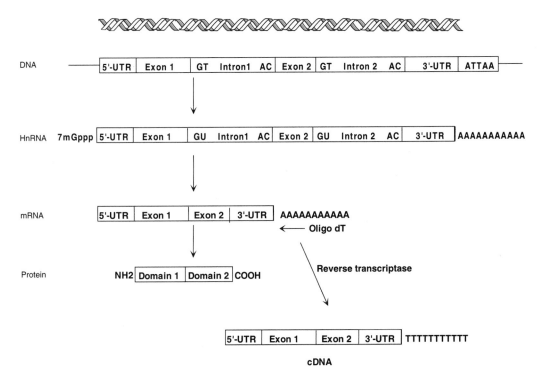

Figure 6.3. A modified central dogma showing RNA capping with 7-methylguanosine (7mG), untranslated regions (UTR), splicing at donor (GU) and acceptor (AG) sites to eliminate introns, and addition of polyA to mature messenger RNA (mRNA). The use of short strings of polyT (oligodT) to initiate a DNA copy of the mRNA (complementary DNA or cDNA) is an important technique for gene cloning and DNA diagnostics. The cDNA will lack introns.

Although determination of the gene sequence is the definitive way of characterizing mutations, antibodies to the normal protein can be used to classify mutations. Proteins containing missense mutations usually cross-react with antibodies (cross-reactive material or CRM), while those with chain terminating or frame shift mutations (*nonsense mutations*) are not recognized by antibodies. A useful notation for gene mutations is shown in the right column of Figure 6.4. The nucleotide or amino acid change is specified and numbered according to its distance from the initiation site. The single letter amino acid codes (Table 6.4) provide a concise notation for amino acid changes, such as the serine deletion in Figure 6.4*F*.

■ 6.4. REGULATION AT THE GENE LEVEL

The flow of genetic information from DNA to protein predicts several ways in which the amount of amount of RNA or protein product from a gene could be regulated. As might be expected, gene regulation in eucaryotes is complex and diverse. Regulatory mechanisms include gene amplifications or losses to alter gene dosage, gene rearrangements to change the amount or type of protein expressed, gene modifications (chiefly DNA methylation) to modulate the accessibility of RNA polymerase, and changes in mRNA production. Excellent summaries of the levels of gene regulation can be found in the classic article by Brown (1981) and in Chapter 7 of Strachan and Read (1996). Although most gene regulation is at the level of RNA transcription, examples at the levels of chromatin structure, RNA and protein processing, or protein translation have been described.

DNA Binding Proteins and Transcriptional Regulation

The ability to isolate eucaryotic genes and to manipulate their DNA sequence content by recombinant DNA technology have revealed many DNA sequence elements that regulate gene expression. Like the classic operon model in bacteria, eucaryotic regulatory elements are often upstream of the gene and operate to increase the frequency of RNA polymerase initiation and chain elongation. Reflecting their higher complexity, eucaryotic regulatory sites occur in modular combinations that allow greater diversity and tissue specificity of expression. Many eucaryotic genes are flanked by arrays of positive and negative control elements that produce different levels of gene activity in particular tissues or in response to hormonal or environmental signals.

Eucaryotic promoters are typically about l00 bp long, occur immediately 5′ to the start of transcription, and mediate selective and stable initiation of RNA polymerase. Within the promoter region are short sequences of 5–12 bp with drastic effects on transcription. These are the TATA box and upstream promoter elements such as the CCAAT box recall that the term "box" refers to a characteristic DNA sequence). *Enhancers* are variably sized DNA sequence elements that act to increase the rate of transcription from promoters. They may enhance transcription from upstream or downstream positions in an orientation-independent manner.

Promoter and enhancer elements serve as binding sites for sequence-specific DNA binding proteins. Several human genetic diseases are caused by deficiencies in these regulatory proteins, as exemplified by Cockayne syndrome in Table 6.2. As might be expected, mutations altering transcription factors produce multiple phenotypic effects as illustrated by the Rubinstein-Taybi syndrome (268600). This disorder produces growth and mental deficiency, broad thumbs and great toes, and a propensity for cancer (Table 6.2).

RNA Splicing and Stability

The events of RNA splicing, RNA transport to the cytoplasm, RNA modification, and RNA stability/degradation offer additional sites at which gene expression may be regulated. The best studied examples concern alternative splicing where different combinations of exons are joined to form unique mRNAs and protein products as in the immune system. Abnormal RNA splicing is a frequent mechanism in human genetic disease, caused by nucleotide replacements that alter splice recognition sites shown in Figure 6.3.

■ 6.5. REGULATION AT THE PROTEIN LEVEL: BIOCHEMICAL GENETICS

Interactions among proteins are major landmarks on the road from genotype to phenotype. Enzymic proteins control the rate of substrate conversions, producing a network known as intermediary metabolism. Proteins and small molecules also provide links among cells and organs, forming the regulated internal environment of each individual that is called *homeostasis*. Many genetic diseases involve altered activity, targeting, or regulation of proteins. These diseases comprise a specialized field within clinical genetics that is called *biochemical genetics*. Laboratory tests involved in biochemical genetics include measurements of enzyme amounts using enzyme activities, quantifying the substrates or products of enzymes, and the direct measurement or cytologic localization of proteins using specific antibodies. The clinical approach to biochemical genetic diseases are discussed in Chapter 12.

Enzymes and Pathways: Intermediary Metabolism

All enzymes act on a range of molecules called *substrates* and facilitate the formation of one or more molecules called *products*. The catalytic activity of individual enzymes can be measured and expressed as standard units. For most medical applications, assay conditions are manipulated so that the enzyme activity is proportionate to the amount of enzyme. An important aspect of enzyme catalysis is the concept of *enzyme reserve*. Most enzymes in cells are present at excess concentration, so that a decrease in enzyme amount does not produce a corresponding decrease in reaction rate. This

explains why many autosomal or X-linked recessive disorders involving genes that encode enzymes exhibit normal phenotypes in heterozygotes.

The regulation of enzyme activity can be complex, involving interactions of subunits, changes in conformation due to interactions with other proteins or small molecules (allosteric changes), and chemical modifications of the enzyme protein molecule. Some enzymes, like pyruvate dehydrogenase that is associated with Leigh's encephalopathy (266150), are complexes of multiple subunit peptides encoded by several genetic loci (Table 6.2).

Allosteric (literally, different shape) interactions are exemplified by the action of calcium and cyclic AMP on enzymes such as the kinases responsible for glycogen release. Chemical reactions also regulate protein activity, exemplified by glycosylation, prenylation, or cross-linking of amino acid residues within proteins. A common form of chemical modification occurs by kinase reactions, in which a phosphate group is added to one or more amino acid side chains.

Protein Processing

In addition to subunit, allosteric, and chemical regulation, many newly translated peptides are tailored by processing enzymes to achieve their mature and active form. Often there are N-terminal regions that serve as leader sequences to target proteins to the correct intracellular compartment. In the case of insulin, the initially translated peptide contains pre- and propeptide sequences that allow the protein to be stored as an inactive form. At least one inherited phenotype results from the alteration of insulin processing (Table 6.2). Hyperproinsulinemia (176730) is caused by a mutation at the site of clevage between the B and C propeptides, resulting in an uncleaved molecule with less insulin activity (hyperproinsulinemia, 176730).

The use of protein processing yields several proteins from one translational product in the case of the pro-opiomelanocortin (POMC)

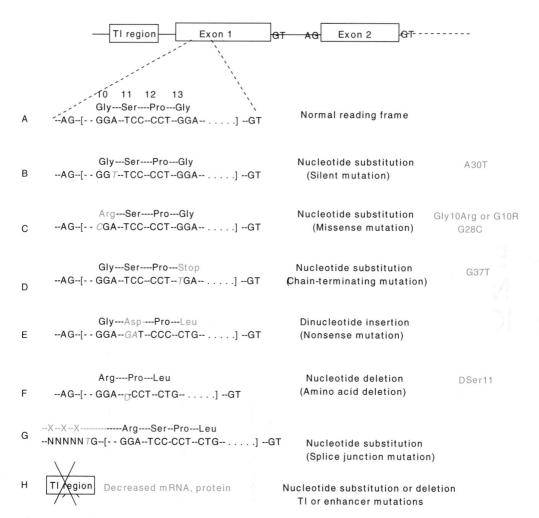

Figure 6.4. Effects of nucleotide sequences within one exon of a gene on the protein products following transcription and translation. TI, transcription initiation.

gene. Variable control of POMC protein processing allows different hormones to be produced in the intermediate and anterior lobes of the pituitary. The proteases that regulate this processing are in turn controlled by extracellular signals, again emphasizing the cascade of regulatory events that occur in complex organisms.

Cell Compartments: Protein Targeting and Transport

Cell membranes also segregate the cytoplasm into compartments or organelles that perform specialized functions. These include the nucleus, endoplasmic reticulum (ER), Golgi apparatus, mitochondrion, peroxisome, and lysosome. Specialized structures for protein synthesis (rough ER) and protein degradation (lysosomes) requires a targeting system for routing proteins to their functional regions (Fig. 6.5). The membranes of these compartments often have different membrane protein components with unique mechanisms for protein uptake or secretion.

Transport into the ER lumen is achieved by means of a leader or signal amino acid domain at the amino-terminus of the targeted protein.

The Z allele of α-1-antitrypsin deficiency (107400) interferes with this targeting process, with the result that α-1-antitrypsin protein is not transported out of liver cells into the blood stream. Homozygous ZZ individuals often develop liver disease in addition to the lung disease that is common with α-1-antitrypsin deficiency. The liver disease is thought to result from abnormal accumulation of α-1-antitrypsin that would normally be secreted outside of the liver cell (Table 6.2).

A genetic disorder called inclusion or I-cell disease (252500) results from a deficiency of glucosamine-N-acetyl-phosphotransferase; absence of the mannose-6-phosphate signal results in abnormal targeting of many proteins destined for the lysosome. The absence of multiple lysosomal enzymes results in the accumulation of abnormal substances in cell from a variety of tissues, producing visible microscopic inclusions. The clinical symptoms of I-cell disease include enlargements of the liver and spleen, severe skeletal deformities, obstruction of cerebrospinal fluid (hydrocephalus), and relentless brain dysfunction that produces neurologic regression and death (Table 6.2). I-cell disease, Hurler syndrome, and glycogen phosphorylase kinase deficiency be-

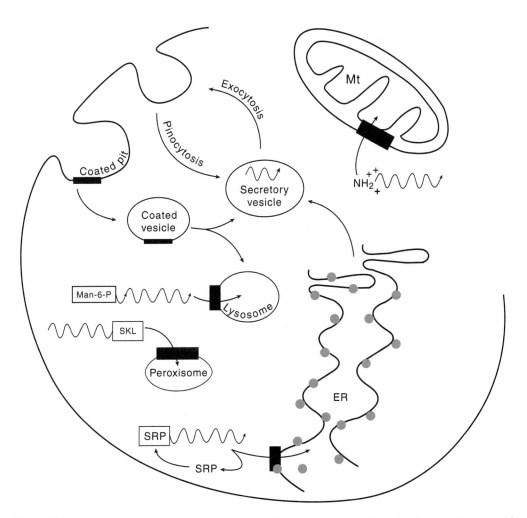

Figure 6.5. Levels of analysis for genetic anemias. Clinical symptoms define the disease category, with possible testing at the cell, protein, and gene levels.

long to a category of biochemical genetic diseases in which substances accumulate to cause pathology. These disorders are called *storage diseases.*

Other cellular compartments that contain specific complements of proteins include peroxisomes and mitochondria. Mitochondria are unique in having a genome, the only other cellular DNA besides that in the nucleus. Like bacterial genomes, mitochondrial DNA lacks introns and encodes peculiar ribosomal and transfer RNAs that resemble those of bacteria. Although a few peptides are encoded by the mitochondrial genome, most are encoded by the nuclear genome and transported into mitochondria. This transport involves a cluster of positively charged amino acids at the N-terminus of proteins destined for mitochondria (Fig. 6.5). A genetic disorder that alters the metabolism of ammonia (urea cycle disorder) involves deficiency of the enzyme ornithine transcarbamylase (OTC—321250). The resulting deficiency of mitochondrial OTC interrupts the flow of conversion of ammonia by the urea cycle, producing hyperammonemia, seizures, coma, and death in untreated children.

Proteins targeted to peroxisomes have specific amino acid signals that lead to transport across the peroxisomal membrane. Some genetic diseases alter the function of peroxisomal membrane proteins, resulting in a deficient peroxisomal matrix that lacks multiple peroxisomal enzyme activities. Because of the vital role of lipid metabolism in the nervous system, patients with generalized peroxisomal deficiencies have severe mental disability, seizures, and hypotonia. Zellweger syndrome (214100) is caused by a heterogenous group of autosomal recessive mutations that affect peroxisomal membrane proteins (Table 6.2).

Cytoskeleton Proteins

Cells of higher animals devote 25–35% of total protein synthesis to construct a cytoskeletal framework that controls cell shape and multiple cellular functions. The cytoskeleton, together with the inner reticulum of cell membranes, provides a network by which regulatory molecules can produce rapid changes in cell growth rates, cell motility and protoplasmic streaming, or cell anchorage and adhesion. The cytoskeleton includes microtubules, intermediate filaments, nonmuscle actin filaments, and coated vesicles that contain the structural protein (clathrin). Dynein is a motor protein associated with microubules in cilia that is deficient in some patients with Kartagener syndrome (244400). Individuals with this condition have sinus infections and infertility due to abnormal ciliary function in the respiratory epithelium and sperm. Unexpectedly, they also exhibit *situs inversus* (reversal of normal sidedness with the heart on the left and liver on the right), presumably because ciliary movement is required to accomplish proper situs in the early embryo.

Extracellular Matrix Proteins

The extracellular matrix is a network of two classes of molecules: fibrillar proteins such as collagens or fibronectins embedded within a glycosaminoglycan (mucopolysaccharide) ground substance. Collagens are the most abundant protein in the extracellular matrix, with more than 15 types that have specific tissue distributions. Mutations in these many collagen genes are responsible for a large and diverse group of genetic diseases such as osteogenesis imperfecta (166200; Table 6.2). The bluish sclerae and weak bones in this condition were discussed in Chapter 1, and its molecular basis is described in Chapter 8.

■ 6.6. GENETIC ANEMIAS: LEVELS OF CELLULAR AND MOLECULAR DELINEATION

Genetic diseases are thus DNA sequence changes that disrupt one or more levels of the genetic hierarchy. Genetic diseases can be defined by laboratory methods that characterize the pathway from genotype to phenotype and establish which processes and molecules are altered. Once a genetic disease is understood in terms of particular molecules and cellular responses, the molecular basis of disease is defined. The cellular and molecular abnormalities can then be used for laboratory diagnosis of the disease. Diseases affecting red blood cell function are now discussed as examples of how the genetic hierarchy serves as a framework for understanding the molecular basis and laboratory diagnosis of genetic diseases (Fig. 6.6).

Genetics of Anemia: The Cellular Level

A deficiency of red blood cells produces numerous clinical manifestations that were recognized early in medical history as anemia. The anemias form a category of disease characterized by pallor in the surface tissues, fatigue and breathlessness due to poor oxygen supply, and progressive heart failure (Fig. 6.6, upper level). The heart failure reflects an attempt to restore homeostasis by more rapid

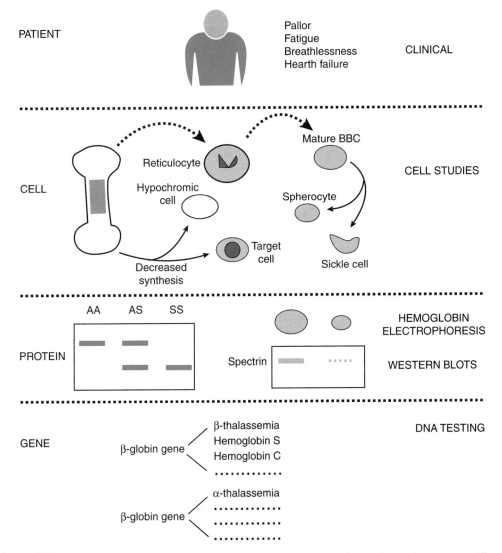

Figure 6.6. Route from globin gene mutations to effects on hemoglobin and vascular structure, illustrated by the sickle cell anemia mutation (S, right panel).

heart contractions and increased blood circulation (increased oxygen delivery). An early clinical distinction separated anemias due to environment influences (e.g., poor nutrition, nitrates in well water) and those exhibiting a familial basis.

The cellular basis for anemias became evident when red blood cells and bone marrow spaces were defined by microscopy. Clinical samples were obtained by blood drawing or bone marrow aspiration, and cellular characteristics were associated with various types of anemia. Some anemias were caused by decreased production of erythrocytes due to defective bone marrow or hemoglobin synthesis; others exhibited increased destruction of erythrocytes with increased reticulocytes (immature red cells) and malformed red cells. Still other anemias became associated with characteristic red cell shapes, exemplified by inherited diseases with spherical, sickle-shaped, or targeted cells (see diagrams in Fig. 6.6, middle level).

Genetics of Anemia: The Protein Level

The first disease to be characterized at the protein level was sickle cell anemia (141900; Fig. 6.6, middle level). Because hemoglobin was abundant in erythrocytes, its subunit α- and β-globin peptides were readily purified and characterized in terms of their amino acid sequences. The laboratory technique of hemoglobin electrophoresis could detect mutations that altered the number of charged amino acids (Fig. 6.6, middle level), and amino acid sequencing demonstrated that patients with sickle cell anemia had a single amino acid difference in their β-globin peptide. The hemoglobin S molecule detected by its abnormal mobility by gel electrophoresis had a valine substituted for glutamine at the sixth amino acid from the amino-terminus of each β-globin peptide (G_6V, Fig. 6.7). Once recombinant DNA technology became available, characterization of the β-globin gene demonstrated that the valine → glutamine amino acid substitution was caused by a point mutation changing

A to T at the 17th base (6th codon) of the first exon ($A_{17}T$, Fig. 6.7).

The missense mutation in β-globin DNA resulted in a β-globin protein that polymerized in deoxygenated red cells, producing sickle-shaped cells that were destroyed more rapidly. The resulting clinical problems included anemia and the occlusion of small blood vessels by sickled cells. These occluded vessels prevented oxygen from reaching nearby tissues, initiating a sequence of tissue hypoxemia, cell death, inflammation, and pain that is known as tissue *infarction*. The bone marrow, lungs, and spleen are particularly susceptible to infarction from occlusion of small blood vessels, leading to the variable combinations of painful organs known as sickle cell crisis. As the patient ages, blood vessel linings (intima) are damaged and accumulate blood clots. The occlusion of larger vessels by clots causes severe complications such as myocardial infarctions (heart attacks), cerebral infarctions (strokes), and splenic infarctions (rendering the patient vulnerable to certain bacterial infections).

As diagrammed in Figures 6.6 and 6.7, the hierarchy of consequences from A or S alleles through protein, cellular, and organ function provides a prime example of the genetic basis of disease. The autosomal recessive inheritance of the SS genotype explained in Chapter 2 can now be visualized in terms of a single nucleotide change that leads to a cascade of cellular and organ abnormalities.

Genetics of Anemia: The Gene Level

Among the genetic causes of anemia are several types of mutations that affect hemoglobin. These mutations form a group of genetic anemias called *hemoglobinopathies*. The spectrum of disease within this group can be explained according to the organization of hemoglobin genes and the type and/or position of the mutation within the α- or β-globin gene. There are two main types of hemoglobinopathies: *thalassemias* with imbalance in the synthesis of α- and β-globin peptides that produce inadequate amounts of hemoglobin, and

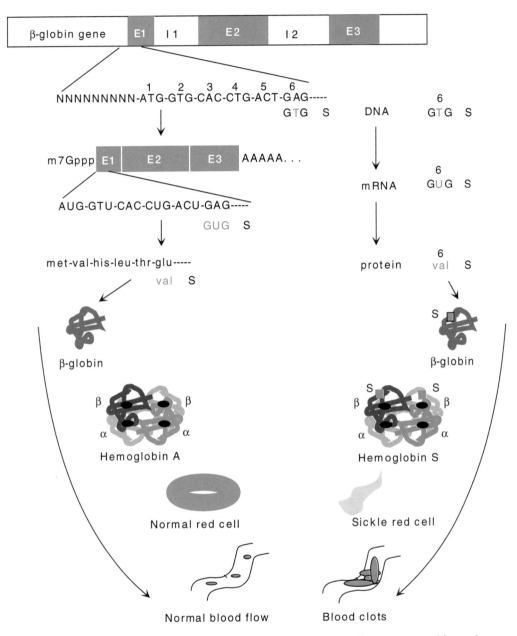

Figure 6.7. Globin gene clusters, α- and β-globin genes with their similar structures with two introns, and the locations of mutations causing thalassemias with targeted cells (T), anemias (A), altered heme binding and oxygen transport (M), or sickle cells (S).

abnormal hemoglobins that are more rapidly degraded or have reduced ability to transport oxygen.

Mutations that produce thalassemia (273500; T in Fig. 6.8) drastically reduce the production of α- or β-globin peptides, resulting in anemia and the presence of depleted cells with hemoglobin only at their centers (*target cells*). Thalassemia mutations can interfere with transcription, splicing, protein coding (e.g., frame

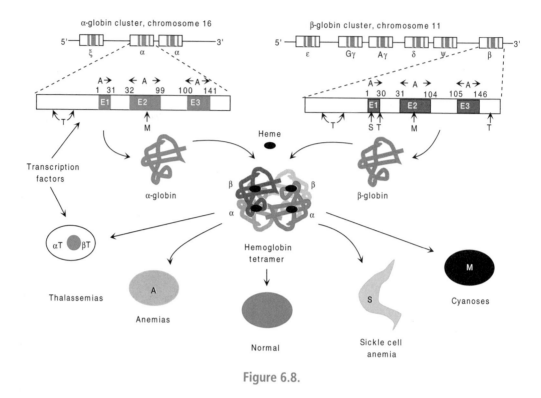

Figure 6.8.

shift mutations), or polyA addition; several sites for thalassemia mutations are therefore diagrammed in Figure 6.8. Mutations reducing the synthesis of α-globin (β-thalassemias) are more common because there is only one β-globin gene in the cluster on chromosome 11 (Fig. 6.8). Mutations producing α-thalassemia must affect both copies of the α-globin gene in the cluster on chromosome 16. Deletions are therefore common causes of α-thalassemia, because mutations that alter the transcription, splicing, or frame of one α-globin gene can be compensated by the presence of the second gene. Individuals with α-globin gene deletions or mutations may have zero, one, two, or three functional genes in diploid cells. Those with two or three functional genes have mild α-thalassemia, while those with one functional gene (hemoglobin H disease) or no functional genes (hydrops fetalis) have severe α-thalassemia. The lack of α-globin chains in these latter diseases lead to the formation of very ab-

normal hemoglobins—hemoglobin H consisting of 4 β-globin chains or hemoglobin Bart's consisting of 4 γ-globin chains.

If mutations in the globin genes do not grossly reduce the amount of α- or β-globin, then balanced globin chain synthesis produces normal amounts of hemoglobin. However, the function of hemoglobin in maintaining red cell structure and, through its heme groups, in transporting oxygen can be compromised by various amino acid changes. Most hemoglobinopathies present as anemia due to mutations (A in Fig. 6.8) that render it or the red cell unstable so that there is increased red cell destruction (hemolysis). Such hemolytic anemias can be distinguished from those due to decreased red cell synthesis by the high numbers of immature red blood cells (erythroblasts or reticulocytes) that are released into the circulation in an attempt to restore homeostasis. As shown in Figure 6.8, missense amino acid changes that produce anemias can occur throughout the exons of the α- or β-globin genes. A special type of missense mutation affects amino acids near the heme binding site, producing M hemoglobins that are poor oxygen carriers (141900). Individuals with M hemoglobins may have bluish discoloration of their lips and other surface tissues that reflects hypoxemia (cyanosis).

The hemoglobinopathies summarized in Figures 6.7 and 6.8 provide an elegant example of the way in which genetic changes can be used to clarify and classify disease mechanisms. Note that the complex array of red cell changes, of symptoms from decreased oxygen to various organs, can be explained by a single concept—the type and position of nucleotide change within the DNA segments that comprise globin genes. The testing for disease also reduces from complex studies of red cell survival, bone marrow synthesis, or cardiopulmonary function to the common medium of DNA analysis; define the gene mutation and the entire cascade of consequences due to the abnormal hemoglobin can be predicted. The mechanisms by which these DNA mutations are detected in hemoglobinopathies and other genetic diseases are presented in Chapter 8.

Genetic Anemias and the Genetic Hierarchy

Other parts of the genetic hierarchy can also be illustrated by the clinical regulation of red blood cell synthesis. Chromatin structure probably mediates the remarkable switch between fetal hemoglobin (γ-globin) and hemoglobin A (β-globin) synthesis that occurs during infancy. There is a locus control region upstream of the α-globin cluster (Fig. 6.8) where specific transcription factors bind to activate globin synthesis in erythroid cells. The red cell also has a cytoskeleton that produces its unique, biconcave shape. Cytoskeletal proteins may be disrupted by genetic diseases such as the spherocytoses (182870; Fig. 6.6). Spherocytosis can be diagnosed from blood smears by noting small, round erythrocytes that are more rapidly destroyed. Several types of spherocytosis have been characterized at the protein level, each involving a cytoskeletal protein such as spectrin (Fig. 6.6, middle level).

Although the repertoire of red cell enzymes is limited due to its large stores of hemoglobin, enzyme deficiencies also come into play as causes of anemia. A key enzyme in red blood cells is the glucose-6-phosphate dehydrogenase (305900) discussed in Chapter 5 as an example of pharmacogenetic variation. Individuals with G6PD deficiency cannot generate sufficient energy and reducing power in their red cells to maintain normal cellular function. When exposed to certain drugs or fava beans, their red cells undergo hemolysis and produce a crisis of anemia and renal failure. Another important enzyme in red blood cells is methemoglobin reductase. Inherited deficiency of this enzyme (250700) leads to increased amounts of underoxygenated hemoglobin (methemoglobin) and produces a bluish appearance of the surface tissues (cyanosis). A phenocopy of the genetic disorder is produced by exposure to well water containing nitrate fertilizers, which inhibit methemoglobin reductase. In contrast to the reductase deficiency, mutations in the β-globin gene also produce methemoglobins by interfering with the heme binding site and oxygenation (Fig. 6.8). The spectrum of genetic anemias from hemoglobinopathies to spherocytosis to red cell enzyme deficiencies thus illustrates the many steps in the genetic hierarchy, each susceptible to disruption by mutation. Genetic diseases can thus be diagnosed and classified according to the level of abnormal gene action, allowing a unifying approach to disease that complements classifications based on organ systems. Additional examples of this molecular approach to disease is found throughout the remaining chapters.

Case 6 Follow-up: A form of X-linked mental retardation has been characterized that would fit the situation of two affected males. This disease results from mutations within an X chromosome locus that encodes a transcription factor. This transcription factor is one of many that acts on the upstream region of the globin genes, particularly enhancing the transcription of α-globin genes. In the presence of the mutation, decreased α-globin production produces mild α-thalassemia and provides a clue to the underlying diagnosis. The two boys had the same hypotonia and somewhat coarsened facial features described in the α-thalassemia-mental retardation syndrome (Gibbons et al., 1992), and red cell studies that confirmed the presence of α-thalassemia suggested the correct diagnosis. Further testing at the DNA level provided additional diagnostic certainty and the chance for the parents to elect prenatal diagnosis in future pregnancies. A specific diagnosis was thus made among many possibilities causing mental retardation, and a beginning of molecular understanding is available for this disease. A search for other genes important for mental function that are regulated by this altered transcription factor is underway in an attempt to explain the molecular basis for the mental retardation.

PROBLEM SET 6
Gene Expression and the Genetic Hierarchy

Questions 6.1–6.2. A hypothetical gene contains two exons that encode a protein of 100 amino acids. They are separated by an intron of 100 bp beginning after the codon for amino acid 10. The gene's messenger RNA (mRNA) has 5′ and 3′ untranslated regions of 70 and 30 nucleotides, respectively. Match the characteristics of the gene with the appropriate measures below.

(A) 500 bp   (D) 100 bp
(B) 400 bp   (E) 70 bp
(C) 300 bp

6.1. Size of nuclear RNA transcript minus added poly(A) tail

6.2. Size of cDNA made from mature mRNA

Questions 6.3–6.5. Recall that adult hemoglobin synthesis requires transcription factors that activate the α- and β-globin genes, splicing to form mature mRNA, balanced globin protein synthesis, and association of the globins with heme to form a functional hemoglobin molecule. Match the phenotypes below with the process(es) affected by mutation:

(A) Severe anemia with targeted cells indicative of imbalanced globin protein synthesis
(B) Mild anemia with no cyanosis
(C) Mild anemia with obvious cyanosis
(D) Mild anemia with small, rounded red cells
(E) Severe anemia with vascular occlusion and thromboses (strokes, heart attacks)

6.3. Deletion in the upstream promoter of the β-globin gene

6.4. Deletion of a 3 bp codon in an β-globin gene

6.5. Frameshift mutation in the β-globin gene

Questions 6.6–6.10. The various types of genetic anemias, like many other genetic disease categories, must be diagnosed by particular laboratory studies. Match the following alterations of β-globin gene expression with the test that will be sufficiently abnormal to allow diagnosis.

(A) Mutation in the upstream region to cause mild thalassemia
(B) Deletion of the second β-globin exon to cause severe thalassemia
(C) Mutation in an RNA splice site to cause severe thalassemia
(D) Amino acid substitution (charged to neutral) to produce an unstable β-globin peptide
(E) Amino acid substitution (neutral to neutral) in the binding site for heme.

6.6. Analysis to detect altered mobility of β-globin protein by electrophoresis

6.7. Analysis to detect decreased oxygen binding by red blood cells

6.8. Analysis to detect altered size of β-globin protein

6.9. Analysis to detect altered DNA sequence of promoter regions

6.10. Analysis to detect altered size of β-globin mRNA

PROBLEM SET 6
Answers

		6.4. B
6.10. C	6.7. E	6.3. A
6.9. A	6.6. D	6.2. B
6.8. B	6.5. A	6.1. A

(Note: answers printed upside-down)

PROBLEM SET 6
Solutions

6.1–6.2. The primary RNA transcript of split genes contains both exons and introns, but the latter are removed by RNA splicing. The 5′ (upstream) and 3′ (downstream) untranslated RNA regions remain in the mature RNA and are thought to regulate RNA transport or translation. A poly(A) tail is added to the primary transcript after transcription, which facilitates transport and processing from the nucleus. The gene under discussion must contain a coding region of 300 bp (100 amino acids × 3 bp per amino acid) plus 100 bp in the intron, plus 70 + 30 = 100 bp in the untranslated regions (total = 500 bp; 6.1-A). The mature RNA contains the same number of bp except for the 100 bp in the intron (500 − 100 = 400 bp; 6.2-B).

6.3–6.5. Mutations that decrease the transcription or translation of β-globin protein lead to a thalassemia phenotype with anemia and target cells that reflect imbalance of globin synthesis (6.3-A, 6.5-A). Mutations that affect one of the two α-globin genes have milder phenotypes with either undetectable or mild anemia (6.4-B). Mutations that affect the heme binding site decrease the ability of hemoglobin to transport oxygen, causing oxygen-depleted tissues and cyanosis (e.g., hemoglobin M, 141900). Mutations in the red cell cytoskeleton, illustrated by spectrin mutations in autosomal dominant spherocytosis (182870), often alter red cell shape and fragility to produce mild anemia. Sickle cell anemia also alters red cell shape because hemoglobin S (141900) polymerizes within the cell, leading to vascular occlusion.

6.6–6.10. Alteration of the β-globin gene promoter region produces decreased amounts of normally sized β-globin mRNA and protein. Such mutations are best detected by DNA analysis (answer 6.9A). Mutations that significantly decrease the amounts of β-globin mRNA or protein produce imbalance of α- and β-globin peptide synthesis, causing thalassemia. Thalassemias due to abnormal mRNA splicing can be detected by altered size of β-globin mRNA (answer 6.10C), while those due to exon deletions have altered size of β-globin protein (answer 6.8B). Substitutions that change charged amino acids like lysine (terminal amino group) to neutral amino acids (like valine with no charged group) alter the mobility of proteins by electrophoresis (answer 6.6D). Those that affect the heme binding site alter the affinity for oxygen (answer 6.7E).

BIBLIOGRAPHY

Gene Structure and Regulation

Alberts B, Bray D, Lewis J, Raff M, Roberts K, Watson JD. 1989. *Molecular Biology of the Cell,* 2nd ed. New York: Garland Publishing.

Benjamini E, Sunshine G, Leskowitz S. 1996. *Immunology: A Short Course,* 3rd ed. New York: Wiley-Liss.

Britten RJ, Kohne DE. 1968. Repeated sequences in DNA. *Science* 161:529–540.

Brown DD. 1981. Gene expression in eukaryotes. *Science* 211:667–674.

Fulton AB. 1982. How crowded is the cytoplasm? *Cell* 30:345–347.

Stellar H. 1995. Mechanisms and genes of cellular suicide. *Science* 267:1445–1449.

Strachan T, Read A. 1996. *Human Molecular Genetics.* New York: Wiley-Liss.

Watson J, Crick. 1953. Molecular structure of nucleic acids. A structure for deoxyribonucleic acid. *JAMA* 269:1966–1969; 1993 (reprinted from *Nature*).

Human Genes and Genetic Disorders

Gibbons RJ, Suthers GK, Wilkie AOM, Buckle VJ, Higgs DR. 1992. X-linked α-thalassemia/mental retardation (ATR-X) syndrome: localization to

Xq12-q21.31 by X inactivation and linkage analysis. *Am J Hum Genet* 51:1136–1149.

Weatherall DJ, Clegg JB, Higgs DR, Wood WG. 1995. The hemoglobinopathies. In Scriver CR, Beaudet AL, Sly WS, Valle D, eds. *The Metabolic and Molecular Basis of Inherited Disease.* New York: McGraw-Hill, pp. 3417–3484.

7

GENETICS AT THE CHROMOSOME LEVEL: CYTOGENETICS

■ LEARNING OBJECTIVES

1. Errors in chromosome segregation and recombination lead to aberrations that cause disease.
2. The organized human chromosome complement is called a *karyotype* and variations can be described precisely using cytogenetic notation.
3. Harmless variations in chromosome structure are called *heteromorphisms*, including particularly the satellite regions (chromosomes 13–15, 21–22) or centromeric heterochromatin (chromosomes 1,9,16).
4. The hallmarks of chromosomal disease are developmental disability and multiple congenital anomalies including an unusual facial appearance.
5. Complete or partial aneuploidy produces distinctive patterns of anomalies (chromosomal syndromes) that require early diagnosis and preventive management.

6. Sex chromosome aneuploidy and certain ring chromosomes produce milder syndromes that present mainly as cognitive and behavioral problems.
7. Smaller interstitial deletions (microdeletions) produce malformation syndromes that reflect haploinsufficiency of specific genetic loci.
8. Chromosome instability occurs because of defective DNA repair, expanding DNA repeats at "fragile sites," and progressive aneuploidy during neoplasia.

*Case 7: **The Undetected Translocation***
A child is evaluated for developmental delay and is noted to have an unusual appearance. The family history is remarkable (Fig. 7.1) in that his mother and maternal grandmother both had several miscarriages; in addition, he has an uncle and cousin who were "slow" on his mother's side. A chromosome study is performed on the child, but is reported as normal.

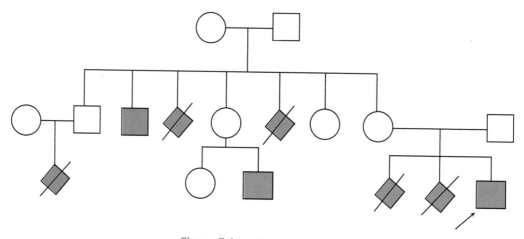

Figure 7.1. Pedigree for Case 7.

■ 7.1. INTRODUCTION: THE SPECTRUM OF CHROMOSOMAL DISEASE

Chromosomal diseases involve extra, missing, or rearranged genetic material, resulting in the abnormal expression of multiple genes. Chromosomal aberrations are associated with medical problems such as spontaneous abortions, children with mental disability and/or congenital anomalies, infertility, and certain cancers. More than one hundred patterns of birth defects due to chromosome anomalies (chromosomal syndromes) have now been characterized, and most types of cancer have been associated with specific chromosome changes. The magnitude of chromosomal disease is illustrated by the fact that at least 50% of spontaneous abortions and 0.5% of live-born children have chromosomal aberrations. Cytogenetics is now a key hospital laboratory service, drawing samples from pediatrics, obstetrics (prenatal diagnosis), and surgical pathology (cancer or abortus tissues).

The ability to analyze human chromosomes using the light microscope ushered in a new era of clinical genetics. Although the human diploid number was repeatedly (and embarrassingly) counted as 48 prior to 1958, a technical advance that utilized hypotonic solutions to spread chromosomes allowed precise inspection and counting. Down and Turner syndromes were rapidly characterized by their extra or missing chromosomes, leading to objective diagnostic tests for children and prenatal diagnosis during pregnancy. The development of banding techniques delineated subtle chromosome changes, and the striking and still unexplained resemblance among children with similar chromosomal changes became appreciated. The merging of chromosome and molecular studies soon promoted a view of chromosomes as road maps for genes, and chromosomal studies became a powerful adjunct for gene localization and isolation. In turn, single copy and repetitive gene probes now provide increased resolution for chromosome studies through the techniques of fluorescent *in situ* hybridization (FISH) and chromosome painting. Modern cytogenetics is thus an important interface between clinical and molecular studies, and the concepts in this chapter lead directly to the principles of molecular genetics discussed in Chapter 8.

■ 7.2. CHROMOSOMES AND CELL DIVISION

Cells undergo cycles of growth and division that are controlled according to their needs and functions. *Cell cycles* can be divided into a stage of growth or quiescence (interphase) and a stage of division (*mitosis* or M phase). Each mitosis involves chromosomal condensation in prophase, alignment of chromosomes at the cell equator during metaphase, centromere division with separation of *sister chromatids* during anaphase, and partitioning of 46 sister chromatids into each daughter cell during telophase and cytokinesis. Unless there are errors in chromosome alignment or DNA replication, mitosis produces daughter cells whose genetic information is identical to that of the parent cell.

Although somatic cells divide by mitosis, germ cells have a special mechanism for cell division that is called *meiosis*. The first meiotic division involves primary spermatocytes or primary oocytes and yields secondary germ cells with 46 chromosomes. The second meiotic division is similar to that of mitosis, with the *centromeres* dividing to produce daughter cells (gametes—eggs or sperm) with 23 chromosomes. Gametes can then fuse together at fertilization to produce a new individual with 46 chromosomes. Greater detail on the differences between mitosis and meiosis is provided on the website (http://www.wiley.com/wilson/).

▪ 7.3. CYTOGENETIC TECHNOLOGY

Chromosomes Are Visualized at Mitotic Metaphase in Diploid Cells

Most human cytogenetic studies are performed on somatic cells at metaphase. In somatic cells, the chromosomes are *diploid* with 22 pairs of autosomes and one pair of sex chromosomes. The diploid chromosome number is described as 2n, where n is the *haploid* number of chromosomes in gametes. For humans, n is 23 and the diploid number (2n) is 46. Additional multiples of the haploid number occur in some cells as *triploidy* (3n) or *tetraploidy* (4n). Cells in which the chromosome count is an even multiple of n are called *polyploid*, while those with uneven multiples of n (i.e., 2n + 1 = 47 chromosomes, 4n − 2 = 90 chromosomes) are called *aneuploid*.

Figure 7.2 illustrates the steps for preparing slides with metaphase spreads of chromosomes from routine samples of peripheral blood. It is important to avoid clotting or freezing of the blood sample, because these events agglutinate or destroy the white blood cells and prevent cell division. The buffy coat or white

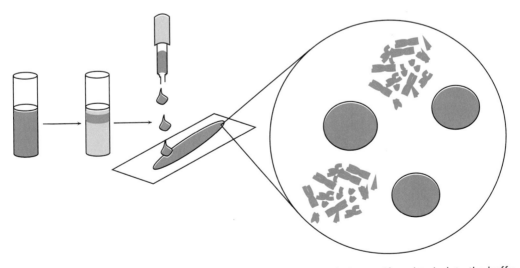

Figure 7.2. Karyotyping from peripheral blood. The blood sample is centrifuged to isolate the buffy coat (white blood cells), which is cultured and arrested in metaphase. After hypotonic treatment, a smear is prepared from the cultured cell suspension and analyzed under the microscope. Successful preparations contain metaphase spreads (right) that can be analyzed and photographed.

blood cell layer is separated from the blood by centrifugation, then incubated with plant lectins such as *phytohemagglutinin;* in rare cases when B rather than T-lymphocytes are the target of analysis, pokeweed mitogen can be added. The cells are allowed to divide for 24–72 hours, then arrested at metaphase with mitotic spindle inhibitors such as colchicine. After cell lysis in hypotonic solution and pipetting onto a glass slide, optimal preparations exhibit a well-separated array of chromosomes from 1–2% of the swollen nuclei (Fig. 7.3A).

Technical judgment and art are still part of the cytogenetic laboratory enterprise. The number of metaphase spreads adequate for analysis depends on the quality of cell culture, the time of hypotonic incubation, the treatment of the glass slide, and the height of the pipette

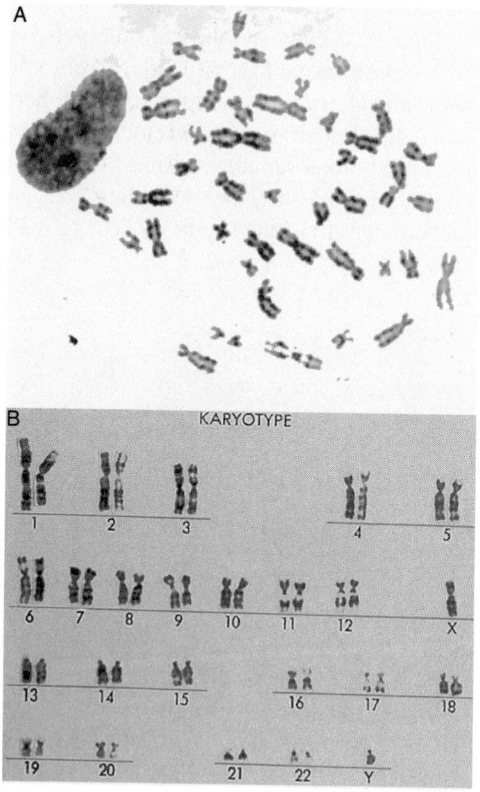

Figure 7.3. *A*, Photomicrograph of a buffy coat smear showing a metaphase spread (left) and intact nucleus (right); *B*, a karyotype arranged from a photomicrograph of a metaphase spread.

from the slide surface. Once dropped and spread, the slides are fixed in successively higher concentrations of alcohol and stained with dyes such as Giemsa (e.g., Fig. 7.3).

Chromosome Banding and Special Stains

Chromosome banding techniques include a variety of acid or heat treatments on slides containing chromosome preparations. The alternation of chromosomal regions with high or low G + C content accounts in part for the banding patterns, although the need for protease treatment indicates a role for chromosomal proteins as well. In any case, standard Giemsa (G) or quinacrine (Q) bands, reverse (R), or centromeric (C) bands can be produced according to the type of heat, acid, protease, or staining treatment employed. Banding using Giemsa dye is now standard, with other techniques reserved for the examination of special chromosomal domains.

Arrest of cells in early metaphase (*prometaphase*) yields more extended chromosomes with over 3000 bands along the 46 chromosomes. The demanding technology of prometaphase analysis has now been modified for routine analysis, making 300–500 bands per karyotype the standard for adequate chromosome analysis. The karyotype shown in Figure 7.3B contains about 300 bands, as can be rapidly estimated by the 9–10 bands visible on each chromosome 10.

Molecular Cytogenetics

Even at optimal resolution, prometaphase banding yields no more than 3000 bands per genome of 46 chromosomes, making the average band equivalent to 2 Mb of DNA or 50 genes of 40 kb in size. This calculation emphasizes why deletions or mutations of single genes are not detected by routine chromosome studies. With the development of recombinant DNA technology and gene cloning, DNA probes could be linked to colored fluorescent tags and hybridized to chromosome preparations (fluorescent in situ hybridization or FISH techniques).

Single-copy FISH DNA probes yield signals in intact nuclei as well as in metaphase spread. In the absence of deletions, the number of fluorescent signals matches the number of chromosomes. Common aneuploidies involving chromosomes 13, 18, 21, X, or Y can thus be detected without the need for laborious counting of metaphase spreads, and results can be provided rapidly because the induction and arrest of cell division is not necessary. *Chromosome painting* techniques use repetitive FISH DNA probes that target repeating DNA segments that are specific for each chromosome. A "chromosome paint" thus causes the entire chromosome to fluoresce with the chosen color, allowing rearranged segments of that chromosome to be visualized where a single chromosome may contain segments of 3–4 other chromosomes. Such changes are common in malignant cells, and related painting techniques called *comparative genomic hybridization* can detect consistent deficiencies or duplications of particular chromosome regions in these complex cells.

■ 7.4. CYTOGENETIC NOTATION

Cytogenetic notation is a standardized code that describes chromosome abnormalities. Health professionals should acquire some familiarity with cytogenetic notation so they can interpret laboratory reports.

The Standard Human Karyotype, Variations, and Aberrations

With a few exceptions, human chromosome structure is the same for all tissues and all individuals. It is thus possible to speak of a standard human karyotype (Fig. 7.3B) and represent it by a diagram called an *idiogram* (Fig. 7.4). The detail and resolution of the idiogram varies according to the methodology for chromosomal analysis, with higher resolution techniques such as prometaphase banding yielding

many more bands per chromosome. Figure 7.4 depicts an idiogram based on a human karyotype obtained under ideal conditions, which should yield about 500 bands per 46 chromosomes or 20–25 bands on each chromosome number 10. Since Giemsa is the usual dye employed for chromosome staining, as in Figure 7.3B, the light and dark bands diagrammed in Figure 7.4 correspond to their appearance after Giemsa banding. Quinacrine or Q-banding techniques would highlight the darker bands as orange fluorescence, while reverse or R-banding techniques would produce the opposite pattern with the lighter bands showing as dark.

Note that the chromosomes are generally placed in order of size and that there are several types of human chromosomes according to the position of the centromere and the lengths of the short and long arms (Fig. 7.4). Symbols have been developed to refer to particular chromosome regions as listed in Table 7.1. By convention, the short arms are represented by p (for *petite*) and always positioned above the centromere in the standard idiogram. The long arms are represented by q (the letter following p) and shown below the centromere. Chromosomes could first be grouped according to their overall shape (Groups A–G), then identified specifically according to their banding pattern (1–22, X, and Y). Groups D (13–15) and G (21, 22, and Y) are notable because of their small p arms consisting of *satellite* DNA; these chromosomes may join to form *Robertsonian translocations*.

Certain chromosome regions exhibit individual variation or *heteromorphism*. These include *heterochromatin* (darkly staining chromatin, h in Table 7.1) surrounding the centromeres on chromosomes number 1, 9, and 16 and the *satellites* (s in Table 7.1) on chromosomes 13–15, 21–22, and Y. The Yq chromosome arm is also highly variable from male to male.

Chromosome aberrations refer to extra, missing, or rearranged chromosomal material that is likely to be associated with disease (Fig. 7.5). The symbols listed in Table 7.1 allow the chromosome aberrations illustrated in Figure

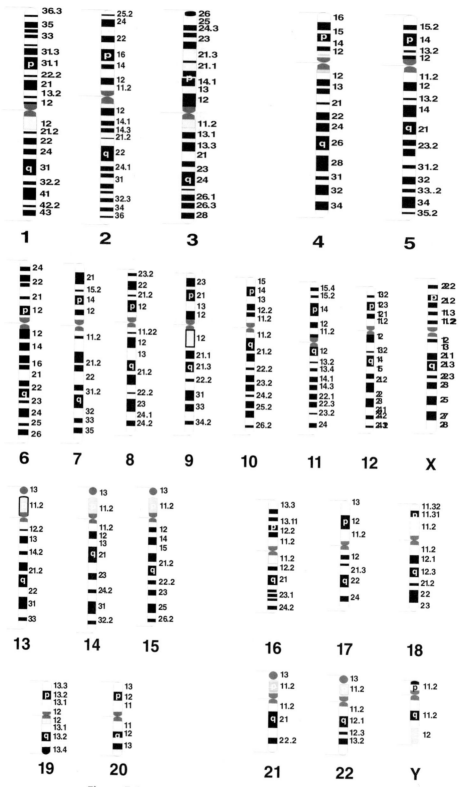

Figure 7.4. Idiogram of the standard human karyotype.

■**TABLE 7.1.** Symbols for Cytogenetic Notation

Symbol	Meaning
cen	Centromere of chromosome
del	Deletion of a chromosome region
der	Derivative chromosome
dup	Duplication of a chromosome region
fra	Fragile site
h	Heterochromatin
i	Isochromosome
ins	Insertion of a chromosome region
inv	Inversion of a chromosome region
mar	Marker chromosome
mat	Maternal origin of chromosome
Minus (-)	Loss of a chromosome
p	Short arm of chromosome
pat	Paternal origin of chromosome
q	Long arm of chromosome
r	Ring chromosome
s	Satellite region of chromosome
Semicolon (;)	Separate chromosome regions
Slant (/)	Separates karyotypes of different cell lines
t	Translocation
ter	Terminus of chromosome

7.5 to be described by specific cytogenetic notation (examples in Table 7.2). An addition of one chromosome to produce 3 rather than the usual 2 in each cell is called a *trisomy* (Fig. 7.5*A*); the loss of one chromosome is called a *monosomy* (Fig. 7.5*B*). Acrocentric D and G-group chromosomes may join together to form Robertsonian translocations (Fig. 7.5*C*), while exchange of material between two different chromosomes is called a *reciprocal translocation* (Fig. 7.5*D*). Individual chromosomes may undergo breakage and reunion with themselves to produce isochromosomes (Fig. 7.5*E*), peri- or paracentric inversions (Fig. 7.8), terminal deletions (Fig. 7.5*F*), or ring chromosomes (Fig. 7.5*H*). Occasionally there is unbalanced rearrangement of chromosomes, as illustrated by extra material on chromosome 20 (Fig. 7.5*G*). Breakage and reunion at homologous sites between sister chromatids is called *recombination* and does not usually produce chromosomal aberrations.

Because every human is a composite of millions of cells derived from one fertilized egg, a karyotype is usually considered typical for every cell in the individual. Occasionally, a chromosomal aberration occurs after fertilization, producing a mixture of normal and abnormal cells called *mosaicism*. Mosaicism can affect the somatic cells, the germ cells, or both depending on the timing of the aberration relative to the derivation of germ cells at about 22–24 days gestation. (See Chapter 10 for discussion of somatic and germ-line mosaicism).

Notation for Chromosomal Aberrations

Cytogenetic notation specifies the number of chromosomes, the sex chromosomes, and, for aberrations, abnormal processes with band positions (Table 7.2). The chromosome number is usually 46 with XX or XY sex chromosomes; a normal karyotype is thus 46,XX or 46,XY. If the karyotype is abnormal, a process is noted that describes what went wrong and band positions are noted to indicate where it went wrong. For clarity, terms within cytogenetic notation are separated by commas but not spaces (Tables 7.1, 7.2). Simple gain (+) or loss (–) of a chromosome is exemplified by the notation 47,XX,+21 (the extra chromosome number 21 in Down syndrome) or 45,XX,–21 (monosomy 21). Trisomy or monosomy for sex chromosomes is listed directly as in the notation 47,XXX (females with trisomy or triple X), 47,XXY (males with Klinefelter syndrome having an additional X chromosome), or 45,X (females with monosomy X or Turner syndrome). Other processes include "r" for ring [e.g., 45,X,rX or 46,XX,r(7)], "i" for isochromosome [e.g., 46,X,iX(q)], or "/" separating the karyotypes of cells in mosaic individuals [e.g., 46,XY/45,XY,–21].

When an aberration involves part of a chromosome rather than the whole chromosome, then its position must be specified. Accordingly, every band in the standard human karyotype is assigned a number (Fig. 7.4). If additional bands are revealed by higher resolution techniques, they are assigned decimal num-

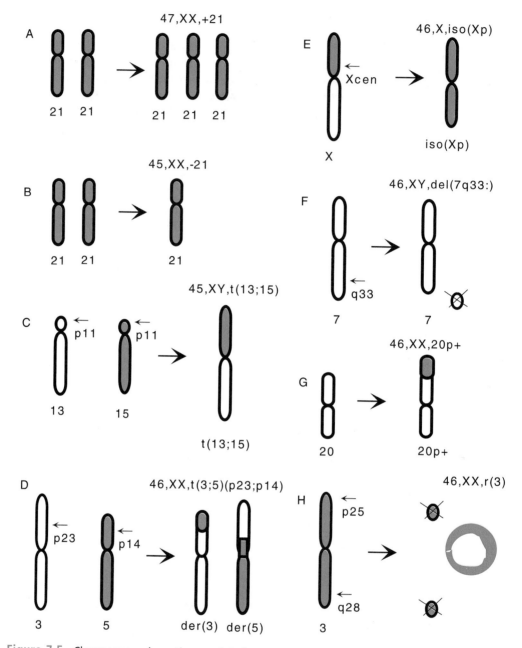

Figure 7.5. Chromosome aberrations and their corresponding cytogenetic notation: *A*, trisomy; *B*, monosomy; *C*, Robertsonian translocation; *D*, reciprocal translocation; *E*, isochromosome formation; *F*, terminal deletion; *G*, duplication with attachment of unknown material to chromosome 20; *H*, ring chromosome.

bers. For example, subbands 18q11.1 and 18q11.2 might be visible within band 18q11). Band numbers allow every cytogenetic rearrangement to be described according to the

segment (i.e., 18q12q14) and process (e.g, *del* or deletion) involved. Cytogenetic abnormalities include "dup" for duplications, "del" for deletions, "inv" for inversions, and "t" for

■ **TABLE 7.2.** Examples of Cytogenetic Notation

Notation	Clinical Phenotype
46,XX or 46,XY	Normal female or male
47,XXY	Male with extra X chromosome (Klinefelter syndrome)
45,X	Female with missing X chromosome (Turner syndrome)
46,X,i(Xq)	Female with isochromosome of two X long arms (Turner syndrome)
47,XY+21	Male with extra chromosome 21 (Trisomy 21, Down syndrome)
45,XX-21	Female with missing chromosome 21 (Monosomy 21)
45,XX/45,X	Female mosaic for monosomy X (mosaic Turner syndrome)
46,XX/46,XY	Individual chimeric for male and female cell lines
46,XX,9qh+	Female with extra heterochomatin on the long arm of chromosome 9
46,X,rY	Male with a ring Y chromosome
45,XY,-14,-21,+t(14;21) or 45,XY,t(14;21)	Male with Robertsonian translocation having a normal phenotype
46,XY,-14,+t(14:21) or 46,XY,t(14;21)	Male with Robertsonian translocation having Down syndrome
46,XY,t(8q24;14q32)	Male with reciprocal translocation, breakpoints at bands 8q24 and 14q32
46,XX,del(5p23:)	Female with deletion from band 5p23 to the 5p terminus (*Cri-du-chat* syndrome)
46,XX,5p+	Female with extra material on the 5p terminus, origin unknown
46,XX,dup(5p)	Female with duplicated material from the chromosome 5 short arm
46,XX,-7,+der(7)(7pter→ 7q32::5p23(5pter)	Female with duplicated material from the chromosome 5 short arm (arising from the long arm of chromosome 7)

translocations (Tables 7.1, 7.2). A colon beside a band number indicates a distal deletion, while a semicolon represents a reunion between chromosome regions (Table 7.2).

For complex chromosome rearrangements, a more detailed terminology is needed. In these situations, the exact composition of a chromosome is specified from the tip of the p arm to the bottom of the q arm. Terms employed for more precise notation include pter for the p arm terminus, qter for the q arm terminus, :: for a site of breakage and reunion, and → for an extent of unbroken chromosome. An example of more detailed notation is 46,XX,−2,+der(2) (2pter → 2q31::7p24 → 7p14::2q31 → 2qter). The notation means that a normal chromosome 2 has been replaced by a derivative chromosome 2 containing a region of chromosome 7 inserted at band 2q31 (see Table 7.2). The identity of the recombinant chromosome is always decided according to the origin of its centromere, which can be specified as "cen" where needed. Another way of describing the rearranged chromosome 2 would use "ins" for insertion, namely 46,XX,ins(2q31)(7p24p14).

There are usually alternative notations for the same chromosomal aberration, and the choice depends on the precision desired. Shorthand notations are preferred for clinical discussion, as in "5p⁻ syndrome" or "46,XX,5p⁻" that denotes deletion of the chromosome 5 short arm in *cri-du-chat* syndrome. Alternatively, the exact band where the deletion begins may be specified as "46,XX,del(5)(p11:)." Sometimes an ambiguous notation such as "46,XX,2q+" may specify additional material on the chromosome 2 long arm that needs additional banding or fluorescent studies for definition. If the extra material were derived from chromosome 7, then a clinical phenotype resembling patients with extra chromosome 7 material would be expected rather than a phenotype resembling patients with chromosome 2 duplications. Such examples illustrate the importance of being able to interpret cytogenetic laboratory reports.

■ 7.5. THE ORIGIN AND TRANSMISSION OF CHROMOSOMAL ABERRATIONS

Nondisjunctions

A principal cause for changes in chromosome number is the process known as *nondisjunction*. Nondisjunction is an error of chromosome sorting that can occur during cell mitosis or meiosis. If the nondisjunction occurs during mitosis, then daughter somatic cells with trisomy and monosomy for the affected chromosome are generated. The resulting degree of mosaicism depends on the timing of the nondisjunction during embryogenesis (early nondisjunctions yield higher numbers of tissues with abnormal cells) and the relative health of cells with the aberration. Monosomic cells often do not survive, because they will have reduced amounts of all proteins encoded by the monosomic chromosome.

If nondisjunction occurs during meiosis, then the derived gametes depend upon whether meiotic division I or II is affected. Figure 7.6 illustrates the possibilities by examining one pair of autosomes during female meiosis. Since the first meiotic division separates homologous chromosomes, nondisjunction at this stage results in secondary oocytes having either an extra autosome or a missing autosome (Fig. 7.6A). Subsequent division that separates the sister chromatids produces ova with 24 or 22 chromosomes, which after fertilization with a normal sperm produces zygotes with 47 or 45 chromosomes (Fig. 7.6A). Note that nondisjunction during the first meiotic division as illustrated in Figure 7.6A can produce a trisomic zygote with both maternal chromosomes; this is an important distinction on occasions where the trisomic zygote undergoes a corrective nondisjunction to produce a disomic individual.

In Figure 7.6B, nondisjunction occurs in the second meiotic division and again produces ova with 24 or 22 chromosomes. The resulting trisomic individuals will have two copies of one maternal homologue, potentially correcting to yield disomic zygotes in which that copy is duplicated. Although correction of trisomic zygotes to mosaic trisomic/disomic individuals as shown in Figure 7.6 is rare, it does occur and is called *uniparental disomy* where both homologues of a chromosome pair derive from one parent. Uniparental disomy has shed light

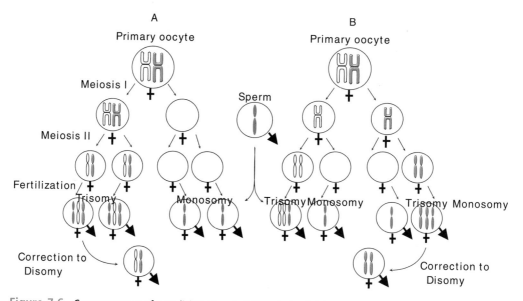

Figure 7.6. Consequences of nondisjunction in (*A*) meiotic division I versus (*B*) meiotic division II. Note that nondisjunction in meiosis II (B) will yield two copies of the same parental chromosome.

on the process known as genomic imprinting that is discussed in Chapter 10.

A particularly instructive distinction between nondisjunction in meiosis I versus meiosis II can be visualized in the case of a 46,XY male. Nondisjunction in meiosis I produces secondary spermatocytes with 47,XY or 45,0 karyotypes, producing 24,XY or 22,0 gametes and 47,XXY or 45,X zygotes after fertilization with a 23,X ovum. Nondisjunction in meiosis II division produces 24,XX, 24,YY, or 22,0 gametes, yielding 47,XXX, 47,XYY, or 45,X zygotes. The 47,XYY karyotype is thus produced only by meiosis II nondisjunction in males, while a 47,XXY karyotype can be produced by meiosis I nondisjunction in males or by meiosis I or II nondisjunction in females

Theories about the cause of nondisjunction include prolonged synapsis that drags both chromosomes to the same daughter cell, or lack of proper synapsis such that the homologues are not lined up on the metaphase plate. Regardless of the primary cause, there is a strong association with maternal age. Pregnant women of age 25 or below have a less than 1 in 1000 risk for nondisjunction, climbing to 1 in 100 at age 37 and almost 1 in 10 by age 45. These risks for nondisjunction are prime factors in eligibility for prenatal diagnosis as discussed in Chapter 15. The lack of genetic factors contributing to the occurrence of nondisjunction is suggested by the low recurrence risk for a second affected pregnancy. Individuals who have had one child with an extra or missing chromosome have a 1% risk for subsequent affected children. This 1% risk must be added to the age-dependent risk for nondisjunction, but is still substantially lower than the risks posed by translocations.

Reciprocal Translocations

Reciprocal translocations involve the equal exchange of material between two chromosomes. The term *balanced translocation* emphasizes the normal phenotype expected in such individuals because they have no extra or missing chromosomal material. There must be two breakpoints to generate a reciprocal translocation as specified by notation such as 46,XX,t(2q24:4p13). Surveys of reciprocal translocations indicate that certain chromosome bands are overrepresented, although a higher frequency of translocation versus better survival of cells with the particular rearrangement cannot be proved. Empirically, 6–10% of individuals with reciprocal translocations have abnormal phenotypes due to gene disruption, subtle imbalance, or other mechanisms. If there is significant extra or missing DNA at one of the breakpoints, then subtle imbalance may cause developmental abnormalities in patients with reciprocal translocations.

A major effect of reciprocal translocations is to generate abnormal gametes after meiosis (Fig. 7.7A). Normal gametes must inherit two translocation chromosomes or two normal chromosomes. Gametes with both translocation chromosomes generate offspring with reciprocal translocations, while those with one translocation chromosome and not the other produce unbalanced offspring with "duplication/deficiency." Although a 50% ratio of balanced versus unbalanced offspring might be predicted from the diagram in Figure 7.7A, the actual frequency of unbalanced offspring at birth is more like 10–20%. These lower risks account for decreased survival of fetuses with chromosome imbalance.

Robertsonian Translocations

Robertsonian translocations result when there is breakage and reunion between the satellite regions of two acrocentric chromosomes. Because satellite regions are near the termini of the acrocentric chromosomes, the translocations appear as though the two chromosomes simply fuse together end-to-end (Fig. 7.7B). In contrast to reciprocal translocations, Robertsonian translocations reduce the chromosome number to 45. Because very little material is lost during the translocation, individuals with Robertsonian translocations have normal phenotypes. Problems arise during meiosis, when segregation of the Robertsonian translocation

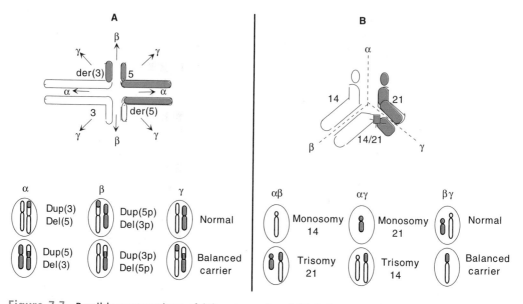

Figure 7.7. Possible segregations of (A) reciprocal and (B) Robertsonian translocations at meiotic metaphase. Pairing of homologues during synapsis leads to chromosome complexes that may segregate in different ways as indicated by the Greek letters. The Greek letters indicate directions in A and lines of division in B.

may lead to imbalance in the gametes. As shown in Figure 7.7B, a translocation carrier may produce a gamete with the translocation chromosome plus one of its normal homologues; fertilization then produces an individual with trisomy. Risks for abnormal offspring vary with the type of Robertsonian translocation, the possibilities for segregation, and the viability of the trisomic fetus. Individuals carrying 13/13 translocations have a 5% risk for chromosomally imbalanced, live-born offspring, while those with 14/21 translocations have a 10–15% risk. Female translocation carriers have slightly higher risks for abnormal live-born offspring than males, and there is an increased risk for spontaneous abortion (miscarriage) as with reciprocal translocations. Carriers of homologous Robertsonian translocations such as 45,XY,t(21/21) may have nearly 100% risks for abnormal offspring. Note that these offspring have karyotypes of 46,XX,t(21/21)or 46,XY,t(21/21)—individuals with extra chromosome material due to a Robertsonian translocation have a normal chromosome number of 46 (Table 7.2).

Pericentric and Paracentric Inversions

People with chromosomal inversions usually have normal phenotypes unless one of the breakpoints interrupts or interferes with a nearby gene. Increased rates of abortion occur because of problems with chromosome alignment during meiosis. As shown in Figure 7.8, inverted chromosomes must undergo contortions in order to synapse with their homologues. The usual crossing over between homologues then produces a rearranged chromosome if the crossover occurs in the mismatched area. Sometimes these crossover products are acentric and sometimes they have two centromeres (Fig. 7.8A). In either case, gametes lacking chromosome material may be produced, and the resulting monosomic fetuses usually present as spontaneous abortions. Crossovers during synapsis of pericentric inversions can produce duplication-deficiencies—that is, extra short arm and no long arm material on one homologue (Fig. 7.8B). Parents with pericentric inversions can thus have surviving offspring with partial aneuploidy. Inversions are very common in the het-

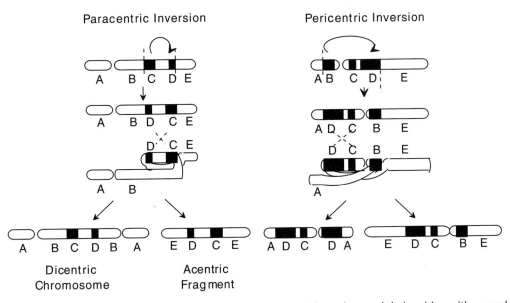

Figure 7.8. The formation of (*A*) paricentric and (*B*) pericentric inversions and their pairing with normal homologues during synapsis of meiosis I. The normal process of homologous recombination can generate aberrant chromosomes if crossovers occur within the inverted segment.

eromorphic, variable chromatin near the centromeres of chromosomes 1, 9, and 16. These inversions may be noted on cytogenetic reports [e.g., 46,XX,inv(9qh)] but are not associated with phenotypic abnormalities.

■ 7.6. KARYOTYPE/PHENOTYPE CORRELATION AND INDICATIONS FOR CHROMOSOMAL STUDIES

The relation between chromosomal aberrations and the abnormal characteristics they produce is called *karyotype/phenotype correlation.* It is an intriguing area of clinical genetics because patients with the same imbalance of chromosomal material tend to resemble each other, illustrated by the recognizable phenotype known as Down syndrome. While striking, this remarkable congruence of signs and symptoms is somewhat diluted by individual variation among patients with the same chromosomal syndrome. Research has focused on the role of duplication/deficiency of specific genes on the aneuploid chromosome segments, but a unifying mechanism by which chromosomal imbalances causes a distinctive yet individually vari-

able phenotype remains elusive. Nevertheless, substantial clinical experience has defined several categories of disease that are likely to reflect chromosomal aberrations. These categories provide a set of clinical indications for chromosomal studies (Table 7.3).

Chromosome Imbalance and Pregnancy Loss

The most severe phenotypes produced by chromosome imbalance cause death during embryonic or fetal life. Improvements in tissue culture have allowed karyotyping of early abortuses, and numerous studies have demonstrated a 50–60% incidence of chromosomal aberrations in first trimester miscarriages. The spectrum of these prenatal chromosomal aberrations is quite different from those documented after birth as shown in Table 7.4. A striking example of this discrepancy is 45,X Turner syndrome that has an embryonic frequency some 300-fold higher than its birth frequency of 1 in 5000 live births. Polyploidy with three (triploidy) or four (tetraploidy) haploid chromosome sets is also much more fre-

■**TABLE 7.3.** Indications for Chromosome Studies

Indications	Tissue	Possible Karyotype Results
Karyotyping of patients		
Mental disability, multiple congenital anomalies	Blood	Polyploidy, aneuploidy, unbalanced chromosome rearrangement
Mild mental disability, behavioral problems, reproductive problems	Blood	Sex chromosome aneuploidy
Selected cancer tissues	Blood, solid tumors	Balanced translocations, aneuploidy
Karyotyping of relatives		
Couples with recurrent abortions, infertility, reproductive problems	Blood	Balanced translocations, sex chromosome aneuploidy
Parent of child with chromosome rearrangement	Blood	Balanced translocation, other chromosome rearrangement
Prenatal diagnosis—fetus at risk for chromosome anomaly	Chorion, amniocytes	Aneuploidy, chromosome rearrangements
Emergent karyotyping of neonates		
Multiple congenital anomalies, urgent medical decisions	Bone marrow	Trisomy 13/18, triploidy, other severe conditions
Ambiguous genitalia	Blood or bone marrow	Male or female sex to guide evaluation and gender assignment

quent in abortus material than in live births. Although prenatal death is the rule in disorders such as trisomy 16, there is increased risk of pregnancy loss even for milder disorders such as Down syndrome, where an estimated 10% of conceptuses present as miscarriages.

The clinical implication of this prenatal toll is to consider chromosomal studies in couples who have had recurrent pregnancy loss (see Chapter 15). Although spontaneous abortion has numerous causes, with an overall frequency of about 15%, two miscarriages confer a 1% risk for a chromosome aberration in one parent and three miscarriages a 3–5% risk. Recurrent miscarriages thus constitute one of the indications for chromosomal studies, particularly if a chromosome rearrangement is identified in one or more abortuses (Table 7.3).

Chromosome Imbalance— Developmental and Growth Delay Plus Congenital Anomalies

The presence of additional or missing chromosomal material usually causes some degree of developmental disability and growth delay. There is a rough correlation with the amount of extra or missing chromosome material and the degree of disability. Triploidy, trisomy 9, and trisomies for chromosomes 13 or 18 all produce severe and lethal phenotypes, while trisomy for the smaller chromosome 21 produces Down syndrome that is compatible with a normal life span. This correlation breaks down with sex chromosome aneuploidy due to mechanisms for dosage compensation that are discussed in section 7.10. There is a definite correlation between the number of extra X chromosomes in females or males and the severity of symptoms (Table 7.4).

When partial aneuploidies are considered—i. e., partial trisomies or monosomies due to an extra or missing segment of one chromosome—it is clear that the quality of imbalanced chromatin is important as well as its quantity. More than 100 chromosomal disorders result from partial trisomy or monosomy of particular chromosome segments. The quantity of extra chromatin certainly influences phenotype as illustrated by the more se-

■**TABLE 7.4.** Incidence of Chromosome Aberrations.

Aberration	Condition	Incidence
Early abortus		
All		1 in 2
69,X__	Triploidy	1 in 10
45,X	Turner syndrome	1 in 17
47,X_,+16	Trisomy 16	1 in 50
Neonate		
All		1 in 200
69,X_	Triploidy	Rare
45,X	Turner syndrome	1 in 5000
47,X_,+16	Trisomy 16	0
47,X_,+21	Down syndrome	1 in 800
47,X_,+13	Patau syndrome	1 in 12,000
47,X_,+18	Edwards syndrome	1 in 6000
46,X_,del(4p)	Wolf-Hirschhorn syndrome	1 in 70,000
46,X_,del(5p)	*Cri du chat* syndrome	1 in 50,000
46,X_,dup(3q)	Dup(3q) syndrome	Rare
47,XXY	Klinefelter syndrome	1 in 900
49,XXXXY	Klinefelter variant	Rare
47,XYY	XYY syndrome	1 in 1000
48,XYYY	XYY variant	Rare
49,XYYYY	XYY variant	Rare
47,XXX	Triple X syndrome	1 in 2500

Source: Schinzel (1984)

Note: 46,X_ represents 46,XX or 46,XY

vere syndrome caused by dup(1)(q25 → qter) than that caused by dup(1)(q32 → qter). However, approximately equal amounts of duplicated chromatin from the chromosome 2 long arm [dup(2)(q21 → q31)] causes a more severe phenotype than equivalent material from the short arm [dup(2)(pter → p23)].

Milder Chromosomal Phenotypes: Behavioral Problems and Reproductive Abnormalities

Some chromosomal aberrations are associated with cognitive and/or behavioral problems rather than obvious congenital anomalies. Patients with Ullrich-Turner syndrome may have anomalies but often retain a normal facial appearance without developmental disability (see Section 7.10). Patients with Klinefelter syndrome and other sex chromosome aberra-

tions in Table 7.4 also lack a distinctively abnormal facial appearance, and may present because of school or reproductive problems. Occasional autosomal aneuploidies have milder features, including trisomy 8 mosaicism, ring chromosome, and certain microdeletion syndromes. Several ring chromosome disorders, including those involving chromosomes 6, 7, 11, and 12, have a similar phenotype of microcephaly (small head), growth delay, and mild cognitive delay. This commonality may relate to the presence of similar repetitive DNA sequences on the telomeric regions of all chromosomes. Smaller ring chromosomes with larger deletions produce more distinctive phenotypes with severe disability and multiple anomalies.

Particularly frequent among the sex chromosome aneuploidies are reproductive abnormalities such as delayed puberty, menstrual abnormalities, or infertility. When other medical causes have been eliminated, and when there are additional harbingers of chromosomal disease such as mental disability or growth delay, these reproductive problems mandate chromosome studies (Table 7.3).

Pedigrees Suggestive of Chromosomal Inheritance

Chromosomal inheritance must be considered in any pedigree displaying several individuals with multiple congenital anomalies, developmental disability, spontaneous abortions, or infertility. The key to recognizing such pedigrees is their discordance with classical Mendelian mechanisms and the presence of multiple miscarriages (Table 7.3).

Case 7 Follow-up: The pedigree in Figure 7.1 is strongly suggestive of chromosomal inheritance because it includes several individuals with disability and/or a pattern of anomalies plus several spontaneous abortions.

Cancers and Syndromes with Chromosome Instability

The ability to detect chromosome instability has come with improvements in cell culture and cytogenetic technology. Constitutional

disorders associated with chromosome instability include Mendelian conditions such as Bloom syndrome (210900) or Fanconi anemia (227650). In Bloom syndrome, malfunction of a gene involved in DNA repair leads to a pattern of growth delay with frequent rearrangements in the chromosomes obtained from peripheral blood leucocytes. In Fanconi anemia, a similar DNA repair defect leads to bone marrow failure, growth delay, and congenital anomalies of the limbs and heart. Both disorders exhibit an increased susceptibility to specific types of cancer, and it has long been postulated that cancer is associated with chromosome aberrations. As expected, specific chromosome translocations have been found in most types of cancer (Table 7.5). Although early stages of cancer often exhibit reciprocal translocations without chromosome imbalance, later stages may develop highly unstable karyotypes with aneuploidy for multiple chromosomes. As discussed further in Chapter 9, balanced translocations in cancer cause neoplasia because their breakpoints disrupt the function of one or more *oncogenes* (cancer genes). Chromosomal studies are thus indicated in a variety of chromosome instability syndromes and cancers (Table 7.3).

Another category of chromosome instability relates to fragile sites that occur at specific

■TABLE 7.5. Examples of Chromosomal Aberrations in Cancer

Chromosomal Aberration	Type of Cancer	Karyotype in Tumor
Translocation	B-cell lymphomas	t(8q24;14q32)
		t(8q24;14q32)
	T-cell leukemias	t(8q24;14q11)
		t(7q35;19p13)
	Breast carcinoma	t(1q21;_)
	Glioma	t (19q31:_)
	Melanoma	t (1q11)
	Ovarian carcinoma	t(6q21;14q24)
	Renal carcinoma	t(3p21;8q24)
Deletions, monosomies	Colon carcinoma	17p, 18q
	Bladder carcinoma	Monosomy 9
	Meningioma	Monosomy 22
	Breast carcinoma	1p, 3p, 17q
	Melanoma	1p, 6q

Source: Solomon et al. (1991).

chromosome regions. Some fragile sites are visible under most cell culture conditions while others, like the fragile X site at band Xq27, are induced by specific culture conditions. Molecular characterization of fragile sites has demonstrated the presence of variable numbers of trinucleotide repeats that can expand or contract during meiosis. Expanding trinucleotide repeats at the Xq27 fragile site cause the fragile X syndrome of mental disability and mild physical abnormalities (see Chapter 10).

■ 7.7. CHROMOSOMAL SYNDROMES: POLYPLOIDY, TETRASOMY, TRISOMY, AND PARTIAL DUPLICATIONS

Polyploidy and Molar Pregnancies

Triploidy is an example of a chromosome aberration that occurs frequently in abortus material but rarely in live-born infants. A frequent presentation of triploidy is a disorganized mass of fetoplacental tissue called a *hydatiform mole* for its grapelike appearance. Note that triploid conceptuses can arise from two maternal and one paternal gamete (69,XXX or 69,XXY) or from two maternal and two paternal gametes (69,XYY). In Chapter 10, the predilection of 69,XYY triploid conceptuses to form hydatiform moles is related to different imprinting of the maternal versus paternal genomes. The presence of four haploid genomes (tetraploidy) is even rarer in live births, and usually presents as mosaicism. Patients with polyploidy mosaicism usually have some degree of developmental disability that correlates with their percentage of polyploid cells. Interestingly, polyploidy is frequent in certain normal cells like those in the hepatic parenchyma.

Autosomal Aneuploidy: Tetrasomies

As illustrated in Figure 7.5*E*, isochromosome formation may produce chromosomes with duplicated short or long arms. When one of these isochromosomes is present in addition to the 46 normal chromosomes, a four-fold dosage or *tetrasomy* for that chromosome arm is present. Tetrasomies for the smaller short arms are most often encountered, including trip(9p), trip(12p), trip(18p), and trip(21q). The phenotypes are usually similar to the corresponding partial trisomies, exemplified by the more severe Down syndrome phenotype associated with tetrasomy for the chromosome 21q region. All of the tetrasomies are extremely rare, with defects of the pupils (colobomata) and growth failure in the cat-eye syndrome [trip(22p)] being the best-known example.

Autosomal Aneuploidy: Down Syndrome

Patients with an entire extra copy of chromosome 21 have Down syndrome. The extra chromosome may arise by nondisjunction (trisomy 21) or translocation (translocation Down syndrome). Patients with mixtures of normal and trisomic cells (mosaic Down syndrome) often have milder phenotypes, but percentages of normal cells among peripheral lymphocytes used for karyotyping may differ from percentages in brain.

The incidence of Down syndrome is 1/650 to 1/1000 live births and shows little variation by ethnic groups. The newborn with Down syndrome is often recognized because of an unusual facial appearance and hypotonia. Characteristic minor anomalies may be needed for diagnosis, including upslanting eyes, epicanthal folds, single palmar creases, and a broad space between the first and second toes. The tongue frequently protudes, more because of hypotonia than true enlargement. As with all syndromes, the pattern of minor and major defects in Down syndrome varies from individual to individual. No physical anomaly is pathognomonic for Down syndrome. Chapter 16 stresses the importance of early diagnosis, parental support, and preventive management of Down syndrome. Improved management has led to an 80% survival to age 30 or beyond in 1991 compared to 50% mortality by age 5 in 1965.

Genetic counseling concerning the 1% recurrence risk for trisomy 21 and the importance of parental chromosome studies in patients with translocations is necessary when the diagnosis of Down syndrome is documented. Genetic counseling for families having children with Down syndrome should also include parental education, social supports, and, most of all, a positive attitude that reflects the ability of most individuals to read, write, participate in sports, hold jobs, and live semi-independently.

Autosomal Aneuploidies: Trisomy 13/18 (Edwards and Patau Syndromes)

Children with extra chromosomal material representing an entire chromosome 13 or chromosome 18 are affected with the trisomy 13 or trisomy 18 syndrome (Fig. 7.9). The extra chromosomal material may arise by trisomy or translocation. Although each syndrome has a distinctive pattern of anomalies, trisomy 13 and trisomy 18 have many overlapping features and a similar natural history.

Trisomy 13 due to nondisjunction or translocation occurs in about 1 in 12,000 live births, with a frequency in miscarriages some hundred-fold higher. Trisomy 18 is slightly more common, with a frequency between 1 in 5,000 and 1 in 7,000 live births. Survival rates are similar with 5% survival at age 1 year in trisomy 18 as compared to 14% surviving 1 year. Each disorder may include early hypertonia (increased muscle tone) with clenched fists, although this sign is more emphasized in

trisomy 18. An important addition to the literature is the study of Baty et al. (1994) that documents some psychomotor development in patients with trisomy 13/18. Older children responded to words or phrases, communicated with simple words or signs, crawled, used a walker, interacted with others, and achieved some toileting skills.

The debilitated state of many patients requires vigilance for respiratory infections and attention to social or local services such as social work, clergy, occupational or physical therapy, respite, and hospice care. The cardiac and brain anomalies often cause respiratory and feeding difficulties, bringing up questions as to the aggressiveness of management. Reasonable strategies include simple surgeries and supportive care that alleviate suffering; more elaborate surgery or prolonged intensive care is usually not recommended.

Autosomal Aneuploidies: Partial Duplications

Partial aneuploidies due to duplication of particular chromosome segments produce syndromes characterized by an unusual facial appearance, developmental disability, growth delay, and congenital anomalies. Resources for predicting common anomalies in specific chromosome duplication syndromes are listed in the Bibliography. Offspring with partial aneuploidy may be produced by parents with bal-

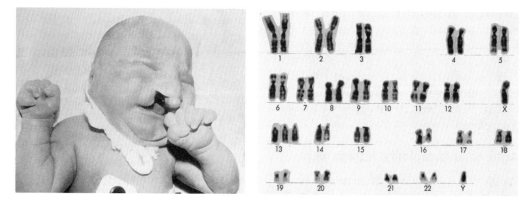

Figure 7.9. *A*, Patient with trisomy 13 showing an abnormal face, small eyes, cleft palate, and extra digits on both hands; *B*, 47,XY,+13 karyotype showing trisomy 13.

anced translocations, emphasizing the need for parental chromosome studies when the diagnosis is made.

■ 7.8. CHROMOSOMAL SYNDROMES: MONOSOMIES AND PARTIAL DELETIONS

Autosomal Aneuploidy: Monosomies

All autosomal monosomies involving the larger chromosomes are prenatally lethal. It is probable that monosomies of chromosomes 21 or 22 also are lethal in utero, because the expected offspring of parents with Robertsonian translocations involving these chromosomes have never been observed (note the expected segregation of monosomic gametes in Fig. 7.7*B*). There are rare reports of patients with monosomy 21 or 22 in the medical literature, but these are now thought to represent subtle translocations rather than true monosomies.

Monosomies occur in cancer cells, where they promote malignant progression by loss of *tumor suppressor* genes. When one dose of a tumor suppressor gene is removed by the acquired monosomy, neoplastic processes are up-regulated to develop more invasive cancers (see Chapter 9).

Autosomal Aneuploidy: Partial Deletions

Terminal deletions of chromosomes 4 and 5 are sufficiently common to produce recognizable phenotypes known, respectively, as the Wolf-Hirschhorn and the *cri du chat* syndromes. Children with del(4p) syndrome usually have low birth weights and exhibit growth delay (failure to thrive). Their facial appearance is often quite typical as illustrated in Figure 7.10, showing prominent brows with a broad nasal root and down-turned corners of the mouth. About one-third of children with the Wolf-Hirschhorn syndrome will die in the first year of life.

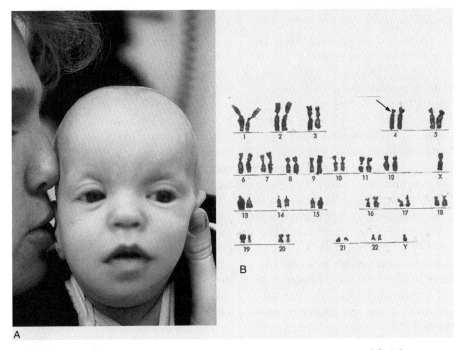

Figure 7.10. *A*, Patient with Wolf-Hirschhorn syndrome showing an unusual facial appearance with a broad nasal root and down-turned corners of the mouth. *B*, 46,XX,del(4)(p11:) karyotype showing deletion of the short arm of chromosome 4.

Patients with the *cri du chat* syndrome are not unique in having an unusual cry, but its resemblance to a cat's cry can be striking. Several families reported being questioned by the neighbors about having a new cat once they brought their child home from the nursery. In addition to changes in the laryngeal anatomy and motor tone that account for the weak, high-pitched cry, the syndrome involves striking microcephaly, cardiac, and genitourinary anomalies. Mental and growth deficiency is usually severe, with most adults having IQ measurements below 20. The incidence of *cri du chat* syndrome, like other rare partial aneuploidy syndromes, is not greater than 1 in 50,000.

■ 7.9. INTERSTITIAL DELETIONS AND MICRODELETIONS

In contrast to the terminal deletions discussed previously, interstitial deletions occur within chromosome segments between the centromere and telomeres. They are described in cytogenetic notation by specifying the borders of the deleted segment [i.e., 46,XY del(3)(q13q25)]. Improved banding and FISH techniques have facilitated recognition of a new cytogenetic category called microdeletions— interstitial deletions that are too small to be visualized by routine karyotyping.

Chromosome *microdeletions* bridge the gap between obvious chromosomal aberrations and mutations in single genes. They can encompass several genes and produce a visible diminution of a chromosome band such that a microdeletion is suspected prior to confirmation using FISH techniques. The appreciation of small deletions and the selection of DNA probes for FISH studies do require a focus on particular chromosome regions as dictated by clinical suspicion. It is therefore important to be aware of common microdeletion syndromes (Table 7.6), because their cytogenetic diagnosis is often dependent on appropriate instructions to the laboratory.

Some microdeletion syndromes can be viewed as aggregate phenotypes, representing the sum of phenotypes expected from *haploinsufficiency* (half dosage) of genes within the deleted region. These aggregate phenotypes have been referred to as *contiguous gene deletion syndromes*. Contiguous gene deletion syndromes are particularly evident when they occur on the X chromosome, because males with one X chromosome are completely deficient for products of genes within the deleted region.

The large Duchenne muscular dystrophy (dystrophin) gene of greater than 2 Mb has been involved in several contiguous gene deletion syndromes (Table 7.6). Duchenne muscular dystrophy (310200), adrenal hypoplasia (300200), and chronic granulomatous disease (306400) had already been described as X-linked recessive disorders before they occurred in the same male patient. The aggregate phenotype of muscle disease, adrenal insufficiency, and phagocyte dysfunction was then explained by the occurrence of a microdeletion in this patient that deleted a portion of the X chromosome containing these three genes.

One of the first contiguous gene syndromes to be recognized, the Wilms tumor-aniridia-genital defect-retardation (WAGR) syndrome, is an example of a more complex microdeletion phenotype. Component defects such as aniridia (106200) and Wilms tumor (194070) had been reported to exhibit autosomal dominant inheritance in selected families, and their combined presence in patients with 11p13 deletions probably reflects haploinsufficiency of their respective genes. The WT-1 gene responsible for Wilms tumor has been characterized as a large tumor suppressor gene that has effects on urogenital development, thus accounting for the genital defect. However, the mental retardation is not usually part of aniridia or Wilms tumor, and its association with the 11p13 deletion remains unexplained. It may derive from an as yet uncharacterized gene within the 11p13 region or relate to other genetic mechanisms such as genomic imprinting.

The recognition of microdeletion syndromes is not only useful for diagnosis, but also provides an approach for understanding the disorder by characterizing genes within the

■ **TABLE 7.6.** Human Microdeletion Syndromes

Disorder	Manifestations	Microdeletion
Williams syndrome	Unusual face, aortic stenosis, joint laxity, mental disability	7q11 (elastin gene)
Langer-Geidion syndrome	Unusual face, cartilaginous exostoses, mental disability	8q23-q24
Wiedemann-Beckwith syndrome	Large size, omphalocele, hypoglycemia	11p11-p15 Dup (p15) also
Wilms tumor-aniridia-genital defects-retardation (WAGR) syndrome	Iris, genital defects, Wilms tumor, mental disability	11p13 (WT-1 Wilms tumor gene)
Prader-Willi syndrome	Unusual face, early hypotonia, later morbid obesity	15q11 pat
Angelman syndrome	Unusual face with prominent jaw, seizures, mental disability	15q11 mat
Rubinstein-Taybi syndrome	Unusual face with broad thumbs, mental disability	16p13.3
Smith-Magenis syndrome	Unusual face, aberrant behaviors, mental disability	17p11
Hereditary neuropathy with predisposition to pressure palsies	Peripheral nerve dysfunction	17p11 (PMP 22 gene) Dup(17p11) causes CMT disease
Miller-Dieker syndrome	Hypotonia, lissencephaly (smooth brain), mental disability	17p13 (LIS-1 gene)
Alagille syndrome	Unusual face, pulmonary artery stenosis, vertebral anomalies, cholestatic liver disease	20p11-p12 (JAG gene)
Shprintzen/DiGeorge/Opitz syndrome	Unusual long face with palatal and speech defects, immune or genital defects	22q11
Duchenne muscular dystrophy, CGD, RP, McLeod phenotype	Muscle weakness, immune dysfunction, vision problems	Xp21 (dystrophin gene, others)
Duchenne muscular dystrophy, acidosis, adrenal insufficiency	Muscle weakness, acidosis, adrenal dysfunction	Xp21(dystrophin gene, others)

Notes: CGD, chronic granulomatous disease; RP, retinitis pigmentosa; PMP, peripheral myelin protein; CMT, Charcot-Marie-Tooth; LIS, lissencephaly; JAG, *jagged* Alagille gene

deleted region. The LIS-1 gene responsible for lissencephaly, discussed in Chapter 9, was discovered after attention was focused on genes in the 17p13 region by study of Miller-Dieker syndrome. Particularly interesting from this perspective of clinical insights are the deletions responsible for the Williams and Shprintzen/DiGeorge syndromes.

Williams Syndrome

Williams syndrome (194050) includes infantile hypercalcemia, stenosis of the aortic, pulmonic, or peripheral pulmonary valves, early feeding and constipation problems, hyperacusis with sensitivity to loud noises, and renal anomalies. Patients have a strikingly happy personality with remarkable musical and language skills that transcend their level of mental function. Genetic linkage studies of families with autosomal dominant aortic stenosis (185500) had localized the causative gene to chromosome band 7q11, paving the way for FISH studies of patients with Williams syndrome (Fig. 7.11). Over 85% of patients with

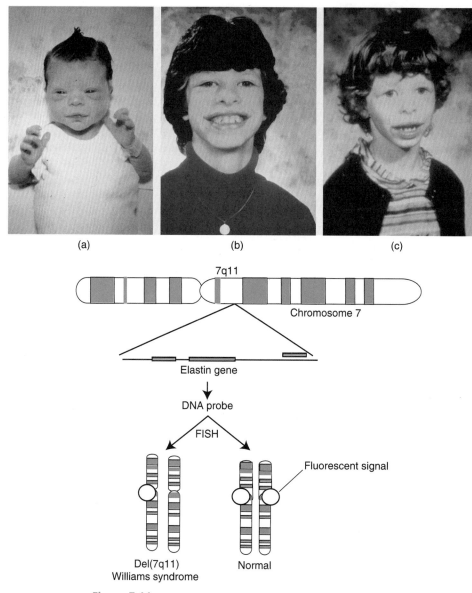

Figure 7.11. Williams syndrome and the 7q11 microdeletion.

Williams syndrome exhibited microdeletions at band 7q11 when an elastin gene probe was used for FISH studies, providing a gateway for characterizing other genes in this region that contribute to the remarkable cognitive phenotype in Williams syndrome. Candidate genes include a DNA replication factor, a syntaxin gene involved in nerve conduction, a protein kinase named LIMK, and a signal transduction receptor homologous to the Wnt-1 receptor discussed in Chapter 9.

Shprintzen/DiGeorge Spectrum and the 22q11 Microdeletion

DiGeorge anomaly (188400) includes several abnormalities including hypoparathyroidism, thymic defects leading to T-cell immune deficiencies, cardiac anomalies including aortic interruptions, and an unusual face with a small jaw. It occurs as a component of several syndromes caused by chromosomal aberrations, teratogen exposure, or single gene mutations. Prominent among these syndromes that may include DiGeorge anomaly is the Shprintzen velocardiofacial syndrome (192430) of growth and developmental delay, unusual facial appearance, cardiac anomalies, palatal and genital defects. When some patients with DiGeorge anomaly were found to have unbalanced translocations involving chromosome 22, attention was focused on the possibility of chromosome 22 microdeletions in both the DiGeorge and Shprintzen phenotypes.

FISH analysis of patients with DiGeorge anomaly and/or Shprintzen syndromes has demonstrated that more than 90% have microdeletions at chromosome band 22q11. Based on the high proportion of conotruncal cardiac defects (tetralogy of Fallot, truncus arteriosus, aortic and pulmonary artery anomalies) in these syndromes, chromosome 22 microdeletions were also found in patients with isolated conotruncal cardiac anomalies. Further heterogeneity was recognized when some patients with Opitz syndrome (145410), a disorder with severe gastroesophageal reflux, conotruncal cardiac defects, and genital anomalies, were found to have chromosome 22q11 microdeletions. The chromosome 22q11 microdeletion has thus unified several disorders (Shprintzen, DiGeorge, Opitz, conotruncal heart defects) which were thought to be separate entities. Genes are now being characterized from the 22q11 region in hopes of explaining the diverse syndrome phenotypes. Interesting candidates include a human homologue of the fly segment-polarity gene *dishevelled,* a protein kinase, a homeotic gene homologous to fly *goosecoid,* and a member of the catenin gene family implicated in colon cancer (see Chapter 9).

Case 7 Follow-up: After the normal karyotype was reported, the parents had another delayed child who resembled their first. A karyotype on this child was sent to a different laboratory, and revealed a subtle deletion on the short arm of chromosome 5 (*cri du chat* syndrome). Analysis of parental karyotypes demonstrated that mother was a 5;6 translocation carrier and allowed a family study to define recurrence risks and explain the spontaneous abortions. Once the familial translocation and higher recurrence risks were recognized, options of prenatal diagnosis were available to interested family members.

■ 7.10. SEX CHROMOSOME ANEUPLOIDY

X Inactivation and the Lyon Hypothesis

Despite the large size of the X chromosome, sex chromosome aneuploidies usually produce milder phenotypes than autosomal aneuploidies. Much of the reason for this difference concerns the mechanism for inactivation of one X chromosome in females. In 1961, Mary Lyon hypothesized a mechanism for dosage compensation regarding genes on the X chromosome so as to equalize their activity between 46,XX females and 46,XY males. She postulated that X inactivation occurred early in embryogenesis, acted randomly in each cell as to whether the paternally or maternally derived X was inactivated, and acted irreversibly. As shown in Figure 7.12, the Lyon hypothesis implies that female tissues will be mosaic with regard to the active X chromosome. Direct confirmation of mosaicism has been possible by examining tissues of females carrying X-linked diseases. For example, carriers of X-linked recessive retinitis pigmentosa (312600) or albinism (300650) exhibit patches of pigment in their retina. These patches correspond to cells deriving from an embryonic precursor cell that inactivated either the X carrying the normal allele (in the case of albinism) or the X carrying the abnormal allele (in the case of retinitis pigmentosa). These and many other observations give Lyon's seminal observation the status of law rather than hypothesis.

The physical correlate of the Lyon hypothesis is a clump of heterochromatin that can be

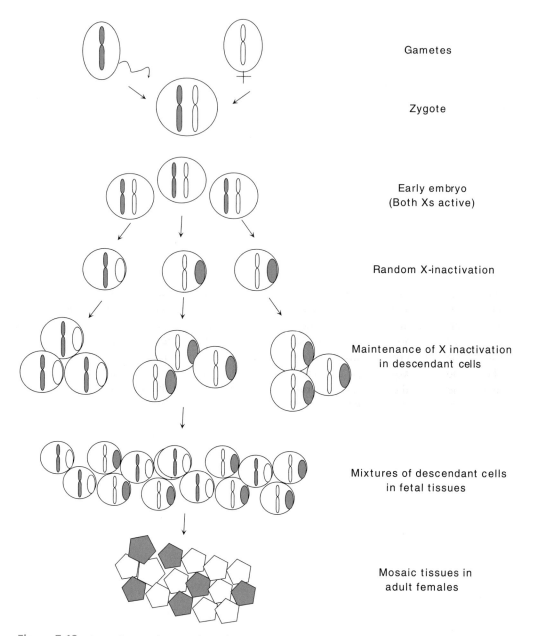

Gametes

Zygote

Early embryo
(Both Xs active)

Random X-inactivation

Maintenance of X inactivation
in descendant cells

Mixtures of descendant cells
in fetal tissues

Mosaic tissues in
adult females

Figure 7.12. According to the Lyon hypothesis, one of the two X chromosomes in females is randomly selected for irreversible inactivation early in embryogenesis. As a result, female tissues are mosaics of cells selecting the paternally (white) or maternally (shaded) derived X chromosome for inactivation.

observed on the nuclear periphery in many cells (Fig. 7.12). This heterochromatin is known as a Barr body after the physician who described it in 1949. It was observed that the number of Barr bodies correlated with the number of inactive X chromosomes. Thus males have no Barr bodies and females one, while patients with multiple sex chromosomes have a number of Barr bodies that is one less than the number of X chromosomes (e.g., 4

Barr bodies in individuals with 49,XXXXX syndrome). It was thus presumed and subsequently proven by in situ hybridization that the Barr body represents an inactive X chromosome. For a time, smears of the buccal mucosa with examination for Barr bodies were used for sex determination in infants with ambiguous genitalia. The buccal smear is now outdated due to unreliability and the advent of superior FISH technology using DNA probes for the X and Y chromosomes.

Two rare consequences derive from the process of X inactivation. One is an exception to Lyon's law that occurs when a female has a structurally abnormal X chromosome. Structurally abnormal X chromosomes such as isochromosomes or large rings are preferentially inactivated, resulting in milder phenotypes than might be expected. Preferential inactivation is reversed when there is a translocation between an X chromosome and an autosome. Because inactivation of the autosomal portion of the translocation would cause a severe deficiency in the affected cells, it is the normal X chromosome that is preferentially inactivated. This process may have a paradoxical result if the translocation breakpoint occurs within a key gene on the X chromosome. Because the normal allele of this gene has been inactivated along with the rest of the normal X chromosome, the woman carrying an X-autosome translocation may be affected with an X-linked recessive disorder such as Duchenne muscular dystrophy.

A second rare consequence arises when the center for inactivation is removed from the X chromosome. The inactivation center was first correlated with a bend on the long arm of one X that was noticed by karyotyping. Later, this center was shown to encode a specific xist-RNA (for X inactivation transcript) that acts along the chromosome to cause chromatin condensation. As mentioned previously, larger ring X chromosomes contain the inactivation center and are preferentially inactivated to produce a milder phenotype. However, small ring X chromosomes have the inactivation center removed and do not undergo normal inactiva-

tion. The duplication of active X material (the ring X together with the normal X) in cells seems to have very severe consequences. Females with small ring X chromosomes have severe mental disability and growth delay.

Ullrich-Turner Syndrome

After the preceding discussion, 45,X females should have normal phenotypes because one X chromosome is inactivated in 46,XX females. The presence of growth delay and congenital anomalies in patients with Ullrich-Turner syndrome indicates that some portions of a second X or Y chromosome must be necessary for function in normal individuals. In fact, molecular studies have demonstrated that some genes on the inactive X, particularly in one region of the short arm, do remain active. This region of residual activity comprises part of the region of X-Y homology that facilitates synapsis of these chromosomes during meiosis (sometimes called the *pseudoautosomal region*). Homologous genes on the Y chromosome must also suppress the phenotype of Ullrich-Turner syndrome, accounting for the low incidence of typical anomalies in 46,XY males.

Females with short stature, immature sexual development, and *webbed neck* exhibit features of Turner syndrome caused by deficiency of all or part of one X chromosome. The majority of patients have a 45,X karyotype or mosaicism with 45,X and 46,XX cell lines. Others have mosaicism involving unusual cell lines—isochromosome Xp or Xq, ring X, Xp or Xq deletion, and even male (46,XY) karyotypes. Rarely, Turner syndrome involves smaller deletions of the X chromosome. The term "male Turner syndrome" has been used imprecisely for a condition called Noonan syndrome that involves a somewhat similar phenotype and a normal karyotype (see Chapter 11).

Klinefelter Syndrome

Males with Klinefelter syndrome have increased stature with gynecomastia and small testes. Most individuals have a 47,XXY karyotype, although "variants" with more severe clinical features due to 48,XXXY, 48,XXYY, or 49,XXXXY karyotypes are sometimes grouped under this term. The classic Klinefelter phenotype has a prevalence of 1.18 per 1000, with 80% having karyotypes of 47,XXY, 10% being 46,XY/47,XXY mosaics, and the remainder having multiple X or Y chromosomes. More than 10% of males presenting with sterility and 3% with breast cancer will have Klinefelter syndrome. The additional X interferes with Leydig cell development in the testis, but the pathogenesis is unknown. The immature body habitus, feminine features (like gynecomastia, high voice, or sparse hair), and incomplete pubertal development reflect androgen deficiency that is partially reversible by hormone supplementation.

Antisocial behaviors including theft or arson, alcoholism, and aggressiveness are described in some reports while others describe XXY men as having similar employment and social status to their peers. Increased frequency of males with 47,XXY and 47,XYY syndrome have been found in mental or penal institutions, but prospective studies to document such associations have been controversial. Psychiatric disorders such as manic-depressive illness, psychosis, depression, and anorexia nervosa may be increased.

47,XYY Syndrome

The 47,XYY syndrome, like Klinefelter syndrome, usually presents with school or behavioral problems. There are few physical anomalies, with tall stature due to long lower legs being a distinguishing feature. Lymphedema (swelling) of the extremities is more common and there is reduced fertility with abnormal spermatogenesis. Most striking are the behavioral abnormalities, which include cognitive disabilities, maladjustment, isolation from peers, disturbed gender identity, and inappropriate sexual activity. Although the incidence of 47,XYY syndrome is increased in institutions for youth offenders, most individuals lead retiring and nonviolent lives.

Other Sex Chromosome Aneuploidies

As listed in Table 7.4, sex chromosome aneuploidies form a continuum from the milder phenotypes of Klinefelter and 47,XXX syndromes to more severe phenotypes when multiple extra chromosomes are present (e.g., the 48,XXXX, 49,XXXXX, 48,XXXY, 48,XXYY, and 49,XXXXY syndromes). The latter syndromes are much more rare, and can involve relatively severe mental and growth deficiency. Interestingly, fusion (synostosis) of the radius and ulna bones of the lower arm is a common anomaly in these sex aneuploidy syndromes. As would be expected, patients with higher numbers of sex chromosomes are infertile.

PROBLEM SET 7
Cytogenetics

7.1. The cytogenetic term "6q+" refers to
  (A) 46,XX,dup(6q)
  (B) extra chromosome material derived from the long arm of chromosome 6
  (C) 46,XX,dup(6p)
  (D) extra chromosome material, origin unspecified, attached to the long arm of chromosome 6
  (E) 47,XX,+6

7.2–7.4. Match each clinical situation below with the appropriate risk figure.
  (A) 1/10,000
  (B) 1/800
  (C) 1/100
  (D) 1/10
  (E) 1

7.2. The risk for a newborn to have Down syndrome

7.3. The theoretical risk for a 21/21 translocation carrier to have a child with Down syndrome

7.4. The risk for parents of a trisomy 21 child to have a second offspring with a chromosomal abnormality

7.5–7.7. Match each of the genetic conditions below with the correct cytogenetic notation.
  (A) 47,XX,+21
  (B) 45,X
  (C) 47,XXX

(D) 47,XY,+21

(E) 45,XX,-21

7.5. Male with trisomy 21 (Down syndrome)

7.6. Female with monosomy X (Turner syndrome)

7.7. Female with monosomy 21

7.8–7.10. Match each cytogenetic description with the appropriate lettered diagram in Figure 7.5.

7.8. Isochromosome

7.9. Terminal deletion

7.10. Ring chromosome

PROBLEM SET 7
Answers

		7.4 C
7.10 H	7.7 E	7.3 E
7.9 F	7.6 B	7.2 B
7.8 E	7.5 D	7.1 D

PROBLEM SET 7
Solutions

7.1. The term "6q+" is shorthand for a karyotype showing extra chromosomal material on the long arm of chromosome 6 (answer D). The origin of the extra material is not specified; therefore, clinical correlation or additional banding and molecular studies are needed to define from which chromosome the extra material is derived. When rearrangements are found, it is necessary to obtain karyotypes from the parents. This may define the extra material if the parent carries a reciprocal translocation (i.e., one of the parental chromosomes is deleted for the material that is attached to 6q). The notation dup(6q) specifies that the extra material is derived from the long arm of chromosome 6. The notation 47,XX+6 implies trisomy for the entire number 6 chromosome.

7.2–7.4. The incidence of Down syndrome at birth is approximately 1 in 800 live-born children with 95% being trisomy 21 (answer B). About 4% of Down syndrome patients have translocations that mandate parental karyotyping to determine if one of the parents is a bal-

anced translocation carrier. The remaining 1% are mosaics, meaning that certain tissues are mixtures of trisomy 21 and normal cells. Translocation carriers have a 5–20% risk for unbalanced offspring with female carriers in general at higher risk than male carriers. Offspring of translocation 21/21 carriers should in theory all have Down syndrome, although some carriers have had normal children (answer E). The empiric risk for parents with a trisomy 21 child is 1/100 for a second child with chromosomal aneuploidy (answer C).

7.5–7.7. Cytogenetic notation provides the chromosome number (e.g., 46), the sex chromosomes, and a shorthand description of anomalies. Examples include the following: 47,XX+21 indicates a female with trisomy 21; 45,X indicates a female with monosomy X; or 45,XX–21 indicates a female with monosomy 21. Note the absence of spaces between symbols and the use of 45,X or 47,XXX for sex chromosomal aneuploidy rather than the more awkward 45,XX2X or 47,XX+X.

7.8–7.10. Isochromosomes (diagram E), terminal deletions (diagram F), and ring chromosomes (diagram H) are examples of intrachromosomal rearrangements in which breaks or crossovers unite different regions of the same chromosome. Translocations (diagrams C and D) are rearrangements that join regions of different chromosomes together. They are reciprocal when there is exchange between two chromosomes and nonreciprocal when there is a one-way transfer of a chromosome fragment. Donor chromosomes may lose material from internal regions (interstitial deletions) or from ends (terminal deletions), just as recipient chromosomes may have insertional or terminal duplications.

BIBLIOGRAPHY

Chromosome Aberrations—General References

Gorlin RJ, Cohen MM Jr, Levin LS. 1990. *Syndromes of the Head and Neck,* ed. 3. New York: Oxford University Press.

Jones, KL. 1996. *Recognizable Patterns of Human Malformation,* 5th ed. Philadephia: WB Saunders.

Schinzel A. 1984. *Catalogue of Unbalanced Chromosome Aberrations in Man.* Berlin: de Gruyter.

Solomon E, Borrow J, Goddard AD. 1991. Chromosome aberrations and Cancer. *Science.* 254: 1153–60.

Trisomy 13/18

Baty BJ, Blackburn BL, Carey JC. 1994. Natural history of trisomy 18 and trisomy 13: I. Growth, physical assessment, medical histories, survival and recurrence risk. *Am J Med Genet* 49: 175–188.

Carey JC. 1992. Health supervision and anticipatory guidance for children with genetic disorders (including specific recommendations for trisomy 21, trisomy 18, and neurofibromatosis). *Pediatr Clin N Amer* 39:25–53.

Trisomy 21

Cooley WC, Graham JM Jr. 1991. Down syndrome—an update and review for the primary pediatrician. *Clin Pediatr* 30:233–253.

Epstein CJ. 1995. Down syndrome (trisomy 21). In Scriver CR, Beaudet AL, Sly WS, Valle D, eds., *The Metabolic and Molecular Bases of Inherited Disease.* 7th ed. New York: McGraw-Hill, pp. 749–794.

Pueschel SM, ed. 1978. *Down Syndrome. Growing and Learning.* Kansas City: Sheed Andrews & McMeel.

Rubin IL, Crocker AC. 1989. *Developmental Disabilities—Delivery of Medical Care for Children and Adults.* Philadelphia: Lea and Febiger.

Sex Chromosome Aberrations

Hall JG, Gilchrist DM. 1990. Turner syndrome and its variants. *Pediatr Clin N Am* 37:1421–1440.

Lyon M. 1961. Gene action in the X chromosome of the mouse (*Mus musculus*). Nature 190: 372–373.

Mandoki MW, Sumner GS. 1991. Klinefelter syndrome: The need for early identification and treatment. *Clin Pediatr* 30:161–164.

Microdeletions

Ewart AK, Morris CA, Atkinson D, Jin W, Sternes K, Spallone P, Stock AD, Leppert M, Keating MT. 1993. Hemizygosity at the elastin locus in a developmental disorder, Williams syndrome. *Nature Genet* 5:11–15.

Fisher E, Scambler P. 1994. Human haploinsufficiency—one for sorrow, two for joy. *Nature Genet* 7:5–9.

McCandless SE, Scott JA, Robin NH. 1998. Deletion 22q11: A newly recognized cause of behavioral and psychiatric disorders. *Arch Pediatr Adolesc Med* 152:481–484.

Schmickel RD. 1986. Contiguous gene syndromes: A component of recognizable syndromes. *J Pediatr* 109:231–241.

8

GENETICS AT THE DNA LEVEL: MOLECULAR GENETICS AND DNA DIAGNOSIS

■ LEARNING OBJECTIVES

1. Human DNA segments can be isolated by restriction endonuclease cleavage, ligation, and cloning in the form of recombinant DNA molecules.

2. Cloned DNA segments can be labeled with radioactive or fluorescent tags and used as DNA probes.

3. Molecular analysis of human DNA reveals variable nucleotides every 200–500 bp that may be used for gene mapping (DNA polymorphisms) or to explain genetic disease (DNA mutations)

4. Variable DNA segments can be isolated using recombinant DNA technology or amplified using the polymerase chain reaction (PCR); DNA mutations are then detected using DNA sequencing, allele-specific oligonucleotide hybridization (ASO), and/or single-strand conformational polymorphisms (SSCP).

5. More than 1000 genetic diseases are now mapped to specific chromosome regions, and more than 300 have been character-ized by defining gene structure and mutant alleles.

6. The human genome project represents an organized strategy to sequence a representative genome of 3×10^9 bp. By the years 2005–2010, every human gene should be mapped and catalogued to facilitate the molecular delineation of genetic disease.

7. Ethical issues concerning the molecular genetic revolution include ownership of cloned DNA segments and DNA samples, confidentiality regarding access to DNA information, and informed consent that accounts for the revelation of unexpected information.

Case 8: **Three Sons with Mental Disability**
A couple requests evaluation because they have three sons with mental retardation (Fig. 8.1*A*). The children have a normal appearance with no obvious congenital anomalies or metabolic aberrations. A chromosome study on individual III-1 has been normal. The family history (Fig. 8.1*B*) reveals many individuals

A

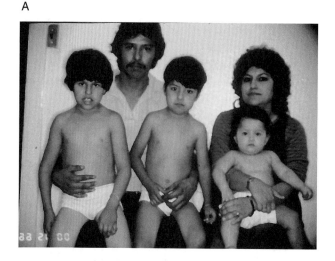

B

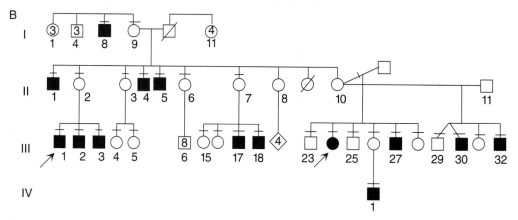

Figure 8.1. *A*, Family and three sons affected with MASA syndrome; *B*, pedigree of family described in Case 8.

with mental retardation, including individuals III-1, III-2, and III-3 illustrated in Figure 8.1*A*. The couple is anxious to know the cause of developmental delay in their three sons, and their risks to have future affected children. The pedigree reveals an obvious inheritance mechanism, and their physician must consider the possibility for additional diagnostic tests in the face of normal chromosomal and metabolic studies.

■ 8.1. DNA AND THE CLINICIAN

The ability to move from the level of visible chromosomes to that of their component genes

was made possible by the field of molecular genetics. Genes could be isolated and manipulated like substances in the chemistry laboratory, and they were defined as concrete DNA segments rather than as abstract "factors" of inheritance. From the viewpoint of molecular biology, genes are contiguous groups of DNA segments that act as a unit to encode a protein and/or RNA molecule. Genes are arrayed on chromosomes like beads on a string and number an estimated 80–100,000 in each cellular genome. The ability to isolate and catalogue genes brought forth a new term called *genomics*, which refers to the analysis of organismal function through study of the structure and interaction of its component genes. Molecular genetics is thus concerned with individual gene action as well as the gene interactions that comprise the *genomics* of cell function.

It is important to recognize that every discovery of human molecular genetics depended on basic research concerning DNA-modifying enzymes in procaryotes. The characterization of reagents like restriction endonucleases, DNA polymerases, and DNA ligases provided methods for engineering DNA. Genetic engineering thus moved from the natural repertoire of living organisms to its scientific uses for isolating genes, characterizing genes, and manipulating genes for functional and therapeutic studies. The first portion of this chapter examines these basic techniques of genetic engineering that employ DNA-modifying enzymes for gene isolation and characterization.

The role of clinicians and allied health professionals in the field of clinical molecular genetics is to ensure that the preliminary diagnosis is correct, to understand and present options for DNA diagnosis to the family, and to explain results of DNA testing in the context of family concerns and values. It is likely that DNA diagnosis will always be directed toward specific genetic diseases rather than performed as a gene-screen in the way that a karyotype can screen for chromosomal abnormalities. Clinicians must therefore understand these limitations and explain the specificity of DNA diagnostic testing to patients and their relatives. Since abnormal alleles may be identified in individuals before they manifest symptoms of disease, clinicians must also be alert to issues of presymptomatic diagnosis. These and other ethical issues concerning molecular genetics are discussed at the end of this chapter and in Chapter 16 concerning genetic counseling.

■ 8.2. IDENTIFYING DNA SEGMENTS IN GENOMIC DNA

The 6×10^9 nucleotides in each diploid human cell are far greater than the 4×10^4 bp DNA region encompassed by the average gene. Exper-

iments to identify and isolate specific genes must overcome this 10^5-fold dilution by other DNA segments in the genome. In fact, this challenge of specificity is even greater because the DNA segments targeted for measurement or isolation are often smaller pieces of genes that measure less than 10 kb in size. To overcome the small concentrations of single copy genes within genomic DNA, methods were developed for synthesizing DNA segments of high radioactivity to serve as *DNA probes,* and for amplifying DNA segments using molecular cloning or chain reaction techniques.

The Isolation of Genomic DNA

DNA can be isolated from peripheral blood leucocytes, cultured cells, or solid tissues. The cells are dissolved in detergent solutions, and the lysate is treated with proteases and RNA-degrading enzymes (ribonucleases or RNases) to purify the DNA. Alcohol is then added to precipitate the genomic DNA as a fibrous thread that can be wrapped around a glass rod. The spooled DNA is dried and suspended in a mildly alkaline buffer for storage in solution or as a frozen sample within a *DNA bank.* Purified DNA is easily transported or stored for long periods in liquid nitrogen, allowing samples from extended families, individuals with similar diseases, or populations to be accumulated for study. Banks of immortalized cells can also be established, providing a continuous supply of DNA for analysis.

DNA Probes and Nucleic Acid Hybridization

The identification of specific DNA segments within genomic DNA utilized the technique of nucleic acid hybridization. Recall that native DNA consists of antiparallel *complementary strands* that separate (*melt*) and reassociate (*hybridize*) spontaneously when placed in appropriate solutions (see Section 6.2 for review). If one strand of duplex DNA is labeled with radioactivity or fluorescence, it becomes a *probe* for its complementary strand in DNA mixtures.

In DNA hybridization experiments, the genomic duplex DNA must first be melted and then incubated with sufficient probe to compete against endogenous complementary strand.

Techniques for making nucleic acid probes included the labeling of abundant RNA molecules using complementary DNA synthesis, or the incorporation of labeled nucleotides via DNA synthesis reactions.

Restriction Endonuclease Cleavage and Gel Electrophoresis—DNA Restriction Maps

The featureless appearance of DNA under the electron microscope contrasts mightily with its wealth of information in terms of nucleotide sequence. *Restriction endonucleases* are bacterial enzymes that recognize sequences on double-stranded DNA and cleave the DNA at those sites. Figure 8.2 shows the *recognition sequences* for two commonly used restriction enzymes as well as their cleavage pattern. Note that the DNA sequence constituting a *restriction site* is a palindrome, with the sequence on one strand being equivalent to that on the other read backward. The pattern of restriction cleavage is also interesting in that it yields overhanging nucleotides at each end (*staggered ends*). These overhanging nucleotides are identical at ends cut by the same restriction endonuclease (Fig. 8.2), a feature that is useful

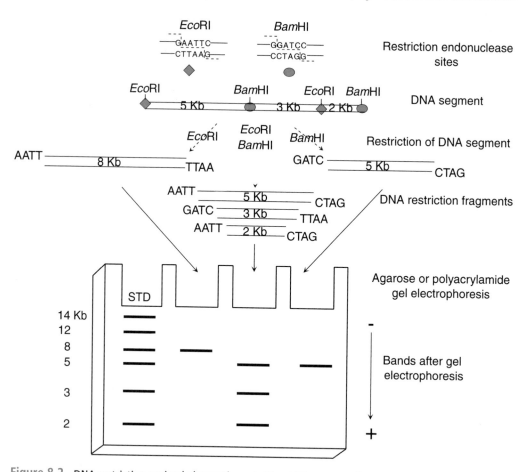

Figure 8.2. DNA restriction and gel electrophoresis. The DNA segment (center) is restricted with the endonucleases *Eco*RI and/or *Bam*HI, then analyzed by gel electrophoreses to reveal the cleaved fragment sizes. A restriction map is deduced from the sizes of restriction fragments visualized on the gel.

for *recombinant DNA cloning*. There are more than 200 restriction endonucleases available commercially, each recognizing different sequences in duplex DNA and yielding different types of blunt or staggered ends after cleavage. Their names reflect their bacteria of origin, exemplified by *Eco*RI from *Escherichia coli* and *Bam*HI from *Bacillus amylofaciens* (Fig. 8.2).

A theoretical experiment using DNA restriction and agarose gel electrophoresis is shown in the lower part of Figure 8.2. Note that the hypothetical DNA segment of 10 kb contains two recognition sites for *Eco*RI and two for *Bam*HI restriction endonuclease, yielding differently sized DNA fragments after restriction with one or both endonucleases. Each aliquot of the targeted DNA segment and its accompanying restriction enzyme(s) is applied to different slots of a molded agarose gel. The DNA fragments produced by each enzyme digest are attracted to the positive pole when an electric current is passed through the gel, with the smaller fragments moving farther due to less obstruction from the agarose pores. The DNA fragments are thus separated according to their size (fragment length), and they are visualized (stained) using fluorescent dyes such as ethidium bromide. The size of each fragment in the mixture can be calculated by noting the position of its band compared with the migration distances of standard fragments (Fig. 8.2). The sizes of DNA segments obtained with different combinations of restriction endonucleases allow the construction of a *DNA restriction map* showing the positions of restriction sites on the original DNA segment. These restriction sites provide identifying landmarks on the DNA segment that differentiate it from other DNA segments. They also provide a method for purifying the DNA segment using the methods of recombinant DNA cloning.

Identifying Gene Fragments in Genomic DNA Samples: Southern Blots

In order to visualize fragments of a particular gene in a restriction digest of genomic DNA, a method for hybridization to gel-separated DNA was required. Figure 8.3 shows the elegant but simple solution to this problem devised by Dr. Ed Southern in Edinburgh, Scotland. After restriction and agarose gel electrophoresis as in Figure 8.2, the gel containing arrays of DNA fragments from the entire genome is placed in denaturing solution. It is then sandwiched between a capillary wick and filter paper in a way that fluid will pass upward through the gel and transfer the denatured DNA onto the filter paper. The filter paper (usually a form of nitrocellulose) then contains an imprint of each restriction sample that has been size-separated on the gel. The stabilized imprint is then placed in hybridization solution with a DNA or RNA probe for the gene of interest, allowed to hybridize, washed free of excess probe, dried, and placed against an X-ray film for autoradiography. Bands on the autoradiogram correspond to fragments of the gene of interest highlighted amid each size-separated array of genomic DNA fragments (Fig. 8.3).

The lengths of restriction fragments displayed by Southern blot and DNA hybridization can then be estimated with reference to standards, and a DNA restriction map can be constructed for the targeted gene as was done for the single DNA segment in Figure 8.2. Note the difference between DNA restriction analysis of a purified DNA molecule (Figure 8.2) compared to Southern analysis of a particular gene segment within a huge excess of genomic DNA (Figure 8.3). The purified DNA segment yields bands that can be viewed directly by fluorescent staining, while the specific gene segment within genomic DNA must be visualized by hybridization with a DNA probe followed by autoradiography. When appropriate probes are available, the Southern blot method can be adapted to study RNA (northern blots) or protein (western blots). The puns on Southern's name reflect their similar techniques for electrophoretic separation of an RNA or protein mixture, followed by the probing of specific molecules within the size-separated array. RNA molecules can be identified by probes derived from the corresponding

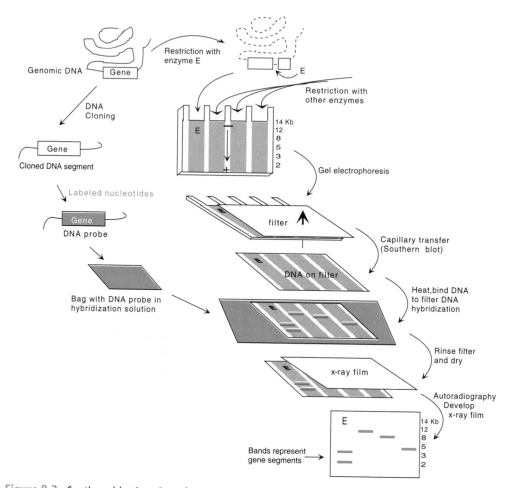

Figure 8.3. Southern blotting. Gene fragments obtained after restriction with enzyme E are visualized by gel electrophoresis, transfer of the DNA to filters, hybridization with the gene probe of interest, and autoradiography. The size of the gene fragments allows construction of a restriction map as shown in Fig. 8.4.

genes and proteins can be identified by labeled antibodies.

The different types of blots allow the basic structure, RNA expression, and protein products of a gene to be defined as a prelude to its molecular characterization. Since each lane of a gel can contain a different restriction enzyme digest or a RNA/protein extract from a different tissue, a DNA restriction map and expression profile can be rapidly defined for any gene for which the appropriate probes are available. The preliminary restriction/expression data provide a map of gene size and organization, allowing the design of gene cloning experiments.

■ 8.3. DNA CLONING AND GENE CHARACTERIZATION

Recombinant DNA cloning uses the uniform ends generated by restriction endonucleases to construct recombinant molecules containing the gene fragment of interest. These recombinant DNA molecules can be isolated free of those containing other genomic DNA fragments and purified to yield large amounts of the targeted gene. DNA cloning is most straightforward when available DNA probes and Southern blots have produced a detailed restriction map for the gene. Other methods for cloning are more indirect, using information about expression or location of the gene.

Cloning Based on Gene Structure

Once a restriction map is available for a portion of a gene, strategies for isolation of the gene can be designed. These strategies initially used plasmid or bacteriophage DNA molecules (*vectors*) that were engineered to accept foreign DNA segments. Both the vector and targeted genomic DNA are restricted with the same endonuclease, then mixed together to form an array of *recombinant DNA* molecules called a *DNA library*. Libraries are constructed with excess vector DNA to maximize the number of genomic DNA fragments incorporated into recombinant DNA molecules. After a library is constructed, two tiers of screening are required to locate the recombinants that contain the gene fragments of interest. First, color reactions are employed to discriminate parent from recombinant vector molecules. Second, recombinant molecules are plated at high density, transferred onto filters using the same methods outlined for the Southern blot, and screened by hybridization to a DNA or RNA probe. Those recombinant molecules that give positive hybridization signals after autoradiography should contain DNA fragments of the targeted gene. These recombinants, having been maintained separately on agar plates, are cultured to large density and harvested to prepare DNA. The particular gene fragment is thus purified from a concentration of about 1 in 100,000 in the genome to 20–30% of the DNA in the recombinant vector.

Many different strategies for DNA cloning have been devised. When a gene probe is available and a restriction map has been characterized, then the appropriate vector and DNA library are selected to provide the gene fragment of interest. Numerous vectors and electrophoretic methods have been developed so that various sizes of DNA fragments can be separated by electrophoresis and cloned. Particularly useful are the yeast artificial chromosome (YAC) vectors that allow cloning of DNA segments as large as 1–3 Mb. If a gene probe is not available, then antibodies to the product protein can be used to screen DNA libraries in vectors engineered for protein expression. Sometimes a portion of the protein's amino acid sequence is known, and oligonucleotide probes (*guessmers*) based on the expected coding sequence can be constructed and used for screening. With the array of cloning vectors and strategies now available, any gene with defined structural or expression properties can be cloned.

Cloning Based on Gene Expression (Functional Cloning)

Certain vectors are engineered to express their cloned genes so that its protein product is present in the bacterial cell. If antibody to the protein is available, then the recombinant DNA library can be screened for the gene of interest based on antibodies to its protein as expressed in the host bacteria. This method requires multiple clones of the gene to ensure that one is inserted in the correct phase so as to express its normal protein product rather than nonsense information.

Other cloning strategies have used cultured animal cells to screen recombinants obtained from a DNA library. If the animal cell is deficient in a particular genetic function, then a strategy can be devised by which a cloned gene will correct the deficient function. Correction is dependent on the techniques of *DNA transformation* or *DNA transfection* that allow recombinant DNA to be internalized and expressed by cultured cells. Successful examples of cloning through correction of deficiencies in cultured cells include the isolation of genes from the xeroderma pigmentosum (194400) and peroxisomal disease (214100) groups.

Cloning Based on Gene Location (Positional Cloning)

Sometimes the chromosomal location of a gene is known from genetic mapping experiments, from its involvement in chromosome

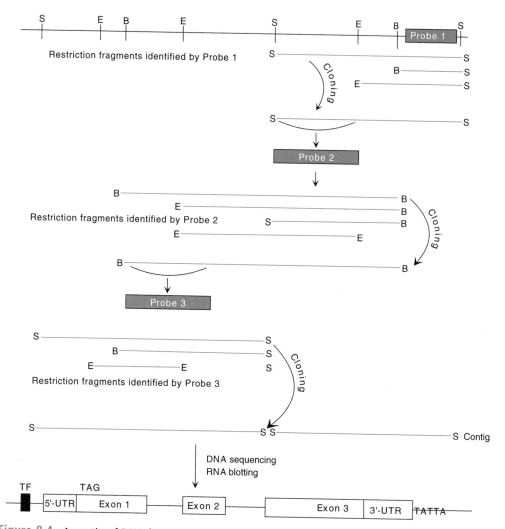

Figure 8.4. A contig of DNA fragments obtained by successive restriction mapping and DNA cloning steps. The contiguous DNA fragments can be characterized by DNA sequencing and RNA blotting to reveal candidate gene regions.

rearrangements or deletions, or from its presence in chromosome-specific recombinant DNA. Cloning strategies can then target the gene by assembling a group of contiguous DNA fragments that bracket the suspected gene location. The assembly of contiguous DNA fragments, known as a *contig*, is a fundamental technique for gene isolation in molecular genetics (Fig. 8.4). The strategy proceeds from a known DNA segment (probe 1 in Fig. 8.4) that is close to the chromosomal locus of interest. The known segment may have been

identified because it encodes a previously known RNA, or it may have been isolated randomly as an anonymous DNA fragment during gene mapping experiments (see section 8.4 below). The available DNA probe is used to construct a restriction map by Southern blotting, highlighting overlapping DNA fragments that allow one to "walk" along the chromosome by successive restriction mapping and cloning. Once an array of contiguous DNA segments have been cloned, they can be characterized by DNA sequencing and RNA blotting experiments to identify genes within the contig region. Such regions become *candidate genes* for the targeted locus, with further genetic and cellular experiments required to ensure that the newly identified gene is responsible for the disease or characteristic of interest. Although more arduous than structural or functional cloning, the pace of positional cloning is increasing rapidly as the human genome project provides gene mapping and sequencing information (see section 8.8 below).

Cloning Using Homologous Gene Motifs

A remarkable fact covered in Chapter 9 is the enormous homology of major genes or gene regions between humans and simpler experimental organisms. It is now recognized that many important genes in yeast, flies, worms, and mice are conserved during evolution, providing an obvious strategy for cloning the homologous genes in humans. Particularly well conserved are key elements within genes called motifs: the homeotic (Hox) and paired (Pax) motifs are examples that allowed genes involved in human development to be cloned and characterized based on knowledge of development in flies. Motifs are typically short DNA segments of 50–200 bp that can be used as probes to identify homologous fragments in human genomic DNA. The motif would function as probe 1 in Figure 8.4, providing a start in isolating a contig that contains the homologous human gene. Once the human gene has been isolated and characterized, it becomes a candidate gene for diseases that map to the particular chromosome region.

Characterization of Cloned Genes

Once a gene or gene fragment is cloned, its organization and DNA sequence must be determined. Northern (RNA) blotting experiments can identify transcribed regions of the gene interval, allowing DNA sequencing experiments to focus on expressed portions of the gene. DNA sequencing strategies involve placing an isotopic or fluorescent label at one end of a

DNA segment, then catalyzing DNA polymerization in the presence of inhibiting nucleotides. After DNA polymerization is allowed to proceed in each of the four reactions, they are applied to a high-resolution electrophoretic gel. Each labeled band is equivalent to a DNA fragment that terminated at the selected nucleotide, allowing the DNA sequence to be read by scanning upward from the bottom of the gel. Once the DNA sequence of a cloned gene is available, RNA splicing sites, intron–exon junctions, and the amino acid sequence of its product protein can be deduced. Genes of unknown function may be matched with other known genes through shared motifs within their protein-coding or upstream regulatory sequences. Examples include the collagen genes to be discussed in Section 8.6, since their repeating (Gly-X-Y) amino acid sequences are very striking and specific.

■ 8.4. GENETIC LINKAGE AND GENETIC MAPS

As discussed in Chapter 6, genes are organized in a standard arrangement called a *genome* that is different for each species and constitutes the major reproductive barrier between species. The visible structures of genome organization are the chromosomes, each containing a linear array of many hundreds of genes. While simpler organisms such as *Drosophila* have only four chromosomes, the larger numbers of genes and chromosomes in the human genome pose a considerable challenge for cataloguing and mapping.

Genetic Linkage Using Protein Polymorphisms

There are two types of gene maps. *Genetic maps* are the traditional maps constructed by observing the segregation of traits in families. Early examples included traits such as hemophilia or X-linked mental retardation, where transmission through females and expression in males established that the responsible loci were on the X chromosome. *Physical maps* localize genes by direct observation (e.g., FISH techniques for visualizing genetic loci on chromosomes) or by defining genes within characterized DNA contigs (e.g., Fig. 8.4). Genetic maps measure distances between genes in terms of the number of recombinations between them, while physical maps associate genes with visible chromosomal landmarks and measure distances in terms of DNA base pairs.

Although the segregation of traits in families allowed a few genes to be mapped, it was rare to find individuals with two inherited traits (e.g., hemophilia and color blindness) where recombination could be used to measure the distance between loci. The ability to characterize gene products at the biochemical or DNA level vastly increased the number of variable alleles at each genetic locus, providing a pow-

erful tool for genetic mapping. Protein polymorphisms provided the first comprehensive approaches to gene maping, illustrated by the pedigree in Figure 8.5. In Figure 8.5*A*, a family with an autosomal dominant disorder called nail-patella syndrome (161200) is shown along with their ABO blood types. Examination of the pedigree to see if the segregation of nail-patella syndrome alleles correlates with that of the ABO blood group alleles is called a *genetic linkage analysis*. Individuals I-2, II-1, II-2, and II-4 are affected with nail-patella syndrome and are blood type A. Since the presumed father was type O and the couple had a child (II-3) who was type O, the type A offspring must all have AO genotypes.

The family exhibits cotransmission of the A allele along with the allele for nail-patella syndrome (N) in three offspring (II-1, II-2, and II-4 in Fig. 8.5*A*), suggesting that the ABO and

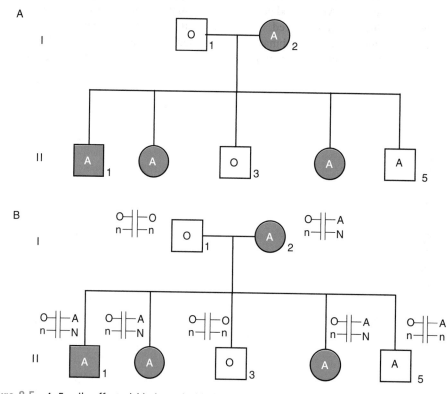

Figure 8.5. *A,* Family affected (dark symbols) or unaffected (light symbols) with nail-patella syndrome together with their ABO blood types (center of symbols); *B,* same family showing alignments of ABO and nail-patella alleles (the paired autosomes for each individual are represented by vertical lines).

nail-patella loci might be located nearby on the same chromosome. In addition, offspring II-3 shows cotransmission of the O allele together with the normal nail-patella allele (n) from his mother. Figure 8.5*B* shows the probable alignments of ABO and nail-patella alleles for this family, using vertical lines to represent each chromosome. The different ABO alleles, detected because they encode different versions of a red blood cell protein, provide information on the clinical status of offspring in Figure 8.5*A*. If evidence for genetic linkage was substantiated, then the ABO blood type could serve as a diagnostic marker for nail-patella syndrome in this family. Also, prior knowledge that the ABO blood group locus is on chromosome 9 would establish this chromosome as the residence for the nail-patella syndrome locus.

Note that individual II-5 in Figure 8.5 is an exception: He is type A but unaffected with nail-patella syndrome. If the ABO blood group and nail-patella syndrome loci are linked, then this individual must represent a recombination during meiosis where the A and n alleles residing on the same maternal chromosome were separated (Fig. 8.5*B*). Study of additional families demonstrated that such recombinations had a frequency of about 10%. Because the frequency of recombination is proportionate to the distance between loci, this 10% frequency can be converted to a relative distance named for the geneticist Thomas Hunt Morgan. Each one percent of recombination between two loci is assigned a distance of one *centimorgan (cM)*, implying that the nail-patella and ABO loci are 10 cM apart. As the genetic distance between two loci increases, they segregate randomly as predicted by Mendel's law of independent assortment (50% recombination frequency is equivalent to a genetic distance of 50 cM).

DNA cloning experiments have established that the physical distance represented by one centimorgan is about one Mb, meaning that genetic linkage cannot be detected unless two loci are less than 50 Mb apart. As might be suspected, frequencies of recombination will vary

somewhat among different chromosome regions and render genetic distances less accurate than physical distances. It is interesting that females exhibit higher recombination frequencies than males, giving them a longer genetic map on the centimorgan scale.

Quantification of Linkage Analysis

Although linkage analysis is an experimental rather than clinical laboratory technique, positive results may lead to tests used in pre- or postnatal diagnosis. For this reason, it is important to appreciate the basis for linkage relationships as they are used in the clinical arena.

Inspection of the family in Figure 8.5 reveals some characteristics crucial to the conclusion that the ABO and nail-patella syndrome loci are linked. First, the transmission of alleles could not be analyzed if the mother were type O (homozygous OO genotype). Such matings are said to be *uninformative,* since it would be unclear which ABO allele traveled with the allele for nail-patella syndrome. The family would also be uninformative if the father and mother were type A heterozygotes, since it could not be determined whether offspring received the maternal or paternal A allele. Second, note that alignment of the A and abnormal N alleles on one maternal chromosome determined that the A allele would be predictive of nail-patella syndrome in this family. The opposite alignment of the O allele with the abnormal N allele in mother would have associated homozygous O genotypes in offspring with the development of nail-patella syndrome. This alignment of alleles is called the *phase of linkage,* and it is important to realize that the phase of alleles in parents determines the scoring of offspring as exhibiting linkage or recombination.

A third attribute of possible linkage in this family concerns the possibility that cotransmission of A and N (or of O and n) maternal alleles may have occurred by chance. Cotransmission in four of five offspring is not very convincing evidence for linkage, because this would be expected to occur two to three in five times by chance alone. Clearly the number of informative offspring observed and the ratio of cotransmission versus recombination influences the odds for linkage between two loci.

The foregoing characteristics have been incorporated into a maximal likelihood strategy for evaluating linkage analyses illustrated in Table 8.1. The number of informative offspring are first tallied, then scored as showing recombination or linkage. The family in Figure 8.5 contained five informative matings of which one (individual II-5) was scored as a recombinant. The odds of observing this result in the family can then be calculated by assuming various recombination frequencies (Θ) between the two loci. If Θ is 0.1 (10% recombination frequency), then the chance of a recombinant occurring is $\Theta = 0.1$ and that of a nonrecombinant occurring is $1 - \Theta = 0.9$. For five offspring, the chance of one recombinant and four instances of cotransmission occurring together is the product of the five probabilities: $\Theta (1 - \Theta)^4 = (0.1)(0.9)^4 = (0.1)(0.66) = 0.066$. In Table 8.1, values for Θ ranging from 0.01 to 0.4 are considered, with the odds for observing one recombinant among five informative offspring being 0.0096 to 0.052. These calculations fulfill the expectation that low recombination frequencies will decrease the odds of observing a recombinant.

In order to calculate the likelihood of linkage based on data from a particular family, the odds for the observed genotypes to occur must be related to the odds if the recombination frequency Θ was 0.5—that is, if there were no linkage at all. For the five informative offspring in Figure 8.5, the odds for 50% recombination at each meiosis is $(0.5)^5 = 1/32$ or 0.031. Now a ratio of the odds can be calculated, as shown in the last column of Table 8.1. For the various assumed recombination frequencies (Θ), the likelihood of linkage (Z) is calculated as the ratio of odds for observing the genotypes in question to the odds of no linkage, or $\Theta(1 - \Theta)^4 / 0.031$ in the case of five offspring with one recombinant. For a 10% recombination frequency, the odds ratio is 0.066/0.31 or 2.13 (Table 8.1). Since these ratios may be large numbers, it is traditional to calculate the logarithm of Z, known as the *logarithm of the odds of linkage* or *LOD score*. By comparing LOD scores for different assumed recombination frequencies, a maximum score can be found that represents the most likely estimate of the true frequency. In Table 8.1, a maximum LOD score of 0.42 is calculated at a Θ of .2, suggesting a true recombination frequency of 20% (and a genetic distance of 20 cM) between the ABO and nail-patella syndrome loci.

Since convincing odds ratios range from 1000 to 10,000, with corresponding LOD scores between three and four, the family in Figure 8.5 does not provide strong evidence for linkage. As mentioned previously, studies of many families estimate the actual recombination frequency between the nail-patella and ABO loci at 10%. More than 15 informative matings with the ex-

■**TABLE 8.1.** Logarithm of the Odds (LOD) Scores as a Function of Recombination Frequency (Θ)

Recombination Frequency (Θ)	Linkage Frequency $(1 - (\Theta))$	$(1 - \Theta)^4$	Odds of 1 Recombinant in 5 Offspring $\Theta (1-(\Theta)^4$	Odds 1 in 5/ Odds No Linkage $\Theta (1-(\Theta)^4/0.031^a$	LOD Score (Z)
0.01	0.99	0.96	0.0096	0.31	−0.5
0.1	0.9	0.66	0.066	2.13	0.33
0.2	0.8	0.41	0.082	2.64	0.42
0.3	0.7	0.24	0.072	2.32	0.37
0.4	0.6	0.13	0.052	1.70	0.23

[a]No linkage implies that $\Theta = 0.5$, which for 5 offspring is $(0.5)^5 = 1/32 = 0.31$.

pected 0–1 recombinants must be observed to obtain an odds ratio (Z) above 1000 at this recombination frequency (Θ). The result would be recorded as a LOD score of 3.0 at a recombination frequency of 0.1.

The two-point linkage analysis between the ABO and nail patella syndrome loci can be rapidly expanded if families can be scored for their inheritance of additional polymorphic alleles at the same time. Multipoint linkage analyses are highly complex because there are many types of recombinants and different possibilities for gene order. For example, a hypothetical locus L might also be located on chromosome 9 and exhibit a 10% recombination frequency with the nail-patella locus and a 20% recombination frequency with the ABO blood group locus. The presumed gene order would then be L-N-ABO, with 10 cM between each locus. Computer analysis is required for such determinations, particularly since the number of possible gene orders rises factorially with the number of loci analyzed.

The result of multipoint analysis is a large linkage group that extends along an entire chromosome. Because portions of chromosomes are conserved during evolution, homologous genes often have conserved distances and orientation when examined among closely related animals. Detailed linkage maps have been constructed in rapidly breeding organisms such as flies and mice, each yielding a number of linkage groups equivalent to their number of chromosomes. In humans, more discriminating polymorphisms were required so that the number of informative matings could be maximized relative to long generations and small family size. These polymorphisms or *DNA markers* were provided by DNA restriction and sequencing.

DNA Polymorphism and Linkage Analysis

During DNA restriction and gene cloning experiments (e.g., Figs. 8.2–8.4), it was realized that certain sites were variable among individuals and constituted polymorphisms. These DNA polymorphisms have two main forms as diagrammed in Figure 8.6. One type is a *single nucleotide polymorphism* or SNP. If this variable nucleotide occurs within a restriction site, then the DNA of some individuals will be cleaved at that site while the DNA from others will not. Because the presence of the restriction site is determined by the length of DNA fragments yielded by restriction and electrophoresis, such polymorphisms are known as *restriction fragment length polymorphisms* or *RFLPs*. In Figure 8.6A, the variable restriction site E_2 results in different DNA fragment sizes after restriction with endonuclease E. These different configurations of restriction sites represent different alleles as determined by the DNA fragments produced. The gel diagrammed in Figure 8.6A shows that individuals can have both alleles (two different DNA fragment sizes) or be homozygous for allele 1 or 2 (single fragment size of double intensity). These RFLP alleles can be used for linkage analysis in the same way as the ABO blood group protein polymorphisms. As DNA sequencing methods have become more rapid, single nucleotide polymorphisms (SNPs) can be evaluated directly by sequence determination rather than by their effects on restriction sites.

In Figure 8.6B, a second type of DNA polymorphism is shown that results from variable numbers of tandem repeats (*VNTRs*) between the restriction endonuclease sites. Here the two restriction sites bracket a variable DNA region that contains different multiples of a nucleotide repeat. Dinucleotide repeats of CA (GT on the opposite DNA strand) are the most common VNTRs, with 3, 4, and 5-mers being occasionally seen. Trinucleotide repeats have been associated with a category of genetic disease, as discussed in Chapter 10. Repeating units with higher numbers of nucleotides are also found in the genome (e.g., satellite or rDNA repeating units discussed in Chapter 6), but these are often clustered together and are less useful as polymorphic markers for nearby genes. Note that the different numbers of repeating units provide a powerful tool for linkage analysis,

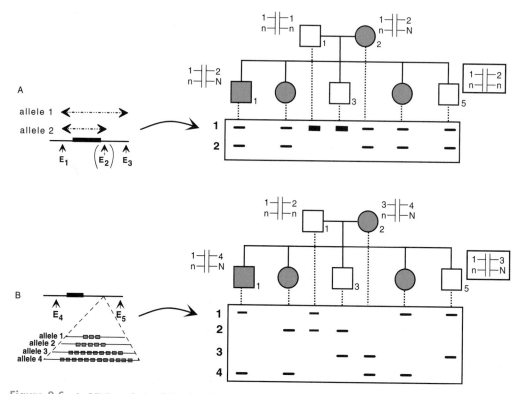

Figure 8.6. A, RFLP analysis of the family in Figure 8.8 showing segregation of the nail-patella allele with the smaller RFLP allele (2); B, VNTR analysis showing segregation of the nail-patella allele with the larger VNTR allele (4).

because each parental chromosome in Figure 8.6*B* has a different allele. Dinucleotide repeating units can also be visualized directly on DNA sequencing gels and are sometimes called *minisatellites*. The presence of SNPs and minisatellites throughout the genome provide useful DNA polymorphisms for linkage analysis and extends the potential for genetic mapping to every chromosome region.

The increased power of DNA polymorphisms for linkage analysis is illustrated for the same family with nail-patella syndrome in Figure 8.6. In Figure 8.6*A*, the smaller restriction fragment (allele 2) exhibits linkage to the abnormal nail-patella allele as shown on the gel beneath the pedigree. In Figure 8.6*B*, allele 4 travels with the abnormal N allele for nail-patella syndrome. In both portions of the figure, individual II-5 exhibits the recombinant genotype of normal nail-patella alleles with al-

lele 2 or allele 4 from the mother. In contrast to the ABO protein polymorphism in Figure 8.5, the VNTR polymorphism in Figure 8.6*B* will be informative for linkage analysis regardless of phase in the mother. The greater number of alleles (four versus three) allows each parental chromosome to be tagged with a unique allele, so offspring can be scored regardless of which parental chromosome carries the abnormal nail-patella allele.

The copious occurrence of DNA polymorphisms establishes a unique "fingerprint" for each individual in terms of DNA sequence. The visualization of VNTR polymorphisms from several chromosomes on the same DNA sequencing gel can be used as a criterion for personal identity or relatedness. These DNA fingerprinting techniques are useful for evaluating paternity or for matching criminals to crime scenes during forensic evaluations. Because each VNTR locus may have tens or hundreds of alleles, the frequency of any one allele can be as low as 1 in 1000 in the population. Matching of three rare alleles between two blood samples can thus lead to very high odds for identity, that is, $(1000)^3$ or 1 billion to one. Such odds offer convincing evidence for paternity or criminal identity.

Linkage Disequilibrium (Allele Association)

A second approach that links protein or DNA polymorphism to disease is called *linkage disequilibrium* or *allele association*. The latter term is preferable, because the relationship between disease and marker alleles does not necessarily involve linkage due to proximity. Allele association may reflect a common genetic background among affected individuals or may occur because the marker locus is somehow involved in pathogenesis. Figure 8.7A illustrates the first case, where a specific alignment of restriction sites has descended through generations along with the mutation for sickle cell hemoglobin (hemoglobin S). The preferred alignment of several mutations on one chromosome, illustrated by the nucleotide changes producing the 13 kb *Hpa*I restriction fragment and S hemoglobin changes is called a *haplotype* or *framework*. A specific haplotype occurs in part because of inheritance from a common ancestor (founder effect, see Chapter 4) and in part because of selective forces acting on that chromosomal region. Despite many generations and opportunities for recombination within the haplotypes, the conjunction of one *Hpa*I pattern with S globin alleles and others with A globin alleles have persisted, presumably driven by the selective advantage of sickle cell heterozygotes against malaria. The resistance of these mutations to the usual equilibrium of recombination accounts for the term *linkage disequilibrium,* just as their tendency to cluster together on the same chromosome accounts for the term *allele association.*

An important distinction between allele association and genetic linkage is shown by the abbreviated pedigree in Figure 8.7A. Note that the *Hpa*I allele 2 and S globin allele will always be in phase, at least to the degree that their allele association holds. Parental phase of these alleles does not vary among different families as was observed for ABO and nail-patella syndrome alleles in Figure 8.5B.

Although the hemoglobin S allele association with *Hpa*I restriction sites concerns alleles that are close together on the chromosome, allele associations can occur between loci on separate chromosomes. Common ancestral inheritance is not a factor in these associations, because the separate chromosomes will sort independently at each meiosis. Allele associations such as those between the HLA B27 allele and the genes predisposing to ankylosing spondylitis (106300) are thought to reflect a common role in pathogenesis (Fig. 8.7B). Ankylosing spondylitis, like type I diabetes mellitus discussed in Chapter 5, is an autoimmune disease where an individual makes antibodies against his or her own tissues. The HLA B27 allele, like certain HLA DQ alleles in diabetes, must interact with genes predisposing to ankylosing spondylitis and facilitate the manufacture of antibodies against the spinal bones (Fig. 8.7B). See Chapter 9 for additional discussion of HLA alleles and their disease associations.

Case 8 Follow-up: The family illustrated by the pedigree in Figure 8.1 exhibits X-linked inheritance of mental disability. Other symptoms in affected males included delayed speech (aphasia), spasticity (tight muscles causing young children to walk on their toes), and adducted or clasped thumbs. This pattern of abnormalities was first recognized by Gareis and Mason, and was described by the acronym MASA syndrome, where each letter stood for a prominent symptom. Because MASA syndrome patients lack distinguishing metabolic aberrations or congenital anomalies, it is classified as a form of nonspecific X-linked mental retardation. Over 40 other examples of nonspecific X-linked mental retardation have been described in the literature, each having subtle differences in ap-

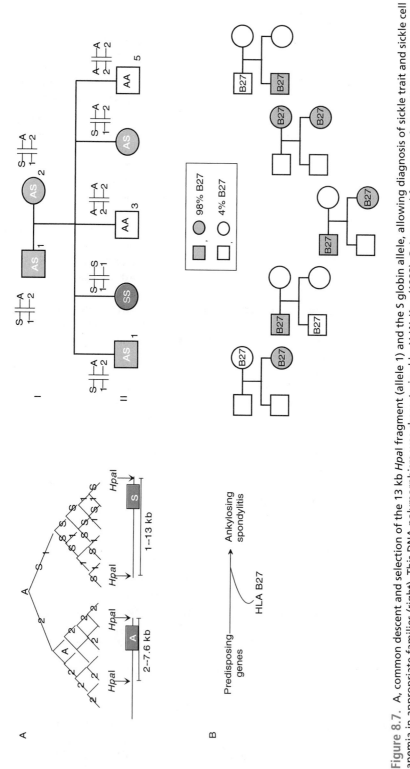

Figure 8.7. A, common descent and selection of the 13 kb *Hpa*I fragment (allele 1) and the S globin allele, allowing diagnosis of sickle trait and sickle cell anemia in appropriate families (right). This DNA polymorphism was characterized by Y. W. Kan (1992). *B*, Increased frequency of HLA allele B27 in association with ankylosing spondylitis, a multifactorial autoimmune disease. The pedigrees demonstrate increased association of the ankylosing spondylitis phenotype and HLA B27 alleles, but they are not always cotransmitted in families.

pearance or neurologic findings to suggest that they are separate disorders. Although relatively few protein polymorphisms had been localized to the X chromosome, the identification of polymorphic DNA markers offered the opportunity to explore whether various disorders with nonspecific X-linked mental retardation were in fact different entities by mapping their causative loci to identical or different loci on the X chromosome. The physician should thus consider DNA linkage analysis since chromosomal and metabolic testing was unrevealing.

The pedigree shown in Figure 8.1 has numerous informative meioses in which carrier females have normal or affected sons. DNA was isolated from multiple family members and analyzed to see if linkage to any of the X chromosome DNA polymorphisms could be demonstrated. Figure 8.8 shows a Southern

blot analysis concerning a portion of the family that defines RFLP alleles at a locus named F8C. Note the cotransmission of the larger RFLP allele from locus F8C with the abnormal allele for X-linked mental retardation, as demonstrated by its presence in DNA from the affected males. Since the marker F8C is located within band Xq28 of the X chromosome, the linkage indicates that the gene for MASA syndrome is near this same position on the tip of the X chromosome long arm. The analysis also demonstrates, to the degree that crossovers can be ruled out, that individual II-3 and her daughters are not carriers for the disorder. If the husband of individual II-2 were homozygous for the smaller allele of F8C, the couple could opt for prenatal diagnosis in their next pregnancy.

Data from several laboratories confirmed this linkage to the Xq28 region with a LOD

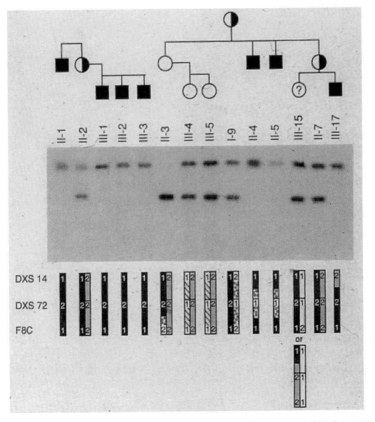

Figure 8.8. Linkage of the larger F8C RFLP allele with the putative mutant allele for MASA syndrome in a portion of the family illustrated in Figure 8.1. (From Macias et al., 1992.)

score greater than 4 and a recombination frequency less than 1%. These results provide prenatal diagnosis with an accuracy of 1% in cases where the parental phase of F8C alleles would allow informative genotypes in the fetus. Linkage to the Xq28 region also established that MASA syndrome was unique from similar types of X-linked mental retardation that mapped elsewhere on the X chromosome and allowed a search for candidate genes.

■ 8.5. CHROMOSOME JUMPING AND PHYSICAL MAPPING

Rapid progress in matching diseases with genes reflects the synergy of genetic and physical mapping techniques. Physical mapping is illustrated by the polytene chromosomes of Drosophila salivary glands that allowed matching of the genetic linkage map with specific chromosomal bands. Physical mapping involves direct localization by molecular analysis (Fig. 8.9).

When an autosomal dominant or X-linked disease is observed together with a reciprocal translocation, the breakpoints become candidate regions for the causative gene. If a cloned DNA segment from the breakpoint region is available, then a contig can be isolated and searched for candidate genes within the region as shown in Figure 8.4. The isolation of a DNA segment from an implicated chromosome region, followed by gradual extension of the cloned region to form a contig, has been called *chromosome walking*. In a sense, one walks along the chromosome until the desired gene is encountered and characterized. In contrast, *chromosome jumping* utilizes the reciprocal

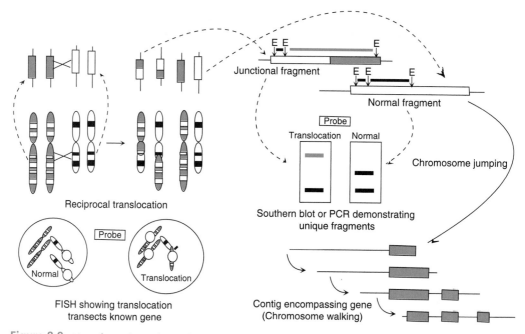

Figure 8.9. Use of a reciprocal translocation to jump from a known gene fragment (light box) to an unknown gene fragment (dark box). Presence of the known gene at a translocation breakpoint is shown by three rather than two fluorescent signals after FISH. Joining of known and unknown gene regions at the translocation breakpoint can be recognized by an altered restriction pattern (right). DNA probes for the known gene fragment can then be employed to isolate a junctional fragment containing the unknown gene (chromosome jumping), followed by the isolation of a contig (chromosome walking) encompassing the entire unknown gene.

translocation to isolate junctional fragments that join characterized DNA segments with new genes. The proximal part of a junctional fragment corresponds to the known restriction map for one chromosome region, while its distal part "jumps" to the map for the other chromosome region. Because characteristic chromosome translocations occur in many cancers, chromosome jumping techniques have been useful for isolating many oncogenes as well as genes causing Mendelian diseases such as neurofibromatosis-1 (162200).

The development of FISH technology has been an enormous aid in localizing genes by physical mapping. Not only does the technique allow for direct mapping of cloned DNA segments to their chromosomal region of origin, it facilitates the characterization of genes at the breakpoints of reciprocal chromosome translocations. If a gene segment is transected by a translocation, its derived fluorescent DNA probe should give two signals in nuclei or cells (one at each breakpoint). When the homologous autosomal locus is taken into account, fluorescent probes for the transected gene give three signals rather than the two expected in cells without the translocation (Fig. 8.9).

8.6. GENE CHARACTERIZATION AND DNA DIAGNOSIS

Once a candidate gene is isolated and characterized, the gene can be "elected" as the etiology for genetic disease by demonstrating the presence of disruptive mutations. Powerful methods are now available for scanning genes for mutations that alter their structure or expression. Because the characterization of gene mutations can establish the presence of genetic disease in an individual, these methods are now incorporated into clinical DNA diagnostic laboratories.

The Polymerase Chain Reaction

The polymerase chain reaction (PCR) again takes advantage of the availability of purified enzymes that act on DNA (Fig. 8.10). The technique exploits heat-resistant DNA polymerases isolated from bacteria living in high-temperature environments. Oligonucleotide primers are synthesized based on the known DNA sequence of a characterized gene region. These primers catalyze replication of a targeted gene segment using the heat-stable DNA polymerase. After replication of the gene segment, the polymerase reaction is heated to denature the DNA and primers, then cooled to allow another cycle of replication. Because each cycle of replication doubles the number of DNA strands synthesized from the targeted region, the technique is a kind of chain reaction that can be performed in automated machines called *thermocyclers*. After 20–30 cycles of replication, heating, and cooling, up to 0.5 μg of a specific gene segment can be isolated from less than 1 μg of genomic DNA. This amount of DNA segment, amplified over one million times from its concentration in genomic DNA, is enough to visualize by gel electrophoresis (as in Fig. 8.2) or to give rapid signals after hybridization with colorimetric, fluorescent, or radioactive DNA probes. If additional cycles are employed, PCR can be used to isolate particular DNA segments from small blood spots or single cells.

Detection of DNA Sequence Variation in Characterized Genes: Mutation or DNA Polymorphism?

Once genetic and/or physical mapping studies lead to the isolation of a candidate disease gene, affected individuals are screened for mutations to "elect" the gene as responsible for the genetic disease. When gene mutations involve deletions, duplications, or rearrangements of nucleotides, their detection is straightforward using PCR or Southern blot analysis. When mutations involve single nucleotides, they must be detected by comparing DNA sequences between normal and affected patients. Once detected, these single nucleotide changes must be further characterized as polymorphisms (SNPs), as silent mutations that do not

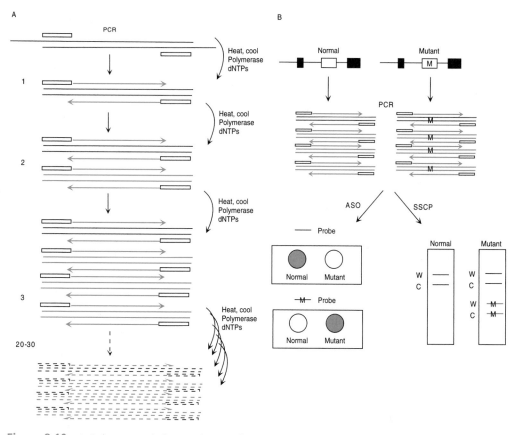

Figure 8.10. *A*, Polymerase chain reaction employing cycles of heating, cooling, and extension of DNA synthesis between oligonucleotide primers. The heat-stable DNA polymerase retains its activity between cycles. B, Use of PCR-amplified DNA to recognize mutations by single-strand conformational polymorphisms (SSCP, right) or to differentiate mutant alleles by allele-specific oligonucleotide hybridization (ASO, left). W, Watson strand; C, Crick strand.

alter the encoded amino acid sequence, or as disease-causing mutations that interfere with expression or function of the gene produce.

Because the DNA sequencing of genes from multiple normal and affected individuals is prohibitively laborious, rapid methods for detecting single nucleotide changes have been developed (Fig. 8.10B, right panel). Labeled gene fragments are amplified using PCR, then subjected to electrophoresis under denaturing conditions. Although the separated DNA strands are complementary, each has a different nucleotide composition that results in a unique shape and mobility during electrophoresis. The differently shaped DNA strands are called single-strand conformational polymorphisms

or SSCP. Using this SSCP technique, homozygous normal individuals will have two bands derived from a gene fragment after gel electrophoresis, while heterozygous individuals will have four bands (Figure 8.10B). Once abnormal SSCP bands are observed, the gene fragment can be sequenced to characterize the single nucleotide difference. The technique is most sensitive for DNA fragments in the 200–500 bp size range, so that complete mutational scanning of a gene region often requires PCR amplification and SSCP analysis of multiple gene segments.

As mentioned previously, single nucleotide polymorphisms occur every 200–500 bp in the human genome. Each SNP detected in a gene must therefore be classified as mutation or polymorphism before a nucleotide mutation is taken as evidence that the gene is responsible for disease. When a single mutant allele predominates, such as the E_6V mutation in the β-globin gene associated with sickle cell anemia, then its presence in patients/relatives and absence in normal individuals makes a compelling case for disease mutation. When most affected individuals have different mutant alleles, as in the genes causing osteogenesis imperfecta, neurofibromatosis, or Marfan syndrome, then the distinction between mutation and polymorphism becomes very difficult. For nucleotide changes within expressed gene regions, the known coding requirements for RNA splice sites or amino acid sequence can be helpful. Nucleotide changes that alter splice sites or produce stop codons are likely to be disease-causing mutations, while those that preserve the amino acid sequence (silent mutations) are likely to be polymorphisms. Sometimes the variant allele can be introduced into cultured cells to demonstrate that it is associated with altered gene expression.

Analysis of Mutant Alleles in the Clinical Laboratory: DNA Diagnosis

Once the range of DNA sequence variation in a gene has been characterized and its principal mutant alleles defined, the detection of mutant alleles can be used for laboratory diagnosis of disease. Gene deletions or rearrangements are easiest to detect, because Southern or PCR analysis visualizes extra, missing, or rearranged fragments. For single nucleotide mutations, a useful technique for DNA diagnosis employs PCR amplification of gene segments and uses allele-specific oligonucleotide (*ASO*) hybridization to discriminate mutant and normal alleles (Fig. 8.10*B*, left panel). In addition to the flanking oligonucleotide primers that allow PCR amplification, allele-specific oligonucleotides are synthesized that match the normal or mutated DNA sequence. These PCR-amplified samples are bound to duplicate or triplicate filters, and each filter is hybridized to

a specific oligonucleotide probe. By comparing the pattern of hybridization on the filters, homozygous normal, heterozygous, or homozygous abnormal individuals can be diagnosed (Fig. 8.10*B*).

■ 8.7. THE MOLECULAR DELINEATION OF GENETIC DISORDERS

The elements of gene isolation, gene characterization, and DNA diagnosis provide an approach to all single gene disorders. If a particular gene or its product protein can be implicated in the disease, then the alteration in gene sequence provides a guide to the molecular pathogenesis. The examples in the following sections illustrate several approaches to gene isolation as summarized in Table 8.2. Each example of molecular delineation has yielded insights into gene structure, biochemical function, and clinical understanding. These characterized diseases emphasize how the genetic approach may resonate between the clinic and laboratory.

Functional Cloning Using a Cellular Phenotype: Familial Hypercholesterolemia

In Chapter 5, familial hypercholesterolemia (143890) was discussed as a Mendelian extreme (early-onset heart attacks) that provided insight into a multifactorial process (coronary artery disease). It is also a classic illustration of how a clinical abnormality, elegantly characterized at the cellular and biochemical level, can be explained by altered gene structure.

The disease has a frequency of 1 in 500 heterozygotes with moderate risk for coronary thrombosis and 1 in a million homozygotes with severe risk and death by the second or third decade of life if untreated. The initial cellular studies focused on the relationship of low-density lipoprotein (LDL), a cholesterol-carrying protein in serum, and intracellular cholesterol synthesis. It was found that LDL was taken up by a specific receptor, imported by a novel endocytosis pathway, and degraded to yield free intracellular cholesterol. The free cholesterol would then inhibit cellular cholesterol synthesis and decrease the number of LDL receptors. Because LDL mediated cholesterol uptake and was repressed by high cholesterol levels, its gene became the target for the molecular analysis of hypercholesterolemia.

Cloning of the LDL receptor gene was accomplished by screening cDNA libraries using antibodies to the purified receptor protein. Characterization revealed that the LDL receptor gene was a composite of several domains, each with unique sequence homology and function (Fig. 8.11). Screening of patients with

homozygous hypercholesterolemia revealed a correlation between mutations in these gene domains and specific steps in cellular cholesterol uptake and/or regulation. A novel type of mutation was also revealed by these studies, because several deletions of the LDL receptor gene occurred by unequal crossing over between Alu repetitive elements. Alu elements occur at thousands of places in the human genome (see Chapter 6), and their presence in several introns of the LDL receptor gene provides a hotspot for mutation by unequal crossover and deletion.

The pivotal role of receptor-mediated uptake in cholesterol metabolism was thus demonstrated through the cellular and molecu-

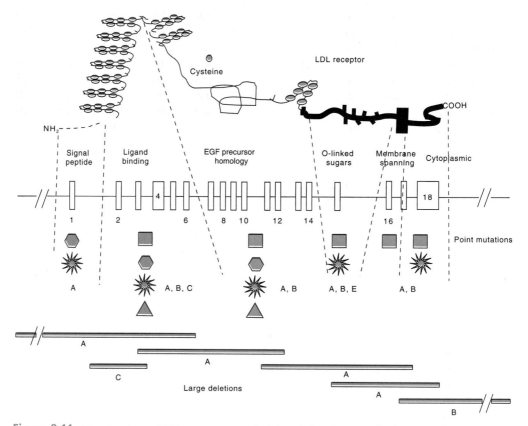

Figure 8.11. The structure of LDL receptor protein (above) showing specific domains with homologies to other genes such as epidermal growth factor (EGF). Multiple units containing cysteine (blue dots) are responsible for LDL binding, while separate regions contain linked sugars required for transport and the hydrophobic, membrane spanning domain. The corresponding LDL gene structure (middle) is shown with representative point mutations (filled symbols) or deletions. Letters correspond to different effects on cellular cholesterol metabolism. (Adapted from Goldstein et al., 1995.)

lar characterization of a genetic disease. The role of LDL receptor defects in causing hypercholesterolemia has been confirmed by altering the gene in transgenic mice, and experiments are underway to correct its deficiency by gene therapy (see Chapter 9). A rare homozygous disorder (hypercholesterolemia) has given insight into a common multifactorial problem (coronary artery disease) and provided immediate (cholesterol-lowering drugs) and future (gene transfer) strategies for treatment.

Functional Cloning Using a Serum Protein: α-1-Antitrypsin Deficiency

Another relatively common autosomal dominant disease is α-1-antitrypsin deficiency (AAT deficiency, 107400). AAT is a major inhibitor of serine proteases that mediate blood coagulation and complement fixation. Despite its location in serum, the main activity of AAT is to inhibit related proteases in the lung. Evidence for this important activity comes from patients with AAT deficiency who develop severe obstructive lung disease (emphysema) because their alveoli are destroyed by uninhibited proteases. Some patients also develop liver inflammation (hepatitis) and scarring (cirrhosis), which may occur in childhood.

The AAT protein could be assayed for its inhibitory activity, identified as a band on gels of serum proteins, purified because of its abundance, and used to construct antibodies for clinical and gene isolation studies. Mutant versions of the AAT protein were identified by their altered mobility on electrophoretic gels, and the more common variants were assigned M, S, and Z letters. Study of the mutant proteins allowed correlation of antitrypsin activity with their respective genotypes. Those with homozygous SS genotypes had 60% inhibitory activity as compared to normal MM homozygotes, those with homozygous ZZ genotypes had 10–15% activity, and MZ or SZ heterozygotes were intermediate between the respective homozygote activities. These reduced activities were because of decreased amounts of the mutant AAT protein in serum. As would be expected, those with SZ and ZZ genotypes have the earliest onset of emphysema and the highest frequencies of liver disease. The aggregate frequency of serious AAT deficiency, accounted for mostly by SZ and ZZ genotypes, is 1 in 2500 Caucasian births. A tragic feature of AAT deficiency is its exacerbation by cigarette smoking, providing a dramatic example of multifactorial disease.

The ready availability of antibodies to the AAT protein allowed cloning of the gene from cDNA libraries and revealed a relatively simple structure with 5 exons and 6 introns spanning 12.2 kb. Its expression is more complex with two upstream promoters and two sites for transcription initiation. One site is used in monocytes and macrophages to produce a longer mRNA than is produced in liver. The AAT gene is located within band 14q32 among a cluster of other serum protease inhibitors (also called *serpins*). It exhibits sequence homology to many of these serpin genes, particularly to those of antithrombin III (28%) and complement 1 inhibitor (27%). The S allele is a Glu264Val (E264V) substitution and the Z allele a Glu342Lys (G342K) substitution in the 394 amino acid protein. These mutant alleles are readily diagnosed using PCR and ASO hybridization as illustrated in Figure 8.10*B*.

As mentioned previously, the Z version of AAT protein has normal inhibitory activity but is present in serum at 15–20% of normal amounts. The amino acid substitution causes decreased secretion of the glycosylated protein from liver cells into the circulation. Accumulation of the unsecreted protein in the endoplasmic reticulum produces microscopic inclusions in liver cells and causes hepatitis and cirrhosis. The glutamic acid residue is located in a key "hinge" region of the protein molecule, and its replacement with lysine by the Z allele changes the conformation and causes aggregation. Although carbohydrate molecules and signal regions are important for protein secretion from cells, the spontaneous aggregation of Z or S variants interferes with AAT secretion (Table 8.2).

■**TABLE 8.2.** Examples of the Molecular Delineation of Genetic Disease

Disease	Cloning Strategy	Type of Gene	Insights
Hypercholesterolemia LDLR, HLC locus at 19p13	Functional—defined cellular phenotype	LDL receptor 45 kb, 18 exons 5.3 kb mRNA 822 amino acids Membrane protein	Gene is composite of functional domains; mutational domains correspond with cellular phenotypes
α-1-antitrypsin deficiency PI, AAT locus at 14q32	Functional—defined serum protein	α-1-antitrypsin 12 kb, 6 exons 1.4 kb mRNA 52 kD protein Serum protein	Novel disease mechanism (Z allele)—instability of protein leads to tissue storage
Osteogenesis imperfecta COL1A1 locus at 7q22, COL1A2 locus at 17q22	Functional—defined tissue protein	α_1, α_2 procollagens 18 kb, 41 exons 7.2, 5.9 kb mRNA 1041 aa protein Matrix protein	Novel disease mechanism—dominant negative (protein suicide)
Neurofibromatosis NF1 locus at 17q11	Positional—gene mapping and translocations	Neurofibromin 300 kb, >100 exons 13 kb mRNA 2818 amino acids Signal transducer	Genes within genes (three genes of opposite orientation in one intron)
MASA X-linked mental retardation L1CAM locus at Xq28	Positional—gene mapping and candidate gene	L1CAM 5.1 Kb, 28 exons 3.8 kb mRNA 1241 amino acids Cell surface protein	Uniting different phenotypes (hydrocephalus, MASA) in one locus
Cystic fibrosis CFTR locus at 7q31	Positional—gene mapping and frequent mutant allele	CFTR 250 kb, 26 exons 6.1 kb mRNA 1480 amino acids Membrane protein	Transport gene family, explanation abnormal sweat test

AAT deficiency contrasts with hypercholesterolemia as a defect in secretion rather than import and degradation. Its molecular pathogenesis also is straightforward with novelty at the level of altered protein conformation rather than diverse mutational mechanisms affecting multiple functional domains. Because of its simple structure and relatively small size, the AAT gene has been the subject of gene therapy studies by injection into lung or liver (see Chapter 9). Some rare mutations in the AAT protein may be useful for therapy, in that a valine for methionine substitution confers 20-fold greater activity against lung proteases. Another mutation substituting arginine for methionine had the unanticipated effect of causing bleeding due to a new inhibitory activity against the blood coagulation protein thrombin. The molecular pathogenesis of AAT deficiency thus illustrates the orchestration of protein function through genetic variation, and its unusual variants provide a glimpse of evolution in action.

Functional Cloning Using a Tissue Protein: Osteogenesis Imperfecta

When an abnormal protein product can be defined in a genetic disease, the protein can lead to the responsible gene. The example of sickle cell hemoglobin leading to characterization of the β-globin gene has been discussed in Chapter 6.

Osteogenesis imperfecta (166240) is a dramatic disease with multiple fractures, unusual skull shape, deafness, and blue sclera of the eyes. Children may sustain hundreds of fractures before puberty, and severe cases produce dwarfism, severe disabity, and death due to mul-

tiple rib and long bone deformities. Because type I collagen was expressed in the afflicted tissues of eye and bone, it became a candidate molecule to explain this autosomal dominant disease. Type I collagen is one of more than 15 types of collagen in humans, and consists of two

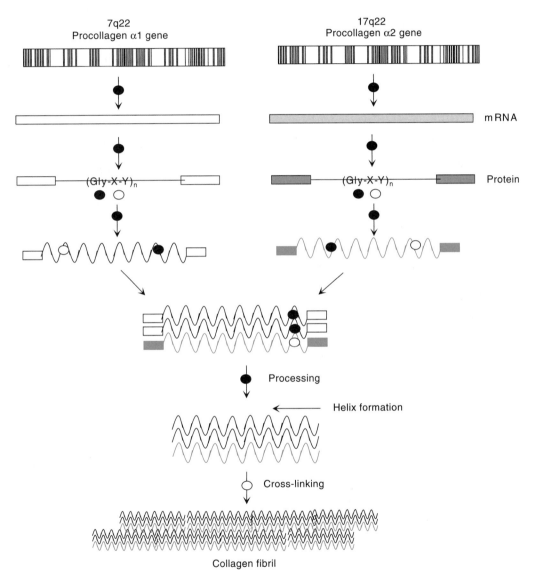

Figure 8.12. Molecular pathogenesis of osteogenesis imperfecta shown by steps in type I collagen synthesis. Severe mutations (filled circles) cause lethal osteogenesis imperfecta as illustrated in Fig. 8.12A, while milder mutations (empty circles) have phenotypes with fewer fractures and a normal lifespan. Severe mutations disrupt RNA splicing or translation, replace glycine with larger amino acids, occur at the carboxy terminus to disrupt triple helix formation, or occur in α1 chains that form 2 of the 3 chains in type I collagen.

polypeptide chains known as α_1 and α_2 (Fig. 8.12). By isolating type I collagen from cultured fibroblasts taken from patients with osteogenesis imperfecta, altered mobility of the polypeptide chains could be demonstrated. These changes suggested that the amino acid sequences of type I collagen polypeptides were different in certain patients with osteogenesis imperfecta, and pointed to type I collagen gene mutations as the cause of disease.

Gene fragments encoding the α_1 and α_2 polypeptides of type I collagen were cloned using antibodies to screen cDNA libraries constructed from human connective tissue. Contigs of the genes were assembled as diagrammed in Figure 8.4, and their organization and DNA sequence were determined. The genes for the α_1 and α_2 chains of type I procollagen are almost identical in containing 41–42 exons, each having a modular structure with units encoding 18 repeating glycine-X-Y amino acid units (54 bp). Glycine is required to allow triple helix formation, and the X and Y are variables standing for any amino acid. After transcription of a large pre-mRNA, the introns are spliced out to yield mRNA of two different sizes. The significance of this alternative

splicing is unknown. Following translation, two α_1 chains associate with one of the α_2 chains to form a triple helix (Fig. 8.12). The triple helix is further processed by removing N- and C-terminal amino acids, secretion into the extracellular space, and cross-linking between lysine residues. The mature, interlaced collagen fibers contribute a major portion of connective tissue strength.

The effects of DNA nucleotide changes on type I collagen, as with any protein-coding gene, depend on the nature of amino acid changes produced, their position within the protein chain, and their effects upon protein function or localization. Some of the mutations affecting type I collagen are diagrammed in Figure 8.12 and summarized in Table 8.3. Because the presence of a small amino acid (glycine) at the beginning of each gly-X-Y repeat in collagen is crucial, mutations replacing glycine are severe, while those substituting amino acids at the X and Y positions are milder. Position of the mutation within the collagen chain is also a factor, because helix formation among the α_1 and α_2 chains is initiated at the C-termini. Mutations affecting glycine residues near the C-terminus are even more se-

■**TABLE 8.3.** Diseases Associated with Collagen Genes

Collagen	Locus	Disease
Type I	COLA1 17q22	Osteogenesis imperfecta types I–IV (166200, 166210, 166220, 166230)
	COLA2 7q22	Ehlers-Danlos syndrome type VII (130060)
		Osteogenesis imperfecta types I–III
		Ehlers-Danlos syndrome type VII (130060)
Type II	COL2A1 12q13	Spondylepiphyseal dysplasia (183900)
		Stickler syndrome (108300)
		Kniest dysplasia (156550)
		Achondrogenesis II (200610)
Type III	COL3A1 2q31	Ehlers-Danlos syndrome, type IV (130050)
Type IV	COL4A3 2q36	Alport syndrome (203780)
	COL4A4 2q36	Alport syndrome (203780)
	COL4A5 Xq22	Alport syndrome (301050)
Type V	COL5A1 9q34	Ehlers-Danlos syndrome type I (130000)
Type VII	COL7A1 3p21	Dystrophic epidermolysis bullosa (226600)
Type X	COL10A1 6q21	Schmid metaphyseal dysplasia (156500)
Type XI	COL11A2 6p21	Stickler syndrome (108300)

vere than those near the N-terminus and cause early neonatal death due to osteogenesis imperfecta with multiple broken bones and chest instability.

Other genotype/phenotype correlations revealed by the molecular delineation of osteogenesis imperfecta include the ability of mutations in one procollagen chain (e.g., α_1) to interfere with function of the other chain (e.g., α_2) by infiltrating the triple helix. This mechanism has been called *protein suicide* and is a specific example of a category known as *dominant negative* mutations (Table 8.3). Molecular analysis also revealed that families with normal parents and affected sibs did not have an autosomal recessive form of osteogenesis imperfecta; the recurrence was due to germinal mosaicism in one parent. Although each mutant allele defined in osteogenesis imperfecta could be used for DNA diagnosis for the family of origin, different families with the disease invariably have different mutant alleles. DNA diagnosis through type I collagen gene analysis is thus not available as a general test for osteogenesis imperfecta due to this allelic heterogeneity. Initial diagnosis still requires the analysis of type I collagen proteins after skin biopsy and fibroblast culture. This example emphasizes that DNA diagnosis must be directed toward specific mutant alleles rather than performed as a general screen that is analogous to a karyotype.

It is also important to appreciate that the molecular characterization of osteogenesis imperfecta became a prototype for understanding other types of connective tissue diseases (Table 8.3). These disorders can be grouped as a connective tissue disease family resulting from a related group of molecules, united by their common molecular pathogenesis. Based on the abnormal tissues involved in each disease, the prevalent type of collagen was examined for abnormalities. Examples of this disease category now include multiple anomaly syndromes (e.g., Stickler syndrome with cleft palate, small jaw, and retinal detachments, 184850), extreme forms of stretchy skin and connective tissue known as the Ehlers-Danlos syndromes (e.g., 130050), and even a common form of degenerative arthritis (Table 8.3).

New types of mutations have also been discovered through study of connective tissue disorders. For example, a point mutation in one of the AG splice donor sites resulted in the deletion of several exons in the type I collagen chain. This exon-skipping mutation was unexpected because analogous mutations in other genes prevented RNA splicing and caused the retention of the intron sequence in mature mRNA. Additional examples of this novel exon-skipping mutation have now been defined in Marfan syndrome (154700) and gyrate atrophy (258870). The molecular analysis of osteogenesis imperfecta has thus clarified clinical classification, defined pathogenesis, and elucidated new mechanisms of mutation.

Positional Cloning Using Chromosome Translocations: Neurofibromatosis

Neurofibromatosis type 1 (NF-1, 162200) is characterized by brown café-au-lait spots on the skin, brown Lische spots in the iris, overgrowths of the neural schwann cells to form neurofibromas, various bony anomalies, and mild mental deficiency in some patients. The disease is relatively common with an incidence of 1 in 3000 births, and the presence of mild symptoms in 85% of patients provided large families for linkage analysis. Genetic linkage to chromosome 17 was refined by the discovery of patients with reciprocal translocations at band 17q11. This breakpoint was common to both patients and became the focus of positional cloning experiments. A contig of cloned DNA segments was therefore assembled from a chromosome 17-specific genomic DNA library. DNA from specific human chromosomes is purified from mouse-human cell hybrids that retain only one human chromosome, from similar hybrids that retain specific fragments of a human chromosome after irradiation, or from actual pieces of chromosome that are cut out from microscope slides.

The contig of cloned DNA segments spanned several Mb along chromosome 17,

■TABLE 8.4. The Identification of Disease Genes by Positional Cloning

Disease	Gene and Mechanism
Duchenne muscular dystrophy	Dystrophin—contractile protein
Cystic fibrosis	Cystic fibrosis transmembrane regulator—transport protein
Wilms tumor	WT-1—developmental protein
Neurofibromatosis-1	Neurofibromin—GTPase activator
Fragile X syndrome	FMR-1—brain protein
Kallman syndrome	KALIG-1—developmental protein
Aniridia	PAX3
X-linked adrenoleukodystrophy	Peroxisomal membrane protein
Huntington disease	Huntingtin—brain protein
Achondroplasia	FGFR3—growth factor
Ataxia-telangiectasia	ATX—DNA repair protein

and there were many candidate genes in the region. Candidate DNA regions could then be tested to see whether they were transected by the chromosome translocation. The chromosome breakpoints occurred within a large, 300-kb region within chromosome band 17q11. The gene for NF-1 was found to encompass this entire region, and a surprise finding was the presence of three other genes within one of its many introns. These genes are of unknown function, and they are transcribed in a direction opposite to the surrounding NF-1 gene. The gene has been named neurofibromin, and its open reading frame predicts a protein of 2818 amino acids. The protein has one domain with similarity to proteins that activate GTP-cleaving enzymes that are important in signal transduction. These GTPase-activating (GAP) proteins are implicated in the regulation of an important cellular oncogene called *p21-ras*. It is also known that neurofibromin associates with microtubules, another indication that it has a role in cell signaling. Although the ras connection may explain the neurofibromas and higher rates of certain cancers that occur in NF-1, other aspects of pathogenesis remain obscure. The large size of the gene, the heterogeneity of mutant alleles so far characterized, and the complexity of its genomic organization limit its usefulness for genotype/phenotype correlation and DNA diagnosis. Diagnosis of NF-1 thus remains clinical, but its molecular characterization has revealed an important ex-

ample of "genes within genes" and should yield insights into pathogenesis and therapy in the future (Table 8.4).

Positional Cloning Using Genetic Linkage: Nonspecific X-Linked Mental Retardation and the MASA Syndrome

As the site of an anciently recognized genetic disease (hemophilia mentioned in the Talmud) and the first example of genetic linkage (color blindness), the X chromosome provides an excellent example for the appreciation of molecular genetic analysis. Explaining the male excess for severe mental retardation are over 80 X-linked disorders that impair mental function. Many of these have dramatic morphologic or metabolic phenotypes with distinctive appearance or congenital anomalies, but the 40 or more with subtle findings ("nonspecific" X-linked mental retardation—XLMR) emphasize the power of genetic linkage analysis. When sufficient families are available, linkage analysis using DNA polymorphisms spanning the X chromosome have demonstrated at least 20 distinct types of XLMR through their distinctive chromosomal locations (Fig. 8.13). An example of this approach was provided in Figure 8.8 showing the linkage analysis of Case 8. Mapping of the MASA syndrome locus to band Xq28 provided a strategy for positional cloning.

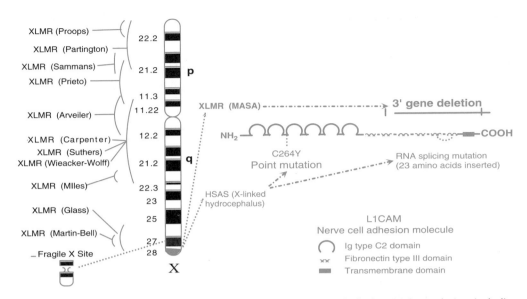

Figure 8.13. Map of the X chromosome showing various loci for X-linked mental retardation, including that for MASA syndrome at Xq28. Screening for candidate genes in the Xq28 region revealed the L1CAM locus, with its immunoglobulin (Ig)-like, fibronectin, and transmembrane domains. X-linked hydrocephalus and MASA syndrome, previously thought to represent separate genetic disorders, are due to mutations in different domains of the L1CAM gene.

Case 8 Follow-up: A contig was assembled in the Xq28 region implicated by linkage analysis and candidate genes were evaluated for a possible relation to the mental disability in MASA syndrome. A candidate L1 cell adhesion (L1CAM) gene was considered, identified based on its homology to a gene in mouse that was expressed in brain. The L1CAM gene was analyzed in several families with MASA syndrome, and a deletion was found in the distal portion of its coding region in the family described in case 8 (Fig. 8.13). This unusual deletion provided strong evidence for a causative role in MASA syndrome, and other L1CAM mutations were soon noted in other families. The L1CAM gene, like that for the LDL receptor, is a composite of different domains, each with unique homology and function. Of particular interest was the finding that a severe form of X-linked hydrocephalus (307000), also linked to the Xq28 region, resulted in mutations in a different domain of the L1CAM molecule. As a result of this work, diseases with separate McKusick numbers (307000 for X-linked hydrocephalus and

303350 for MASA syndrome) have been unified as McKusick number 307000.

Molecular analysis of MASA syndrome has allowed distinction between *syndrome variability* and *genetic heterogeneity,* two types of phenotypic variation in clinical genetics. Linkage analysis refined clinical delineation by distinguishing MASA syndrome from other X-linked mental retardation disorders with spasticity, and mutational analysis substantiated clinical suspicion that MASA and X-linked hydrocephalus could result from mutations at the same genetic locus. Study of the developmental expression and cerebral distribution of the *L1CAM* molecule should now give insights into the hydrocephalus and spasticity associated with these mutant alleles.

Positional Cloning Using Genetic Linkage and a Common Mutant Allele: Cystic Fibrosis

Cystic fibrosis (219700) is an autosomal recessive disease that produces pulmonary and gastrointestinal symptoms. It was first diagnosed based on excess sodium and chloride concentration in sweat. The high incidence of the disease in Caucasians (1 in 1600) provided abundant families for linkage analysis, and the gene causing cystic fibrosis was localized to chromosome band 7q31. The lack of translocations or deletions in patients with cystic fibrosis necessitated an exhaustive approach toward positional cloning of the gene. A large contig from the chromosome 7q31 region was isolated, then characterized to identify candidate genes. An initial candidate with homology to the Wnt-1 group of developmental proteins (see Chapter 9) stimulated a flurry of excitement, but screening of patient DNA for mutations was not revealing. The successful candidate gene attracted interest because it contained the DNA signature of transmembrane regions (repeating units that could encode hydrophobic amino acids suitable for the interior of a lipid membrane). As might be predicted for a disease with altered sodium concentration in sweat, the candidate molecule showed homology to a family of membrane transport proteins called the ABC transporters (A stands for ATP, which provides the energy needed for transport).

The crucial piece of evidence that identified the cystic fibrosis transmembrane regulator (CFTR) as the molecule defective in cystic fibrosis was an unexpected type of mutation. A 3-bp deletion was found in the CFTR gene of numerous patients with cystic fibrosis but not in their normal relatives. The deletion neatly excised the codon for phenylalanine (F), and was dubbed ΔF508 as befitted its position in the 1480 amino acid CFTR protein. The CFTR gene is very large, spanning 250 kb of DNA with 26 exons. The case for the ΔF508 deletion being a disease-causing mutation rather than an unusual polymorphism was strengthened by its presence in the binding site for ATP. More than 20 other mutant alleles have been characterized, and DNA diagnosis is routinely performed for cystic fibrosis using direct analysis for the ΔF508 deletion. Point mutations can be recognized by PCR and ASO tests analogous to those in Figure 8.10. The sensitivity of cystic fibrosis DNA testing varies for different ethnic groups, and particular allele frequencies determine the feasibility of population screening as discussed in Chapters 4 and 12.

The isolation of the CFTR gene by positional cloning, despite primitive knowledge about its possible mode of action, was a dramatic success that paved the way for similar successes with other disease-causing genes (Table 8.4). Many genetic diseases can now be matched with their causative genes, allowing new pathways of molecular pathogenesis to be defined. Table 8.4 llustrates how the same steps in DNA technology can clarify the pathogenesis of diseases as diverse as Duchenne muscular dystrophy and hemochromatosis.

■ 8.8. THE HUMAN GENOME PROJECT

The ability to map and isolate genes led to the concept of characterizing an entire genome using recombinant DNA technology. Although considerable progress has been made by targeting individual genes, as shown in Table 8.4, this bottom-up strategy lacks economies of perspective and scale that might be attained through an organized project to characterize the entire genome. The human genome project was therefore conceived as a top-down strategy that would strive to isolate and sequence every DNA segment in the genome, then to explore individual genes. Systematic identification of every gene in the genome would be accomplished by noting their DNA signatures of upstream regulatory sequences, open reading frames, and so forth. Once a map of all human genes is available, appropriate candidates should be easily evaluated for causative mutations when a suspect DNA region is implicated in disease. It is hoped that an organized human genome project will greatly expand the human gene map by providing a complete catalogue of mapped anonymous genes that can be matched up with their respective genetic phenotypes or predispositions.

The whole-scale assault on the human genome involves some unique considerations that are different from those relevant to the cloning of individual genes listed in Table 8.4. These considerations have been tested in smaller genome projects concerning organisms of biological interest. Genomes of the bacteria *Hemophilus influenza* (genome size 1.8 Mb) and *E. coli* (genome size of 4.6 Mb) have been completely sequenced, and their entire set of genes are now available for analysis and experimentation. Genome projects are underway for yeast (genome size 14 Mb), the nematode *Caenorhabditis elegans* (genome size 100 Mb), and the classic model organism *Drosophila melanogaster* (genome size 165 Mb). Random cloning of DNA segments is a key strategy in all of these projects, placing emphasis on the sequencing and ordering of these randomly cloned DNAs. Vectors that incorporate large fragments of DNA, such as yeast artificial chromosomes, greatly facilitate the attainment of what is essentially a contig of the entire genome. The ability to minimize duplicate studies on the same DNA fragment and the rapidity and economy of DNA sequencing become key issues for characterizing the 3000 Mb genomes found in humans, mice, and rats.

The human genome project was initiated in 1990 with a goal of obtaining an entire genome sequence by 2005. The project has spawned a special institute at the National Institutes of Health and genome centers at several universities in the United States. Genome centers have also arisen in other countries, including those at several large industries. Controversy has surrounded industrial involvement because of patent rights to characterized DNA segments that have commercial applications. The strategies of these diverse genome centers differ somewhat, but mainly involve random cloning (*shotgun cloning*) as utilized in the projects for model organisms. Although random strategies are most efficient in the long run, they involve a delayed payoff because a complete repository of important genes will not be provided until the project is almost complete. For this reason, several centers have modified the ran-

dom approach by targeting DNA segments that are known to produce RNA in one or more human tissues. Commercial laboratories in particular have been interested in expression libraries of cloned DNA segments and have assembled maps *of expressed sequence tags* (ESTs). ESTs are DNA polymorphisms that reside within DNA segments that are transcribed into RNA. Expressed DNA segments can be isolated from cDNA libraries or identified in randomly cloned DNA libraries through hybridization with RNA. The focus on expressed sequences, combined with random DNA cloning, should provide the interim dividend of clinically important genes before the complete human sequence is assembled. One commercial company plans to sequence 99% of the human genome, including all expressed regions, for $300 million over five years. This amount would represent a fraction of the $3 billion price tag estimated for the government-sponsored human genome project.

■ 8.9. ETHICAL ISSUES IN MOLECULAR GENETICS

Recombinant DNA technology has numerous clinical and commercial applications that pose new ethical concerns. Although human DNA segments can be viewed as a natural resource, their source and characterization through cloning experiments bring up issues of ownership. DNA diagnosis is rapidly expanding the scope of genetic testing, providing a uniform technology for recognizing mutant alleles. These concerns have sparked debates and conferences and resulted in ethical guidelines published by governmental and professional organizations.

Ownership of Materials

In the course of research studies, DNA may be collected from individuals with the purpose of diagnostic test development or the isolation of new genes. In a few instances, individuals whose cells or genetic material have become valuable reagents have requested recompense for their contribution. Of more general concern is the confidentiality of the patient's cell or DNA sample once it is banked for possible future study. As emphasized by Annas (1993), these samples are like future diaries that contain information about a person's family and their predisposition for certain diseases. The ethical principles of patient autonomy and nonmalificence dictate that thorough counseling and consent accompany any collection of blood samples for the purpose of cell and/or DNA banking. It is widely accepted that consent forms should include specific provisos that a patient's sample will not be tested without consent, and that any information from testing remains confidential as part of the medical record.

Less clear are the implications of patenting DNA samples or the patenting of human genes and repositories derived from DNA samples. Some companies have tried to patent gene constructs used to manufacture rare proteins or DNA libraries that can be used for gene isolation. Some religious thinkers have argued strongly against the patenting of materials used for genetic engineering, stating that humans and animals are creations of God, not humans (Cole-Turner, 1995). The potential medical uses of recombinant DNA technology ensure that patenting of genetically engineered products will be an active area of debate.

Genetic Discrimination

The ability to diagnose diseases with specific liabilities for employment or health insurance poses significant concerns about discrimination against individuals with these diseases. In some cases, knowledge about predisposition could provoke beneficial changes in a worker's environment—that is, emphasis on prohibitions against cigarette smoking for workers with α-1-antitrypsin deficiency. Conversely, transfers away from more lucrative positions (e.g., dye workers with glucose-6-phosphate dehydrogenase deficiency) could result in conflicts between autonomy and benefi-

cence. For company-funded health plans, workers with certain genetic diseases can become significant economic burdens. Court decisions have affirmed the rights of one employer to limit health benefits for employees with AIDS (Holtzman and Rothstein, 1992).

As genetic testing has become more widespread, several organizations have argued that prior legislation protecting individuals with disabilities can be utilized for patients with genetic disease. The Rehabilitation Act of 1973, which prohibited discrimination against individuals with disabilities at federally funded workplaces, and the Americans with Disabilities Act of 1990, which extended this law to all workplaces with more than 15 employees, provide sufficient legal precedent to fight genetic discrimination. The potential for discrimination again emphasizes the need for counseling to ensure informed consent and the maintenance of strict confidentiality for genetic samples and genetic tests.

Eugenics and Reductionism

As discussed in Chapter 1, a principal fallacy of the eugenics movement early in this century was the assumption that complex traits could be attributed to single hereditary factors or genes. Even worse was the corollary that hereditary factors were simply transmitted, meaning that all descendants of the unfortunate individual would be similarly affected. Although multifactorial determination of complex traits and the complexities of inheritance ratios have eliminated these simplistic fallacies from intelligent discourse, a tendency to define people by their diagnosis or to define a disease in terms of an abnormal gene can still occur. Despite the predictive power of DNA diagnosis, it is still important to keep in mind the many other characteristics of an individual outside of his disease and to acknowledge the many modifiers of gene expression. Fundamental to the ethical principal of patient autonomy is respectful treatment with "people-first" language and the avoidance of pejorative terms for disease. Also important is the avoidance of discriminatory or fatalistic attitudes toward individuals recognized by DNA diagnosis to have predisposition for disease, but who do not yet have symptoms. See Chapters 14 and 16 for additional discussion of ethical issues regarding presymptomatic diagnosis.

Case 8 Follow-up: The discovery that both X-linked hydrocephalus and Gareis-Mason or MASA syndrome were due to alternative expression at the L1CAM genetic locus provided an exciting avenue for research. Unfortunately, the name CRASH syndrome was then proposed for these disorders, representing an acronym for Clasped thumb, Retardation, Absent corpus callosum, Spasticity, and Hydrocephalus. While this term does indicate the overlap between MASA syndrome and X-linked hydrocephalus, its negative connotation for parents and affected individuals makes it use undesirable in clinical settings. This example illustrates how the benefits of research findings can be diminished if they are isolated from clinical perspective.

PROBLEM SET 8:
Molecular Genetics

Pick the single best answer to the following questions:

8.1. Which characteristic best refers to single nucleotide substitutions in human DNA?

(A) They are rarely seen in introns.

(B) They usually result in disease.

(C) They may create a restriction fragment length polymorphism (RFLP).

(D) They may create a VNTR allele.

(E) They may delete a codon.

Questions 8.2–8.4. A family with autosomal dominant retinitis pigmentosa and blindness requests counseling for their current pregnancy. DNA studies have been performed as shown in Figure 8.14A, and they wish to know the risk for their fetus to develop retinitis pigmentosa.

8.2. The bands below the pedigree in Figure 8.14 refer to:

(A) Restriction enzymes of different electrophoretic mobility

(B) DNA restriction fragments from a locus that may be linked to that for retinitis pigmentosa

(C) PCR-amplified DNA fragments from the abnormal allele for retinitis pigmentosa

(D) Allele-specific oligonucleotides (ASO) that hybridize to normal or mutant alleles at the retinitis pigmentosa locus

(E) Single strand conformational polymorphisms (SSCP) that reveal variation at the retinitis pigmentosa locus

8.3. If the bands below the pedigree in Figure 8.14A represent DNA segments from an RFLP locus, then use of this DNA marker for diagnosis of future retinitis pigmentosa in the fetus must be validated by:

(A) DNA analysis of many unrelated individuals with retinitis pigmentosa

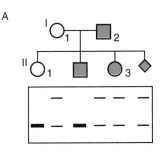

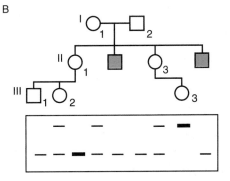

Figure 8.14.

(B) DNA analysis of individuals with retinitis pigmentosa from many ethnic groups

(C) DNA analysis of several families with unknown types of retinitis pigmentosa

(D) DNA analysis of several families with autosomal dominant retinitis pigmentosa

(E) DNA analysis of twin pairs with late-onset retinitis.

8.4. If the bands beneath the pedigree represent DNA alleles from a locus within 0.1 cM of the locus for autosomal dominant retinitis pigmentosa, what is the risk that the fetus will be affected?

(A) 100%

(B) 99%

(C) 50%

(D) 1%

(E) virtually 0%

Questions 8.5–8.8. A family requests prenatal diagnosis for an X-linked recessive form of retinitis pigmentosa with onset in adulthood (pedigree in Fig. 8.14*B*). Individuals in generation III are all less than 15 years old. DNA analysis is performed with marker DSX255, known from prior linkage analysis to be within 1 cM of the retinitis pigmentosa locus on the X chromosome (Fig. 8.14*B*).

8.5. What is the risk that individual II-1 is a carrier?

(A) 100%

(B) 99%

(C) 50%

(D) 1%

(E) Unable to determine from the data

8.6. What is the risk that individual III-1 will develop retinitis pigmentosa?

(A) 98–100%

(B) 50%

(C) 25%

(D) 1–2%

(E) Unable to determine from data

8.7. What is the chance that individual III-2 is a carrier?

(A) 98–100%

(B) 50%

(C) 25%

(D) 1–2%

(E) Unable to determine from data

8.8. What is the risk that individual III-3 is a carrier?

(A) 98–100%

(B) 50%

(C) 25%

(D) 1–2%

(E) Unable to determine from data

8.9. Which of the following statements regarding genetic linkage analysis are not true?

(A) The probability of linkage can be expressed as a LOD score that is the logarithm of a ratio.

(B) The higher the LOD score, the more likely that there is linkage.

(C) The recombination fractions between multiple loci can be used to order the loci on chromosomal DNA.

(D) The larger the number of informative meioses, the higher the potential LOD score.

(E) A recombination fraction of 50% is common when there is strong evidence for linkage.

8.10. Which of the following methods could not be used to detect the point mutation in the β-globin gene that causes sickle cell anemia?

(A) Polymerase chain reaction with allele-specific oligonucleotide hybridization

(B) Southern blot analysis

(C) DNA sequencing

(D) Polymerase chain reaction with restriction enzyme digestion

(E) Northern blot analysis

PROBLEM SET 8
Answers

		8.4. C
8.10. E	**8.7.** B	**8.3.** D
8.9. E	**8.6.** B	**8.2.** B
8.8. D	**8.5.** B	**8.1.** C

PROBLEM SET 8
Solutions

8.1. DNA polymorphisms, including single nucleotide substitutions, occur every 200–500 nucleotides in human DNA. The single base change may create a new restriction site and thus a new RFLP (restriction fragment length polymorphism, answer C), but it will not create an additional repeat that comprises a VNTR (variable number of tandem repeats). Point mutations do not delete entire codons and cause disease only if they occur within exons and alter function of the expressed RNA and protein.

8.2–8.4. The bands beneath the pedigree in Figure 8.14A are arranged beneath the pedigree symbols as would be appropriate for electrophoresis of samples from each individual. Restriction endonucleases are enzymes that cleave DNA at specific nucleotide sequences; it is the cleaved DNA segments rather than the enzymes that are subjected to electrophoresis (answer B). ASO provides direct detection of mutant and normal alleles, while SSCP is a screening technique for DNA variation. The bands could represent PCR-amplified DNA fragments, but they would be identical if they originated from the same abnormal allele. Use of a DNA polymorphism (DNA marker) for prenatal testing requires the demonstration of genetic linkage between marker and disease loci. Linkage analysis must evaluate segregation of the markers in families with the same type of disease (answer D), requiring cosegregation in 10–15 meioses before a LOD score above 3 is obtained that is significant for linkage. Analysis of unrelated normal and affected individuals with retinitis pigmentosa might demonstrate association between one of the marker alleles and the disease allele. Analysis of identical twins alone might be useful for demonstrating allele association but not for the establishment of genetic linkage (they will have identical alleles). The RFLP pattern in individual II-2 indicates that the smaller (lower) RFLP allele in the father is segregating with the allele for autosomal dominant retinitis pigmentosa. It is not clear whether the smaller allele in the fetus was inherited from mother or father, making the risk for being affected 50% (answer C—same as before the analysis). In any case, a distance of 0.1 cM corresponds to a recombination frequency of 0.1% rather than 1%, so answers B and D would not be correct.

8.5–8.8. The smaller (lower) RFLP allele in I-1 is in phase with the abnormal allele for re-

tinitis pigmentosa, as shown by the single allele in her two affected sons. Individual II-1 received the smaller allele from her father and the smaller allele from her mother, meaning that she has a 100%—the chance for recombination = 99% chance of being a carrier (answer 8.5B). Individual III-1 is too young to manifest the disease, so his status must be determined by DNA analysis. It is not possible to decide which smaller allele he has inherited from his carrier mother, so his risk is 50% to be affected (answer 8.6B). Similarly, individual III-2 has a 50% risk to be a carrier since it cannot be determined which smaller allele she received from her mother (answer 8.7B). Individual II-3 did not receive the smaller allele from her mother and is thus not a carrier within the limits of recombination. Therefore, individual III-3 cannot be a carrier (answer 8.8D).

8.9. A logarithm of the odds of linkage (LOD) score (Z) assesses the transmission of alleles in one or more families and is a ratio: the odds that the segregation pattern reflects linkage over the odds that it occurred by chance. The higher this ratio, the better the odds for linkage, with LOD scores greater than 3 (1000 to 1 for linkage) considered significant. The fraction of recombinations observed in the families (Θ) reflects the genetic distance between loci in centimorgans (cM, 1% recombination = 1 cM). For multipoint linkage analysis, the recombination fractions can be used to order the loci along the chromosome. A recombination fraction of 50% reflects random assortment and not genetic linkage (answer E).

8.10. The answer is E. A point mutation is a change in one nucleotide. Point mutations that alter RNA synthesis or alter the protein product of a gene can cause disease. The point mutation responsible for sickle cell anemia could be detected by Southern blot analysis if it altered a restriction site or was associated with an altered restriction site pattern (as with the HpaI polymorphisms shown in Figure 8.7A). DNA sequencing or hybridization with allele-specific oligonucleotides would provide direct detection of the altered nucleotide. Northern blot analysis is analogous to Southern blot analysis but detects RNA products rather than DNA fragments. Since the point mutation causing sickle cell anemia does not alter the size of β-globin mRNA, northern analysis would not be useful in detecting the mutation (answer E).

BIBLIOGRAPHY

General Texts and References

Guyer MS, Collins FS. 1993. The human genome project and the future of medicine. *Am J Dis Child* 147:1145–1152.

Guyer RL, Koshland DE Jr. 1989. The molecule of the year (PCR). *Science* 246:1543–1546.

Lander ES. 1996. The new genomics: global views of biology. *Science* 274:536–538.

Schuler GD et al. 1996. A gene map of the human genome. *Science* 274:540–545.

Strachan T, Read AP. 1996. *Human Molecular Genetics.* New York: Wiley-Liss.

Specific References

Adams MD et al. 1991. Complementary DNA sequencing: expressed sequence tags and the human genome project. *Science* 252:1651–1656.

Annas GJ. 1993. Privacy rules for DNA databanks. *JAMA* 270:2346–2350.

Botstein D, White RL, Skolnick M, and Davis RW. 1980. Construction of a genetic linkage map in man using restriction fragment length polymorphisms. *Am J Hum Genet* 32:314–331.

Byers PH. 1995. Disorders of collagen biosynthesis and structure. In Scriver CR, Beaudet AL, Sly WS, Valle D, eds. *The Metabolic and Molecular Bases of Inherited Disease,* 7th ed. New York: McGraw-Hill, pp. 4029–4077.

Cole-Turner R. 1993. Religion and gene patenting. *Science* 270:52.

Cox DW. 1995. α1-antitrypsin deficiency. In Scriver CR, Beaudet AL, Sly WS, Valle D, eds. *The Metabolic and Molecular Bases of Inherited Disease,* 7th ed. New York: McGraw-Hill, pp. 4125–4158.

Friend SH, Oliff A. 1998. Emerging uses for genomic information in drug discovery. *N Eng J Med* 338:125–126.

Goldstein JL, Hobbs HH, Brown MS. 1995. Familial hypercholesterolemia. In Scriver CR, Beaudet AL, Sly WS, Valle D, eds. *The Metabolic and Molecular Bases of Inherited Disease,* 7th ed. New York: McGraw-Hill, pp. 1981–2030.

Gutmann DH, Collins FS. 1995. von Recklinghausen neurofibromatosis. In Scriver CR, Beaudet AL, Sly WS, Valle D, eds. *The Metabolic and Molecular Bases of Inherited Disease,* 7th ed. New York: McGraw-Hill, pp. 677–696.

Holtzman NA, Rothstein MA. 1992. Eugenics and Genetic Discrimination. *Am J Hum Genet* 50:457–459.

Jacenko O, Olsen BR, Warman ML. 1994. Of mice and men: Heritable skeletal disorders. *Am J Hum Genet* 54:163–168.

Kan YW. 1992. Development of DNA analysis for human diseases: sickle cell anemia and thalassemia as a paradigm. *JAMA:*1532–1536.

Macias VR, Day DW, King TE, Wilson GN. 1992. *Am J Med Genet* 43:408–14 (figure on p. 411)

Rommens JM et al. 1989. Identification of the cystic fibrosis gene: chromosome walking and jumping. *Science* 245:1059–1065.

Wulfsberg EA, Hoffmann DE, Cohen MM. 1994. α-1-antitrypsin deficiency: Impact of discovery on medicine and society. *JAMA* 271:217–220.

9

GENETICS AT THE CELLULAR LEVEL: DEVELOPMENTAL, CANCER, AND IMMUNOGENETICS

■ LEARNING OBJECTIVES

1. Cell interactions are involved in embryonic development, in cell growth regulation that is deranged to produce cancer, and in the immune response. Cell interactions involve extracellular matrix and surface molecules that comprise signal transduction pathways.

2. Developmental processes include those of cell growth, cell differentiation, and pattern formation.

3. Insights into developmental processes have been provided by genetic analysis, including mechanisms for early pattern formation in the model organisms *D. melanogaster* and *C. elegans.*

4. Genes important for early development in simpler organisms often have homologues in complex organisms like mouse and man; these genes become candidates for human developmental genetic disorders.

5. The ability to delete or "knock out" genes in model organisms provides a powerful tool for studying genes involved in development and neoplasia. Transgenic and natural mouse mutations have been particularly useful.

6. Human development involves essential stages of blastogenesis and gastrulation to form an oriented embryo with three germ layers. Specific genes involved in these processes have now been defined through their roles in human disease.

7. A relatively small set of proto-oncogenes and tumor suppressor genes are now recognized as causes for most human cancers. These genes are altered in inherited and sporadic cancers, providing laboratory tests for cancer susceptibility and cancer progression.

8. Genes that have early roles in developmental anomalies often have later roles in the transformation of somatic cells into malignancies.

9. Genetic immune deficiencies illustrate major components of the immune response.

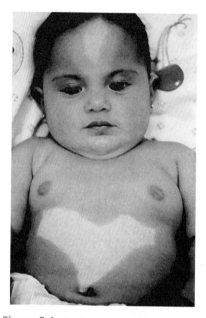

Figure 9.1. Patient described in Case 9.

Case 9: ***Mother and Child with a***
White Forelock

A newborn female is referred for evaluation because of the depigmented regions pictured in Figure 9.1. Her mother also has a central white patch on her chest and a white forelock of hair. There are two normal siblings and the remainder of the family history is not revealing. Physical examination discloses no abnormalities aside from the pigmentary changes. The skin lesions are typical of a disorder called piebald trait (172800), implying autosomal dominant inheritance and a 50% recurrence risk. The parents were interested in why the depigmented spots occurred on the front of the body and whether their child would be at risk for other medical problems.

■ 9.1. INTRODUCTION

As various tissues and organs arise from a fertilized egg during development, a network of cellular relationships is established that is a key component of normal homeostasis and function. Cellular interactions include growth, differentiation, adhesion, migration, and com-

munications that are mediated by cascades of proteins and small molecules. Genetic mutations can derange these interactions, producing altered embryonic development, altered somatic cell growth or differentiation (cancer), and altered cell lineages exemplified by defective immune function. Although the study of these inherited defects may be denoted, respectively, as developmental genetics, cancer genetics, or immunogenetics, they each involve abnormalities of cell networks produced by alterations in growth-regulating and/or signaling molecules. Recent progress of vital importance to clinical genetics has involved the use of model organisms and cell culture techniques to clarify the genetic basis of developmental and neoplastic diseases.

■ 9.2. REGULATION OF CELL GROWTH, DIFFERENTIATION, AND COMMUNICATION

Cell Growth and Death

The cell cycle involves a stereotypic sequence of events that results in the doubling of cell structures (chromosomes and cytoplasm) followed by mitotic division. A search for factors controlling the cell cycle was initiated using a powerful technique for genetic research called *somatic cell hybridization.* Chemical reagents or viruses are used to join the membranes between two cell types, producing *heterokaryons* with two nuclei and shared cytoplasm. The tetraploid cells, with two sets of diploid chromosomes, allow experiments that examine the ability of alleles in one nucleus to modify expression of alleles in the other nucleus (*genetic complementation analysis).* If mutant alleles in one nucleus cannot restore function of mutant alleles in the other nucleus, then it can be assumed that the respective mutations are at the same genetic locus. If mutant alleles in one nucleus do restore function (i.e., gene product expression) in the presence of mutant alleles in the other nucleus, then they complement alleles in the other nucleus, showing that the mutations affect different genetic loci. Modern technology now allows direct complementation analysis through adding mutant alleles to cells in the form of DNA, either by direct uptake (*DNA transformation*) or conveyed into the cell in a recombinant virus that integrates with the cellular genome (*DNA transfection*).

Genetic analysis of cell cycle regulation was performed by fusing cells in one cell cycle phase with those in another. When cells in M (mitotic) phase were fused with cells in G1 (early interphase), substances in the M cell would accelerate mitosis in the heterokaryons. These experiments led to the characterization of *cyclins* that wax and wane during particular phases of the cell cycle. Cyclins in turn stimulate cyclin-dependent protein kinases (CDKs) that regulate these cell cycle phases (Table 9.1). Particular cyclins and their targeted protein kinases are now associated with particular steps in the S (DNA replication) and M (mitotic) phases. These cyclin signals initiate processes such as DNA replication, chromosome condensation, and so forth, and are balanced by inhibiting proteins that ensure the coordination and fidelity of cell cycle events. For example, cell division is arrested if sufficient damage to DNA or chromosomes has occurred. These inhibitory proteins led to the concept of *cell cycle checkpoints* where division and proliferation can be delayed, arrested, or even diverted to a specific program of cell death known as *apoptosis*.

The cell cycle can also be regulated by factors external to the cell as listed in Table 9.1. Many are proteins that stimulate or suppress growth. Sometimes the same protein acts as a stimulant to one cell type and a suppressor for other cell types (e.g., transforming growth factor-β listed in Table 9.1). Many of these factors act by a general mechanism called *signal transduction*. The growth factor binds to a cell surface receptor, followed by transduction of its signal to coordinate changes in gene expression or protein activity. As would be expected, genetic alterations of growth or signal transduction pathways may disrupt cellular interactions and lead to developmental abnormalities or cancer.

■ **TABLE 9.1.** Proteins Acting on the Cell Cycle

Protein	Activity
Internal to cell	
M-phase cyclin	Activates CDK1[a]
CDK1	Induces M phase
S-phase cyclin	Activates CDK2
CDK2	Activates S phase
ATM[b]	Blocks S phase if DNA damage
Ubiquitin-coupled proteases	Inactivates cyclins
Interleukin-1β converting enzyme (ICE)	Initiates apoptosis
BCL2 gene	Inhibits apoptosis
Caspases	Apoptosis cascade
External to cell	
Platelet-derived growth factor	Stimulates fibroblast cell growth
Transforming growth factor-β	Stimulates fibroblast, inhibits epithelial cell growth
Insulin-like growth factor I	Stimulates fat cell growth
Insulin-like growth factor II	Stimulates fat cell growth
Nerve growth factor	Stimulates neural cell growth
Interleukin-2 (IL-2)	Stimulates T-lymphocyte growth

Source: Nasmyth (1996); Barinaga (1998).

[a]Cyclin-dependent kinases.

[b]Ataxia-teleangiectasia mutated.

Cell Communication: Growth Factors, Hormones, and Signal Transduction

Cell growth and death is modulated by signals from distant or neighboring cells. Signal molecules may be secreted into the extracellular matrix or bloodstream, extruded onto the cell surface, or transported through gap junctions that unite groups of cells into a single functional unit. Endocrine signals (hormones) travel through the bloodstream to influence diverse and distant cell populations, while paracrine signals (certain growth factors, matrix molecules) exert transient influences at distances of 1 mm or less. Specialized types of signaling occur across the synapses of nerve cells and among the syncytial cells of heart or skeletal muscle.

Cell signals often act by binding to specific molecules called *receptors* (Fig. 9.2). Signals like steroid hormones that are fat soluble (hydrophobic) can cross cell membranes and bind to intracellular receptors, while those that are water soluble (hydrophilic) act by binding to receptors on the cell surface. Often, binding of a signaling molecule to its receptor changes the shape of the receptor protein and initiates a cellular response. The signal molecule (e.g.,

a steroid hormone) often elicits changes in different types of molecules (e.g., altered amounts of nuclear proteins that control transcription (transcription factors). Coupled with this signal transduction are various mechanisms that amplify the cellular response so that small concentrations of hormones or ligands can produce dramatic changes in cell shape and function.

There are four major mechanisms by which cell receptors act to produce a cellular response. Activated steroid hormone receptors often travel from the cytosol to the nucleus, where they bind directly to enhancer DNA sequences and activate transcription. Cell surface receptors are involved in the other three

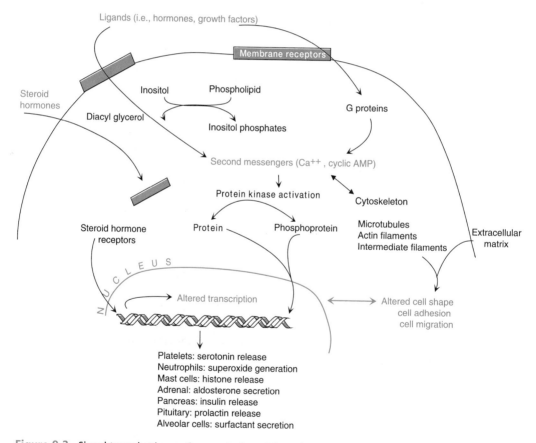

Figure 9.2. Signal transduction pathways. Action of ligands at cell surface receptors, of hormones from distant tissues, and of "second messengers" such as cyclic AMP are shown. Signal transduction often involves the covalent modification of proteins (e.g., phosphorylation by protein kinases) and/or nuclear trafficking to alter gene expression.

mechanisms. They include channel-linked receptors that enhance ion transport through channels in the cell membrane, catalytic receptors that extend across the cell membrane and act as kinases to activate intracellular proteins, and G-protein-linked receptors that act indirectly by modulating channel-linked or catalytic receptors. The latter group often activates a chain of events through their GTP-binding or *G proteins,* using intracellular messengers such as cyclic AMP or calcium ions.

An example of G-protein-linked receptor action is the ability of epinephrine to initiate glycogen degradation. Release of epinephrine from the adrenal gland raises its concentration in the blood stream and activates epinephrine receptors in liver cells. The activated receptors then transduce their signal by activating a G protein, initiating a chain of events that includes activation of adenylate cyclase enzyme, production of intracellular cyclic AMP, activation of glycogen phosphorylase enzyme, and release of glucose from liver glycogen as discussed in Chapter 6. Certain glycogen storage diseases, like deficiency of glycogen phosphorylase (232700), interfere with transduction of the epinephrine signal that coordinates glycogen degradation and glucose release. Advances in developmental and cancer genetics have defined analogous signal transduction pathways that are important regulators of cellular growth, differentiation, and pattern formation. Reviews of signal transduction pathways and their effects on cell differentiation can be found on the companion website (http://www.wiley.com/wilson/) or in the reference section.

■ 9.3. DEVELOPMENTAL GENETICS: ANIMAL MODELS

Perhaps the most complex level of genetic and cellular regulation concerns the evolution of a human being from a fertilized egg. As with other biological processes, genetic techniques have been powerfully revealing in the area of human development. These genetic advances began with observations of inherited anomalies and syndromes in humans, then blossomed elegantly with molecular analysis in simpler organisms. The emerging field of developmental genetics is concerned with the role of genes in embryogenesis and the mechanisms by which gene mutations produce developmental anomalies. It is not surprising that many genes acting during embryogenesis regulate cell growth and differentiation and that they are similar or identical to those acting after birth to cause cancer. The similarities among developmental and cancer genes, and the surprising homology among developmental genes among all animals, have allowed rapid progress in matching inherited anomalies with their causative genes (Table 9.2).

The advantages of model organisms lie in their short life cycles, their observable and manipulable embryos, and/or their accommodation to breeding schemes necessary for genetic analysis. In animals with long laboratory histories like fruit flies or mice, spontaneous mutations were observed that then "bred true" to produce a recurring source of mutant organisms for analysis. Animals can be inbred to make spontaneous mutations homozygous and crossbred to obtain genetic backgrounds that maximize the effects of mutation. Animals can also be treated with mutagenic chemicals to produce mutant embryos, as highlighted in the Nobel prize-winning work of Nusslein-Volhard and Weischaus (1980). Mutagenesis has produced a useful compendium of inherited anomalies in organisms as diverse as worms, fruit flies, zebrafish, and mice.

The fruit fly, so useful for matching genes with chromosomal bands by virtue of its giant polytene chromosomes, has proved to be a premier model for early embryonic development or *pattern formation.* More recently, the same strategies for comprehensive mutagenesis and screening of embryos have moved closer to mammals by their application to roundworms and zebrafish. Numerous genes associated with remarkable developmental phenotypes in simpler organisms are now available for knockout in mice or matching with known genetic disorders in humans. Model systems for

■ **TABLE 9.2. Model Organisms in Developmental Genetics**

Organism	Genome Size	Advantages	Relevant Molecules
C. elegans (nematode worm)	8×10^7 bp ~ 4000 genes	Visible cell lineage Hermaphroditic	*Lin* (lineage) mutants—homology to vertebrate growth factors *Ced* (cell death) mutants—homology to vertebrate apoptosis genes
D. melanogaster (arthropod fly)	1.65×10^8 ~10,000 genes	Extensive genetics Large chromosomes Body segments Homeotic transformations	Maternal mutants affecting A-P and D-V axes—homology to vertebrate oncogenes Segmentation mutants *paired, wingless*—homology to vertebrate *PAX, Wnt-1* genes Homeotic mutants like *antennopedia*—homology to vertebrate *HOX* genes
Zebrafish (fish vertebrate)	1.7×10^9 ~100,000 genes	Accessible embryos Haploid embryos	Systematic mutagenesis in progress Mutations affecting axes and gastrulation
Frog (amphibian vertebrate)	3×10^9 ~100,000 genes	Accessible embryos Large oocytes	TGF-β homologue controls induction *Wnt-1* and *Hox* homologues induce axis duplications
Chicken (vertebrate)	3×10^9 ~100,000 genes	Accessible embryos Visible gastrulation Visible limb buds	Fly *hedgehog* homologue (*sonic hedgehog*) controls lateral axis, limb bud polarity FGF homologue controls limb extension Retinoic acid and *Hox* homologues control limb patterning
Mouse (mammalian vertebrate)	3×10^9 ~100,000 genes	Extensive genetics Transgenic techniques	Natural mutants like *splotch* (*PAX* homologue) or *dominant spotted* (c-*kit* homologue—see Case 9) Transgenic knockouts—*Hox* knockouts cause facial and limb defects
Human (mammalian vertebrate)	3×10^9 ~100,000 genes	Documented phenotypes (human syndromes)	c-*kit* mutants cause piebald trait (see Case 9) *PAX* mutants cause aniridia and Waardenburg syndrome *HOX* mutants cause limb defects *Sonic hedgehog* mutants cause holoprosencephaly Retinoic acid exposure causes limb and facial defects *FGFR3* mutants cause achondroplasia

Notes: A-P, anteroposterior; D-V, dorsoventral; TGF, transforming growth factor; FGF, fibroblast growth factor; FGFR3, fibroblast growth factor receptor 3; see text for explanations of genes and diseases.

animal development are briefly reviewed because of their growing application to human genetic disease (Table 9.2).

Roundworms: Cell Growth, Death, and Lineage

The nematode *C. elegans* is a small (1 mm in length), rapidly developing (16 hours) and hermaphroditic organism, making it easy to breed. A major advantage is its transparent cuticle, which has allowed mapping of the lineage of all 959 of its somatic cells (Fig. 9.3). The organism has an estimated 4000 genes distributed over 6 chromosomes, and a genome project is underway because of its utility in developmental analysis (Table 9.2).

A key developmental mechanism illustrated by *C. elegans* is that of cytoplasmic determinants (Fig. 9.3A). P granules become visible in the *C. elegans* zygote, then segregate with the first division to establish P1 cells. Continued segregation of the P granules with the P lineage directs these cells to become eggs and sperm. The segregation of particular cytoplasmic structures, illustrated by presumed mRNA molecules within the P-granules, thus confers a particular phenotype on descendent cells. This mechanism for cytoplasmic determination is often called *mosaic development,* and it is used by many types of animals including perhaps the determination of germ cells in humans.

A contrasting developmental mechanism involves interactions among cells rather than the segregation of cytoplasmic determinants and is called *regulative development.* The P lineage that gives rise to germ cells also produces the vulva (female genital organ) of *C. elegans.* If one cell (the *anchor cell*) in the later P lineage is ablated by laser, the surface cuticle cells are not influenced to transform into vulva cells (Fig. 9.3). Genetic mutations were then found that lacked anchor cells and consequent vulvae formation. Certain genes targeted by these mutations were called *lin* genes, named for their effects on cell lineage, and many have homology to mammalian growth factor genes, including the gene for epidermal growth factor

(Table 9.3). Laboratory manipulation of *lin* gene activity causes deficiency or excess of anchor cells or their equivalents, regulating genital development to produce absent or multiple vulvae. Overactivity of a *lin* growth factor seems to inhibit normal mechanisms for cell death, resulting in excess cells and multiple vulvar structures.

Because the origin and fate of every cell in the *C. elegans* embryo could be visualized, it was recognized that programmed cell death, or *apoptosis,* is a regular and normal process that shapes multiple cell lineages in the worm embryo. (The word *apoptosis* is derived from the Greek words *apo* for apart and *ptosis* for fallen) More than 14 different genes influencing cell death in *C. elegans* (*ced* genes) were identified, some with homology to human cancer genes like *BCL-2* gene (see Table 9.1). These studies promoted a view of cell regulation by signal pathways that mediate a choice between growth through cell cycles or cell death.

Fruit Flies: Cell Differentiation and Pattern Formation

The first fly mutants to draw attention to early pattern regulation had dramatic changes that replaced one body part with another, exemplified by the *antennapedia* mutation that replaced antennae with legs (Fig. 9.4). This process was named "homoeosis" because it replaced one body part with a homologous one. Two major complexes of genes called *bithorax* (*BX*-C) and *antennapedia* (*ANT*-C) were found to be responsible for homeotic mutations. These gene complexes determine the identity of segments in the fly embryo, causing them to become head, thorax, or abdomen (Fig. 9.4A). Molecular cloning experiments revealed that the genes within the *BX*-C and *ANT*-C complexes shared a striking DNA motif called the *homeobox.* Homeoboxes are 180-bp stretches of DNA that encode a 60-amino acid domain that allows their product proteins to bind to DNA. Homeotic proteins function as transcription factors, regulating the expression of other

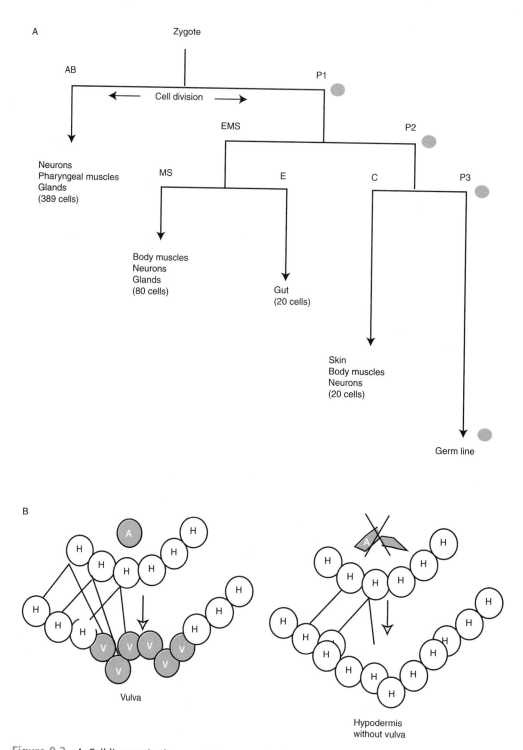

Figure 9.3. *A*, Cell lineage in the nematode worm *C. elegans* illustrating how segregation of a cytogenetic determinant (the P granule symbolized by the shaded dot) produces the germ cell lineage. *B*, Key role of the anchor cell (A) in inducing hypodermis cells (H) to divide into one hypodermal cell and one vulval (V) cell (left). Laser ablation of the anchor cell causes each hypodermal cell to divide into equivalent cells (right) that do not form the vulva. (See Wilkins, 1986, pp. 194–9.)

■ **TABLE 9.3.** Gene Families in Development

Gene Family	Worm	Fly	Chick	Mouse	Human
Hedgehog		+ *hedgehog*	+ limb	+ brain	+ brain
Wingless/int		+ *wingless*	+ *Wnt*-1	+ *Wnt*-1 brain	+ *Wnt*-1
Paired		+ *paired*	+	+ (*Pax*) eye	+ (*PAX*) eye
GLI		+ *Krüppel*	+	+ toes	+ face, limb
Homeotic	+	+ *antennapedia* *bithorax*	+ limb	+ (*Hox*) face, limb	+ (*HOX*) limb
Cell death	+ *ced*	+ caspases	+ caspases	+ caspases	+ caspases
TGF	+	+	+ laterality	+	+
EGF	+ *lin*	+ *notch*	+	+	+
FGF	+	+	+ limb	+ limb	+ skeleton

Notes: TGF, transforming growth factor; EGF, epidermal growth factor; FGF, fibroblast growth factor; + indicates a homologue is present in the genome.

genes that produce specific head, thoracic, or abdominal structures. The homeobox sequence of 60 amino acids is highly conserved among different homeotic genes, suggesting that this gene family arose by duplications of an ancestral gene.

It was soon realized that the homeotic genes act at the end of a regulatory cascade that divided fly embryos into compartments. By studying nonviable mutant embryos, workers (Nusslein-Volhard and Wieschaus, 1980; Nusslein et al., 1987) defined the genes in this regulatory cascade and initiated a Copernican revolution in development. Instead of describing developmental processes according to the position and timing of derived structures, a central patterning process was delineated that could predict future position and structure. In Figure 9.5, key characteristics of the gene mutations affecting early embryos are shown. The earliest genes acted to demarcate large regions of the embryo, exemplified by *dorsal* mutations that produce nonviable embryos with exaggerated dorsal and absent ventral structures. Later genes demarcated the pattern of segments, exemplified by gap phenotypes caused by *Krüppel* gene mutations, pair-rule phenotypes caused by *paired* gene mutations, and segment polarity phenotypes caused by *hedgehog* or *wingless* gene mutations (Fig. 9.5). Note that the genes are named according to the appearance of anomalous embryos produced by their mutations, including rather fanciful comparisons like *Krüppel* (a German pastry) or *hedgehog*.

After the early maternal genes demarcate the anteroposterior and dorsoventral embryonic regions, and after the segmentation genes produce the appropriate number and orientation of segments, the homeotic genes act to give each segment its identity. In Figure 9.4, it can be seen that the striking *antennapedia* mutation causes the identity of head segments (antennae) to be replaced by that of thoracic segments (limbs). There is a correlation between the regions in which genes are expressed and the pattern of the phenotype produced. Gap genes are expressed in the middle embryonic segments, which are absent in the presence of gap gene mutations. Segment polarity genes are expressed in the distal half of each segment and produce aberrant segment pattern (hedgehog) or absent wings (wingless) when the segments are not properly oriented. The antennapedia homeotic genes are expressed in head segments, while the bithorax homeotic genes are expressed in thoracic and abdominal segments. Segment identity is determined by the number of homeotic genes expressed in each segment, with progressively more genes expressed as one reaches the distal abdominal segments. Because the order of the genes within the homeotic loci corresponds to the anatomic order of the segments they regulate,

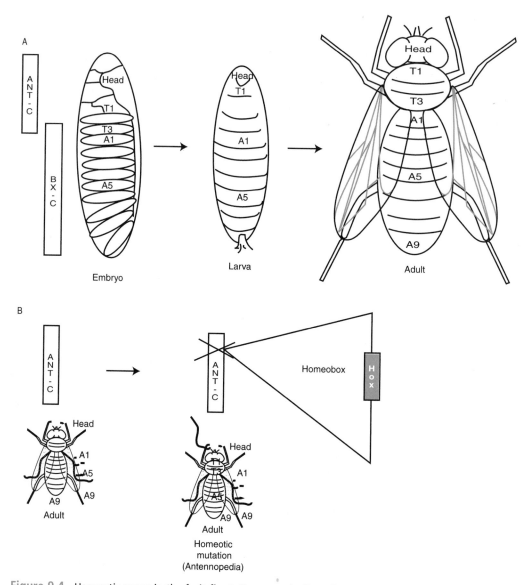

Figure 9.4. Homeotic genes in the fruit fly. *A,* Segments in fly embryos, larvae, and adult controlled by homeotic genes in the antennapedia (*ANT-C,* head and thoracic segments) or bithorax clusters (*BX-C,* thoracic and abdominal segments); *B, antennapedia* mutation substituting a leg segment for antenna segment and its molecular characterization to reveal the homeobox (*Hox*) domain. (See Wilkins, 1986, pp. 275–87.)

mutations in these genes produce simple anatomic transformations—that is, abdominal into thoracic, thoracic segment 3 into thoracic segment 2. The latter genetic change transforms a fly with two wings into one with four, emphasizing the remarkable effects of fly patterning genes on morphogenesis.

The sequential sculpturing of the fly embryo by the action of related sets of genes thus provides an impressive example of developmental genetics. Each set of gene products is restricted to a particular embryonic compartment by the actions of preceding genes, and acts to further regulate and restrict the expres-

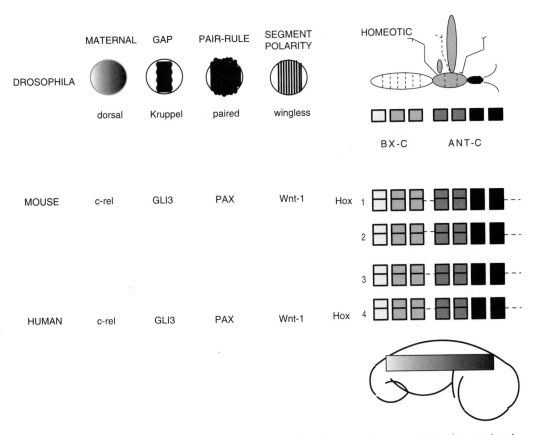

Figure 9.5. Genes regulating fly segmentation, consisting of maternal, segmentation (gap, pair-rule, segment polarity), and homeotic categories. Homologues from each category have been defined in mammals, including four major cluster of homeotic genes in mouse and man. The homeotic genes exhibit anteroposterior patterns of expression in embryos that correlates with their 5′ to 3′ location in each homeotic gene cluster (right of figure)

sion of its following genes. As the cascade of gene expression proceeds, cells undergo differentiation to produce regional differences in phenotype that are perceived as morphologic pattern. The products of early maternal genes are present in graded concentrations across the entire embryo, stimulating regional differences according to their local concentrations. Although fly embryos are unique in forming as a large, continous cell (syncytium) with multiple nuclei, later cellular interactions establish the segmentation process as a regulative form of development. Similarities of fly segmentation to pattern formation in more complex organisms is now supported by the finding that many fly genes have relatives in vertebrates.

Because the fly homeobox was such a characteristic marker for developmentally important genes, it was natural to examine more complex animals and humans for homologues of these genes. The use of radioactive homeobox DNA probes from the fly has identified related genes in all animals examined, with hundreds of homologues in humans and mice (Fig. 9.5). Mammals have four major clusters of homeotic genes and many isolated homeotic genes scattered throughout the genome. The clustered homeotic genes are given letters to denote their cluster and numbers to denote their order within the cluster, exemplified by the *HOXD13* gene that is mutated in a human limb defect syndrome (Table 9.2). Homologues of other fly segmentation genes are also abundant in the mouse and human genomes as illustrated by the *PAX* (*paired*) gene family or the sonic hedgehog (*hedgehog*) gene (Fig. 9.5).

Amphibia and Zebrafish: Genes Controlling Gastrulation

After the specification of the early body plan, the next great event of animal embryogenesis is gastrulation. Gastrulation refers to the establishment of the three germ layers—endoderm, mesoderm, and ectoderm—that are the foundations of organ development. Frog embryos have been the organism of choice for studying gastrulation because of their relatively large size, accessibility, and tolerance of tissue manipulations. The classic experiments of Spemann defined the phenomenon of induction in the frog, showing that tissue from the dorsal lip of the blastopore (an opening in the spherical frog blastocyst) would produce mesoderm when transplanted next to susceptible tissue (Fig. 9.6A). The dorsal lip clearly contained tissue with special regulatory properties, because it also could induce a second body axis when transplanted onto early embryos.

The next step was to isolate the responsible molecules that directed these striking inductions. Unfortunately, frogs are like sea urchins in yielding accessible embryos without the convenience of easy breeding and genetics.

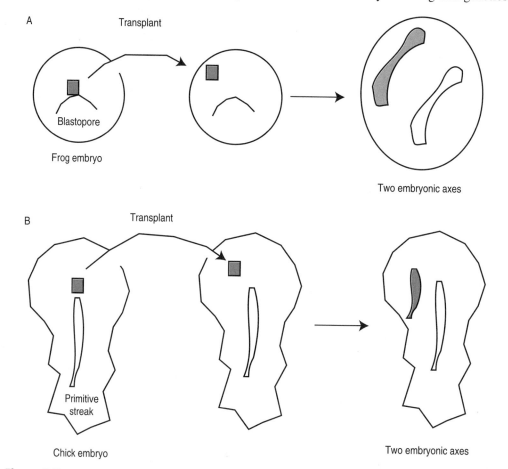

Figure 9.6. Gastrulation in the frog (*A*) and chick (*B*). Transplant of material from a region anterior to the gastrulation structure (blastopore in frogs, primitive streak in chicks) will induce a second embryonic axis.

Rather than isolating mutants defective in dorsal lip action, experiments focused on the extraction of various molecules from the dorsal lip and testing to see which had inductive activity. A major determinant was found to be a gene for activin, a member of the transforming growth factor-β family. Thus a growth factor is again implicated in an embryonic event controlling cell differentiation. Similar inductive activity can be seen by transplanting a region of the chick embryo called the primitive node (Fig. 9.6*B*). When the primitive node region anterior to the primitive streak region of one embryo is transplanted onto another, it induces a second embryonic axis in the recipient embryo. *Activin* gene homologues have also been implicated in chick axis formation (see the next section), emphasizing the recurring use of similar molecules in animal development.

One aspect of dorsal lip inducing activity in the frog has been simulated by relatives of fly segmentation genes. If the frog homologue of fly *wingless* (called *Wnt-1* based on homology to vertebrate *int-1* genes) was injected, it produced duplications of the anterior axis and yielded embryos with two heads (Table 9.3). This alteration was also produced by a frog homologue of fly homeotic genes called *Xhox*. Homologues of fly patterning genes can thus produce dramatic alterations of pattern in an amphibian, supporting their importance in vertebrate development (Fig. 9.5).

Adding the power of genetics to the tractable embryos of simpler vertebrates is the zebrafish (Table 9.2). This organism can reproduce parthogenetically as a diploid, yet produce haploid embryos when eggs are fertilized with irradiated sperm. Haploid embryos, like human males with X-linked diseases, show the effects of any abnormal alleles because there is no paired allele to compensate. Transgenic animals can also be produced in zebrafish, and an extensive genetic linkage map has already been assembled.

The zebrafish exhibits classical phenomena like embryonic induction, and its embryos can be manipulated surgically to allow transplants or explants to produce cultured cells. A saturation approach for characterizing mutations affecting early embryogenesis has been initiated, simulating that for the fruit fly, and many interesting mutant phenotypes have been produced for genetic study. Several of these, like *trilobite* (resembling a fossil) or *half-baked,* have alterations in gastrulation. The zebrafish thus combines the advantages of developmental genetics with an embryo that is much more similar to that of humans than is the fruit fly (Table 9.2).

Chickens: Genes Controlling Laterality and Limb Patterning

As with frogs, genetic analysis has not been emphasized in chickens. The chick embryo does allow easy visualization and manipulation, and it provides a primitive streak stage of gastrulation very similar to that of humans (Table 9.2). Recent experiments with chick embryos have defined molecules that contribute to the third embryonic axis—that for right-left differences or laterality. By using probes for gene expression during the early primitive streak stage, certain gene products were found exclusively on the right or left side of the primitive streak. Shortly after the primitive streak stage, the heart tube and then the body axis loop to the right in chicks, mice, and humans (Fig. 9.7*A*). Genes that exhibited side-specific expression included those for an activin receptor, *nodal* (a member of the transforming growth factor-β family), and a relative of the fly *hedgehog* gene that was playfully named *sonic hedgehog* after the video game (Table 9.3). Activin receptor expression was noted on the right side of the chick primitive streak (dotted line in Fig. 9.7*A*), followed shortly thereafter by expression of *nodal* and *sonic hedgehog* on the left side (solid line in Fig. 9.7*A*). The asymmetry of gene expression guides rightward looping of the heart and leftward rotation of the neural axis to produce the characteristic chick embryo.

Sequential action of these genes to produce differences between the right and left sides is reminiscent of the fly genes that produce an-

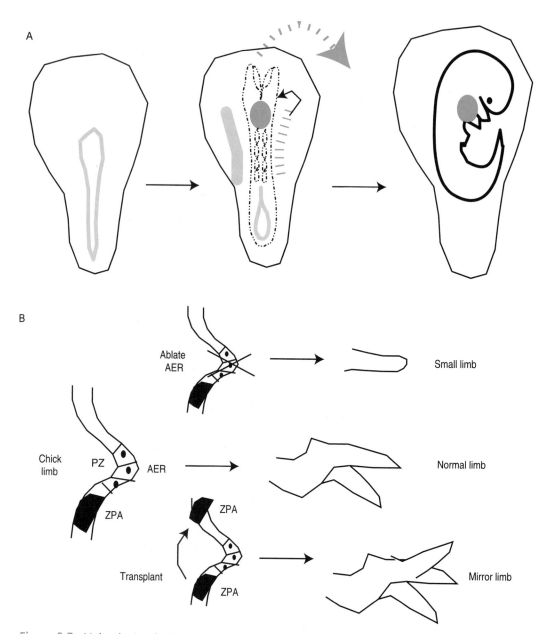

Figure 9.7. Molecules involved in chick laterality (*A*) and limb patterning (*B*). *A*, Nodal and activin gene products are expressed on the right (solid line), *sonic hedgehog* on the left (dotted line) of the neuraxis in symmetrical chick embryos prior to the asymmetric folds that place the heart on the left. *B*, The zone of polarizing activity (ZPA) controls the positioning of digits as shown by mirror anomalies when it is transplanted (lower diagram). These mirror anomalies can be mimicked by injection of *sonic hedgehog* gene product or retinoic acid. The apical epidermal ridge (AER) secretes molecules such as transforming growth factor-β and stimulates cells in the proliferating zone (PZ) to promote limb elongation.

teroposterior and dorsoventral differences. Note that the same gene families—activin, activin receptor, transforming growth factor-β, *hedgehog*—are involved in early patterning of flies, frogs, and chicks (Table 9.3). These findings emphasize the way in which molecular genetic analysis is unifying the approach to developmental mechanisms in diverse organisms.

Another valuable contribution of chick embryology has been in the analysis of limb patterning. After a primary embryonic pattern with three major axes and three germ layers is determined, secondary patterning processes sculpt the forms and relationships among particular organs. The limbs are prime examples wherein an early limb bud translates anteroposterior (shoulder-fingertip), dorsoventral (back of hand-palm) and right-left (thumb versus little finger) information into segmented and bilaterally symmetrical limbs. The accessibility of chick embryonic limbs provided an excellent experimental system where final form could be related to particular tissue and molecular manipulations (Fig. 9.7*B*).

The developing chick limb bud contains an apical ectodermal ridge (AER) that stimulates cells in the progress zone (PZ) to proliferate, and a zone of polarizing activity (ZPA) that patterns or organizes the emerging limb. One of the molecules used by the AER to stimulate proliferation is the chick homologue of fibroblast growth factor-1. This family of molecules has also been implicated in human skeletal development (Table 9.2).

The patterning or organizing activity of the ZPA was recognized by surgical manipulation of this region. When tissue from the ZPA is transplanted anterior to the limb bud, a mirror-image duplication results (Fig. 9.7*B*). This organizing activity is mimicked by adding solutions of certain molecules to the same anterior region. One of these molecules is the *sonic hedgehog* gene product mentioned previously regarding laterality. The same genes may thus control embryonic patterning at early and later stages, producing multiple effects when they are mutated. Such *pleiotropic* effects are rele-

vant to humans with patterns of anomalies called *syndromes*. Also interesting are regional differences in chick homeotic gene expression in the limb. Relatives of the homeotic genes that regulate fly segment identity are also involved in later limb patterning in the chick. Once again a cascade of cellular interactions is regulated by successive gene activation through the timed expression of transcription factors like the *sonic hedgehog* and vertebrate *Hox* gene products (Table 9.3).

Retinoic acid is another molecule that can produce mirror image limb anomalies when added to the anterior limb bud (Fig. 9.7*B*). Retinoids have been defined as morphogens in several experimental organisms, and their activity in the chick correlates with the patterns of birth defects in children exposed prenatally to retinoids such as the antiacne medicine Accutane.

Mouse Models of Genes Controlling Human Development

The mouse offers a mammalian model for development with a long history of genetic analysis. The mouse gene map is extensive and shows similarities to the gene map of humans, in that the same genes tend to be grouped (*syntenic*) in both organisms. Similarities in gene organization between mouse and man are paralleled by similarities in the phenotypes produced by homologous gene mutations. Table 9.4 shows examples of several human genetic disorders that have homologous phenotypes in the mouse. Genetic disorders altering the development of the neural tube, limbs, craniofacies, and skin have been described in both species. In some cases, homologous location implies that the mutant genes are the same, as is the case for X-linked disorders such as chondrodysplasia punctata (humans) and *bare patches* (mice), ornithine transcarbamylase deficiency (humans) and *sparse fur* (mice), or anhidrotic ectodermal dysplasia (humans) and *Tabby* (mouse). Homology has been proved by molecular cloning of the genes involved in a growing list of disorders, exemplified by cau-

■**TABLE 9.4.** Homologous Disorders of Mice and Men

Malformation Type	Mouse	Human
Neural tube/sacral defects	*Splotch (Sp)*	Spina bifida
	Curly tail (ct)	Caudal regression
Axial defects	*Rib fusion (Rf)*	Jarcho-Levin syndrome (277300)
	Malformed vertebrae (Mv)	Spondylocostal dysplasias (122600,
	Amputated (am)	271520)
Limb defects	*Limb deformity (ld)*	Cenani-Lenz syndactyly (212780)
	Luxoid (lu)	Synpolydactyly type II (186000)
	Strong's luxoid (lst)	Acrorenal syndromes (e.g., 102520)
	Oligosyndactyly (Od)	
Craniofacial defects	*Extra toes (Xt)*	Greig syndrome (175700)
	First arch (Far)	Hemifacial microsomia (e.g., 141400)
Pigmentary anomalies	*Dominant spotted (Ds)*	Piebald trait (172800)
	Piebald (s)	Waardenburg syndrome (193500)
Laterality defects	*Situs inversus viscerum (iv)*	Kartagener syndrome (244400)
	Visceral inversion (vi)	Polysplenia/asplenia (e.g., 208530)
Ectodermal defects	*Bare patches (bpa)*	Chondrodysplasia punctata (302960)
	Tabby (Ta)	Ectodermal dysplasia (305100)
	Sparse fur (spf)	OTC deficiency (311250)

Notes: Mouse loci are capitalized when autosomal or X-linked dominant, lower case when recessive; *Bare patches*, *Sparse fur*, and *Tabby* are X-linked; recall that the McKusick number begins with 1 for autosomal dominant, 2 for autosomal recessive, and 3 for X-linked human disorders; *Extra toes* and Greig (GLI3), *Dominant spotted* and piebald trait (*c-kit*; Case 9), *Tabby* and ectodermal dysplasia, *Sparse fur* and OTC deficiency are known to involve homologous loci.

sation of both *extra toes* (mice) and Greig syndrome (humans) by mutations in the *GLI3* gene that is homologous to the fly segmentation gene *Krüppel*. Once a homologous developmental disorder has been identified in the mouse, the relevant embryonic mechanisms and even potential therapies can be explored in the model system.

Another vitally important role for mouse genetics lies in attacking complex phenotypes produced by multifactorial inheritance. Examples include cleft palate or neural tube defects. Specific mouse strains have higher rates of cleft palate, and these rates can be increased when the mice are exposed to steroids during gestation. The genetic tendency for cleft palate has been further dissected by finding strains with different types of predisposing variations. Some strains have broader heads with longer distance for the palatal shelves to travel, while others have smaller jaws that obstruct palatal shelf fusion. These predisposing genetic factors can be investigated by utilizing another advan-

tage of mouse genetics, the recombinant inbred strain. After some 20 generations of brother-sister mating, inbred mice are produced with virtually identical genotypes like human monozygous twins. The significance of single locus or environmental differences can be assessed in the inbred strains with the assurance that all other genetic modifiers are identical.

The mouse has also provided several interesting mutations that are relevant to neural tube defects such as human anencephaly and spina bifida (Table 9.4). Examples include the *splotch* gene, which produces defects in the dorsal neural tube in homozygous mutant mice. Although initially identified because of a depigmented splotch of fur, the splotch gene is now known to be a mouse version of the fly *paired* gene called *PAX3*. This gene and the depigmented fur are homologous to the human Waardenburg syndrome that is also caused by *PAX3* mutations. The *splotch* mutation illustrates the interaction of genes and environment in birth defects such as those of neural tube closure. It is known that folic acid supplementation can lower neural tube defects in human populations by one-third and that *splotch* mouse mutants are deficient in the supply of folic acid needed to synthesis pyrimidines (Fleming and Copp, 1998).

Case 9 Follow-up: The ventral depigmentation of the patient shown in Case 9 was noted to be very similar to that in a mouse mutation called *dominant spotted*. The *dominant spotted* phenotype in mice also produced white spots on the front (ventral) side of the body, and its autosomal dominant inheritance made it an attractive model for piebald trait in humans.

Engineering Development with Transgenic Organisms: Mouse Knockouts

Although the characterization of mouse mutants obtained through breeding or mutagenesis experiments has been very useful, a much more powerful technology was developed using recombinant DNA technology. The ability to inject DNA into mouse oocytes and to create transgenic breeding lines has vastly increased the ability to create mice with genetic diseases and developmental abnormalities (Fig. 9.8). Although the transgenic approach was initially compromised by aberrant or multiple insertions of genes, homologous recombination techniques were developed that could exactly excise and replace an endogenous gene segment. Transgenic mice allow vertebrate embryos or adults to be obtained in which a particular gene has been altered for increased or decreased expression. When the genetic alteration is lethal to embryos, carrier mice can be bred and the abnormal embryos harvested for analysis prior to birth (Fig. 9.8).

One example of the utility and complexity of mimicking human genetic diseases in mice concerned replacement of the mouse β-globin genes with the sickle globin gene from humans. Mice with sickle cell anemia would be extremely useful for testing potential therapies.

Unfortunately, replacement of both mouse β-globin genes with the human mutant genes was required before the vascular obstructions characteristic of sickle cell anemia were observed. Additionally, the human γ-globin genes encoding fetal hemoglobin also had to be placed in the mouse so that they underwent a fetal-to-adult hemoglobin switch during neonatal life as humans do. Otherwise, the neonatal mice with sickle cell anemia died from vascular obstructions before therapies could be attempted. Construction of a mouse model for sickle cell anemia thus required three separate gene replacement steps to obtain mice with similar genotypes and phenotypes to those of affected humans.

A great advantage from the developmental genetic perspective is the ability to use transgenic mice to assess the effects of new genes on mammalian development. As mentioned previously, genes defined in simpler organisms like worms and flies often have relatives in mammals that can be identified by DNA hybridization and isolated by recombinant DNA cloning. Over- or underexpression of the homologous gene in transgenic mice can then be arranged to evaluate the role of this gene in mouse development. Most often the normal copies of the mouse gene are replaced or knocked out by mutant copies, and *mouse knockouts* have produced several revealing developmental phenotypes.

One of many interesting lines of investigation targeted the mouse homologues of fly homeotic genes. Mice, like humans, contain more than 300 genes that contain the homeobox motif, including four major clusters of 10 genes each (*HOX* in humans, *Hox* in mice). The *Hox* genes in each of the four clusters are reminiscent of the *Antennapedia* and *bithorax* loci in flies, with similar 5′ to 3′ orientation of the clustered genes (see Fig. 9.5). As a generalization from many complex phenotypes (see Table 9.4), knockout or overexpression of *Hox* genes toward the 5′ end of the cluster tend to affect anterior (head) structures in the mouse, while alteration of *Hox* genes toward the 3′ end of the cluster affect posterior structures.

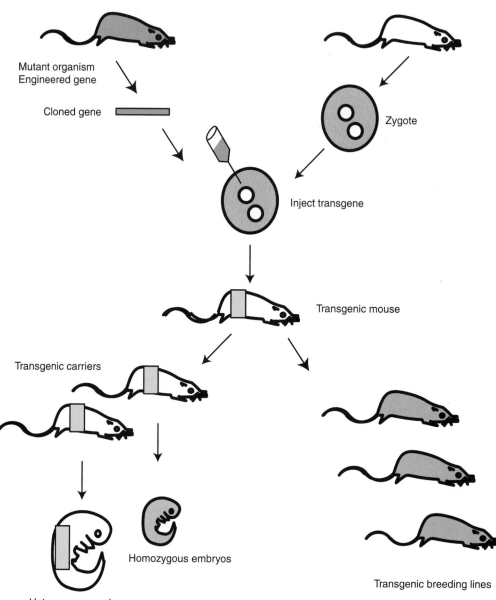

Figure 9.8. Generation of transgenic mice. Genes isolated from mutant mice or other organisms are injected into normal mice oocytes. The mutant genes are placed into vectors that facilitate homologous recombination with oocyte DNA, allowing normal genes to be precisely excised and replaced with their homologous mutant gene. The oocytes with transgenes are placed into surrogate mothers to produce heterozygous offspring and transgenic breeding lines. Effects of homozygous mutations can be assessed by breeding carriers and inspecting the affected embryos.

One particular example concerns the development of mice with knockouts of the *Hox* 1.1 gene. These mice have altered facial development with small jaws and altered maxillae reminiscent of a human disorder called Treacher-Collins syndrome (Table 9.2). Not only has the clustered structure of homeotic genes been conserved from flies to mammals, but the same correlation between 5′ to 3′ location within *Hox* clusters and effects on patterning is observed. This correlation suggests that the clustered homeotic genes have retained similar developmental functions during more than one million years of metazoan evolution.

■ 9.4. HUMAN DEVELOPMENTAL GENETICS

Overview of Human Developmental Anomalies

During the first 2 weeks of human development, the fertilized egg proliferates rapidly to form the morula and blastocyst. Major axis orientation must be specified before the blastocele forms to demarcate a bilaminar embryo that is oriented dorsoventrally with amniotic cavity above and yolk sac below. Gastrulation begins as epiblast cells migrate through the primitive streak to become mesoderm, and the notochord forms to demarcate the midline. Major embryonic regions are already differentiated shortly after gastrulation, including anterior structures (forebrain, primitive heart), dorsal structures (neural tube and neural crest), ventral structures (foregut that will generate lungs and thyroid), and posterior structures (hindgut and allantois that will generate the urogenital system). The human body plan is thus complete by 19 to 20 days after conception, a time when the possibility of pregnancy may just have occurred to the mother because of delayed menstruation. Many early embryonic defects in humans may pass unnoticed because their demise is not distinguished from menstruation.

Once the primitive streak stage and gastrulation have occurred, the germ layers of endoderm, mesoderm, and ectoderm give rise to all ensuing structures of the embryo. The ectoderm develops into skin, teeth, sweat glands, and neural tissue that includes the ventrally migrating neural crest cells. Neural crest contributes not only to many facial and nerve ganglion structures but also to the pigmented skin cells (melanoblasts), explaining why interference with neural crest transformation and migration may cause ventral patches of white skin (see Case 9 follow-up at the end of this section). The mesoderm is partitioned into paraxial mesoderm that forms the internal skeleton, muscle, and dermis; intermediate mesoderm that forms urogenital tissue; and lateral mesoderm that forms the heart, limbs, and lateral body wall. Endoderm forms the gastrointestinal system that gives rise to the pharynx, trachea, and lungs at its anterior end and cloaca and urogenital system at its posterior end.

After specification of the primary body plan and the germ layers in the first month of gestation (the period of blastogenesis), organ systems are formed by additional steps of cell growth/death, cell differentiation, and cell movements. Once basic organ structure is specified in the period of organogenesis, occupying approximately the second month after conception, there is continued tissue maturation necessary for independent function after birth (the period of phenogenesis). The embryo-fetal periods of blastogenesis (primary pattern formation), organogenesis, and phenogenesis are useful to bear in mind when considering the effects of mutant genes on human embryonic development. Multiple major anomalies like limb and kidney defects can result from alterations of blastogenesis, single major anomalies like absent kidney from alterations during organogenesis, and minor anomalies such as a single palmar crease from alterations during phenogenesis. More detailed discussion and illustration of human embryogenesis can be found at the companion website (http://www.wiley.com/wilson/) or in the references. Some examples of genetic alterations of human development are now presented.

Human Developmental Genes: Overgrowth Disorders

A group of human developmental genetic disorders that clearly reflect abnormal growth regulation are the overgrowth disorders. Affected children often have large birth weights, reflecting increased fetal growth, and show rapid, proportionate growth after birth. One example of this category is the Simpson-Golabi-Behmel syndrome (312870) with affected males exhibiting gigantism, a characteristic facial appearance with large mouths, and postaxial polydactyly (extra fingers on ulnar side). The X-linked pattern of inheritance allowed mapping of the causative locus to chromosome band Xq26, and two X;autosome translocations in affected boys led to the identification of the responsible gene. The gene encoded a glycoprotein called glypican 3 that extends from the cell membrane to the extracellular matrix. The glypican 3 protein is thus an integral membrane protein in part, serving as a cell surface receptor that connects with the extracellular matrix. It is expressed in most mesodermal tissues including lung, liver, and kidney, and exhibits increased levels in rapidly growing tissues (e.g., embryonic tissues). One of the growth factors that interacts with the glypican 3 protein is insulin-like growth factor-2, a growth factor with increased activity in another overgrowth syndrome called Beckwith-Wiedemann syndrome. Simpson-Golabi-Behmel syndrome thus exemplifies a pattern of overgrowth and developmental abnormalities that derive from enhanced signaling for cell growth (Table 9.5).

Human Developmental Genes: Skeletal Disorders

During the discussion of chick limb morphogenesis, the role of fibroblast growth factors in signaling limb bud proliferation was mentioned. This family of molecules has diverse roles in inducing growth or differentiation of embryonic ectoderm and mesoderm. The fibroblast growth factors act through a signal transduction pathway involving receptor binding, activation of GTP-binding proteins, and a series of kinase reactions that alters nuclear transcription factors and gene expression. The receptors for fibroblast growth factors are also widely distributed in embryos, particularly in mesodermal tissues contributing to the axial or appendicular skeleton. The cloning and characterization of fibroblast growth factor receptor (*FGFR*) genes revealed a closely knit family of related structures with immunoglobulin-like (Ig), transmembrane (TM), and tyrosine kinase (TK) domains (Fig. 9.9). Mutations in the *FGFR* gene family have now been related to particular forms of craniosynostosis or skeletal dysplasia (Table 9.5).

Patients with skeletal dysplasias have short stature due to undergrowth of the proximal limb segments (rhizomelic limb shortening), prominent foreheads (frontal bossing), and narrowing of the foramen magnum due to aberrant cranial growth, and midface hypoplasia with a shallow nasal bridge. Hypochondroplasia (146000), achondroplasia (100800), and thanatophoric (death-loving) dysplasia (187600) were initially characterized as separate diseases with mild, moderate, and severe skeletal changes, respectively. In neonates with thanatophoric dysplasia, the ribs are so severely shortened that they cannot breathe. As shown in Figure 9.9, these three types of skeletal dysplasia are all caused by mutations in the *FGFR3* gene. Allelic versions of mutations in a growth factor receptor gene thus produce different degrees of skeletal dysplasia. The most dramatic alterations are produced by mutations in the stop codon for *FGFR3*, which result in elongated and severely dysfunctional receptor proteins. As expected, these stop codon mutations produce the severe clinical phenotype of thanatophoric dysplasia.

Human Developmental Genes Causing Brain Anomalies

Three types of human brain anomalies have been related to specific genes active in development—the *sonic hedgehog* gene associated with holoprosencephaly, the *LIS-1* gene associ-

■ TABLE 9.5. Human Genetic Disorders Affecting Development

Disorder	Phenotype	Cause
Simpson-Golabi-Behmel syndrome (312870)	Overgrowth, facial changes, extra digits	*Glypican-3* gene encoding membrane, ECM protein; interacts with IGF-2
Crouzon syndrome (123500) Apert syndrome (101200) Pfeiffer syndrome (101600)	Cranial suture fusion with or without fused or broad digits	Different domains of *FGF receptor-2* gene
Achondroplasia (100800) Hypochondroplasia (146000) Thanatophoric dysplasia (187600)	Cranial changes, short limbs, skeletal dysplasia	Different domains of *FGF-receptor-3* gene
Holoprosencephaly (e.g., 157170)	Abnormal face due to absent forebrain	*Sonic hedgehog* gene, interacts with *patched* receptor
Lissencephaly (e.g., 247200)	Smooth brain without convolutions	*LIS-1* gene encoding GTP-binding protein homologous to fly *Groucho*
Kallman syndrome (308700)	Anosmia, genital defects	*KAL* gene encoding cell adhesion molecule involved with axonal growth
Greig syndrome (175700)	Cranial changes, extra digits	*GLI3* transcription factor homologous to fly *Krüppe*l
Waardenburg syndrome (193500)	Cranial changes, white hair, bowel stenosis	*PAX3* transcription factor homologous to fly *paired*
Aniridia (106200)	Absent iris of the eye	*PAX2* transcription factor homologous to fly *paired*
Synpolydactyly (186000)	Extra digits, fused digits	*HOXD13* transcription factor homologous to fly homeotic genes
Retinoic acid embryopathy	Craniofacial, brain, limb defects	Retinoic acid exposure during pregnancy; retinoids activate homeotic genes

ated with lissencephaly, and the *KAL* gene associated with the Kallmann syndrome of olfactory and genital defects.

The *sonic hedgehog* gene, a relative of the *Drosophila* segmentation gene *hedgehog* (Fig. 9.5), was discussed with regard to chick laterality (Fig. 9.7). If the mouse version of *sonic hedgehog* is disrupted by a transgene, mice with defective brain and facial development

are produced. The mouse anomalies are similar to a human brain anomaly known as holoprosencephaly (Fig. 9.10). Holoprosencephaly is caused by a failure of mesoderm near the anterior end of the notochord to induce differentiation of the primitive forebrain. As a result of this failure, several midline events that produce symmetrical structures of the brain and face do not occur. The spectrum of anomalies

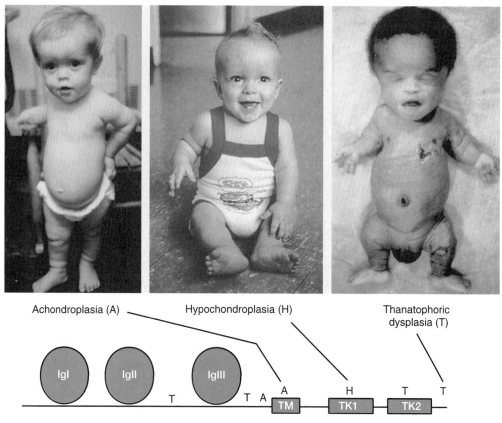

Figure 9.9. Skeletal dysplasias of variable severity (achondroplasia, left; hypochondroplasia, middle; thanatophoric dysplasia, right—photograph by Dr. Mason Barr, U. of Michigan) correlating with mutations at various positions in the *fibroblast growth factor receptor-3* gene. As would be expected, chain-terminating mutations that produce severely truncated *FGFR-3* molecules cause the lethal thanatophoric dysplasia phenotype.

in holoprosencephaly include single eye (cyclopia), absent nose (premaxillary agenesis), midline cleft lip/palate, single cerebral ventricle (rather than two), and absent olfactory lobes. The human *sonic hedgehog* gene is located at chromosome band 7q36 that corresponds to one of many chromosome deletions associated with holoprosencephaly. It is thus likely that inactivation of one copy of the *sonic hedgehog* gene is one of several causes for defective forebrain differentiation and holoprosencephaly.

Strengthening the association between *sonic hedgehog* gene deficiency and holoprosencephaly are characteristics of the signaling

pathway. S*onic hedgehog* protein acts on a receptor called *patched,* named for its knockout phenotype in the fly. Activation of the *patched* receptor requires that the *sonic hedgehog* protein be cleaved and bound covalently to cholesterol. Holoprosencephaly and related brain anomalies occur in human disorders with defective cholesterol synthesis like the Smith-Lemli-Opitz syndrome (270400). Defective cholesterol synthesis appears to interfere with *sonic hedgehog* action on prechordal mesoderm and to produce holoprosencephaly in patients with Smith-Lemli-Opitz syndrome.

A second defect of brain differentiation to be explained by a specific genetic alteration is

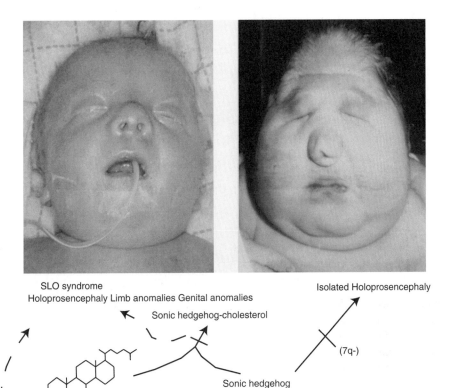

SLO syndrome
Holoprosencephaly Limb anomalies Genital anomalies

Sonic hedgehog-cholesterol

cholesterol

HO

7-dehydro
cholesterol

Isolated Holoprosencephaly

(7q-)

Sonic hedgehog
7q33

Limb anomalies

Fly hedgehog

Figure 9.10. Smith-Lemli-Opitz syndrome (left photograph), a condition with brain, limb, and genital anomalies, is caused by inadequate conversion of 7-dehydrocholesterol to cholesterol in certain tissues. Holoprosencephaly (right photograph) is associated with deletions of chromosome 7 that knock out one copy of the *sonic hedgehog* gene. Since the activity of *sonic hedgehog* protein requires covalent linkage to cholesterol, the brain defects in Smith-Lemli-Opitz syndrome (which sometimes include holoprosencephaly) may result from deficient *sonic hedgehog* protein activity.

lissencephaly (smooth brain). In patients with lissencephaly, the absence of normal brain convolutions produces severe developmental disability and seizures. A specific chromosome deletion at band 17p13 was shown to occur in many patients with lissencephaly, and a *LIS-1* gene with homology to GTP-binding proteins was characterized within the deletion interval. The *LIS-1* gene has homology to cyclins (cell cycle stimulators, Table 9.1) in yeast and to a gene called *Groucho* in the fly that is important for brain development. Once the *LIS-1* gene was characterized, patients with lissencephaly who had no obvious chromosome deletions were explained by finding point mutations within the gene.

A third defect of brain differentiation also affects the differentiation of genital structures from the intermediate mesoderm. The X-linked disorder called Kallmann syndrome

(308700) involves defective anterior brain differentiation with absent olfactory lobes and genital defects due to gonadotrophin deficiency. The genital defects include cryptorchidism (undescended testes) or small testes, and relate to defective gonadotrophin synthesis by the hypothalamus. Other symptoms of abnormal brain development occur in Kallmann syndrome, including mirror movements of the hands, deafness, spasticity, and mental retardation. Obvious deletions of chromosome band Xq22 in rare patients with Kallmann syndrome led to the discovery of a *KAL* gene with homology to other molecules important in brain development. One portion of the gene encodes a protease inhibitor domain that is seen in other molecules like neurophysin that influences axon elongation. Another portion encodes a domain of fibronectin-like repeats that are found in cell adhesion and extracellular matrix molecules. The *KAL* gene appears to be a specific growth regulator that modulates axonal growth and brain differentiation, just as the glypican-3 gene mentioned previously acts as a general growth regulator at mesoderm-derived cell surfaces (Table 9.5).

Human Developmental Genes: Limb and Skin Pigmentation Defects

The early segmentation genes of the fruit fly have already been discussed with regard to the role of *hedgehog* homologues in chick limb and human brain defects. Other homologues of the segmentation genes shown in Figure 9.5 have also been implicated in human developmental anomalies (Table 9.5). One of these is the human *GLI3* gene that is a homologue of the fly *Krüppel* gene. This gene was defined at chromosome band 7p13 that was disrupted by a balanced translocation in a patient with Greig syndrome (175700). Greig syndrome includes a large head, a broad nasal root with increased distance between the eyes (hypertelorism) and polydacty of the little fingers (postaxial) and the great toes (preaxial). Greig syndrome has a homologous phenotype in the mouse that is called extra toes (Table 9.4), and this pheno-

type is caused by the mouse version of the *GLI3* gene. The *GLI3* and *Krüppel* genes encode proteins with zinc finger motifs and polyalanine tracts that emphasize their likely roles as DNA-binding proteins that regulate transcription.

Waardenburg syndrome (193500) is caused by mutations in human homologues of the fly *paired* genes (Fig. 9.5). *Paired* genes were first identified because some contain a homeobox, then characterized by a similar type of DNA binding domain called the *paired* box. Waardenburg syndrome, like Greig syndrome, involves alterations in midline development to produce a broad nasal root and hypertelorism (Table 9.5). It also involves eye anomalies (differently colored eyes or heterochromia) and midline pigmentary defects of the hair (poliosis). The pigmentary anomalies, like those in piebald trait discussed in Case 9, may relate to abnormal neural crest migration known to be responsible for defects in colon function that occur in Waardenburg syndrome. The absence of posterior colonic ganglion cells produces chronic colon contraction and constipation called *Hirschsprung anomaly*. Waardenburg syndrome is caused by mutations in the *paired* homologue called *PAX3*, one of many *PAX* genes in the human genome. Similar defects are found in mice with *PAX3* mutations. Mutations in other *PAX* genes cause human iris or anterior eye chamber defects (aniridia, 106200; Peters anomaly with corneal clouding) and produce a corresponding mouse phenotype called *small eye*.

As would be expected, homologues of fly homeotic genes have also been related to human developmental anomalies. Homeotic mutations in humans have been difficult to identify, perhaps because many *HOX* mutations produce severe and lethal abnormalities that present as miscarriages. The regulated patterns of homeotic gene expression in chick limb (Fig. 9.7) predicted that homeotic gene mutations would be responsible for human limb defects. Mutations in the *HOXD13* gene are responsible for alterations of limb pattern in a disorder called type II synpolydactyly

(186000). Fusions (syndactyly) and extra digits (polydactyly) occur in the hands with no other anomalies. The mutations affect a region of the *HOXD13* gene that encodes a stretch of alanine residues. This stretch is greatly lengthened in mammalian *HOXD13* genes as opposed to the chick and zebrafish homologues, suggesting that they are necessary for the adaptable digits of many mammals. Other transcriptional regulators such as the fly *Krüppel* gene contain similar polyalanine tracts, suggesting that they function in DNA binding.

A final example of human genes acting during embryonic developmental does not concern a genetic disorder. Retinoic acid was mentioned as a key morphogen that influences chick limb development (Fig. 9.7*B*). Retinoic acid is known to activate homeotic genes and to interact with a family of diverse receptors specific for particular tissues. The chemical also has medical uses such as the suppression of acne, and has been marketed as a pharmaceutical product called Accutane. Despite warnings, women have taken Accutane while pregnant and produced children with severe patterns of anomalies that are referred to as retinoic acid embryopathy. The affliction of ears, eyes, jaw, and limbs in retinoic acid embryopathy is reminiscent of craniofacial defects in mice with *Hox* gene overexpression. The embryopathy undoubtedly reflects the importance of early patterning genes in human development, although it is not known whether the mechanisms involve increased *HOX* gene expression or other actions mediated by retinoic acid receptors.

Case 9 Follow-up: Although the diagnosis of piebald trait in this family seemed likely, other disorders such as Waardenburg syndrome (193500, discussed previously) or tuberous sclerosis (191100, with seizures, mental retardation, heart and kidney problems) also are associated with depigmented spots and need to be eliminated as diagnostic possibilties. Matching of the piebald trait with a specific gene might allow DNA diagnosis and explain the origin of depigmented spots. Rare patients with piebald trait were described with deletions of the chromosome 4q12–15 region, and this led to a search for genes in this region that could cause the phe-

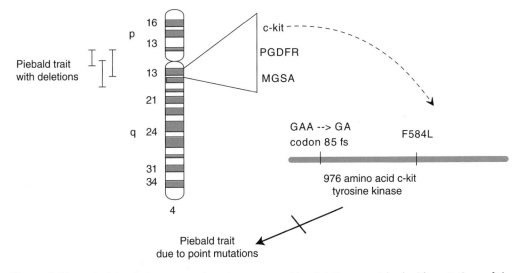

Figure 9.11. Piebald trait first mapped to chromosome 4 by deletions, matched with mutations of the signal transducing c-*kit* proto-oncogene. (GAA to GA frameshift, fs, or F84L phenylalanine to leucine).Homologous gene mutations cause the similar dominant spotted phenotype in mice. Ventral patches of depigmentation shown in Figure 9.1 would be expected if the ventral migration of dorsal neural crest/melanoblast cells were inhibited because of decreased c-*kit* activity.

notype (Fig. 9.11). A gene called *c-kit* had been recognized through its involvement in certain cancers, and was screened for mutations in patients with piebald trait. The *c-kit* gene is involved in a signal transduction pathway that appears to be necessary for normal melanoblast migration. Since melanoblasts differentiate from ventrally migrating neural crest cells, defective signal transduction and migration would account for the occurrence of depigmented spots in ventral regions. The piebald trait is thus a vivid illustration of a patterning defect, explained by a developmentally active gene that modulates signal transduction. The *c-kit* gene is also mutated in the *dominant spotted* mouse that has similar ventral spots. Mouse experiments defined the ligand for the *c-kit* gene to be mast cell growth factor, and a knockout of this ligand produces hypopigmentation of the entire coat (Steel trait). As with other examples previously given, defects in a gene acting earlier in the signal transduction pathway produce more generalized alterations of development.

■ 9.5. CANCER GENETICS

Cancers as Diseases of Cell Growth and Communication

At the beginning of this century, Theodor Boveri predicted that cancer would be explained by excess or deficient action of genetic factors. An exciting aspect of modern genetics has been the confirmation of Boveri's hypothesis by defining specific chromosomal and/or genetic changes in many types of cancer. The numbers of molecular changes causing sporadic or inherited cancers are now sufficiently great that they can be gathered under a new field called *cancer genetics.*

The first discovery leading to the recognition of genetic mechanisms in cancer involved cancer-causing viruses in various birds and mammals. These viruses, exemplified by Rous sarcoma virus in chickens, were often retroviruses that integrated their DNA or RNA genome into the chromosome(s) of host cells.

By dissecting the viral RNA or DNA, it was realized that certain viral genes were responsible for inducing the tumors in animals or cultured cells. A great deal of effort was then expended in looking for viruses or viral molecules in human cancers, but none have been successful. It is known that some viruses like herpes or hepatitis virus may chronically damage tissues and produce secondary cancers.

Evidence that single mutant genes could cause human cancers came from genetic complementation assays similar to those involved in the discovery of cyclins described previously. Cancer cells were fused with normal cells to form somatic cell hybrids, and the heterokaryons acted like cancer cells. A dominant-acting cancer gene seemed to be influencing the cytoplasm and/or nucleus of the normal cell to produce a rapidly proliferating heterokaryon. The dominant-acting cancer genes (*oncogenes*) were identified further by injecting DNA from cancer cells into normal cells (Fig. 9.12*A*). If injection of the genomic DNA transformed the normal cells into tumor cells, then the DNA was fractionated until a single segment could be associated with the tumor-inducing activity. Once these cellular oncogenes (*c-onc*) were isolated, they were found to be mutant versions of normal cellular genes (*proto-oncogenes*).

The startling fact that every cell contained genes that could mutate and cause cancer was soon reconciled with previous work on cancer-causing viruses. It was known that viral infection or transformation of cells with viral DNA could produce cancer cells (Fig. 9.12), and that many of these tumor viruses inserted their DNA into the host cell nucleus. If the virus integrated near a cellular gene active in signal transduction or growth regulation, then chance uptake of the regulatory gene would confer advantages for cell growth and viral replication. Under the relaxed constraints of viral DNA replication, the cellular gene could mutate rapidly and optimize its effects on viral replication. Viral oncogenes (*v-onc*), like cellular proto-oncogenes (*c-onc*), were normal cellular genes excised from their regulatory context and selected for their growth-promoting activ-

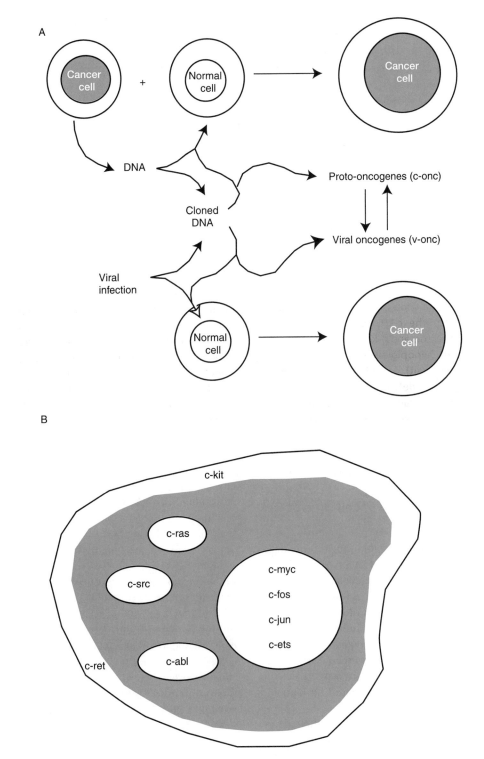

Figure 9.12. *A*, Transformation or transfection of normal cells with DNA from cancer cells or cancer-causing viruses can produce cancer cells. The cancer cell transformation can be used as an assay to isolated cloned genes that produce the cancer phenotype. The cancer-promoting genes from cellular (c-*onc*) or tumor viruses (v-*onc*) are mutated versions of normal cellular genes (proto-oncogenes) active in signal transduction and cell growth regulation. *B*, Cellular locations of selected oncogene products.

ity during multiple viral replication cycles. Homology among cellular and viral oncogenes genes was quickly demonstrated, explained by the fact that viruses acquired the same proto-oncogenes that occasionally mutated internally to become cellular oncogenes (Fig. 9.12A). Whether by viral uptake or spontaneous mutation, proto-oncogenes are subverted to escape normal constraints on cellular interaction and produce immortal cells that proliferate without regard for organismal function.

More than 40 cellular or viral oncogenes have now been characterized, each derived from a cellular proto-oncogene with a key role in signal transduction or growth-regulating pathways. As illustrated in Figure 9.12B, some proto-oncogenes encode surface proteins and receptors (e.g., *c-kit* or *c-rel*) while others encode cytoplasmic (*c-ras, c-abl*) or nuclear (e.g., *c-myc, c-fos*) proteins. The cytoplasmic proteins are often protein kinases and the nuclear proteins are often DNA-binding transcription factors (Fig. 9.12B). The names of oncogenes are condensed from the tumors or viruses from which they were characterized.

A second category of cancer genes was predicted by Knudson in his two-hit hypothesis (Fig. 9.13). Knudson studied the epidemiology of retinoblastoma, a tumor of retinal cells that exhibits autosomal dominant inheritance in some families (180200). Inherited eye tumors were predominantly bilateral (e.g., individuals II-2 and III-2 in Fig. 9.13A), while sporadic, noninherited cases of retinoblastoma were predominantly unilateral (e.g., individual I-2 in Fig. 9.13A). The inherited tumors often had multiple foci in each retina, as if multiple cells had independently become cancerous. Knudson explained this data by a model that attributed the retinoblastoma phenotype to two genetic mutations (two hits). The first mutation was a predisposing one, while the second converted a predisposed cell to frank retinoblastoma (Fig. 9.13B). The gene inherited in autosomal dominant retinoblastoma was transmitted to all cells in the body, but its presence in retinal cells predisposed them to cancer. When second mutations occurred in these pre-

disposed retinal cells, they became overtly cancerous and formed retinoblastomas.

The Two-Hit Hypothesis

Individuals without mutant retinoblastoma (*Rb*) alleles (individual I-2 in Fig. 9.13A) will be unlikely to develop retinoblastomas, since it is unlikely that two genetic mutations (two hits) will occur in the same retinal cell. Those tumors that do occur will present in older individuals (the chance of rare events increases with time) and will be isolated (i.e., unilateral and unifocal). Individuals who inherit mutant retinoblastoma alleles (individuals II-2 and III-2 in Fig. 9.13A) will have a predisposing mutation (first hit) in every retinal cell. Second mutations will be much more likely in these individuals, producing multifocal, bilateral tumors of earlier onset (Fig. 9.13A). Since every retinal cell contained the first mutation or hit, many different retinal cells were likely to sustain second mutations and become cancerous (Fig. 9.13B).

Subsequent characterization of the genetic "hits" revealed that they occurred at a locus on chromosome 13. The retinoblastoma or *Rb-1* locus prevented tumor development in retinal cells when it contained two normal alleles. If one allele was mutated by DNA or chromosomal change, this first hit predisposed that individual cell to become a tumor. When the homologous allele was inactivated by a second mutation, no normal *Rb-1* gene product was available to suppress tumor development. The *Rb-1* gene is now known to encode a cyclin type of protein that regulates the cell cycle. If both copies of the *Rb-1* gene are inactivated, then the cell cycle winds out of control and causes dysfunctional proliferation. It is not known why this proliferation is limited to retinal cells in most patients, although some patients also develop osteosarcomas (tumors of bone).

Once the *Rb-1* gene was characterized, individuals and their retinal tumors could be studied to define *Rb-1* mutant alleles (Fig. 9.13C). Predisposing mutations (first hit) were usually point mutations that disrupt *Rb-1* function, al-

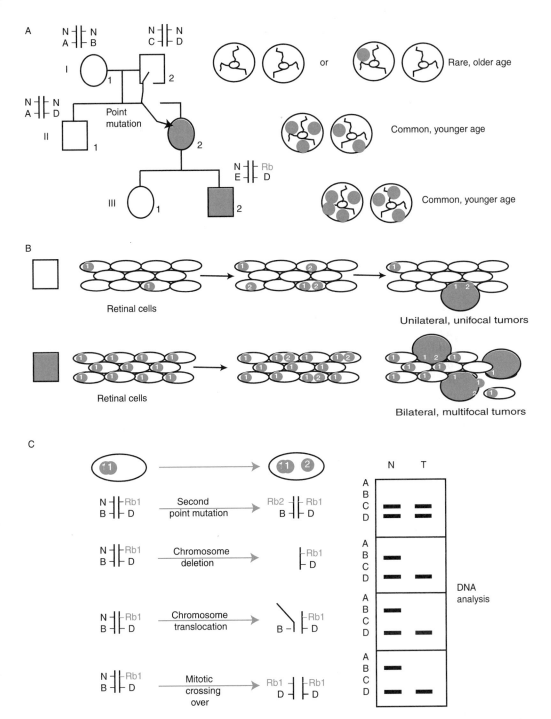

Figure 9.13. *A, B,* Family with autosomal dominant retinoblastoma showing rare, unifocal tumors in the retinae of individuals without the predisposing *Rb-1* gene mutation (individual I-2). Individuals with predisposing mutations (first hit—II-2, III-2) incur secondary mutations (second hit) in susceptible retinal cells that result in frequent, bilateral, and multifocal retinal tumors. *C,* Second-hit mechanisms that knock out the remaining *Rb-1* allele in susceptible retinal cells. These mechanisms may be distinguished by their impact on a neighboring polymorphic locus with alleles A–D as revealed by the companion Southern analyses. Note that chromosome deletion or rearrangment removes the neighboring locus and produces loss of heterozygosity as revealed by the presence of D but not DB genotypes in the tumor cells.

though small chromosome 13 deletions may remove one copy of the *Rb-1* locus in rare patients. Once the predisposing mutation occurs, a variety of second mutations have been identified in cancerous retinal cells. Interstitial deletions of chromosome 13, translocations that disrupt the *Rb-1* gene, and even loss of an entire chromosome 13 to produce monosomy are all mechanisms that can remove the second *Rb-1* allele (Fig. 9.13*C*). Other patients incur a second, independent point mutation that inactivates the second *Rb-1* allele in their tumor cells, or produce homozygous abnormal *Rb-1* alleles through mitotic recombination. Note that these mechanisms can be distinguished by analyzing DNA polymorphisms near the *Rb-1* locus (markers A–D in Fig. 9.13*C*). If analysis of DNA from individual II-2 in Figure 9.13*A* is performed using PCR or Southern blotting methods, then neighboring marker alleles will be retained with secondary point mutations but lost with secondary chromosome 13 deletions. Translocations will disrupt the second *Rb-1* allele but preserve nearby markers (Fig. 9.13*C*). It can be appreciated that similar types of DNA analysis can be used to isolate the causative tumor suppressor gene in families that inherit tumor predisposition. Once a candidate gene is available, its alteration in particular tumor types can be explored by looking for disruptions in translocations or loss in deletions and monosomies.

Numerous tumor suppressor genes like *Rb-1* are now defined, including the neurofibromin gene that is mutated in neurofibromatosis-1 (162200). Note that the predisposition to tumors is an autosomal dominant phenotype as illustrated by familial retinoblastoma or neurofibromatosis. However, acquisition of the cancer phenotype by predisposed cells is an autosomal recessive phenotype that requires inactivation of both autosomal alleles. The general phenomenon by which predisposed cells undergo a second mutation at a tumor suppressor locus to produce cancer is called *loss of heterozygosity*. As shown in Fig. 9.13*C*, loss of heterozygosity can be demonstrated by the absence of DNA marker alleles

in tumor cells. As with dominant-acting oncogenes, many tumor suppressor genes normally participate in growth-regulating or signal transduction pathways. Cancer genes, like the genes responsible for abnormal development, have illuminated new mechanisms that regulate cellular growth and interaction.

Cancer as a Multistep Process

Although tumor suppressor genes were elegantly anticipated by the two-hit hypothesis, cancer actually progresses through multiple genetic and cellular stages. The initial step is often a specific genetic aberration that produces an abnormal allele through mutation or chromosomal rearrangement. Additional mutations and chromosomal aberrations are then acquired to produce the grotesquely aberrant cells of advanced cancer. This sequential process has been defined for certain types of colon cancer, involving changes in the adenomatous polyposis of the colon (*APC*) gene, receptors for transforming growth factor-β (*TGF*-β), and other loci.

The sequential progression of cancer can certainly include environmental agents that promote carcinogenesis. Examples include cigarette smoking and asbestos exposure that are known carcinogens predisposing to lung cancer. Cancer is thus a multifactorial disease, where genes and environmental agents interact to initiate carcinogenesis in certain tissues. The genetic component is emphasized not only by the specific oncogenes and tumor suppressor genes listed in Table 9.6, but also by genetic diseases with high rates of cancer.

■ 9.6. INHERITED CANCERS AND CANCER SYNDROMES

Skin cancer is the most common cancer in the United States (>750,000 new cases per year), followed by lung, colon, and breast cancer (150,000 new cases) and prostate cancer (100,000 new cases). Agents of the external or internal environment have been emphasized in the causation of these cancers, exemplified re-

■ **TABLE 9.6.** Hereditary Cancers

Cancer	Causative Locus	Function
Retinoblastoma (180200)	*Rb-1* tumor suppressor gene	Transcription factor
Adenomatous polyposis coli (175100)	*APC* tumor suppressor gene	Regulates the *c-myc* proto-oncogene through interaction with *Wnt*-1 and β-cadherin
Lynch colon cancer (114500)	*MSH2* tumor suppressor gene	Involved in DNA repair
Chromosome 18 deletion colon cancer	*DCC* tumor suppressor gene	Homologous to FGF receptors, regulates cell growth
Breast cancer	*BRCA-1* tumor suppressor gene	Transcription factor
Li-Fraumeni syndrome (114480 breast, brain, blood cancers)	*p53* tumor suppressor gene	Cell cycle regulator
Ataxia-telangiectasia (208900) with lymphoid cancers	*ATM* tumor suppressor gene	Involved in DNA repair
Gorlin syndrome (109400) with basal cell carcinomas	*patched* tumor suppressor gene	Represses TGF-ß
Leukemias	*trithorax* proto-oncogene	Homeotic transcription factor activated by translocations
Lymphomas	*BCL-2* proto-oncogene	Cell death inhibitor

Notes: TGF, transforming growth factor; FGF, fibroblast growth factor; see text for descriptions of genes.

spectively by sunlight, tobacco, high fat and low fiber diet, estrogens, or testosterones. Genetic factors in these cancers have only recently been emphasized, since few cases were familial. This emphasis on environment changed as alterations of oncogenes and tumor suppressor genes were defined in diverse tumor tissues. Aiding this appreciation of genetics was the delineation of genetic diseases that showed high rates of cancer (Table 9.6). Frequently these genetic syndromes involve developmental anomalies, as illustrated by Down syndrome and its high incidence of leukemia. The characterization of genes responsible for familial cancers or for cancer syndromes has provided insights into the mechanisms of carcinogenesis and the possibilities of screening to identify high-risk individuals. Often the same genes are identified in early embryonic defects or later cancers, reflecting the dependence of both processes on transcriptional regulation and signal transduction pathways.

Inherited Cancers: Colon Cancer

Adenomatous or familial polyposis coli (APC—175100) provided evidence for an im-

portant colon cancer gene through its autosomal dominant inheritance. The disease begins as multiple benign tumor growths (polyps), mostly in the large intestine, that appear during the childhood and teenage years. About half of the individuals have bony tumors in the facial region and patches of hypertrophied retina that has been called Gardner syndrome. Each polyp has a risk for transformation to malignant colon cancer, causing a 100% incidence of colon cancer in affected individuals by age 50. Because of this high cancer risk, prophylactic removal of the colon is recommended in these individuals. Rare persons with deletion of chromosomal bands 5q15–5q22 provided a candidate gene region for familial polyposis, and this region was searched by positional cloning to isolate the adenomatous polyposis coli (*APC*) gene. In line with the general rule for Mendelian disorders as extreme phenotypes was the finding that mutant alleles of the *APC* gene also occur in sporadic cases of colon cancer. About 80% of colon cancers that occur in individuals without a family history and without manifestations of Gardner syndrome have mutations at the *APC* locus.

The *APC* gene is a tumor suppressor gene, and the inactivation of both normal alleles in intestinal cells initiates a cascade of genetic changes. The direct action of *APC* occurs through a cell junction molecule named β-cadherin, which is a homologue of the fly segmentation gene *armadillo*. The *APC*/β-cadherin complex is normally destroyed in the cytoplasm of colonic epithelial cells, but some complex remains active in the presence of an *APC* mutant allele. This active complex in turn signals the nucleus to transcribe the growth-promoting proto-oncogene *c-myc*, contributing to polyp formation. The fly *wingless* gene product interacts with *armadillo* product to produce segmentation, and the human homologue *Wnt*-1 protein interacts with *APC* and β-cadherin proteins to regulate the cellular production of *c-myc*. This example is one of many that illustrate the overlap between genes mediating altered cell communications in both cancer and development.

Hereditary nonpolyposis colon cancer or Lynch syndrome (114500) is another disease predisposing to colon cancer that is not associated with multiple colon polyps. Lynch syndrome is caused by a gene called *MSH2* that repairs mismatched DNA sequences on homologous chromosomes. The lack of one *MSH2* allele increases the mutation rate of susceptible tissues, particularly those at the bowel surface that undergo rapid turnover. Genes like *MSH2* (and the *ATM* gene responsible for ataxia-telangiectasia described in the section on Disorders of DNA Repair) have been called caretaker genes by Kinzler and Vogelstein (1998), because they indirectly suppress neoplasia by maintaining the integrity of the genome. A third gene involved in colon cancer was defined by study of cancer tissue rather than families. The deleted in colon carcinoma (*DCC*) gene was detected by noting frequent deletions at chromosomal band 18q21 in colon cancers. The *DCC* gene encodes a transmembrane protein with immunoglobulin-like regions similar to those of the fibroblast growth factor receptors diagrammed in Figure 9.9. There is also a domain characteristic of cell adhesion pro-

teins, suggesting that the *DCC* protein acts as a signal transducing receptor that conveys growth-regulating signals from extracellular matrix molecules. The progression of colon cancer may thus proceed through the loss of a tumor suppressor activity (*APC*), enhancement of mutations (*MSH2*), to decreased cell growth control (*DCC*). When one defective *APC* or *MSH2* allele is inherited through the germ line, then a large number of polyps or unstable cells will arise in the colon and have a virtual 100% chance for tumor progression. When no predisposing mutations are inherited in the germ line, then cumulative effects of aging and diet may produce a colon cell that progresses to a unifocal, sporadic cancer.

Inherited Cancers: Breast Cancer

Breast and prostate cancer are sufficiently frequent that all individuals may be affected if they live long enough. Familial breast cancer is much less common, but enough families were identified to show genetic linkage of breast cancer susceptibility to a locus on chromosome 17. The isolation of candidate genes from this region revealed a gene called *BRCA1* (breast cancer-1) that was mutated in families with high frequencies of breast cancer. *BRCA-1* is a large gene spread over 100,000 bp with 22 exons encoding a protein of 1863 amino acids. The coding sequence contains a prominent motif known as a RING domain that is typical of proteins that bind to DNA, suggesting that *BRCA-1* acts as a transcription factor. Families with *BRCA-1* mutations have higher frequencies of ovarian as well as breast cancer, emphasizing the potential value of this gene for screening of high-risk individuals. Complicating the use of screening are the many *BRCA-1* mutations that occur, the prospect of prophylactic mastectomies in women who test positive, and the age at which testing should occur. These complications of genetic screening are discussed more extensively in Chapter 12.

The contribution of *BRCA-1* to breast cancer is emphasized by the odds for its detection. Twelve percent of woman under 30 who develop breast cancer will have mutations in *BRCA-1*, as opposed to 3% who are over age 40. In families with 3 or more affected individuals, 40% will have *BRCA-1* mutations, rising to 91% where 2 or more individuals have breast cancer and 2 or more have ovarian cancer. Additional genes predisposing to breast cancer, including the *BRCA-2* and *p53* genes (see next section), should increase the sensitivity of genetic screening for women who have relatives with early-onset breast cancer. The serious consequences of positive screening (bilateral mastectomy) and the significant possibility of false negative results in breast cancer screening require considerable expertise for appropriate counseling and interpretation (see Chapter 14).

Cancer Syndromes: Li-Fraumeni Syndrome

In a review of 648 children with a rare muscle tumor called rhabdomyosarcoma, Li and Fraumeni (1969) identified four families in whom a relative had sarcoma. These families also contained individuals with breast, brain, and blood cancers, suggesting that they were affected with a hereditary cancer syndrome. The syndrome was to be explained by the examination of a gene encoding a 53 kD protein that was initially classified as an oncogene. The *p53* gene was first characterized based on the elevation of its protein product in cells transformed by oncogenic viruses like simian virus 40. The *p53* genes isolated from such cells appeared to be oncogenes, because they could be injected along with other oncogenes and cause cancer transformation as in Figure 9.12. Then it was realized that these *p53* genes were mutated, and that normal *p53* genes were in fact tumor suppressor genes. In Li-Fraumeni syndrome (114480), individuals receive a mutant copy of *p53* that predisposes them to second hits in susceptible tissues. The *p53* gene is somewhat unique in that the protein produced by certain mutant alleles can interact with that produced by normal alleles and render it inactive. This dominant-negative effect of certain

p53 alleles is similar to that discussed in Chapter 8 for type I collagen mutations that cause osteogenesis imperfecta. Individuals with Li-Fraumeni syndrome have *p53* mutations without this dominant negative effect, since such actions would probably disrupt early embryonic development and result in spontaneous abortion.

In addition to its involvement in Li-Fraumeni syndrome, the *p53* gene is mutated in more than 50 types of cancer, including cancers of the lung, breast, lymphnodes, esophagus, brain, pancreas, prostate, and stomach. Often the mutation in *p53* occurs in a sequence of cancer progression, and its laboratory detection is frequently used as a marker for tumor metastasis and poor prognosis. The *p53* gene acts by turning on a second gene that encodes a *p21* protein. The *p21* protein binds to a cyclin-dependent kinase like those listed in Table 9.1 and slows down the cell cycle. The *p53* protein also rises significantly in cells with damaged DNA. If the *p53* gene is knocked out in these cells, then their normal progression through apoptosis and cell death does not occur. The *p53* protein is thus a damage control agent as well as a cell growth suppressor, emphasizing again the close link between cell growth and cell death. It is understandable why mutation of one *p53* allele increases susceptibility to several types of cancer as in the Li-Fraumeni syndrome, and why *p53* mutations crop up frequently during the analysis of sporadic cancers. Restoration of *p53* activity in cancer cells should correct these deficits in growth or damage control, and therapeutic trials using *p53* gene therapy are underway.

Genetic Syndromes with Cancer Predisposition: Disorders of DNA Repair

The conjunction of DNA damage and cancer discussed with the *MSH2* and *p53* genes also occurs in several genetic syndromes that exhibit DNA repair defects and higher incidences of cancer (Table 9.6). One example is ataxia-telangiectasia (208900), which produces an abnormal gait due to neurologic damage (ataxia) and dilated blood vessels (telangiectasias) in the conjunctiva of the eyes. Ataxia-telangiectasia is due to mutation in the *ATM* (ataxia-telangiectasia mutated) gene, which acts to arrest division of cells with damaged DNA. Like the *p53* gene, the failure of *ATM*-mediated damage control renders patients with ataxia-telangectasia susceptible to cancers such as T-cell leukemia, Hodgkin's lymphoma, stomach, brain, liver, ovary, and breast cancer. Correlating with the high rate of lymphatic malignancies is a defect in immune function represented by defective T-cell response and thymic hypoplasia. There is also a high rate of chromosome breakage, usually involving translocations of chromosomes 7 and 14 that led to the identification of the *ATM* gene. The association of developmental abnormalities (cerebellar atrophy, blood vessel dilations), chromosome breakage, and cancer is seen in several other DNA repair defects as listed in Table 9.6. Bloom syndrome, a disorder with growth failure, cancer predisposition, and increased sister chromatid exchange, was discussed in Chapter 7.

Overlap Between Developmental Genes and Oncogenes

As mentioned for the *APC* gene above, many cancer genes are developmental genes in disguise. Examples include the fly maternal gene *dorsal* and the fly segmentation gene *wingless* (see Fig. 9.5), which are respectively homologous to the c-*rel* proto-oncogene and the *int*-1 (now called *Wnt*-1) gene found as the integration site for a mouse mammary tumor virus. A striking example of this overlap is afforded by the *patched* gene product that was discussed as the receptor for the *sonic hedgehog* gene product. Recall that the *sonic hedgehog* gene has been implicated in chick wing development (Fig. 9.7) and in human holoprosencephaly (Fig. 9.10). The human homologue of *patched* is now known to be responsible for the basal cell nevus or Gorlin syndrome (109400), a condition with multiple skeletal anomalies, dental cysts, and skin moles or nevi that

progress to become basal cell carcinomas. In the fly, *patched* acts to repress the transcription of transforming growth factor-β family members. Its inactivation in Gorlin syndrome may thus be accompanied by increased growth factor expression and conversion of nevi to basal cell skin cancers. As mentioned previously, basal cell carcinomas are very common in temperate climates. Mutational analysis of the *patched* gene may prove extremely useful in distinguishing these tumors from normal nevi and in measuring their invasiveness.

Another correlation of cancer genes with developmental genes occurs in the leukemias. Leukemias derive from the uncontrolled proliferation of leukemoid (white blood) cells due to failures of stem cell differentiation. Many types of leukemia are associated with specific chromosome translocations, allowing researchers to define the genes involved at the translocation breakpoints. Several of these genes proved to be human homologues of fly homeotic genes, including members of the four human homeotic clusters (A–D) and isolated genes with homeoboxes such as the homologue to fly *trithorax*. Although the precise mechanisms by which translocated *HOX* genes cause cancer are not defined, it has been shown that overexpression of specific *HOX* genes in transgenic mice can cause the proliferation of white cells and the development of leukemia.

Another group of genes located at leukemia translocation junctions are the retinoic acid receptors. As discussed previously, retinoic acid acts through its receptors to activate homeotic genes in various model organisms, and this important developmental pathway seems to have been subverted in white blood cells to produce malignancy. As with previous examples, the common themes in these developmental and neoplastic transformations are transcriptional regulation and signal transduction.

Programmed cell death is also a prominent feature of white cell development. More than 75% of B-cell and 95% of T-cell precursors undergo cell death, so it is not surprising that certain lymphoid cancers interfere with this process of selection and differentiation. One of the genes implicated by translocation break-points in leukemia is the *BCL2* proto-oncogene that was discussed as a cell death inhibitor in *C. elegans*. In this case, disruption of *BCL2* gene activity seems responsible rather than the overexpression implied for *HOX* genes. Discussion of white cell lineage sets the stage for the final example of cell interaction discussed in this chapter, that of the immune system.

Case 9 Follow-up: The proto-oncogene *c-kit* was identified as an oncogene that was activated in certain leukemias (Fig. 9.12*B*). It was then found to have a role in melanoblast development, illustrated by its causation of piebald trait in humans. Common involvement of the *c-kit* gene in the control of white blood cell proliferation and the regulation of neural crest and melanoblast migration illustrates that the same genes may go awry in developmental abnormalities and neoplasia.

■ 9.7. IMMUNOGENETICS

The immune system is an example of tissues that continue development after birth. Like the gonads, skin, and blood, stem cells of the immune system undergo constant cycles of differentiation to provide defense against invasion. The study of immune function has provided many insights into genetics, illustrated by its importance in genetic diagnosis, its relevance to transfusion and transplantation, and its utility in establishing markers for autoimmune diseases such as diabetes mellitus. Because excellent references are available in immunology (see next section), discussion here is limited to genetic diseases causing immunodeficiency. Some additional information is included on the companion website (http://www.wiley.com/wilson/).

The Two Types of Immune Response are Illustrated by Genetic Immunodeficiencies

The cellular and humoral immune responses arise as separate lineages from the same stem cell (Fig. 9.14), as illustrated by their derangements in particular genetic diseases. Severe combined immune deficiency (SCID) diseases involve the inability of stem cells to proliferate and form T- or B-cell precursors. Some types of SCID are caused by cellular defects in nucleotide salvage, illustrated by adenosine deaminase (102700) and nucleoside phosphorylase (164050) deficiencies. The inability to salvage nucleotides from nucleic acid degradation impairs tissues such as immune stem cells that require rapid expansion for function. In adenosine deaminase deficiency, the growing points of bone (metaphyses) are also affected due to inability of chondrocytes to proliferate. The result is deficiency in both Bursa- and thymus-derived lymphocytes (B- and T-cells), producing deficiency of immunoglobulins and low numbers of lymphocytes. Affected patients with SCID face recurrent bacterial infections due to immunoglobulin deficiency plus recurrent viral and fungal infections due to defective cellular immunity. Until recently, therapy for SCID was possible only by immunoglobulin infusions and bone marrow transplant to reconstitute the defective stem cells. Unfortunately, the transplanted bone marrow cells would recognize the host as foreign and initiate an immune response known as the graft-versus-host reaction. Recent approaches to children with SCID have attempted enzyme or gene replacement therapy as discussed in Chapter 10.

Other genetic diseases illuminate the separate functions of the humoral and cellular arms of the immune response (Fig. 9.14). Bruton's agammaglobulinemia (300300) involves defective differentiation of primitive B-cells into mature B-cells that synthesize immunoglobulins (plasma cells). The defective gene encodes a tyrosine kinase that allows a particular B-cell to expand after contacting a specific antigen on its cell surface. In the absence of this signal to the nucleus, the B-cell DNA does not rearrange constant, joining, and variable regions in a way that promotes specific immunoglobulin synthesis. As with development and cancer, a defect in a signal transduction pathway leads to

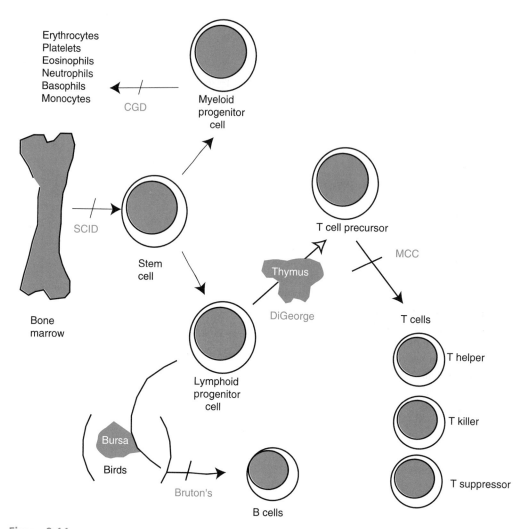

Figure 9.14. B- and T-cell lineages illustrated by examples of genetic disease. Severe combined immune deficiency (SCID) interferes with stem cell production, while DiGeorge syndrome with thymus deficiency interferes with T-cell formation. Mucocutaneous candidiasis (MCC) interferes with T-cell maturation, Bruton's agammaglobulinemia with B-cell maturation, and chronic granulomatous disease (CGD) with phagocyte function.

specific immune disease. Patients with agammaglobulinemia can fight off viral or fungal infections, but develop recurrent bacterial infections at age 4–8 months when their maternal immunoglobulins are deplected.

Cellular immune deficiencies often produce syndromes with multiple medical problems, perhaps because the diversity of T-cells means that many signal transduction pathways may be impacted that are shared by other organ systems. One group of T-cell deficiencies results from a failure of the thymus to develop, including the DiGeorge anomaly of branchial arch defects (Fig. 9.14). Abnormal development of branchial arches I–II may produce an unusual facial appearance with down-turned corners of the mouth, abnormal ears and a small jaw, while defective development of arches III and IV can produce cardiac anomalies, thymic hypoplasia, and parathyroid hormone deficiency with low serum calcium levels. The children have milder cellular immune deficiencies than those with SCID, but are susceptible to chronic yeast and severe viral infections. One form of DiGeorge anomaly is associated with deletions of chromosome 22 as discussed in Chapter 7.

Other cellular immune deficiencies may affect interactions of T-cell subpopulations, producing susceptibility to particular fungal or viral agents. Chronic mucocutaneous candidiasis (114580, 212050) exhibits extreme susceptibility to candidal (yeast) infections of the mouth and skin, while Duncan syndrome (308240) involves susceptibility to Epstein-Barr viral infections that cause diseases such as infectious mononucleosis. The complexity of T-cell interactions is also illustrated by infections diseases such as the acquired immune deficiency syndrome (AIDS), because the ratio of CD4 (helper cell) to CD8 (killer cell) surface antigens on the patient's lymphocytes are important indicators of disease progress.

A last category of immune deficiencies involves the white blood cells that engulf foreign antigens or cells after they have been aggregated by immunoglobulins or killer T-cells. White blood cells with a single nucleus (monocytes or phagocytes) must be able to respond to immune complex signals and to destroy the antigens with lysosomal hydrolases. A prototypic disease in this category is chronic granulomatous disease (306400), where the gene encoding cytochrome b245 is defective. Males with this deficiency cannot generate hydrogen peroxide in their phagocytes that is essential for bacterial killing. Affected patients develop chronic skin infections (boils, pustules) with layers of inflamed tissue (granulomas) due to persisting infections with staphylococcus and other bacteria. Several autosomal recessive types of chronic granulomatous diseases have also been described (233690, 233700, 233710) that inhibit the ability of phagocytes to adhere to the offending antigen or to activate the appropriate cytochrome. These diseases illustrate the cascade of signal transduction pathways involved in immune cell stimulation and function (Fig. 9.14).

PROBLEM SET 9
Developmental Genetics

9.1–9.5 Match the following human developmental disorders with their causative gene families
  (A) Simpson-Golabi-Behmel overgrowth syndrome
  (B) Crouzon craniosynostosis syndrome
  (C) Holoprosencephaly
  (D) Lissencephaly
  (E) Kallman anosmia-genital hypoplasia syndrome

9.1. fibroblast growth factor receptors

9.2. extracellular matrix-membrane molecules

9.3. cell adhesion molecule

9.4. G-protein signal-transducing molecule

9.5. fly segmentation homologue

9.6–9.10. Match the following neoplastic disorders with the relevant gene families
  (A) Li-Fraumeni syndrome
  (B) breast cancer
  (C) Gorlin basal cell nevus syndrome
  (D) ataxia-telangiectasia
  (E) lymphomas

9.6. tumor suppressor gene active in DNA repair

9.7. tumor suppressor gene that regulates the cell cycle

9.8. tumor suppressor gene with homology to fly *patched*

9.9. tumor suppressor gene that acts as transcription factor

9.10. proto-oncogene that regulates cell death

PROBLEM SET 9
Answers

9.6 D; 9.7 A; 9.8 C; 9.9 B; 9.10 E
9.1 B; 9.2 A; 9.3 E; 9.4 D; 9.5 C

PROBLEM SET 9
Solutions

9.1–9.5. Table 9.5 summarizes fibroblast growth factor receptor mutations in Crouzon syndrome (answer 9.1B), glypican-3 extracellular matrix molecule defects in Simpson-Golabi-Behmel syndrome (answer 9.2A), *KAL* cell adhesion molecule mutations in Kallman syndrome (answer 9.3E), *LIS-1* G protein mutations in lissencephaly (answer 9.4D), and *sonic hedgehog* mutations in holoprosencephaly (answer 9.5C).

9.6–9.10. Table 9.6 summarizes *ATM* mutations in ataxia-telangiectasia (answer 9.6D), p53 mutations in Li-Fraumeni syndrome (answer 9.7A), *patched* mutations in Gorlin syndrome (answer 9.8C), *BRCA-1* mutations in hereditary breast cancer (answer 9.9B), and *BCL-2* mutations in lymphomas (answer 9.10E).

BIBLIOGRAPHY

General References

Benjamini E, Sunshine G, Leskowitz S. 1996. *Immunology: A Short Course,* 3rd ed. New York: Wiley-Liss.
De Pomerai D. 1990. *From Gene to Animal: An Introduction to the Molecular Biology of Animal Development.* 2nd ed. Cambridge: Cambridge University Press.
Gilbert SF. 1988. *Developmental Biology,* 2nd ed. Sunderland, MA: Sinauer.
Wilkins AS. 1986. *Genetic Analysis of Animal Development.* New York: John Wiley & Sons.

The Cell Cycle

Jacks T, Weinburg RA. 1998. The expanding role of cell cycle regulators. *Science* 280:1035–1036.
King RW, Deshaies RJ, Peters J-M, Kirschner MW. 1996. How proteolysis drives the cell cycle. *Science* 274:1652–1658.
Nasmyth K. 1996. Putting the cell cycle in order. *Science* 274:1643–1645.

Cell Death

Barinaga M. 1998. Death by dozens of cuts. *Science* 280:32-34.
Stellar H. 1995. Mechanisms and genes of cellular suicide. *Science* 267:1445–1449.
Thompson CT. 1995. Apoptosis in the pathogenesis and treatment of disease. *Science* 267:1456–1462.

Signal Transduction

Darnell JE Jr. 1997. STATs and gene regulation. *Science* 277:1630–1635.
Edelman GM. 1983. Cell adhesion molecules. *Science* 219:450–457.
Gilman AG. 1989. G proteins and regulation of adenylyl cyclase. *JAMA* 262:1819–1824.

Early Patterning in Flies and Worms

Anderson K. 1995. One signal, two body axes. *Science* 269:489–490.
Nusslein-Volhard C, Weischaus E. 1980. Mutations affecting segment number and polarity in Drosophila. *Nature* 287:795–801.
Nusslein-Volhard C, Frohnhöfer HG, Lehmann R. 1987. Determination of anteroposterior polarity in Drosophila. *Science* 238:1675–1681.
Peifer M. 1994. The two faces of *hedgehog. Science* 266:1492–1493.
Robertson EJ. 1997. Left-right asymmetry. *Science* 275:1280–1281.

Vertebrate Embryology

Duboule D. 1994. How to make a limb? *Science* 266:575–576.
McMahon AP, Moon RT. 1989. Ectopic expression of the proto-oncogene *int-1* in Xenopus embryos leads to duplication of the embryonic axis. *Cell* 58:1075–1084.
Nusslein-Volhard C. 1994. Of flies and fishes. *Science* 266:572–574.
Weeks DL, Melton DA. 1987. A maternal mRNA localized to the vegetal hemisphere in *Xenopus* eggs codes for a growth factor related to TGF-β. *Cell* 51:861–867.

Mouse Genetics

Fleming A, Copp AJ. 1998. Embryonic folate metabolism and mouse neural tube defects. *Science* 280:2107–2109.
Martin G. 1996. Pass the butter. *Science* 274:1996.
Murray JC. 1995. Face facts: Genes, environment, and clefts. *Am J Hum Genet* 57:227–232.
Ryan TM, Ciavatta DJ, Townes TM. 1997. Knockout-transgenic mouse model of sickle cell disease. *Science* 278:873–878.

Human Developmental Genetic Disorders

Barsh GS. 1995. Pigmentation, pleiotrophy, and genetic pathways in humans and mice. *Am J Hum Genet* 57:743–747.

Fleischman RA, Saltman DL, Stastny V, Zneimer S. 1991. Deletion of the *c-kit* proto-oncogene in the human developmental defect piebald trait. *Proc Natl Acad Sci USA* 88:10885–10889.

Muragaki Y, Mundlos S, Upton J, Olsen BR. 1996. Altered growth and branching patterns in syn-polydactyly caused by mutations in *HOXD13*. *Science* 272:548–551.

Park W-J, Bellus GA, Jabs EW. 1995. Mutations in fibroblast growth factor receptors: Phenotypic consequences during eukaryotic development. *Am J Hum Genet* 57:748–754.

Proto-oncogenes and Growth Factors

Culotta E, Koshland DE Jr. 1993. *p53* sweeps through cancer research. *Science* 262: 1958–1961.

Davies DR, Armstong JG, Thakker N, Horner K, Guy SP, Clancy T, Sloan P, Blair V, Dodd C, Warnes TW, Harris R, Evans DGR. 1995. Severe Gardner syndrome in families with mutations restricted to a specific region of the *APC* gene. *Am J Hum Genet* 57:1151–1158.

Tumor Suppressor Genes

Friend S. 1994. *p53*: A glimpse at the puppet behind the shadow play. *Science* 265:334–335.

Hansen MF, Cavenee WK. 1988. Retinoblastoma and the progression of tumor genetics. *Trend Genet* 4:125–128.

Li FP, Fraumeni JF Jr. 1969. Soft tissue Sarcomas, breast cancer, and other neoplasms. A familial syndrome? *Am Intern Med* 71:747–752, 1969.

Malkin D, Li FP, Strong LC, Fraumeni JF Jr, Nelson CE, Kim DH, Kassel J, Gryka MA, Bischoff FZ, Tainsky MA, Friend SH. 1990. Germ line *p53* mutations in a familial syndrome of breast cancer, sarcomas, and other neoplasms. *Science* 250:1233–1238.

Weinberg RA. 1991. Tumor suppressor genes. *Science* 254:1138–1146.

Human Cancers

Fearon ER. 1997. Human cancer syndromes: Clues to the origin and nature of cancer. *Science* 278: 1043–1050.

Goodrich LV, Milenkovic L, Higgins KM, Scott MP. 1997. Altered neural cell fates and medulloblastoma in mouse *patched* mutants. *Science* 277: 1109–1114.

Hoskins KF, Stopfer JE, Calzone KA, Merajver SK, Rebbeck TR, Garber JE, Weber BL. 1995. Assessment and counseling for women with a family history of breast cancer: A guide for clinicians. *JAMA* 273:577–585.

Kinzler KW, Vogelstein B. 1998. Landscaping the cancer terrain. *Science* 280:1036–1037.

Overlap of Cancer and Developmental Genetics

Johnson RL, Rothman AL, Xie J, Goodrich LV, Bare JW, Bonifas JM, Quinn AG, Myers RM, Cox DR, Epstein EH Jr, Scott MP. 1996. Human homolog of *patched*, a candidate gene for the basal cell nevus syndrome. *Science* 272: 1668–1672.

Look AT. 1997. Oncogenic transcription factors in the human acute leukemias. *Science* 278: 1059–1064.

Peifer M. 1996. Regulating cell proliferation: As easy as *APC*. *Science* 272:974–975.

Pennesi E. 1998. How a growth control path takes a wrong turn to cancer. *Science* 281:1438–1441.

Immunogenetics

Alt FW, Blackwell TK, Yancopoulos GD. 1987. Development of the primary antibody repertoire. *Science* 238:1079–1087.

Ward PA. 1995. Cytokines, inflammation, and autoimmune diseases. *Hosp Pract* May 15:35–41.

NEW APPLICATIONS OF CLINICAL GENETICS: ATYPICAL INHERITANCE MECHANISMS AND GENE THERAPY

■ LEARNING OBJECTIVES

1. X-linked inheritance was the first violation of Mendelian laws; somatic or germ-line mosaicism, chromosome microdeletions, genomic imprinting, triplet repeat expansion, and mitochondrial inheritance are additional examples.

2. Identical microdeletions with different parental origins cause the Prader-Willi and Angelman syndromes, revealing the operation of genomic imprinting in humans.

3. Genomic imprinting produces different DNA methylation and gene expression patterns within certain chromosomal regions according to their origins in maternal or paternal gametes.

4. Uniparental disomy refers to the inheritance of two homologous chromosomes from one parent, frequently causing disease because of abnormal genomic imprinting.

5. Triplet repeat expansion diseases produce anticipation in pedigrees and unusual inheritance patterns.

6. Genetic engineering allows the production of rare proteins; enzyme therapy involves the intravenous administration of purified enzymes to correct genetic enzyme deficiencies.

7. Gene therapy employs cloned genes in specially constructed vectors to alter gene expression in patients with genetic diseases. Somatic gene therapy is a reality but germ-line therapy remains a controversial possibility.

Case 10A: *A Child with Morbid Obesity*

An 11-year-old male (Fig. 10.1A) is evaluated because of mild obesity and hypogonadism. His past medical history reveals that he had severe hypotonia and failure to thrive with hypogonadism in early life. In the past few years, he has gained more than 100 lbs with unusual eating behaviors. Often he will raid the kitchen at night, making unusual snacks on counters and on the floor. He has not slept well for the past 2 years, and his height growth is actually below normal centiles despite his large weight. He now has difficulty

227

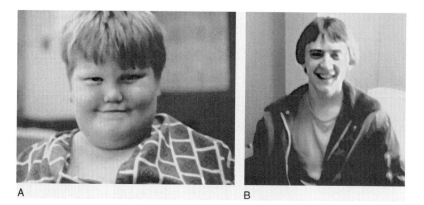

Figure 10.1.   *A*, Case 10A; *B*, case 10B.

walking without respiratory distress and cannot participate in sports or physical education at school.

■ 10.1. INTRODUCTION—EARLY EXCEPTIONS TO MENDEL'S RULES

The ability to isolate and manipulate genetic material has led to new applications in clinical genetics. For many Mendelian disorders in humans, gene isolation has confirmed Mendel's principles and given physical definition to his concept of hereditary factors. For other disorders, gene characterization has revealed atypical inheritance mechanisms that are outside the scope of Mendel's experiments. In addition, new approaches for recombining and injecting genes or enzymes is expanding the passive model of genetics as diagnosis and counseling to include active modes of therapy. As expressed by a pioneer in this transformation, the geneticist has changed from being a "bookie" giving odds to a "fixer" that changes them (Schmickel, 1974).

Segregation of independent and paired alleles (A, a) was Mendel's premier hypothesis, with the ratios of offspring being simply derived (AA, 2Aa, aa). Allele interaction accounted for dominant versus recessive inheritance, whereas extrapolation to multiple alleles or loci accommodated the behavior of metric (e.g., height, blood pressure), multifactorial (e.g., schizophrenia, diabetes), or threshold traits (e.g., common birth defects). Physical evidence for chromosomes explained why independent assortment was occasionally violated by linkage, and why some traits exhibited strong sex preference (X-linkage). Triumphs of the Mendelian model include Garrod's inborn error, Beadle's one gene-one enzyme hypothesis, and the route from inherited trait to DNA diagnosis that is now possible.

Molecular technology combined with improved phenotypic delineation has catalyzed a genuine scientific revolution in clinical genetics. The simple rules for loci, alleles, and segregation derived by Mendel have been outgrown; a new genetic paradigm has emerged. Although Mendelian reasoning could be stretched to include multifactorial and threshold traits, newer embryologic and genetic findings can no longer be accommodated. Contiguous gene deletions, altered gene dosage, gene expression differences based on parent of origin, and expanding triplet repeats have transcended Mendelian boundaries. These new mechanisms provide many additional reasons why the patient with no family history may reflect a genetic change and add new applications of genetics to clinical practice.

■ 10.2. SOMATIC AND GERM-LINE MOSAICISM

The origin of human individuals from a fertilized egg involves an enormous number of cell

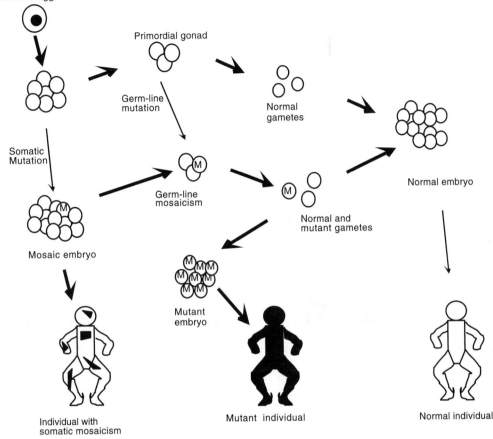

Figure 10.2. Somatic versus germ-line mosaicism. A fertilized egg (zygote, upper left) develops into a morula and blastocyst before a separate cell lineage derives from the yolk sac to form the primordial gonad and germ cells. Mutations occurring in these germ cells will produce germ-line mosaicism that can be transmitted to offspring, while mutations in somatic cells can produce affected body regions without germ-line transmission.

divisions and a split between two major cell lineages (Fig. 10.2). Most cells form the body or soma, and these somatic cells arise from the three germ layers as described in Chapter 9. A minor cell lineage with major import for reproduction are the primordial germ cells that arise from the yolk sac. The germ cells acquire special properties, including the capability for meiotic division and attendant features such as the erasure of genomic imprints (Section 10.4 below). If a mutation M occurs early in embryogenesis, it may be transmitted to somatic cells that will comprise particular regions of the body. The individual will then be a com-

posite of cells containing normal and mutant alleles, a combination known as *somatic mosaicism*. The occurrence of somatic mosaicism for chromosomal anomalies was mentioned in Chapter 7, and the occurrence of somatic mutations in adults to cause cancer was discussed in Chapter 9. Somatic mutations are not transmitted to descendants unless their distribution includes the primordial germ cells.

Visible examples of somatic mosaicism have been documented for diseases such as neurofibromatosis-1 (162200), in which the distinctive café-au-lait spots and neurofibroma tumors may occur in one limb or one body region. A recently recognized category of diseases that are caused by somatic mosaicism are those classified under the term hypomelanosis of Ito (146150). The distinctive lesions in these patients are hypopigmented spots, which sometimes follow an autosomal dominant form of inheritance. Recent analysis of skin biopsy tissue has shown that most patients are mosaic for chromosomal aberrations; the reason for hypopigmentation is not clear, but it may represent delayed melanoblast migration of aberrant cells as discussed for piebald trait in Chapter 9.

As discussed in Chapter 7, females are normally mosaic for cells that inactivate one or the other X chromosome. In female carriers of X-linked disorders with visible phenotypes, patches of affected tissue alternate with patches of unaffected tissue depending on whether the X chromosome carrying the normal allele is inactivated. A special class of X-linked dominant diseases are particularly striking in this regard. X-linked dominant forms of certain skin and skeletal diseases (e.g., incontinentia pigmenti, 308300, X-linked chondrodysplasia punctata, 302960) show asymmetric lesions in females with one normal allele due to mosaicism for X inactivation. Often the dominant allele is lethal when transmitted to affected males, so that patchy expression in females with increased miscarriages (aborted males) are hallmarks for these X-linked dominant diseases.

Germ-line mosaicism does not produce identifiable physical features and must be recognized based on the family history. For autosomal dominant or X-linked diseases, the characteristic of germ-line mosaicism is multiple affected offspring with normal parents. For autosomal dominant disorders, correct paternity must be proved before germ-line mosaicism can be assumed. Examples demonstrated by molecular analysis include achondroplasia (100800), osteogenesis imperfecta (166240), and tuberous sclerosis (191100). Although germ-line mosaicism is rare, its frequency in disorders with high mutation rates may be significant enough to be taken into account for genetic counseling. In osteogenesis imperfecta, for example, a recurrence risk of 5–6% is given to normal parents who have an affected child with this autosomal dominant disease. Germ-line mosaicism is even more exceptional in X-linked disorders, recognized when females having more than one affected offspring lack mutant alleles in their skin or blood.

■ 10.3. PRADER-WILLI SYNDROME AND THE RECOGNITION OF GENOMIC IMPRINTING

Chromosomal microdeletion syndromes were discussed in Chapter 7 as subtle deletions that require high-resolution banding or FISH techniques for diagnosis. Particularly interesting were the Prader-Willi and Angelman syndromes, each described with apparently identical deletions affecting chromosome band 15q11. Despite their identical deletions, patients with Prader-Willi and Angelman syndromes had consistently different phenotypes that were not easily explained by variable effects of haplo-insufficient genes. Patients with Prader-Willi syndrome begin as hypotonic infants who may require tube feeding, then mature into morbidly obese individuals who compulsively overeat. They also have subtle changes in their facial appearance, with almond-shaped eyes and down-turned corners of the mouth (see Fig. 10.1). In contrast, patients with Angelman syndrome have prominent jaws with severe seizures and mental retardation. Their seizures often included unusual laughter (gelastic seizures) that, when combined with their jerky, ataxic movements, prompted the inappropriate name of "happy puppet" syndrome. Patients with Angelman syndrome usually have normal eating behaviors and are rarely obese. Now it is known that the differences in these two syndromes relate to different parental origins of the 15q11 deletion (Fig. 10.3).

DNA polymorphisms from the 15q11 region were used to determine the parental origin of the deleted chromosome 15 in patients with

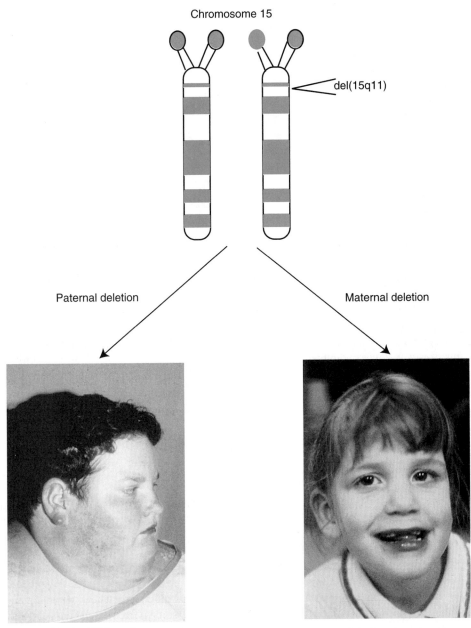

Figure 10.3. Different parental origin of 15q11 microdeletions in the Prader-Willi and Angelman syndromes.

Prader-Willi or Angelman syndrome. Prader-Willi patients always had deletions in the paternally derived chromosome 15, while Angelman patients always had deletions in the maternally derived chromosome 15 (Fig. 10.3). Despite the presence of apparently identical deletions in these vastly different clinical syndromes, the source of the genetic material proved to be as important as its content. These differences relate to the mechanism of genomic imprinting (see Section 10.4) and emphasize that the phenotypes caused by microdeletions may not relate simply to haploinsufficiency of genes in the deleted region. The genes within this region are still being characterized, and include a nuclear protein expressed in neurons (necdin) as well as a UBE3A gene that is involved in the ubiquination of proteins.

10.4. UNIPARENTAL DISOMY AND GENOMIC IMPRINTING

The different phenotypes produced by identical deletions in the Prader-Willi or Angelman syndromes correlated with pioneering experiments in mice that identified the phenomenon known as genomic imprinting. Genomic imprinting is a mechanism that modifies the phenotype of several neoplastic and developmental diseases, and it will undoubtedly be important in many others.

Genomic Imprinting

The concept of genomic imprinting suggests that identical genes may be marked differently during maternal versus paternal germ cell development. Evidence for this phenomenon, named by analogy to observations in animal behavior, was first provided by studies in mice.

Shortly after fertilization, the male and female pronuclei within mouse oocytes can be manipulated under a microscope. Replacement of the female pronucleus with a male pronucleus (i.e., two male pronuclei without maternal contribution) produces a placenta but no embryo; those produced from two oocyte pronuclei (i.e., no paternal contribution) develop embryos without placentas (Fig. 10.4). In these experiments, a normal mouse genome is present but its usual biparental source is altered. The lethality of uniparental inheritance of a normal genome explains why parthenogenesis (female conception without fertilization) does not occur in mammals.

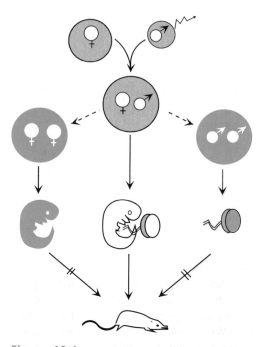

Figure 10.4. Pronuclear manipulation in the mouse. Normal development requires that a male-derived and female-derived pronucleus be present in the zygote (central pathway). Manipulation to produce zygotes with two female-derived pronuclei results in embryos that lack placentas (left pathway), while two male-derived pronuclei result in placentas that lack embryos (right pathway). Biparental origin of the genome is thus essential for mammalian development.

An analogous situation to mouse pronuclear experiments has been observed in certain human tissues. Molar pregnancies are extremely abnormal conceptions in which the entire uterus is filled with placentalike tissue. The molar tissue is often triploid (69 chromosomes), as would occur when a diploid gamete (46 chromosomes) from one parent is fertilized with a normal haploid gamete (23 chromosomes) from the other. Despite the alternative possibility, molar placental tissue always has two sets of male-derived chromosomes as would be predicted from the fates of mice with two male-derived pronuclei. The opposite experiment is also simulated by human tissues, because ovarian teratomas that consist of embryonic cells but not placental tissue also may be triploid. The triploid teratomas have two female-derived haploid sets that are analogous to mouse embryos with two female-derived pronuclei. In both species, genetic material with predominance of female origin produces embryonic tissue without placenta.

Evidence for genomic imprinting from human disorders includes the example of Prader-Willi and Angelman syndromes mentioned previously (Fig. 10.3). The Wilms tumor-aniridia-genital anomaly-mental retardation syndrome also provides evidence for the operation of genomic imprinting within its characteristic 11p13 deletion. Sporadic cases of Wilms tumor may exhibit molecular deletions or acquired homozygosity in this 11p13 region. Interestingly, it is always the maternal 11p region that is deleted or lost in Wilms tumor. Nearby the 11p13 band is a region associated with Wiedemann-Beckwith syndrome, a condition with hypoglycemia, omphalocele, increased prenatal growth, and variable mental retardation. Predominance of female transmission in familial cases of Wiedemann-Beckwith syndrome suggests possible imprinting effects, and it is notable that the 11p region is homologous to a demonstrably imprinted region of mouse chromosome 17. This mouse region is well known because of reciprocal imprinting of the insulin-like growth factor-2 gene and its receptor—only the paternal copy of the former is expressed in embryos and only the maternal copy of the latter. These opposing effects may provide insight into the biological reasons for genomic imprinting.

Haig (1992) has suggested that imprinting mediates a maternofetal tug of war by which maternally and paternally derived genes have opposing effects on fetal growth. Maternally derived genes would optimize their presence in descendants by balancing growth and survival of the current fetus against the need to conserve resources for future pregnancies. Paternally derived genes, with their ability to transmit through many different females, could maximize transmission by enhancing growth of every fetus. For growth-regulating genes such as insulin-like growth factor-2, mater-nally derived genes are often programmed for decreased expression and growth restriction in the fetus, while paternally derived genes are programmed for increased expression and growth enhancement. When there is normal biparental origin, the imprinting effects are balanced and normal fetal growth ensues. When there is a failure of imprinting or uniparental origin, then enhanced or inhibited fetal growth can occur as exemplified by the Wiedemann-Beckwith syndrome.

Regardless of whether fetal growth regulation was a factor in the evolution of genomic imprinting, the imprint laid down during gametogenesis correlates with DNA methylation in regulatory regions of genes. Increased DNA methylation in gene regions that promote RNA transcription will decrease levels of gene expression, while decreased DNA methylation will do the opposite. A current research question is to understand the mechanisms by which DNA methylation is altered during maternal and paternal gametogenesis and how it is erased in the zygotes that migrate into the yolk sac of the embryo and become primordial germ cells. Although every other cell in the embryo bears the maternal and paternal imprint on its chromosomes, germ cells erase this imprint and replace it with the appropriate maternal or paternal imprint according to the sex of the fetus.

Uniparental Disomy

Uniparental disomy refers to the inheritance of two chromosomes from one parent, rather than the usual inheritance of one chromosome from each parent. Despite having no extra or missing chromosome material, uniparental disomies may be associated with an abnormal phenotype if the relevant chromosome region is imprinted. The consequences of uniparental disomy were systematically explored in mice by breeding parents with balanced translocations. A certain percentage of offspring undergo nondisjunction with correction to produce uniparental disomy for a specific chromosome or chromosomal region (Fig. 10.5A, B).

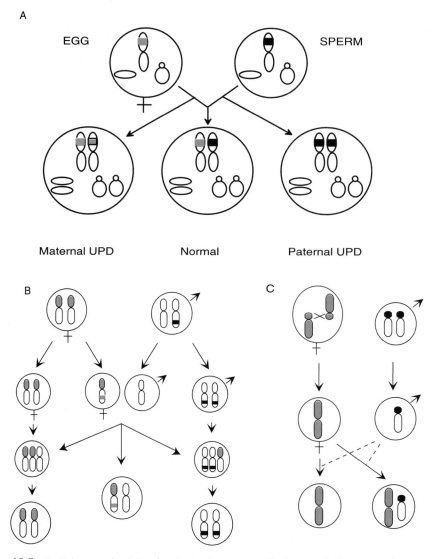

Figure 10.5. *A*, Uniparental origin of a single chromosome (uniparental disomy, UPD) can produce abnormalities due to lack of imprints or homozygosity for recessive alleles (shaded boxes). *B*, Paternal (right) or maternal (left) uniparental disomy is thought to originate by correction of trisomic zygotes, with one-third retaining both chromosomes from one parent. *C*, Chromosome imbalance or rearrangements may produce abnormalities due to imprinting effects, as illustrated by the balanced Robertsonian translocation 22 (left) in which both chromosomes 22 derive from one parent. The patient with trisomy (gamete at lower right) may exhibit different phenotypes according to whether the extra chromosome is maternally or paternally derived.

Such experiments have demonstrated that uniparental disomy for chromosomes 2, 6, 7, 11, and 17 are associated with abnormal phenotypes in mice, frequently showing different effects according to whether the chromosome pair derives from mother or father. Fetal growth retardation is a common finding in mice with uniparental disomy. Now human chromosomal diseases are being scrutinized for imprinting effects to discern how many human chromosomes will be imprinted. Results so far implicate human chromosomes 7, 11, 16, and 22 in addition to the chromosome 15 region dramatized by Prader-Willi and Angelman syndromes.

Evidence from chromosome 16 aberrations illustrates how uniparental disomy may occur. When chorionic villus sampling is performed at 8–10 weeks of pregnancy for prenatal diagnosis (see Chapter 15), chromosome mosaicism may be detected. Since chorionic villi are derived from placental tissue, this mosaicism may be confined to the placenta (*confined chorionic mosaicism*) or distributed throughout the fetoplacental unit (Kalousek, 1993). In several pregnancies, chorionic mosaicism for trisomy 16 was followed by demonstrating uniparental disomy for chomosome 16 in fetal tissue (amniotic cells or fetal blood). These fetuses had marked growth retardation, suggesting that chromosome 16 is imprinted and requires biparental inheritance for normal outcomes. Such observations further suggest that uniparental disomy can occur by correction of zygotes conceived as trisomies; Figure 10.5*B* illustrates that loss of a zygotic chromosome produces uniparental disomy on one of three occasions. As would be expected, confined chorionic trisomy 15 mosaicism with correction to paternal uniparental disomy 15 has also been demonstrated in Angelman syndrome.

Figure 10.5*A* and *B* diagram another potential effect of uniparental disomy that depends on whether one or both chromosomal homologues from one parent are transmitted. If the homologous chromosomes in offspring both derive from a single parental homologue (isodisomy), then a mutant allele on that chromosome can become homozygous in the offspring. This effect was first observed during genetic testing for cystic fibrosis, where a father was found not to be a carrier for this autosomal recessive disorder. Tracking of parental chromosomes using DNA polymorphisms revealed that the affected offspring had received

two copies of a maternal chromosome 7 that carried a mutant allele for cystic fibrosis. The carrier mother had thus conceived an affected offspring through uniparental isodisomy despite the fact that father was not a carrier for cystic fibrosis (see the problem set for detailed discussion of this case). In addition to cases of cystic fibrosis (Spence et al., 1988; Voss et al., 1989), uniparental disomy has now been demonstrated as a cause of 18 different autosomal or X-linked recessive diseases involving 11 different chromosomes. If the chromosome is imprinted, then the phenotype in offspring with uniparental disomy may represent a combination of effects from imprinting and homozygosity. The patients with cystic fibrosis due to uniparental disomy for chromosome 7 had some features that were atypical for cystic fibrosis such as fetal growth retardation.

Broader Effects of Imprinting

Genomic imprinting is a potential influence on phenotype that should be considered in many Mendelian and chromosomal diseases. Diseases worth studying for imprinting effects include dominant disorders where homozygous and heterozygous expression are similar (i.e., Huntington disease), disorders with more than one locus (i.e., tuberous sclerosis or polycystic kidney disease), disorders with early onset forms (i.e., Huntington disease), and disorders with differences based on parental tranmission (i.e., Huntington disease, myotonic dystrophy, diabetes mellitus, psoriasis). Since mice with uniparental disomy of the same chromosomal region exhibit variable phenotypes according to their strain and genetic background, variability among human individuals and families regarding the degree of imprinting effects can be expected.

Imprinting effects on the phenotypes of chromosome disorders are still being defined. Uniparental disomy of chromosome 21 has been reported without phenotypic consequences, and two unrelated normal females have received balanced, uniparental 22/22 Robertsonian translocations from their mothers. (See Fig. 10.5*C*). In contrast, a paternally derived 14/14 translocation (paternal uniparental disomy) was associated with mental retardation and minor anomalies in one female, and maternal uniparental disomy 14 was associated with minor anomalies but normal intellect in a male. As mentioned previously, autosomal recessive rod monochromacy has also been reported with maternal uniparental disomy of chromosome 14, emphasizing again that imprinting effects must be dissociated from homozygosity for recessive loci when isodisomy is found.

A final and important example of genomic imprinting may concern X chromosome inactivation. It is known that X-chromosome inactivation involves increased degrees of DNA methylation at many X chromosome genes, and that the DNA methylation shuts down activity in most genes. In marsupial mammals, the paternal X contributed to females is always inactivated while the maternal X remains active. This pattern of DNA methylation and inactivation of the X chromosome in gametes according to sex of the parent is exactly that seen in autosomal examples of genomic imprinting. It is possible to view imprinting and X-inactivation as mechanisms for cell memory, with changes in DNA methylation functioning secondarily to "lock in" changes in gene activity and maintain them through subsequent cell divisions (Migeon et al., 1991).

In contrast, mammals such as humans and mice exhibit random inactivation of the maternally or paternally derived X in early female embryos as emphasized by the Lyon hypothesis (see Chapter 7). It may be that the imprinting mechanism has been modified for X chromosome inactivation in humans, perhaps to allow more flexibility of X-chromosome gene expression. In line with the randomness of X inactivation are the similar phenotypes of women with 45,X Turner syndrome (monosomy X) regardless of whether the single X is maternally or paternally derived. The influence of gene methylation and possibly of genomic imprinting is also seen in the next category of atypical inheritance, disorders of expanding triplet repeats exemplified by the fragile X syndrome.

Case 10A Follow-up: The patient in Figure 10.1*A* had many manifestations of the Prader-Willi syndrome, but no chromosome 15 deletion was revealed by FISH analysis. It was then postulated that the patient had inherited two chromosomes 15 from his mother, with resulting absence of the paternal imprint in the 15q11 region, but analysis with DNA polymorphisms showed biparental origin of his chromosomes 15. Finally, analysis of the DNA methylation patterns of a small nuclear riboprotein (SNURP) gene in the 15q11 region revealed that he had only the methylation pattern characteristic of maternal origin for this gene. The lack of the paternal methylation pattern thus supported a diagnosis of Prader-Willi syndrome. Current studies of Prader-Willi syndrome show that about 60% of patients have deletions, 30% uniparental disomy, and the remainder abnormal DNA methylation patterns that presumably reflect failures of the imprinting mechanism.

■ 10.5. DISORDERS DUE TO DNA DUPLICATION: MICRODUPLICATIONS AND EXPANDING TRIPLET REPEATS

The idea of "selfish DNA" was proposed to explain the significant fraction of the human genome that is repetitive and apparently nonfunctional. Replication advantage through polymerase affinity, replication slippage, and such could amplify DNA copy number without requiring phenotypic advantage. Molecular technology has fulfilled this expectation by demonstrating numerous examples of DNA duplication that underlie polymorphisms (e.g., VNTRs, CA repeats discussed in Chapter 8). However, DNA duplications also account for new categories of disease: subtle chromosomal duplications that may not be detected by routine karyotyping (microduplications) and several diseases caused by expanding triplet repeats.

Small Gene Duplications

An interesting form of gene duplication is responsible for one type of Charcot-Marie-Tooth disease. Charcot-Marie-Tooth disease involves peripheral nerve abnormalities that lead to a characteristic "foot drop" on walking with atrophy of the hands and feet. Although Charcot-Marie-Tooth disease is genetically heterogenous (118200, 214400, 302800) with three types of Mendelian inheritance, most cases are autosomal dominant (118200). Over 70% of unrelated type I patients and up to 90% of sporadic cases have exhibited duplication of a 1.5-Mb DNA segment at chromosome band 17p11. Molecular FISH analysis must be used to demonstrate this duplication because it is not visible on a routine karyotype. An attractive candidate gene was present in the duplicated region that encodes a 22 Kd peripheral myelin protein (PMP22) that is mutated in a mouse with peripheral nerve problems (the *trembler* mouse). A pivotal role for this duplicated gene is suggested by the fact that some human Charcot-Marie-Tooth patients without 17p duplications have point mutations in the *PMP22* gene. The mutant allele, whether duplicated or changed by point mutation, must interfere with normal allele function to produce abnormal myelin and nerve conduction. Mechanisms relating extra gene dosage to phenotypic abnormalities have relevance to larger chromosomal aneuploidies such as Down syndrome, and it is likely that more examples of microduplication will be defined as FISH technology becomes more widely used.

Disorders with Unstable Triplet Repeats

Case 10B. Developmental Delay and Large Testes

The young man in Figure 10.1B had developmental delay and was placed in special education classes in school. On physical examination, he had large ears, lax joints, and large testes. Note that his face is somewhat narrow with a prominent jaw. A family history showed normal parents and a normal sister. Routine chromosomal analysis was normal.

Dramatic examples of DNA duplication have been defined in disorders caused by unstable and expanding triplet nucleotide repeats. The appreciation of this disease category began with a form of X-linked mental retardation known as the Martin-Bell syndrome. Martin and Bell had described males with moderately severe mental disability, severe speech delay, unusual behaviors, and physical abnormalities including large ears, prominent jaw, joint laxity, and megalotestes (illustrated in Fig. 10.1B). They recognized that the disorder was X-linked recessive, and Martin-Bell syndrome became known as one of more than 40 "nonspecific" X-linked mental retardation disorders that lacked defining morphogenetic or metabolic features. The breakthrough toward molecular understanding came in 1969, when Lubs observed an unusual X chromosome in a male with Martin-Bell syndrome. This "marker X" chromosome had a gap at its long arm telomere that prompted its identification as a "fragile X." Although ignored because of its inconsistency, the fragile X marker was eventually recognized to depend on culture of cells in low folic acid medium prior to karyotyping. Fragile X chromosome testing then allowed diagnosis of affected males, but was often unrevealing in carrier females. This inconsistency, together with some features of transmission that were unusual for X-linked disorders, was explained by cloning of the responsible gene.

A first round of studies utilized genetic linkage analysis to demonstrate that the causative gene for fragile X syndrome was located at chromosome band Xq27 where the fragile site was expressed. The usual progression for isolating progressively smaller DNA segments from this region gave an unexpected result: A particular DNA segment exhibited size variation among normal individuals and dramatic size increase in individuals with fragile X syndrome. This size variation was shown to be due to different numbers of trinucleotide repeats within the cloned DNA segment. The variation in numbers of triplet repeats was similar to that in CA repeat polymorphisms, except that this variation could become extreme and result in disease.

Additional gene characterization revealed that the region of triplet repeat variation was upstream of an open reading frame called the fragile X mental retardation-1 or FMR-1 gene. Amplification of the triplet CGG repeats caused increased DNA methylation in the upsteam promoter region and led to decreased FMR-1 gene expression. Since the FMR-1 gene is expressed in brain and testes, its lack of expression correlated with the phenotype of mental retardation and megalotestis in fragile X syndrome.

The analysis of fragile X syndrome families also explained the unusual inheritance patterns that had been noted from clinical studies. Using PCR primers that bracketed the triplet repeat region, numbers of triplet repeats upstream of the FMR-1 gene could be measured in various individuals (Fig. 10.6). Normal individuals had between 6 and 59 repeats, female carriers 60 to 200 repeats, and males with full clinical and cytogenetic expression of fragile X syndrome from 500 to 1500 repeats. A surprise was the finding of asymptomatic males with 60–200 repeats that could transmit the disease. This triplet repeat amplification in "transmitting males" was called a *premutation*—it did not cause symptoms in the transmitting male or his obligate carrier daughters, but could become unstable during female meiosis.

Carrier females thus had offspring with dramatically expanded numbers of triplet repeats, producing affected carrier daughters or affected males. Fragile X syndrome is thus a disease that worsens in subsequent generations, a phenomenon known as *anticipation.* Once the number of triplet repeats expands over a threshold of 60, it becomes unstable during female meiosis to cause symptoms in females or males who receive that X chromosome. The disease is worse in affected males with the triplet repeat expansion, because they will not have a companion X chromosome with normal numbers of triplet repeats as will carrier females (Fig. 10.6).

The expanded triplet repeat region is also unstable in early embryogenesis in both males and affected carrier females. These individuals are thus mosaics of cells containing different numbers of repeats, so that a broad band of variably sized DNA fragments is seen after PCR or Southern analysis (Fig. 10.6). The long string of cytosines in CCG repeats is thought to explain the fragile X site because salvage of pyrimidines requires folic acid as a cofactor. Depletion of the vitamin in cultured cells may thus decrease cytidine supplies and produce breaks during DNA synthesis that are recognized as a fragile site. It is still not known why there is initial amplification of trinucleotide repeats in transmitting males, but such premutations may be important causes of genetic disease.

Triplet repeat amplification in Fragile X syndrome is now a prototype for several diseases, meaning that DNA diagnosis analogous

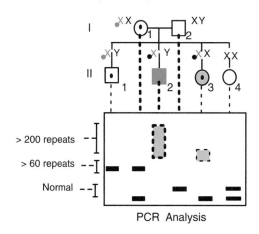

PCR Analysis

Figure 10.6. DNA diagnosis of fragile X syndrome. Two normal alleles (upper and lower bands in normal molecular weight range) are shown in the normal female (individual II-4), with a higher molecular weight allele (> 60 repeats) in the carrier female without symptoms (individual I-1). The affected male (II-2) and the carrier female with symptoms (II-3) have abnormal alleles with > 200 repeats that are unstable during embryogenesis and yield a broad range of fragment sizes (enclosed with dotted lines). Individual II-1 could be a "transmitting male" with slightly elevated allele size and no symptoms.

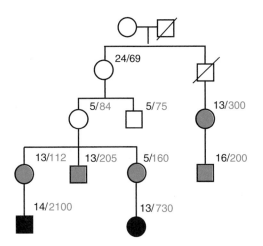

Figure 10.7. Inheritance of unstable repeats in myotonic dystrophy. The number of repeats in each myotonic dystrophy allele on chromosome 19 is shown beside each pedigree symbol. Amplification above 70 repeats produces instability, with congenital (dark) or adult-onset (shaded) myotonic dystrophy occurring in descendants. (Modified from Redman et al., 1993).

to that in Figure 10.6 is available. Steinert myotonic dystrophy (160900) is a disorder of muscle function with decreased muscle tone (hypotonia), difficulties in muscle relaxation (myotonia), and physical findings such as frontal baldness, cataracts, and an elongated face. The handshake is characteristic in this disease, since the affected person cannot release his grip. Myotonic dystrophy exhibits autosomal dominant inheritance with similar anticipation (increasing severity in subsequent generations) to that in fragile X syndrome.

DNA probes targeting the Steinert gene on chromosome 19 disclosed a variable CTG repeat near a protein kinase gene that was expressed in muscle. The CTG repeats, present in the 3'-untranslated mRNA from this gene, were shown to range from 5 to 37 in normal people and 44–3000 in myotonic dystrophy patients (Fig. 10.7). The repeats often increased in number with subsequent generations and were particularly susceptible to expansion during female meiosis. Even females with fewer than 80 repeats (asymptomatic) could undergo sufficient meiotic expansion to cause severe congenital myotonic dystrophy in their offspring (Figure 10.7). In infants with congenital disease, muscle dysfunction and hypotonia are so severe that their respiratory dysfunction and pneumonias are usually lethal.

Unstable trinucleotide repeats have been found in several neurodegenerative diseases such as Huntington chorea (143100), Friedreich ataxia (229300—recall Case 1), and spinocerebellar ataxias (e.g., 183050, Table 10.1).

■ **TABLE 10.1.** Disorders Due to Expanding Triplet Repeats

Disorder	Manifestations	Locus: Causative Mutation
Huntington chorea	Adult onset neurodegeneration, chorea	4p16: CAG repeats > 37 (Huntington gene)
Spinocerebellar ataxia	Adult onset, abnormal gait and coordination	6p24: CAG repeats >43
Dentatorubral pallidolysian atrophy (DRPLA)	Abnormal movements, chorea, seizures, dementia	12p13: CAG repeats > 40
Mercado-Joseph disease	Adult onset, neurodegeneration	14q: CAG repeats > 65
Friedreich ataxia	Adult onset, abnormal gait, neurodegeneration, heart disease	16p: GAA repeats > 27 (frataxin gene)
Steinert myotonic dystrophy	Juvenile or adult onset, myotonia, baldness, cataracts	19q13: GCT repeats > 37 copies (myotonin protein kinase gene)
Spinobulbar muscular atrophy	Adult onset, peripheral nerve and muscle dysfunction	Xq21: CAG repeats >30 (androgen receptor gene)
Fragile X syndrome	Childhood onset, subtle facial anomalies, joint laxity, megalotestis, mental disability	Xq27 CGG repeats > 60 (fragile X mental retardation FMR-1 gene)

In Huntington disease, during male meiosis triplet repeats may dramatically expand to produce severe, congenital disease in young daughters of affected fathers. Because most cases of Huntington disease have onset in middle age or later, diagnosis of triplet repeat expansion using testing similar to that in Figure 10.6 establishes a presymptomatic diagnosis with gruesome implications. The complex issues raised by presymptomatic diagnosis of Huntington disease are discussed in Chapter 14.

DNA probes have been used to detected more than 40 loci in the human genome that contain triplet DNA repeats. It is thus likely that many more diseases will be discovered that involve triplet repeat expansion. This disease mechanism must be suspected when any disease shows unusual transmission patterns, particularly when there are worsening symptoms in subsequent generations.

Case 10B Follow-up: A DNA test for fragile X syndrome was performed, confirming the diagnosis of fragile X syndrome. A careful cardiac examination was followed by echocardiogram to demonstrate mitral valve prolapse that occurs in these patients. The patient's mother was shown to be a carrier with > 60 triplet repeats, making his apparently normal sister at risk. She refused DNA testing.

◾ 10.6. GENE TARGETING AND GENE THERAPY

Spatiotemporal Targeting of Gene Products: The Challenge of Gene Therapy

The ability to isolate genes and to place them within recombinant genomes provides an opportunity for gene therapy. Several types of genetic therapy can be imagined, including the replacement of deficient gene products, the down-regulation of overexpressed gene products, the repair or replacement of defective genes, and the design of novel genes that restore defective functions. Many of these ap-

proaches have been the subject of preliminary experiments, and there are more than 100 gene therapy protocols underway in humans (see Table 10.2 for a small selection). A website is maintained with current protocols and resources concerning gene therapy (Wiley, 1998).

Three scientific principles are crucial in preparation for gene therapy:

1. The gene or gene product must be distributed into sufficient cells for sufficient times to effect a change in phenotype.
2. The gene or gene product must be targeted to the appropriate genomic and cellular compartments.
3. The gene or gene product must not disrupt other functions.

In addition to these scientific concerns, ethical issues of ownership of genetic material, costs versus benefits of therapy, and the rights to tamper with the essence of human inheritance (the genome) are relevant to enzyme and gene therapy.

Despite these scientific and ethical barriers, it can be imagined that gene therapy will effect changes in medicine that are analogous to those witnessed by Lewis Thomas (1983) as the era of antibiotics began:

The two great hazards of life were tuberculosis and syphilis. These were feared by everyone, in the same way that cancer is feared today. There was nothing to be done for tuberculosis except to wait it out, hoping that the body's own defense mechanisms would eventually hold the tubercle bacillus in check. . . . For most of the infectious diseases on the wards of the Boston City Hospital in 1937, there was nothing to be done beyond bed rest and good nursing care. . . . I remember the astonishment when the first cases of pneumonia and streptococcal septicemia were treated [with sulfanilimide] in Boston in 1937. The phenomenon was almost beyond belief. Here were moribund patients, who surely would have died without treatment, improving in their appearance within hours of being given the medicine and feeling entirely well within the next day or so. . . . For an intern, it was the opening of an entire new world. We had been raised to be ready

■ **TABLE 10.2.** Gene Transfer Experiments

Approach	Methods	Results
Genetic engineering		
Growth hormone in bacteria	Growth hormone gene insertion	Abundant growth hormone
Growth hormone in mice	Growth hormone gene insertion	Larger mice
Growth hormone in livestock	Growth hormone gene insertion	Larger livestock
Myostatin gene knockout in cows	Mimic "double-muscled" cow	Livestock with more meat
Cloning of sheep expressing human factor IX genes	Transfection of sheep fibroblasts, nuclear transfer to oocytes	Sheep making factor IX protein to use in hemophilia B patients
Gene Therapy		
Replace cystic fibrosis gene in mice with lethal homozygous CF	Gene replacement with human CF gene and intestinal promotor	Cure of mice with homozygous CF using human CFTR gene
Reverse familial hypercholesterolemia in the FH rabbit	Retroviral LDLR gene insertion into hepatocytes	Transplanted hepatocytes lowered cholesterol levels
Therapy of ADA deficiency (SCID)	Retroviral infection of patient's own stem cells	Several patients with improved immune status and persistence of ADA transgene
Therapy of Gaucher disease	Glucocerebrosidase enzyme therapy, bone marrow transplant with transgene	Improved bone disease Decreased size liver and spleen
Therapy of familial hypercholesterolemia	Retroviral infection of hepatocytes with LDLR gene	Partial correction of lipid abnormalities
Therapy of cystic fibrosis	Adenoviral infection of nasal epithelium with CFTR gene	Partial correction transport abnormality in nasal membrane
Therapy of cystic fibrosis	Deoxyribonuclease enzyme inhaled into lung	Pulmonary function improvements
Cancer therapy	Plasmid-liposome complex delivering HLA B27 antigen	Altered surface antigen of tumor cells, improved immune response
Cancer therapy	Retroviral infection of neuroblastoma with IL-4 gene	Higher interleukin levels in tumor, enhanced immune response

for one kind of profession, and we sensed that the profession itself had changed at the moment of our entry.

Genetic Engineering for Therapeutic Products and Agricultural Benefits

An overview of the approaches to genetic engineering and gene therapy is shown in Figure 10.8. The technology is similar to that discussed in producing transgenic mice in Chapter 9. Retroviruses that have the ability to integrate within host DNA are redesigned to replace certain genes for viral functions with a gene of interest. The recombinant retroviral DNA is then added to cultured cells that contain competent retroviral genes, allowing the transgene to be packaged and exported within the retroviral capsule. This recombinant virus can enter the cell and integrate into the cellular

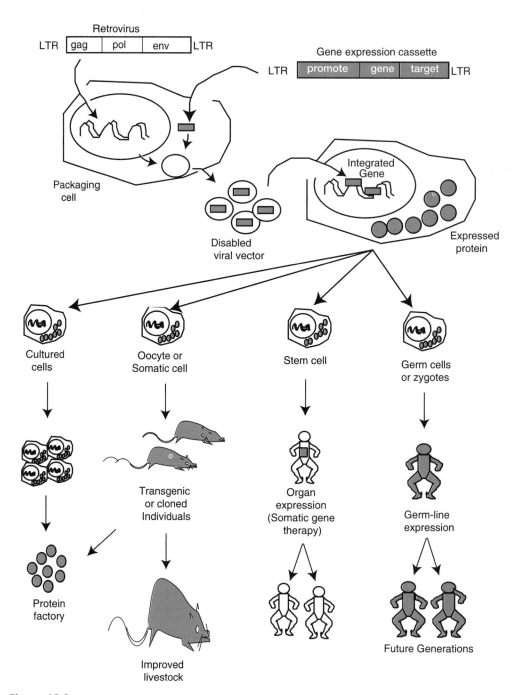

Figure 10.8. Strategies for genetic engineering and gene therapy. Genes of interest are combined with DNA regions that promote expression and proper targeting within a viral DNA that can insert the gene into foreign genomes (expression cassette or construct, upper part of figure). The most common strategy uses disabled retroviral vectors that pass through a packaging cell with intact retrovirus (above), then transfect a host cell. The host cell may be cultured to produce rare proteins (left), or it may be cloned to produce transgenic animals with desired properties (left center). Transgenes may also be placed in stem cells for somatic gene therapy (right center) or in germ cells that will produce individuals that contain the transgene in all tissues (germ-line therapy—right).

genome, but the absence of key viral genes prevents infection and damage to the cell. The transferred gene is also bracketed by DNA that ensures adequate expression and targeting of gene product to the necessary cell compartments and/or tissues. This *expression cassette* is the most essential design for gene therapy experiments, because the timing, targeting, and tissue distribution of gene product is essential for producing a protein or changing an organism's phenotype.

As shown in Figure 10.8, left panel, the first applications of genetic engineering concerned the manufacture of rare human proteins with medical uses. A premier example was the cloning and expression of genes for human growth hormone in bacteria, allowing this scarce protein to be manufactured for use by growth hormone-deficient children. The bacterial synthesis of human growth hormone replaced the laborious isolation of the protein from cow pituitaries and conferred three important advantages. First, the human protein did not provoke immune reactions. Second, it did not have risks for transmitting a rare but devastating virus that caused Creutzfeld-Jacob disease that was sometimes present in calf brain. Third, growth hormone was now sufficiently abundant to treat all deficient children plus others with various forms of short stature. For example, girls with Turner syndrome due to monosomy X have responded to synthetic growth hormone, increasing their height 4 to 6 inches, from the $4^1/_2$–5 feet range to normal. The synthetic hormone has also been tried in other dwarfing conditions, but its use is limited by its high cost of about $30,000 per year. The abundant supply of growth hormone has also been used as a high-cost treatment for normal children whose parents desire extra growth for athletic or social reasons. Such treatments raise ethical questions regarding distribution of resources and consents of minors that may apply broadly to scarce proteins manufactured through genetic engineering.

Bacterial synthesis of coagulation factors has also been possible by inserting the appropriate human transgenes, and this has been valuable for treating diseases such as hemophilia A (306700). Prior to the manufacture of factor VIII in bacteria, these children were administered plasma concentrates that had high frequencies of contamination with AIDS virus. Transgenic or animal cloning technologies may also be useful for generating novel animals that express human proteins (Fig. 10.8, left panels). Cultured somatic cells from sheep can now be injected with transgene vectors and selected for cells containing the desired genes. These genetically identical nuclei from transgenic cells can then be placed into enucleated sheep oocytes for propagation of adult sheep. One example of this strategy employed an expression cassette for the factor IX transgene (defective in hemophilia B—306900) that prompted its antihemophilia protein to be secreted in sheep milk (Schnieke et al., 1997). The flexibility of gene transfer techniques allows harnessing of bacteria, cultured cells, or various animals to produce needed human proteins. These techniques also allow the manipulation of specific gene expression in diverse animal species, providing a new and powerful discipline of experimental genetics.

Human Enzyme Therapy

Because many metabolic disorders involve enzyme deficiencies, the ability to purify enzymes from human tissues provided an obvious strategy for therapy. Enzyme therapy has been tried for several genetic diseases but is most effective for lysosomal enzyme deficiencies. As reviewed in Chapter 6, lysosomal enzymes contain a mannose-6-phosphate ligand that targets them to lysosomal membranes containing a mannose-6-phosphate receptor. When administered into the blood stream, lysosomal enzymes are taken up by cells and targeted to the lysosomal compartments where they are needed. Other types of enzyme or protein therapies may be limited by formidable difficulties in targeting the gene product to its necessary cellular location.

Enzyme therapy has been most successful for lysosomal enzyme deficiencies like type 1

Gaucher disease (230800) that do not affect the central nervous system. In this form of Gaucher disease, glycolipid accumulates in liver, spleen, and bone but not in brain. The patients may develop painful fractures and hypersplenism with bleeding or disfiguring abdominal enlargement. The glucocerebrosidase that is deficient in Gaucher disease has been purified by pharmaceutical companies and modified to expose or increase its targeting mannose residues. Administration of Ceredase (alglucerase) has been effective in treating the disease, but its cost for adults approaches $300,000–400,000 per year.

Gene Therapy

As illustrated in the right panels of Figure 10.8, genes may be introduced into somatic or germline cells of experimental animals. Somatic gene therapy has already become a reality in humans, while germ-line therapy has been deferred for technical and ethical reasons. The first successful instance of somatic gene therapy utilized retroviral vectors to replace the adenosine deaminase (ADA) gene in patients with severe combined immune disease due to ADA deficiency. These patients were already being treated successfully with purified ADA enzyme, allowing a trial of gene therapy that could be assessed without concern about dire outcomes. The ADA gene was placed in a disabled retrovirus as shown in Figure 10.8 and added to peripheral blood leucocytes from the ADA deficient patient. T-cells within these leucocytes were then expanded by treatment with interleukins, and the enhanced T-cells expressing ADA were transfused back into the patient. The use of the patient's own cells prevented immune reactions, and the treatment of cells early in the immune cell lineage provided a continuous and expanding source of ADA competent cells. Several patients have now demonstrated sustained synthesis of ADA with immunocompetence after somatic gene therapy. The gene therapy has not been more successful than enzyme therapy, but maintenance of the gene in stem cells has decreased the need for repetitive transfusions.

Other gene therapy trials have targeted liver or lung cells (Table 10.4). Familial hypercholesterolemia has been ameliorated by retroviral transfection of the LDL receptor gene into patient hepatocytes. The hepatocytes were obtained from the patient by partial liver resection, then reinfused after LDL receptor gene transfer into the liver via the portal vein. Decreased blood cholesterol and low density lipoprotein levels were noted. The cystic fibrosis transmembrane regulator (CFTR) gene has also been inserted into nasal mucosal cells in patients with cystic fibrosis. An adenoviral vector with affinity for respiratory epithelium was used as the vector, and uptake CFTR genes into nasal mucosa was demonstrated. In addition, improved conductance of the mucosa was shown using measures analogous to the sweat test that examines sodium and chloride ion levels. Since respiratory epithelium extends from the nasal mucosa to the bronchi and lungs, it is hoped that the same vector will improve lung function after delivery via inhalers. Despite the expectations for gene therapy, it is important to realize that dramatic improvements in outcome have been obtained using enzyme, pulmonary, antibiotic, and deoxyribonuclease therapy for cystic fibrosis. Other medical approaches should not be ignored in the anticipation of gene therapy.

The greatest number of somatic gene therapy protocols concern cancer, as illustrated by two examples in Table 10.2. By delivering a transgene for a foreign HLA antigen into the tumor, the patient can mount a stronger immune response to produce tumor regression. Another approach inserts genes for interleukins into tumors such as neuroblastoma. Interleukins are powerful transducers of immune signaling pathways that offer another way of stimulating host responses to tumor cells. The important roles of genes in cancer as summarized in Chapter 9, together with the many gene therapy protocols now underway, suggest that cancer therapy will be the first area in which gene transfer becomes a routine part of medical care.

PROBLEM SET 10
New Applications of Clinical Genetics

Provide the single best answer to the following questions:

10.1. The discovery of genetic disases due to expanding triplet repeats validated the concept of:
  (A) Variable expression
  (B) New mutation
  (C) Genomic imprinting
  (D) Anticipation
  (E) Mitochondrial inheritance

10.2. A child has symptoms of neurofibromatosis-1 (NF-1; 162200), including café-au-lait spots and neurofibromas, but they are confined to his right leg and inguinal region. The family history is normal. This is most consistent with:
  (A) Mitochondrial disease
  (B) Triplet repeat disease
  (C) Gene expression influenced by parent of origin (imprinting effects)
  (D) Somatic mosaicism
  (E) Germ-line mosaicism

10.3. In a large family, disease A occurs in offspring when their mother is affected, while disease B occurs in offspring when their father is affected. This pattern is suggestive of:
  (A) Mitochondrial disease
  (B) Triplet repeat disease
  (C) Gene expression influenced by parent of origin (imprinting effects)
  (D) Somatic mosaicism
  (E) Germ-line mosaicism

10.4. A DNA methylation analysis is performed on a gene region known to be imprinted in the mouse. The finding of identical DNA methylation patterns on alleles from both homologous chromosomes would occur in which tissue?
  (A) Male gametes
  (B) Heart tissue in adult females
  (C) Liver tissue in adult males
  (D) Male primordial germ cells
  (E) Female neural crest cells

10.5. Atypical inheritance mechanisms have been revealed by molecular genetic technology, including all of the following except:

  (A) Sporadic mutation
  (B) Uniparental disomy and genomic imprinting
  (C) Mitochondrial inheritance
  (D) Trinucleotide repeat amplification
  (E) Maternal inheritance

10.6. Normal grandparents have a grandson with the fragile X syndrome. Their daughter has had learning differences in school, but is otherwise normal. The grandfather is most likely:
  (A) An affected male with incomplete penetrance
  (B) A transmitting male
  (C) A son of a fragile X carrier
  (D) Not the real father of his daughter
  (E) Mosaic in his germ-line tissue

10.7–10.8. Match the following diseases with the genetic mechanisms indicated below:
  (A) Huntington chorea
  (B) Prader-Willi syndrome
  (C) Angelman syndrome
  (D) Myotonic dystrophy
  (E) Hypomelanosis of Ito

10.7. Triplet repeat expansion during male meiosis

10.8. Triplet repeat expansion during female meiosis

Provide short answers to the following questions:

10.9. Testing of a child with chronic infections reveals adenosine deaminase (ADA) deficiency (102700). It is known that ADA deficiency prevents maturation of immune stem cells into functional T- and B-cells, producing severe combined immune deficiency. Discuss possible treatments for this disease.

10.10. Discuss why diseases with triplet repeat expansion may worsen in subsequent generations.

PROBLEM SET 10
Answers

10.9–10.10	See short answers in Solutions	
10.3 C	**10.6**	B
10.2 D	**10.5** A	**10.8** D
10.1 D	**10.4** D	**10.7** A

PROBLEM SET 10
Solutions

10.1. Disorders caused by expanding triplet repeats may show worsening symptoms with successive generations (anticipation, answer D). Variable expression occurs in autosomal dominant as well as expanding triplet repeat diseases, as do new mutations. Mitochondrial disorders are associated with maternal inheritance, while genomic imprinting would be related to parent of origin effects.

10.2. Somatic mosaicism is caused when a mutation occurs in a tissue outside of the germ line (answer D). The child presumably sustained a neurofibromin gene mutation in cells surrounding the lower right limb bud, producing characteristic findings of NF-1 in one body region. Mitochondrial disease can exhibit tissue specificity due to heteroplasmy, but NF-1 is not a mitochondrial disease phenotype.

10.3. Genomic imprinting, named by analogy to behavioral imprinting of offspring on their mothers, refers to different expression of genes according to whether they were transmitted from males or females (answer C). Sex-specific differences in transmission can occur in mitochondrial (maternal inheritance) or triplet repeat expansion (instability during male or female meiosis), but they would not be evident from males and females in the same family. The "imprint" can be defined experimentally in the form of DNA methylation in regulatory regions, causing that allele to be up- or downregulated. The imprint is erased in embryonic cells that begin the germ line, then reestablished in primordial germ cells according to fetal sex. In all somatic tissues, homologous chromosomes have different methylation patterns in imprinted regions according to whether that chromosome arose from the mother or father. In humans, it is thought that five to seven of the autosomes contain imprinted regions.

10.4. Only in primordial germ cells will imprinted regions exhibit equivalent methylation patterns on a pair of homologous chromosomes (answer D). Imprint erasure must occur in primordial germ cells in order to reset the imprint according to fetal sex. All somatic cells, whether embryonic or adult, have different methylation patterns on imprinted chromosomes that reflect their transmission from mother or father.

10.5. New mutations have been recognized as a cause of isolated (sporadic) cases of diseases known to exhibit autosomal or X-linked inheritance (answer A). Usual mutation rates were approximately one mutation per 10^6 individuals per locus per generation. Molecular analysis has revealed new inheritance mechanisms such as uniparental disomy with imprinting effects, mitochondrial diseases with maternal inheritance, and disorders due to unstable trinucleotide repeats. Trinucleotide repeat instability provided a new mechanism for mutation with unprecedented rates of up to one mutation per individual per generation.

10.6. Fragile X syndrome is a disorder involving triplet repeat expansion within the Xq27 chromosome region. As with other triplet repeat disorders, an initial or premutation that causes the number of triplet repeats to rise above the normal range of variation may occur. Once this number of repeats occurs, there is further instability with the potential for expansion during male or female meiosis. In fragile X syndrome, premutations may occur in males and be transmitted to their obligate carrier daughters (transmitting males, answer B). The daughters may have severely affected sons after their premutation becomes amplified in oocytes during meiosis.

10.7–10.8. Some disorders associated with unstable triplet repeats exhibit instability during male meiosis (e.g., Huntington chorea, answer 10.7A), while others exhibit instability during female meiosis (e.g., Mytonic dystrophy, answer 10.8D and fragile X syndrome). The basis for these differences is not known.

10.9. Standard modes of therapy would include avoidance of infection, chronic antibiotic treatment, and drugs that stimulate the immune response (e.g., interferons, gammaglobulins).

The famous bubble boy was a patient with ADA deficiency who did well when insulated from microorganisms in the environment. Other than this extreme isolation, standard therapies were not effective. Replacement of the missing enzyme could be done by infusing normal cells (e.g., bone marrow transplant), infusing enzyme, or insertion of a functional ADA gene. Bone marrow transplantation is hazardous in any case (10–15% mortality), especially in an immunodeficient patient where the grafted cells will attack the defenseless host. Enzyme administered in polyethylene glycol beads was successful in the disease, but gene therapy using retroviruses containing a functional ADA gene produced longer benefits. The patient's own white cells were removed, transfected with the recombinant retrovirus, and returned to the patient so that cross-reactions were avoided.

10.10. Worsening with succeeding generations is called *anticipation,* an early clinical observation that was dismissed as an artifact by the famous geneticist L. S. Penrose. Anticipation was validated by the discovery of expanding trinucleotide repeats, where a certain theshold repeat number causes instability during male or female meiosis. Once unstable, repeat numbers can amplify dramatically during each generation, producing more severe symptoms in affected individuals. Steinert myotonic dystrophy is caused by unstable trinucleotide repeats near a muscle protein kinase gene on chromosome 19; the repeats are particularly unstable during female meiosis and may cause a severe syndrome of fetal muscle weakness and joint contractures called congenital myotonic dystrophy.

BIBLIOGRAPHY

General References

Schmickel RD. 1974. Genetic counseling as a form of medical counseling. *Univ Michigan Med Center J* 40:38–43.

Thomas L. 1983. *The Youngest Science.* New York: Bantam.

Expanding Triplet Repeats

Lubs HA. 1969. A marker X chromosome. *Am J Hum Genet* 21:231–44.

Martin JB. 1993. Molecular genetics of neurological diseases. *Science* 262:674–678.

Miwa S. 1994. Triplet repeats strike again (DRPLA). *Nature Genet* 6:3–4.

Redman JB, Fenwick RG, Fu Y-H, Pizzuti A, Caskey CT. 1993. Relationship between parental trinucleotide GCT repeat length and severity of myotonic dystrophy in offspring. *JAMA* 269:1960–1964.

Sutherland GR, Richards RI. 1992. Anticipation legitimized: Unstable DNA to the rescue. *Am J Hum Genet* 51:7–9.

Gene and Enzyme Therapy

Barranger JA, Bahnson AB, Nimbaonkar MT, Ball ED, Robbins P, Boggs SS, Ohashi T. 1995. Gene therapy for genetic disease. *Int Pediatr* 10:5–9.

Chowdhury JR, Grossman M, Gupta S, Chowdhury NR, Baker JR, Wilson JM. 1991. Long-term improvement of hypercholesterolemia after ex vivo gene therapy in LDLR-deficient rabbits. *Science* 254:1802–1805.

Crystal RG. 1995. Transfer of genes to humans: Early lessons and obstacles to success. *Science* 270:404–410.

Dickman S. 1997. More meat on the hoof. *Science* 277:1922–1923.

Glasbrenner K. 1986. Technology spurt resolves growth hormone problem, ends shortage. *JAMA* 255:581–587.

Schnieke AE, Kind AJ, Ritchie WA, Mycock K, Scott AR, Ritchie M, Wilmut I, Colman A, Campbell KHS. 1997. Human factor IX transgenic sheep produced by transfer of nuclei from transfected fetal fibroblasts. *Science* 278:2130–2133.

Wiley. 1999. *The Wiley Gene Therapy Website.* http://www.wiley.co.uk/genetherapy/

Wivel NA, Walters L. 1993. Germ-line gene modification and disease prevention: Some medical and ethical perspectives. *Science* 262:533–538.

Genomic Imprinting and Uniparental Disomy

Engel E. 1998. Uniparental disomies in unselected populations. *Am J Hum Genet* 63:962–966.

Haig D. 1992. Genomic imprinting and the theory of parent-offspring conflict. *Semin Devel Biol* 3:153–160.

Hall JG. 1990. Genomic imprinting: Review and relevance to human disease. *Am J Hum Genet* 46:857–873.

Kalousek DK. 1993. The effect of confined placental mosaicism on development of the human aneuploid conceptus. *Am J Med Genet* 45:13–22.

Migeon BR, Holland MM, Driscoll DJ, Robinson JC. 1991. Programmed demethylation in CpG islands during human fetal development. *Somat Cell Mol Genet* 17:159–68.

Spence JE, Perciaccante RG, Greig GM, Willard HG, Ledbetter DH, Hejtmancik JF, Pollack MS, O'Brien WE, Beaudet AL. 1988. Uniparental disomy as a mechanism for human genetic disease. *Am J Hum Genet* 42:217–226.

Voss R, Ben-Simon E, Aviatl A, Zlotogora Y, Dagan J, Godfry S, Tikochinski Y, Hillel J. 1989. Isodisomy of chromosome 7 in a patient with cystic fibrosis: Could uniparental disomy be common in humans? *Am J Hum Genet* 45:373–380.

Microdeletions

Kubota T, Sutcliffe JS, Aradhya S, Gillessen-Kaesbach G, Christian SL, Horsthemke B, Beaudet AL, Ledbetter DH. 1996. Validation studies of SNRPN methylation as a diagnostic test for Prader-Willi syndrome. *Am J Med Genet* 66:77–80.

MacDonald HR, Wevrick R. 1997. The necdin gene is deleted in Prader-Willi syndrome and is imprinted in human and mouse. *Hum Mol Genet* 6:1873–1878.

Schmickel RD. 1986. Contiguous gene syndromes: A component of recognizable syndromes. *J Pediatr* 109:231–241.

Somatic and Germ-Line Mosaicism

Hall BD. 1989. Invited editorial: Of mice, persons, and pigment. *Am J Hum Genet* 45:191–192.

Hall JG. 1988. Review and hypothesis: Somatic mosaicism: Observations related to clinical genetics. *Am J Hum Genet* 43:355–363.

Part III

CLINICAL GENETICS

PEDIATRIC GENETICS:
BIRTH DEFECTS AND SYNDROMOLOGY

■ LEARNING OBJECTIVES

1. The morphologic examination consists of gestalt inspection, analysis of major and minor anomalies, and interpretation of primary cause.
2. The morphologic examination can distinguish between isolated congenital anomalies and the patterns of minor and major anomalies known as syndromes.
3. Isolated anomalies usually imply a low (2–3%) recurrence risk, whereas syndromes may arise from Mendelian or chomosomal mechanisms with higher recurrence risks.
4. Generalists should use the morphologic examination to assign a syndrome category, then obtain a precise diagnosis by specialty referral and laboratory testing.
5. A syndrome diagnosis allows genetic and prognostic counseling with the anticipation of specific complications at particular ages.
6. Preventive management based on syndrome complications can enhance parent adjustment and patient outcome.

Cases 11A, 11B, and 11C: ***Three Faces***

A plastic surgeon working on a craniofacial surgery team encounters three children with identical anomalies consisting of a small jaw and posterior cleft palate (Fig. 11.1*D*). Patient 11A (Fig. 1.11*A*) was a 3-month-old male whose facial appearance, gestational history, and family history were normal. Patient 11B (Fig. 11.1*B*) had additional anomalies of the heart and radial aplasia (absent radius in the arm) together with his jaw and palatal defect. Her heart anomaly led to death at age 3 months, and her parents were first cousins. Patient 11C (Fig. 11.1*C*) also had additional anomalies including an unusual facial appearance with down-slanting palpebral fissures and hollow cheeks (malar hypoplasia). Patient 11C had respiratory problems in association with his oral anomalies, and his problem was said to have occurred previously in the family. These three patients required assessment to determine the genetic and medical risks implied by their small jaw and posterior cleft palate shown in Figure 11.1*D*.

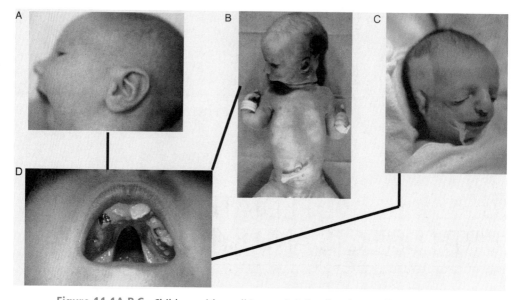

Figure 11.1A,B,C. Children with small jaw and cleft soft palate as illustrated in D.

■ 11.1. INTRODUCTION

Pediatric genetics is a subspecialty of pediatric medicine that is relevant to every health professional who deals with children or reproduction. By design or default, the field of pediatric genetics can be divided into the three major categories of dysmorphology, metabolism, and counseling. *Syndromology* or d*ysmorphology* (*dys* = painful or abnormal, *morph* = shape) is the most abundant category, including the 3–5% of all newborn children that have congenital malformations. Among these malformation are those due to maternal environmental or drug exposure, emphasized by the related term of *teratology* (*terata* = monstrosities). *Inborn errors of metabolism* are much rarer than congenital anomalies or birth defects, but their aggregate 1 in 600 birth frequency is amplified by the frequent visits needed by these patients for dietary and medical management.

Technically within the field of pediatric genetics is a third category of activity that encompasses general genetics and counseling. Genetic diseases such as cystic fibrosis or sickle cell anemia are encompassed by the field of pediatric genetics, but their diagnosis and counseling is usually managed by other subspecialties. The management of cystic fibrosis by pulmonologists, of sickle cell anemia by hematologists, of spina bifida by developmental pediatricians, or of cleft palate by craniofacial surgeons emphasizes the importance of clinical genetic principles in various medical specialties. If these specialists are well informed, then the pediatric genetic specialist is required only for unusual or complex cases of these genetic diseases. Other pediatric genetic categories are discussed in Chapter 12 (inborn errors of metabolism) and Chapter 13 (isolated congenital anomalies), while general principles relevant to Mendelian and multifactorial disorders were discussed in Chapters 2 and 3.

The focus on congenital malformations in this chapter is based on knowledge of morphology, a branch of biology that concerns the form, formation, and transformation of living beings (Opitz and Wilson, 1997). Because human morphology is inherently variable and the subject of numerous medical diagnoses, its wide spectrum of syndromes and minor anomalies may be intimidating to health professionals. Simple principles are therefore emphasized in this chapter, all pointing toward the goal of placing the child into a diagnostic category. The genetic approach summarized in Figure 1.1 is focused in Figure 11.2 to emphasize an approach to dysmorphology.

The morphologic evaluation begins with a gestational and family history, where certain findings are red flags for the occurrence of congenital anomalies (Table 11.1). Breech presentation, intrauterine growth retardation, and altered intrauterine head growth are typical of children with malformation syndromes, and these problems are frequently revealed prior to birth by modern obstetrical practice. The hours after birth provide an important opportunity for supportive counseling (Fig. 11.2), where simple explanation of anomalies and an outline of the proposed evaluation may be all the parents are ready to hear. Feeding problems, seizures, or hypotonia during the neonatal period are other harbingers of anomalous birth, and these factors can accentuate neonatal jaundice. Later signs of growth or developmental delay may prompt morphologic evaluation, and there are even some syndromes with early gigantism or obesity. An unrevealing family history will be documented with sporadic

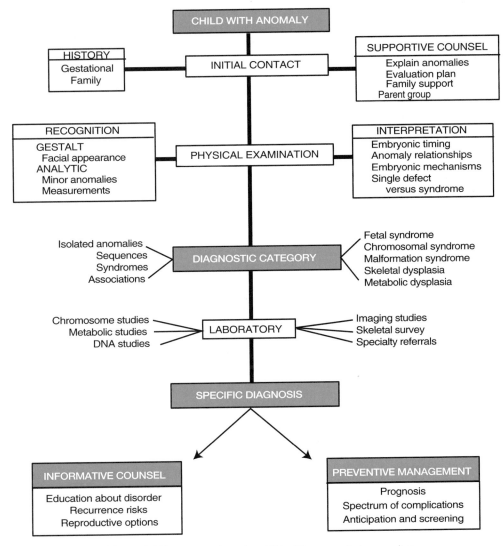

Figure 11.2. Approach to the child with congenital anomalies

■ TABLE 11.1. Red Flags for Congenital Malformations and Syndromes

Multiple spontaneous abortions (miscarriages)
Breech presentation
Advanced maternal age (chromosomal aberrations)
Advanced paternal age (new mutations)
Intrauterine growth retardation
Altered intrauterine head growth (e.g., microcephaly)
Postnatal growth retardation
Postnatal growth acceleration
Disproportionate growth (e.g., short limbs)
Several minor anomalies
Microcephaly (small head)
Mental disability (developmental delay)

anomalies or new mutations, but multiple miscarriages, advanced parental ages, or consanguinity will sometimes alert the examiner to the possibility of chromosomal or Mendelian disease (Table 11.1).

The next step in the morphologic evaluation is physical examination (Fig. 11.2). After utilizing the gestalt and analytic approaches described in the following paragraphs, the examiner attempts to interpret the morphologic findings, translating them into a meaningful syntax of genetic and embryonic mechanism.

Usually it is possible to fit the child into a diagnostic category such as cleft lip/palate or skeletal dysplasia, and this interpretation can guide medical management. Additional laboratory studies or specialty referrals are often needed as in Figure 11.2, ideally resulting in a specific diagnosis and etiology. Once a cause is defined or a syndrome is confirmed, then informative genetic counseling and preventive management can begin. The stepwise approach outlined in Figure 11.2 is available to all health professionals; it demystifies facial recognition that is given too much prominence in dysmorphology and avoids the need to memorize hundreds of syndromes and eponyms. The generalist can link hands with laboratory and specialty services, supporting the family until definitive answers are found.

The ability to interpret dysmorphology allows a practitioner to bring valuable gifts to the family. There is first the role of parental advisor and counselor, facilitating the acceptance of a child's handicaps and fostering a realistic but positive attitude. There is also the importance of genetic counseling, since many congenital anomalies and syndromes have significant recurrence risks with implications for future pregnancies. There is finally the benefit of early diagnosis and preventive management, allowing the patient to avoid complications that add insult to injury. Despite the lack of cures or treatments for most congenital anomalies and syndromes, the management of children with disabilities often brings great rewards. It is surprising how often the child saved from infection elicits parental relief with no thanks, while the family supported through the crisis of birth defects expresses unending gratitude and loyalty.

■ 11.2. APPROACH TO THE CHILD WITH CONGENITAL ANOMALIES— CATEGORIES AND TERMINOLOGY

Congenital anomalies may be classified according to their mechanism and distribution. Isolated or single anomalies such as cleft palate affect a single body region and are commonly associated with sporadic occurrence or multifactorial determination. Multiple congenital anomalies or malformation *syndromes* affect several body regions and are sometimes associated with a characteristic facial appearance. Syndromes are more likely to exhibit chromosomal or Mendelian inheritance than single anomalies, and they obviously imply more medical complications with a greater need for preventive management. Discrimination between the isolated anomaly and the multiple anomaly syndrome is the most important step in the morphologic evaluation.

As individual anomalies are encountered during physical examination, they can also be classified according to type and mechanism. These classifications guide the examiner toward interpretation of mechanism and the as-

signment of a defect category, the primary goal for generalists. The classification of anomalies described in the following sections is supported by consensus recommendations (Spranger, et al., 1982). Examples of birth defect categories are summarized in Table 11.2.

Isolated Anomalies

The characterization of *anomalies* as "abnormal" distinguishes them from *normal variants* (e.g., Mongolian spot). Normal variants are more frequent (arbitrarily, > 4% of the popula-

■ **TABLE 11.2.** Categories of Birth Defects

Category	Subcategory	Definition	Example
Isolated defect			
Normal variant		Present in > 4% of population, not abnormal	Mongolian spot
Anomaly		Deviation from expected or average type in structure, form and/or function which is interpreted as abnormal	Bifid toe
	Major anomaly	Anomaly of surgical or cosmetic consequence	Cleft palate
	Minor anomaly	Diagnostically helpful, little impact on individual well-being	Low-set ear
	Malformation	Morphological defect resulting from an intrinsically abnormal developmental process	Radial aplasia (absent radius)
	Dysplasia	Abnormal organization of cells into tissues	Hemangioma
	Disruption	Extrinsic breakdown or interference with an orginally normal developmental process	Amniotic band
	Deformation	Abnormal form, shape, or position of a part of the body caused by mechanical forces	Plagiocephaly (lopsided head)
	Sequence	Pattern of anomalies derived from a single known or presumed prior anomaly or mechanical factor	Pierre Robin malformation sequence Potter deformity sequence
Multiple defects			
	Syndrome	Multiple anomalies thought to be pathogenetically related and not representing a sequence	Zellweger malformation syndrome Skeletal dysplasia syndromes
	Association	Nonrandom occurrence in one or more individuals of several morphologic defects not identified as a sequence or syndrome	VATER association
	Developmental field defect	Reactive unit of morphogenesis—a set of embryonic primordia that react identically to different causes	Holoprosencephaly spectrum Polyasplenia spectrum

tion) and less significant than anomalies (Table 11.2). *Major anomalies* are those with cosmetic or surgical consequences—e.g., an amputated limb or a duplicated great toe. *Minor* *anomalies,* despite their diagnostic importance, have little impact on individual well-being—for example, the epicanthal fold, prominent occiput, preauricular pit, toe syndactyly,

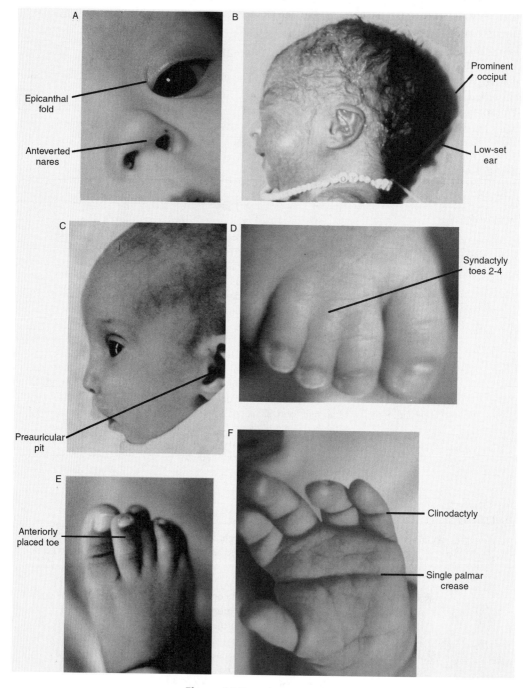

Figure 11.3. Minor anomalies

anteriorly placed toe, and clinodactyly, and the single palmar crease shown in Figure 11.3.

In addition to their distribution, anomalies may be classified according to their mechanisms and causes (see Tables 11.2 and 11.3). As discussed in Chapter 9, abnormalities occurring during the period of blastogenesis (approximately 1–4 weeks after fertilization) affect entire embryonic regions and produce multiple major anomalies (e.g., the VATER association discussed in Section 11.10). Abnormalities that occur during organogenesis (approximately 5–8 weeks after fertilization) affect specific organs and produce single major

anomalies (e.g., congenital heart defects or spina bifida). Abnormalities that occur after the major body regions and organs are formed (9–40 weeks after fertilization) alter the fine tuning of embryonic structure (phenogenesis). These later derangements produce more subtle defects including minor anomalies and normal variants (e.g., single palmar crease). An interesting type of anomaly is the *developmental arrest* that resembles more primitive embryonic structures. Examples include cleft palate, webbing of the digits, bicornuate uterus, single brain ventricle (holoprosencephaly), and persistence of the tail—all normal structures at

■ **TABLE 11.3.** Causes of Congenital Anomalies

Category	Types	Usual Characteristics	Example
Chromosomal abnormalities	Polyploidy	Multiple defects, mental retardation	Triploidy
	Aneuploidy		Down syndrome
	Mosaicism		Hypomelanosis of Ito
	Uniparental disomy		Angelman syndrome
	Microdeletions		Williams syndrome
Mendelian abnormalities	Autosomal dominant traits	Vertical patterns	Achondroplasia (100800)
	Autosomal recessive traits	Horizontal patterns	Zellweger syndrome (214100)
	X-linked dominant traits	Oblique pattern, male lethality	Incontinentia Pigmenti (308300)
	X-linked recessive traits	Oblique pattern, males affected	Coffin-Lowry syndrome (303600)
	Y-linked traits	Vertical pattern, males affected	None
Atypical inheritance	Mitochondrial diseases	Maternal inheritance	MELAS syndrome
	Disorders of imprinting	Parent-of-origin effects	Prader-Willi syndrome
	Triplet repeat expansion	Anticipation	Fragile X syndrome
Multifactorial abnormalities	Common birth defects	Empiric recurrence risk	Hydrocephalus
		Sex predilection	Spina bifida
		Lower twin discordance	Cleft palate
			Pyloric stenosis
			Heart defects
Environmental abnormalities (teratogenic syndromes)	Chemicals	Sporadic occurrence	FAS
	Physical agents	High twin concordance	Hyperthermia
	Infectious agents	Low recurrence risk	Congenital rubella
	Maternal metabolism	Gestational exposure	Maternal PKU, maternal DM

Notes: MELAS, mitochondrial encephalopathy with lactic acidosis and strokes; FAS, fetal alcohol syndrome; PKU, phenylketonuria; DM, diabetes mellitus.

earlier developmental stages. These anomalies are "frozen in time" at the moment when their development became overtly abnormal.

Further classification of anomalies can be made according to embryonic mechanism. Extrinsic developmental injuries interrupt normal embryonic processes in contrast to intrinsic developmental injuries where the primordial structure (anlagen) is abnormal from the beginning. An example is cleft palate caused by hydantoin therapy in women with seizures. Palate development is normal until the drug interferes with (disrupts) its formation, an extrinsic process known as *disruption.* Another extrinsic process is that of *deformation,* illustrated by clubfeet (*talipes equinovarus*) that occur in fetuses born to a mother with uterine anomalies or fibroids. Constriction of the uterine cavity exerts pressure on the developing limb, resulting in inadequate movement and limb deformation to produce clubfoot.

Intrinsic developmental abnormalities are exemplified by abnormal connective tissue (dysplasias) or malformations such as an extra finger (polydactyly). Some dysplasias, like those affecting the blood vessels (hemangiomas) or bones (skeletal dysplasias), extend throughout the body in the appropriate tissue regions. Others, like lymphatic enlargements of the neck called *cystic hygromas,* occur in one location. Malformations involve abnormal primordia like the embryonic limb bud that results in polydactyly. Each of these categories—deformations, disruptions, dysplasias, and malformations—can occur in combinations known as syndromes.

Because the precise details of development are rarely known in detail, overlap among these mechanistic categories can certainly occur. For example, clubfoot may occur as a secondary deformation in certain syndromes involving uterine constriction or fetal immobility and as a primary, isolated malformation in other individuals. Any particular anomaly is often causally heterogenous, illustrated by the many genetic and chromosomal syndromes that can produce a duplicated great toe or radial aplasia.

Dysplasias include disorders such as achondroplasia (100800), osteogenesis imperfecta (166240), or Marfan syndrome (154700) because the abnormalities in each condition can be reduced to a defect in connective tissue (Table 11.2). Disruptions may be extended to include anomalies produced by teratogens, because these interfere with normal development. Deformations can include lopsided head shapes (plagiocephalies), wry or tilted neck (torticollis), scoliosis (curved spine) in the absence of vertebral anomalies, single palmar crease, and bowing of the legs.

Sequences: Single Anomalies with Multiple Consequences

A *sequence* represents a cascade of primary and secondary events that are consequences of a single primary malformation or a disruption. Sequences, like isolated malformations, are most often associated with sporadic or multifactorial inheritance. Examples include the sequence of lower limb immobility and atrophy with bladder dysfunction produced by denervation secondary to lower spina bifida. Another would be the defective sacrum, imperforate anus, and urinary tract obstruction produced by a caudal fetal tumor called sacrococcygeal teratoma. Sequences are often mixtures of anomaly types, exemplified by the renal malformation in Potter sequence that produces sparse amniotic fluid (oligohydramnios) with secondary deformations including flattened face and club feet. Affected fetuses also have dysplasia of skin elastic tissue, producing redundant skin and wrinkles.

A dramatic phenotype is produced by the fetal akinesia or immobility sequence, in which decreased breathing and limb movements produce lung hypoplasia with multiple limb contractures (arthrogryposis). Milder disorders with fetal hypotonia or immobility produce bitemporal hollowing, down-turned corners of the mouth, chest concavity due to increased flexibility (pectus excavatum), single palmar creases, and undescended testes (cryptorchidism), and constipation due to abdominal muscle weakness.

Multiple Congenital Anomalies

The distinction between patients with isolated versus multiple congenital anomalies is fundamental for classifying anomalies by type and possible cause (Tables 11.2 and 11.3). Crucial for this distinction is the recognition of minor anomalies such as those in Figure 11.3 that may shift the patient with one major defect into the syndrome category. It is also important to distinguish *associations* from syndromes. Associations are relatively common and usually have more optimistic medical and genetic prognoses than do syndromes.

When the term *syndrome* is employed, a lower level of embryologic understanding is implied than that for a sequence. Sequences presume the operation of an initiating event and an ensuing cascade of secondary effects that can be predicted. Syndromes either are not understood as patterns of secondary effects, or are suspected to extend beyond the effect of any one organ or body region. As human embryology becomes better defined, some syndromes may become sequences. Syndromes often imply greater genetic and medical risks that require more complex counseling and management.

Associations consist of major anomalies with similar embryologic timing. The VATER association of *V*ertebral, *A*norectal, *T*racheo-*E*sophageal, *R*adial and *R*enal defects involves mesodermal derivatives that begin differentiation at 20–25 days of embryogenesis. Associations have few minor anomalies, because there is no persistent influence like an extra chromosome to alter fine-tuning of development. Individuals with associations do not have a characteristic facial appearance. One tabulates the defects, then appreciates the association as opposed to recognizing a typical face and anticipating the defects in a syndrome. Radial aplasia, if associated with tracheo-esophageal atresia and renal defects, immediately suggests a diagnosis of VATER association. Unfortunately, patients with trisomy 18 may have the same major defects. Suspicion of the more devastating syndrome requires attention to minor anomalies such as the disproportionately small face, prominent occiput, clenched fist, and convex feet that are illustrated in Figure 11.3*B*.

A final type of anomaly is more theoretical and is known as a *developmental field defect*. Developmental field defects affect a reactive unit of the embryo such that a consistent pattern of major anomalies are produced by different genetic or environmental agents. The concept is similar to Spemann's organizer in frog embryos that was discussed in Chapter 9. Tissue in the dorsal lip of the blastopore had the potential to induce a second embryonic axis when explanted to frog embryos, suggesting that defects in this region might produce a spectrum of craniospinal anomalies. An example in humans is the holoprosencephaly spectrum of anomalies that varies from midline cleft palate (premaxillary agenesis) to severe cyclopia (single eye) with absence of the forebrain. Holoprosencephaly can be produced by toxins in sheep, defective *sonic hedgehog* gene product in the mouse (see Chapter 9), and by numerous Mendelian, microdeletion, or aneuploid genetic changes in humans. The value of recognizing developmental field defects is similar to that of recognizing sequences: the realization that several consequences are a reproducible response to a single embryonic injury allows them to be viewed as a single anomaly rather than an anomaly pattern. Field defects such as the holoprosencephaly spectrum often have the lower recurrence risks of isolated anomalies unless they are part of an expanded syndrome like that caused by trisomy 13 (see Chapter 7) or Smith-Lemli-Opitz syndrome (270400, see below and Fig. 9.10 of Chapter 9).

Case 11 Follow-up: In patient 11A, the absence of additional major or minor anomalies, together with knowledge of branchial arch development, suggests an isolated anomaly of the jaw with excellent prognosis and low recurrence risk. This anomaly is known as Pierre Robin sequence, involving small jaw (micrognathia), protuberant tongue (glossoptosis), and a posterior, U-shaped cleft palate. These anomalies are related as a sequence in which the small jaw prevents tongue descent and interferes with fusion of the palatal shelves. Because the cleft palate and abnormal tongue are secondary effects of the small jaw, Pierre Robin sequence can be viewed as a single anomaly. This view is supported by the low recurrence risk of less than one percent and the excellent prognosis for Pierre Robin sequence. Neonates with Robin anomaly do have increased risk for respiratory obstruction when placed on their backs, so prone positioning is recommended. This is an exception to the recent "baby on back" recommendations that recognize a higher risk for sudden infant death with prone positioning.

The more extensive anomalies in patients 11B and 11C (Fig. 11.1) are suggestive of malformation syndromes. Patient 11B had the Nager syndrome (154400) of branchial arch anomalies including Robin sequence, absence of the radius with wrist deviation, and cardiac anomalies. This syndrome is listed as an autosomal dominant condition in the McKusick catalogue, but many cases have exhibited autosomal recessive inheritance. Suspicion of a syndrome by the managing physician led to specialty evaluation and a diagnosis with a

potentially significant (25%) recurrence risk as outlined in Figure 11.2. Had the diagnosis been recognized in the nursery, preventive management of Nager syndrome would have included cardiac assessment with possible surgical or medical therapy. In this case, the Robin sequence occurred as one among several anomalies known as Nager syndrome.

Patient 11C has facial anomalies in addition to those of the small jaw and cleft palate that again suggest a malformation syndrome. The facial appearance is characteristic of the autosomal dominant Treacher Collins syndrome (154500) with down-slanting palpebral fissures and malar hypoplasia. Suspicion of a syndrome led to documentation of the family history in which the father and two brothers were had similar manifestations (Fig. 11.4). The diagnosis of Treacher Collins syndrome allowed genetic counseling reinforcing the 50% recurrence risk for affected individuals and preventive management concerning the risks for feeding problems, deafness, and respiratory problems due to the small jaw and pharynx. Although patients with Treacher Collins syndrome have the same small jaw and risk for cleft palate as in Robin sequence, the actual mechanism is probably different. Once again, the small jaw

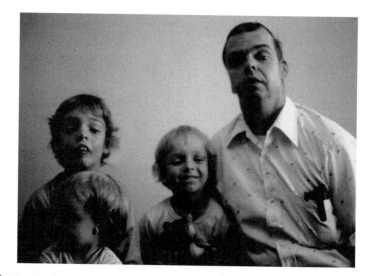

Figure 11.4. Family of Case 11C. The father and one brother of the patient have down-slanting palpebral fissures, malar hypoplasia, and small jaws characteristic of the Treacher Collins syndrome.

and cleft palate occur within a larger pattern that suggests a malformation syndrome with higher recurrence and complication risks.

■ 11.3. THE DYSMORPHOLOGY EXAMINATION: GESTALT, ANALYTIC, AND INTERPRETIVE APPROACHES

Despite advances in chromosomal and DNA analysis, most congenital anomalies and anomaly patterns must be diagnosed by physical examination. The systematic gathering of gestational and family history data, followed by a careful physical examination, usually allows placement of the anomalous child into a particular diagnostic category (Fig. 11.2). The recognition and interpretation of anomalies during physical examination is essential to this categorical approach, and it is necessary to be familiar with minor anomalies such as those illustrated in Figure 11.3. As emphasized previously, children that fall into the category of single anomalies have lower risks for complications than do those with multiple anomalies. Individuals with isolated anomalies have a more optimistic prognosis for function and quality of life unless the anomaly involves the brain. If a major anomaly is diagnosed without appreciation of subtle facial or minor anomalies, then the pattern indicative of a syndrome may be missed. The examples of cases 11B and 11C show that misdiagnosis of these syndromes as isolated Robin sequence would lead to inappropriate genetic counseling and missed opportunities for early recognition and treatment of complications.

The Gestalt Approach— Facial Recognition

The gestalt approach takes advantage of the stereotypic facial appearance of many malformation syndromes that is illustrated in Figure 11.5. Gestalt recognition draws upon the innate ability of human beings to recognize and recall thousands of faces. This skill probably evolved along with the higher brain functions that led to complex social interactions among primates, including pair bonding and dominance hierarchies. It was by gestalt recognition that the "funny-looking kid" became identified for morphologic evaluation, now better expressed as the child with unusual facial appearance. The value of gestalt recognition is recognized in syndrome nomenclature, illustrated by the fetal face (Robinow—180700) or whistling face (Freeman-Sheldon—193700) syndromes. It is highlighted in certain atlases of syndromes like those of Jones (1997), Gorlin et al. (1990), or visual databases like that of Winter and Baraitser (1998) or Bankier (1998).

As useful as gestalt recognition may be in disorders like Down syndrome, its limitations include bias by past experience and the rush to a snap diagnosis before a thorough evaluation has taken place. Familial features may underlie the resemblance of a patient to syndrome photographs, and significant clinical problems may be ignored in the attempt to match a face with published pictures. A quotation from Gor-

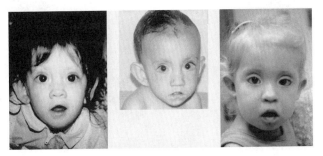

Figure 11.5. Three children with Niikawa-Kuroki syndrome that illustrate a stereotypic facial appearance.

lin (1980) emphasizes the bias endemic to gestalt diagnosis as taken from the principles of gestalt psychology: "We, as dysmorphologists, can learn much from the psychiatrists: why we see what we do and fail to see what we should."

Syndrome variability is another limitation of gestalt recognition, reflecting variable severity, family background, age, and ethnicity. A helpful way of differentiating syndrome gestalt from family background is to inspect the family photograph albums. The examiner can establish rapport by sharing a pastime with pleasant connotations, providing the opportunity to differentiate variant from familial features. The utility of inspecting parental baby pictures emphasizes that many syndromes have a natural history with different facial characteristics at different ages. This natural history has been elegantly defined for Noonan syndrome (Fig. 11.6). The examiner is like the audience in John Barth's novel *The Floating Opera:* A complete story unfolds as the boat moves along the river, but those at any one place are limited to a single scene.

The Analytic Approach—Minor Anomalies and Measurements

A second aspect of the morphologic examination can be described as the analytic approach (Fig. 11.2). The unusual face is described in terms of particular minor anomalies like the down-slanting palpebral fissures mentioned in Figures 11.1*B* and 11.1*C*. Unlike the inspection that promotes gestalt recognition, the patient is gone over thoroughly to find each variation in morphology, however subtle. The distinction between qualitative and quantitative traits mentioned in Chapter 1 comes into play in the morphologic examination. Some anomalies, like the prominent occiput or syndactyly in Figure 11.3*D*, are subjectively assessed as present or absent. Other anomalies such as decreased height or head circumference (microcephaly) are objectively determined using measurements and age-appropriate standards. For these quantitative traits, deviation by more than two standard deviations from the age-appropriate norm (below the 3rd or above the 97th centile) is scored as abnormal. Still other anomalies may be recorded either as subjective all-or-none judgments or based on objective measurements. Patients with increased distance between the eyes (hypertelorism) may be identified by gestalt recognition or by measured deviation beyond the 97th centile for age. Experience of the examiner often determines whether subjective inspection or measurements are used.

The analytic approach stems from physical anthropology and can utilize numerous measurement standards accumulated for human growth and development (e.g., Saul et al., 1988). Although these objective measures may be useful in certain clinical situations, they may require training to use properly and are mostly in the domain of clinical genetic spe-

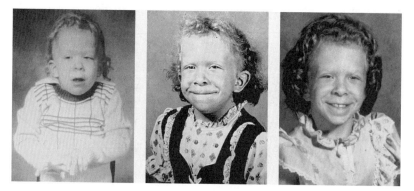

Figure 11.6. Different facial appearances in a child with Noonan syndrome at ages 3, 10, and 12 years.

cialists. Radiology is of particular value in the analytic approach, and a skeletal survey often reveals valuable information in any syndrome with bony abnormalities. Several textbooks provide standard measurements for such radiographic traits as bone age, limb lengths, skull size, acetabular angles, or hand bone length profiles as mentioned previously. All measurements must be used in the context of overall patient evaluation, because no set of measurements can replace clinical judgment in assessing the presence and significance of morphologic variations.

A useful adjunct to the analytic morphologic examination is a checklist to ensure complete ascertainment. Checklists are particularly useful in training, because they force novice examiners to become familiar with the many types of minor anomalies. The value of checklists has been demonstrated in several studies, exemplified by the lack of findings in infants exposed to cocaine (Little et al., 1996) or the use of minor anomaly clusters to predict the presence of major anomalies (Leppig et al., 1987). In the latter study of 4305 infants, a 114-item checklist was used to demonstrate a 19.6% risk for major anomalies in infants with three or more minor anomalies compared to 3.7% in the screened population. These and other studies dramatize the value of minor anomalies in recognizing children at risk for major anomalies and syndromes.

An additional task of the analytic approach is to determine which tissues and body regions are affected by a particular anomaly pattern. The distribution and type of anomalies has played a major role in syndrome nomenclature, illustrated by the prefixes acro- (terminal), meso- (middle), or rhizo- (proximal) to describe limb shortening. Other prefixes useful for describing skeletal dysplasias include spondylo- (spinal), costo- (ribs), or coxo- (hips) for body parts, or epiphyseal (epiphysis), metaphyseal (growth plate), or diaphyseal (shaft) for regions of long bones. Spondyloepiphyseal dysplasia describes a category of skeletal dysplasias that involve the spine and long bone epiphyses, typified by spondyloepiphyseal dysplasia congenita (183900) with

early onset. Other concessions to geographic description without knowledge of cause include otopalatodigital (Taybi) syndrome (311300), oculodentodigital syndrome (164200), and the group of orofaciodigital syndromes. The ability to define particular anomalies or affected body regions also promotes the use of syndrome databases with search functions (Jones, 1997; Gorlin et al., 1999; Winter and Baraitser, 1998; Bankier, 1998).

A last but extremely important aspect of the analytic approach is the preservation of material for subsequent evaluation. Anomalous children may be encountered as stillbirths, autopsy specimens, or as patients in remote or noncompliant settings. These encounters still provide opportunities for diagnosis if appropriate photographs, radiographs, and/or tissue specimens are preserved. As emphasized in Chapter 5, the stillborn or expiring infant with an unusual appearance or multiple anomalies should have photographs, full-body radiographs (babygram), and possibly tissue preserved for later analysis. Skin biopsy for subsequent fibroblast culture and metabolic or chromosomal analysis can be preserved in tissue culture medium at room temperature, as can heparinized peripheral or cord blood. As illustrated by patient 11B, photographs can lead to postmortem diagnoses with substantial genetic implications.

Interpretation of Anomalies: The Transcendental Approach

A third aspect of the morphologic examination consists of interpretation. Here, one attempts to go beneath the surface pattern, the quantitative profile, the organ distribution, and acquire insight into the primary etiology. This process of interpretation might be termed the transcendental approach (Fig. 11.2) in homage to the transcendental morphologists of the nineteenth century. These morphologists, exemplified by Etienne Serres, labored to relate congenital anomalies to fundamental principles like "ontogeny recapitulates phylogeny." The transcendental morphologists were fascinated by anomalies such as holoprosencephaly (Fig. 11.1; Fig. 9.10) that mimicked the organ structures of simpler animals. As Serres expressed in 1866:

> I did not know how to express the feeling of admiration I had for the grandeur of creation in general and for that of man in particular, when I saw that, at a first stage [of ontogeny], the human brain resembled that of a fish, that at a second stage it resembled that of reptiles, at a third, that of birds, and at a fourth, that of mammals, in order finally to elevate itself to that sublime organization that dominates all nature. (Gould, 1977).

Anomalies were viewed as arrests in this evolutionary process that gave insights into both embryogenesis and comparative anatomy.

Once a facial resemblance is considered, and the number and types of anomalies documented, the transcendental or interpretive aspect of the morphologic examination attempts to weave these findings into a chain of etiology and diagnosis. Anomalies are interpreted according to the timing and mechanism of altered development, to their status as primary or secondary effects, and, most importantly, to their distribution as isolated anomalies or syndromes (Fig. 11.2). As particular examples of syndrome categories are discussed in Sections 11.4–11.10, the role of the gestalt, analytic, and interpretive approaches are illustrated in marking the path to etiology. The modern equivalent of transcendental morphology is the relation of syndrome patterns to particular developmentally active genes as discussed extensively in Chapter 9. The discovery of homologous developmental genes that direct the embryology of organisms as diverse as fruit flies and humans would have brought great pleasure and vindication to morphologists of the nineteenth century.

■ 11.4. CLINICAL PROBLEMS WITH HIGH RISKS FOR SYNDROMES

Before considering examples of different syndrome categories, clinical problems associated with increased risk for syndromes is discussed. Some of these problems are listed in Table 11.1.

Mental Disability

The multiple anomalies in malformation syndromes are evidence of abnormal embryonic processes. Because abnormal developmental processes tend to affect the most complex organs, brain structure and function is often impacted in these disorders. Mental retardation or, to use terminology with a less negative connotation, mental disability is present in almost 40% of Mendelian syndromes but in only 3% of inherited single anomalies (Wilson, 1992). The greater risk for mental disability as the number of congenital anomalies increases is also supported by its presence in 95% of chromosome disorders, which average 11 defects per syndrome compared to 3.5 defects per syndrome for Mendelian disorders. Mental disability is thus present in about one-half of children with multiple congenital anomalies, and its presence should be considered and anticipated by referral for early intervention services.

The correlation between multiple malformations and mental disability also works in reverse, evidenced by frequent referral of children with developmental delay for morphologic evaluation. Often these delayed children are seen by specialists in neurology, developmental pediatrics, and genetics/dysmorphology for consideration of etiologies within each specialty domain. Children with obvious brain malformations, particularly when accompanied by seizures, are often followed by neurology. Children with cerebral palsy, hydrocephalus, or spina bifida, plus those with autistic or hyperactive behaviors, are often followed by developmental pediatricians with expertise in rehabilitative services. Many, if not most, of these children have an underlying genetic disorder with or without obvious anomalies. Genetic etiology is easy to recognize in disorders with obvious anomalies such as Treacher-Collins syndrome (Fig. 11.1C) but difficult or impossible to recognize in children with subtle anomalies or no anomalies at all. Some children with disabilities and no dysmorphology have metabolic diseases, while others have so-called nonspecific mental retardation without any obvious morphologic or metabolic changes.

The prediction that many or most children with nonspecific mental retardation have underlying genetic disease comes from the work on X-linked mental retardation. As mentioned in Chapter 10 concerning fragile X syndrome, more than 40 types of nonspecific X-linked mental retardation have been recognized because of the obvious inheritance pattern in families. If one extrapolates from the X chromosome to 22 autosomes, and recognizes that simpler organisms such as the worm *C. elegans* have 120 types of cells in their brains, then it is easy to visualize the multiple genes and cell types that must be necessary for human brain function. Mutations in these genes may present as sporadic cases of mental disability with or without additional anomalies. It is likely that the human genome project (see Chapter 8) will eventually provide panels of neurally expressed genes that can be tested in such children. Until such screening is available, the examiner should look for minor anomalies that will aid syndrome identification but never eliminate the possibility of genetic causation when this search is unrevealing. Fetal alcohol syndrome, discussed in Section 11.9, provides an example of how children with mental disability may be assigned a specific diagnosis by noting subtle morphologic alterations.

Parts of the Elephant: Cerebral Palsy, Autism, and Pervasive Developmental Disorder

The rule emphasizing overlap between malformation syndromes and mental disability must also be extrapolated to other types of mental dysfunction. Using again the analogy of the blind men and the elephant, particular developmental or behavioral features may be noted without appreciating the entire spectrum of abnormality. It is important to realize that terms such as cerebral palsy, autism, or pervasive de-

velopmental disorder are really adjectives rather than nouns, descriptions rather than designations of primary cause. The "syndrome" of increased reflexes, toe-walking, and incoordinated movements (spasticity), coupled with oromotor problems concerning swallowing and speech, may provide a clinical diagnosis of cerebral palsy that is quite useful for anticipation and management. However, it does not imply a specific etiology even though brain insults in the perinatal period have been emphasized. Despite the propaganda of wrongful birth lawsuits, many genetic disorders such as the Lesch-Nyhan syndrome (308000) include spasticity and abnormal movements that may be called cerebral palsy until the appropriate metabolic studies are performed. Spasticity is also a common symptom in several types of nonspecific X-linked retardation, mandating careful morphologic examination, gestational, and family histories in all children with a diagnosis of cerebral palsy.

Autism is also a symptom complex that occurs in many children with mental disability. Avoidance of gaze, poor interactions, and self-preoccupation are seen in many genetic disorders such as fragile X syndrome, although specialty evaluation may distinguish these "autistic features" from true autism. Pervasive developmental disorder that tends to involve children with large head circumference (macrocephaly), autistic features, inappropriate play (as in lining up rather than playing with toy cars) also is heterogenous. Children with these diagnoses, however useful they may be for behavioral and school management, must always be suspected of genetic etiology and have thorough morphologic assessments. When several minor and/or major anomalies are found in children with nonspecific mental retardation, with or without symptoms of spasticity or autism, then a genetic evaluation including chromosome studies is mandated.

Growth Abnormalities

The most common abnormality of growth in children is undergrowth or *failure to thrive,* with rare children exhibiting overgrowth or *gigantism.* Malformation syndromes with both types of abnormal growth have been described, as summarized in Table 11.4. Growth failure can be due to inadequate calories (starvation), inadequate feeding (behavioral problems, multiple types of oromotor dysfunction or blockage), inadequate absorption (intestinal defects such as celiac disease or lactase deficiency), inadequate metabolism due to hormonal deficiencies (e.g., thyroid hormone deficiency), or inadequate growth response to normal food intake. Children with syndromes often fail to grow because of oromotor problems or because their tissues simply do not respond to normal food intake. This abnormal growth response is a striking feature of many children with malformations, and it often cannot be defined in terms of specific gastrointestinal defects or hormonal deficiencies.

■**TABLE 11.4.** Syndromes with Growth Delay

Syndrome (inheritance)	Incidence	Frequent Abnormalities
Growth delay, often with low BW and/or microcephaly		
Russell-Silver (sporadic; 312780)	~150 cases reported	Normal head size, triangular face, hemihypertophy, clinodactyly
Fetal alcohol (teratogen)	1 in 1000 births	Low BW, microcephaly, thin upper lip, absent philtrum, cardiac defects, mild DD
Cockayne (216400)	~50 cases reported	Low or normal BW, microcephaly, accelerated aging, severe DD
Smith-Lemli-Opitz (270400)	~100 cases reported	Low BW, microcephaly, brain anomalies, hypertelorism, GI defects, severe DD
Brachmann-de Lange (sporadic, 122470)	1 in 10,000 births	Low BW, microcephaly, hirsutism, glaucoma, cardiac defects, severe DD
Noonan (sporadic, 163950)	1 in 2500 births	Normal BW, ptosis, webbed neck, cardiac defects, cryptorchidism, mild DD
Aarskog (100050)	~100 cases reported	Normal BW, hypertelorism, lax finger joints, saddle-bag scrotum, mild DD
Niikawa-Kuroki (sporadic, 147920)	~150 cases reported	Normal BW, microcephaly, cardiac defects, renal defects, moderate DD
Williams (microdeletion, 194050)	1 in 25,000 births	Normal BW, microcephaly, aortic stenosis, renal anomalies, mild DD
Skeletal dysplasias, usually with normal BW and normal head size		
Thanatophoric dwarfism (187600)	1 in 25,000 births	Short limbs, small thorax, cleft palate, neonatal death
Achondroplasia (100800)	1 in 25,000 births	Short limbs, frontal bossing, spinal compression, hypotonia
Cleidocranial dysplasia (119600)	~ 700 cases reported	Macrocephaly, large fontanelle, absent clavicles, dental anomalies
Cartilage-hair hypoplasia (250250)	~ 100 cases reported	Short limbs, immune deficiency, Hodgkin's disease, lymphomas
Osteogenesis imperfecta type I (166200)	1 in 20,000 births	Multiple fractures, blue sclerae, hearing loss, bowed limbs

Notes: BW, birth weight; DD, developmental disability; GI, gastrointestinal.

As part of routine pediatric care, growth is monitored using charts for expected height, weight, and head circumference (Fig. 11.7). Growth abnormalities can be categorized according to their deviation from these normal growth charts as illustrated in Figure 11.7. In contrast to child A whose height, weight, and head circumference are in the normal range, child B has proportionate decreases in all three measurements. Child B has the classic profile of failure to thrive that can represent inadequate intake (e.g., neglect, poverty) or a myriad of medical diseases. Child C, on the other hand, has disproportionate growth with decreased height (short stature) and increased head circumference (macrocephaly). This

growth profile suggests a skeletal dysplasia, because the limb bones are shortened but the head circumference, driven by brain growth, is less affected. Child D has decreased height and weight with even greater decrease in head circumference (microcephaly). Since there is usually "head sparing" when calories are inadequate, the disproportionately small head circumference suggests abnormal brain development common in many teratogenic (e.g., fetal alcohol), chromosomal (e.g., Down), and other malformation syndromes.

Patterns of overgrowth are also suggestive of certain syndrome categories, as summarized in Table 11.5. Proportionate overgrowth as in child E of Figure 11.7 occurs in disorders such as the Wiedemann-Beckwith or Sotos syndromes (see Section 11.8), while the disproportionate head growth in child F is common in benign tumor (hamartosis) syndromes (Table 11.5) like neurofibromatosis-1 (162200) or tuberous sclerosis (191100). Child G exhibits marked weight increase (obesity) that is seen in the Prader-Willi or Cohen (216550) syndromes, while child H shows the tall stature and lower weight (thin habitus) that would be typical of syndromes with connective tissue laxity (e.g., Marfan syndrome, 154700). Growth failure or acceleration, particularly if there is disproportion between head circumference and stature, is a strong indicator for genetic evaluation.

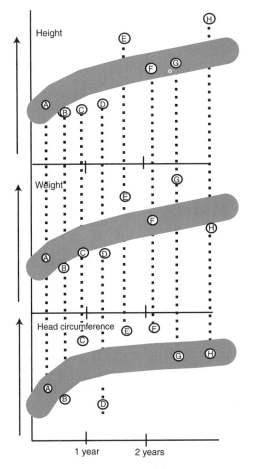

Figure 11.7. Patterns of abnormal growth. Each letter represents the height, weight, and head circumference measurements of a particular child.

Hypotonia with or Without Congenital Contractures (Arthrogryposis)

A common early symptom of abnormal brain development is decreased muscle tone or hypotonia. Hypotonia may be striking in disorders such as Zellweger syndrome (214100), producing characteristic facial manifestations (see Section 11.7). The facial manifestations include concavities at the temples (bitemporal hollowing), down-turned corners of the mouth, and an expressionless, masklike face. Children with severe hypotonia have impaired oromotor strength during infancy and may require tube feedings. They may exhibit proportionate failure to thrive as in profile B of Figure 11.7.

■ **TABLE 11.5.** Overgrowth and Hamartosis Syndromes

Syndrome (inheritance)	Incidence	Frequent Abnormalities
Overgrowth syndromes, often with large BW and large head size (macrocephaly)		
Wiedemann-Beckwith (sporadic)	1 in 17,000 births	Large tongue, omphalocele, renal anomalies, neonatal hypoglycemia
Sotos (cerebral gigantism) (sporadic)	> 200 cases reported	Macrocephaly, hypotonia, accelerated osseous maturation, moderate DD
Weaver (sporadic)	~ 20 cases reported	Macrocephaly, accelerated osseous maturation, joint contractures, hernias
Simpson-Golabi-Behmel (312870)	~ 30 cases reported	Macrocephaly, polydactyly, GU anomalies, early death, moderate DD
Hamartosis (benign tumor) syndromes, often with large head size (macrocephaly)		
Basal cell carcinoma (Gorlin—109400)	~ 500 cases reported	Nevoid basal cell carcinomas, jaw cysts, scoliosis, other cancers
Bannayan-Ruvalcaba-Zonana (153480)	~ 100 cases reported	Macrocephaly, lipomas, hemangiomas, intestinal polyps, penile spots, mild DD
Gardner (APC—175100)	1 in 12,000 births	Skin cysts, bony osteomas, colonic polyps, colon cancer, other cancers
Klippel-Trenauney-Weber (sporadic)	~ 1000 cases reported	Hemangiomas, skeletal asymmetry, limb anomalies
Neurofibromatosis-1 (162200)	1 in 2500 births	Café-au-lait spots, neurofibromas, skeletal anomalies, seizures, mild DD
Neurofibromatosis-2 (101000)	1 in 100,000 births	Acoustic neuromas, deafness
Peutz-Jeghers (175200)	~ 300 cases reported	Skin and mouth pigmentation, intestinal polyposis, cancer
Tuberous sclerosis (191100)	1 in 10,000 births	Hypopigmented spots, angiofibomas, brain, cardiac and renal tumors

Notes: APC, adenomatous polyposis coli; BW, birth weight; GU, genitourinary; DD, developmental disability.

Children with Prader-Willi syndrome usually exhibit marked hypotonia and feeding problems in the neonatal period, then undergo a remarkable transition to overeating and obesity in later childhood.

When hypotonia is severe during fetal life, the immobility of limb and chest muscles may produce changes that have been called the fetal akinesia sequence. The limbs become flexed and immobile, presenting as congenital contractures that are known as *arthrogryposis* (*arthro* = joint, *gryp* = contracture). Because the lungs require chest wall movement and fetal breathing for development, there is pulmonary hypoplasia that may be lethal. The fetal akinesia sequence can be produced in rats by administering the paralyzing agent curare during gestation.

Although fetal immobility is known to result in arthrogryposis, there are many syndromes with various patterns of arthrogryposis due to neuropathic, myopathic, or positional causes (Table 11.6). Severe impairment of the central or peripheral nervous system can lead to arthrogryposis because of impaired limb innervation, as illustrated by the Pena-Shokeir (208150) or severe Werdnig-Hoffman spinal nerve atrophy (253300). The clubfeet in Zellweger syndrome occur because of abnormal brian function and hypotonia. Impaired muscle function can cause decreased movement and arthrogryposis as in the Marden-Walker syn-

■ **TABLE 11.6.** Syndromes with Congenital Contractures or Joint Laxity

Syndrome	Incidence	Complications
Disorders with Congenital Contractures		
Amyoplasia (sporadic)	1 in 10,000 births	Limb contractures, small jaw, muscle atrophy
Multiple pterygium (265000)	~ 60 cases reported	Limb and digital contractures, pterygia (webbing) of neck and limbs, cleft palate, scoliosis, genital anomalies, DD, FTT
Popliteal pterygium (119500)	~ 80 cases reported	Limb and digital contractures, popliteal pterygia, cleft palate, genital anomalies, DD, FTT
Beals congenital contractural arachno-dactyly (121050)	~ 100 cases reported	Digital contractures, unusual ears, Marfanoid habitus, aortic dilatation, scoliosis, optic lens dislocation
Pena-Shokeir type I (208150)	1 in 10,000 births	Digital contractures, clubfeet, hypertelorism, cardiac anomalies, urogenital anomalies, DD, FTT
Pena-Shokeir type II (214150)	~ 25 cases reported	Hip and knee contractures, microcephaly, brain anomalies, cataracts, DD, FTT
Whistling face (Freeman-Sheldon) (193700)	~ 65 cases reported	Distal limb contractures, microstomia and "whistling face," facial immobility, deviated ("windvane") fingers, DD, FTT
Disorders with Joint Laxity		
Cutis laxa (123700)	~ 100 cases reported	Lax skin and joints, pulmonary disease, dilated arteries, hernias, diverticula
Ehlers-Danlos type I (130000)	1 in 10,000 births	Lax joints, "cigarette paper" scars, scoliosis, hernias, prematurity
Larsen (150250)	~ 200 cases reported	Lax joints, dislocations, cleft palate, laryngeal stenosis, spinal anomalies
Marfan (154700)	1 in 10,000 births	Tall stature, lax joints, optic lens dislocation, aortic aneurysm, hernias
Stickler syndrome (108300)	~ 200 cases reported	Lax joints, Marfanoid habitus, myopia, retinal disease, cleft palate

Notes: DD, developmental disability; FTT, failure to thrive.

drome (248700), as can fetal constraint exemplified by the Potter sequence. Contractures due to fetal constraint by extrinsic forces in the uterus are called *deformations*. In Potter sequence, the oligohydramnios resulting from decreased fetal urine constrains fetal limb motion and produces lower limb contractures (clubfeet, immobile hips). Although congenital contractures can be associated with nongenetic causes such as the presence of uterine fibroid tumors, the presence of arthrogryposis is another strong predictor of a malformation syn-

drome (Table 11.6). These children need careful morphologic and genetic evaluation.

Connective Tissue Laxity

Lax joints are in a sense the opposite of arthrogryposis, and they constitute another risk factor for malformation syndromes. Increased joint flexibility occurs as a nonspecific feature in children with hypotonia but is more striking in disorders with abnormal connective tissue (Table 11.6). A striking example is Marfan syndrome (Fig. 2.2, 154700), now known to result from deficiency of the extracellular matrix protein fibrillin. The decreased connective tissue strength results in increased stature as shown in Fig. 11.7*H*, as well as tissue defects in the eye (dislocated lens), heart (aortic dilation), chest (pectus excavatum), trunk (inguinal hernia), and limbs (flat feet, joint dislocations). Certain of these problems are general features of syndromes with connective tissue weakness as summarized in Table 11.6. When the lax connective tissue occurs in the skin, an aged appearance (e.g., cutis laxa—123700) or unusual scarring (e.g., Ehlers-Danlos syndromes—130000) may result. Many children with diverse chromosomal or malformation syndromes may have lax joints, blue sclerae (decreased connective tissue in the white of the eye as with osteogenesis imperfecta—166200), and loose or redundant skin as nonspecific manifestations.

Apparently Isolated Congenital Anomalies

The category of single congenital anomalies is discussed extensively in Chapter 13 concerning surgical disorders; it is mentioned here as

■ TABLE 11.7. Single Anomalies That May Predict Syndromes

Anomaly	Associated Syndromes	Additional Findings
Hydrocephalus	Walker-Warburg (236670)	Lissencephaly, retinal detachment, severe DD
	Pallister-Hall (146510)	Pituitary tumors, polydactyly, genital anomalies, anal atresia, severe DD
	Hydrolethalus (236680)	Small jaw, heart defects, cleft palate, polydactyly, severe DD
Dislocated lens	Marfan syndrome (154700)	Tall stature, lax joints, arachnodactyly, aortic aneurysm, hernias, flat feet
	Homocystinuria (236200)	Marfanoid habitus, clotting diathesis, elevated blood homocystine
	Beals contractural arachnodactyly (121050)	Digital contractures, unusual ears, Marfanoid habitus, scoliosis
Cleft lip/palate	Rib gap (CCM, 117650)	Small jaw, abnormal ribs, respiratory difficulties
	EEC (129900)	Absent digits, conical teeth, sparse hair, decreased sweating, hyperthermia
	Larsen (150250)	Lax joints, flat face, joint dislocations
	Meckel (249000)	Encephalocele, renal defects, severe DD
Robin (small jaw, cleft palate)	Treacher-Collins (154500)	Branchial defects, abnormal ears, deafness
	Nager (154400)	Branchial defects, abnormal ears, radial aplasia
	Stickler (108300)	Lax joints, Marfanoid habitus, shallow midface, retinal detachment, arthritis
Radial aplasia	VATER association	Vertebral, anal, tracheoesophageal, renal anomalies
	Holt-Oram (142900)	Cardiac defects
Potter sequence	Branchio-oto-renal (113650)	Small jaw, ear pits
	Cryptophthalmos (Fraser—219000)	Skin over eyes, syndactyly, genital defects, severe DD
Micropenis	CHARGE association (sporadic, 214800)	Eye coloboma, choanal atreaia, heart defects, moderate DD
	Prader-Willi (microdeletion)	Hypotonia, obesity, moderate DD
	Smith-Lemli-Opitz (270400)	Microcephaly, polydactyly, cardiac defects, severe DD

Notes: CCM, cerebro-costo-mandibular; EEC, ectrodactyly-ectodermal dysplasia-clefting; DD, developmental disability.

another reminder that discovery of minor anomalies may unmask the syndrome disguised as single defect (Table 11.7). Dramatic examples include the presence of supravalvular aortic stenosis in Williams syndrome and the presence of conotruncal heart defects in DiGeorge/Shprintzen syndrome. As illustrated in Chapter 7, children with Williams syndrome may be difficult to recognize, appreciated only by their characteristic facial appearance in addition to other minor anomalies. The presence of one anomaly must therefore be considered a risk to have additional anomalies, and children with anomalies such as cleft palate or congenital heart disease must be examined and followed carefully to rule out accompanying signs of syndromal disease (Table 11.7). If additional major and minor anomalies are discovered, particularly in the presence of developmental delay, then a genetic evaluation is mandated. Although a karyotype is usually included in this genetic evaluation, the presence of microdeletions in Williams and Shprintzen syndromes emphasize that a normal routine karyotype does not eliminate the possibility of a genetic syndrome.

■ 11.5. MEDICAL MANAGEMENT OF MALFORMATION SYNDROMES

A remarkable change in the approach to patients with mental disability and congenital anomalies has occurred. Individuals with Down syndrome that were often placed in mental institutions two decades ago are now receiving the benefits of medical intervention and inclusive education. The Baby Doe law written to ensure the provision of basic feeding and comforts of children with disabilities now seems anachronistic when most children with Down syndrome are having curative surgery for congenital heart disease. Guidelines for the anticipation syndrome complications are now available for many diseases, making family support, care coordination, and preventive management essential for the management of congenital anomalies (see Chapter 16 also).

Family and Social Support

As illustrated in Figure 11.2, family support can begin as soon as the affected child is evaluated and the parents are present. When the diagnosis is obvious, explanation and education can begin immediately with the realization that parents may absorb little in this moment of crisis. When the diagnosis is obscure, as is often the case on first encounter, then the wait for laboratory and specialty results can parallel the resolution of parental anger and denial that is required before they can absorb medical information. Explanation of the anomalies and a plan for evaluation is often sufficient medical information when coupled with a positive attitude and the company of friends, relatives, clergy, ancillary professionals and/or parent group representatives.

Early intervention services comprise a first level of family support that can be emphasized for children likely to have developmental delay or disability. Often these services are provided by regular home visits and accompanied by assistance with health management, access to information, transportation, and respite care. Health professionals should ascertain whether families have resources to deal with multiple health visits and/or medical technology and ensure that the individual family plan designed by the early intervention team takes these factors into account. Social risk factors should also be evaluated, and include very young parents or those with developmental disabilities, risk factors such as HIV exposure, low birth weight, histories of abuse or neglect, and low socioeconomic status (Cooley, 1994). A team of providers including social workers, nurses, and therapists is ideal for coordinating family support as discussed in Chapter 16.

Contrary to prior assumptions, numerous studies have demonstrated that most families cope well even when children have severe disabilities or malformations. When supportive and anticipatory care is provided, the parents usually do not have increased rates of divorce or mental illness. Some families describe their adjustment in terms of enrichment, empowerment, and spiritual growth, providing strong incentives for supportive initial contacts (Cooley, 1994). It should be recognized that parents are very sensitive to dated or obsolete terms that can damage perceptions and undermine their confidence in professionals. People-first language is an important aspect of parental counseling, referring to the child before the disease (e.g., the child with Down syndrome, not the Down's child).

Preventive Management and Checklists as a Strategy

The central rationale for preventive management is that each syndrome or anomaly places a patient at higher risk for particular complications as compared to the general population. Preventive screening or evaluation for these complications is then justified by criteria of cost-effectiveness (selection of high-risk patients) and ethics (improved quality of life for the patient). This strategy of ameliorating complications is one of secondary or tertiary rather than primary prevention, since few congenital disorders can be prevented or cured. Each syndrome has a list of potential complications that form the basis for preventive management guidelines. Examples of detailed management guidelines are provided in Chapter 16. Well-documented complications of Down syndrome, such as cardiac, thyroid, vision, and hearing problems, led to the formulation of a Down syndrome checklist by Dr. Mary Coleman in 1963. The checklist consisted of specific recommendations at particular ages, exemplified by an echocardiogram during infancy, hearing and vision screening by age 8–10 months, and yearly thyroid function measures. The Committee on Genetics, American Academy of Pediatrics (1994) has endorsed these consensus recommendations for Down syndrome, and similar checklists have been formulated for more than 30 other syndromes (Cassidy and Allanson, 1999, Wilson and Cooley, 1999).

Several studies have documented that checklists improve compliance with recommended guidelines. Although there is a clear rationale

for alerting practitioners to the complications of a disorder, the nature and timing of intervention often requires clinical judgment. Some children with severe dysfunction may benefit more from palliative care than the inconveniences of medical intervention. Decisions about screening measures must be balanced against the need for anesthesia (e.g., brain imaging) or the accuracy of positive results (e.g., cervical spine radiographs for atlantoaxial instability in Down syndrome). An example of preventive management checklists and health-care supervision for children with congenital anomalies is presented in Chapter 16.

General Medical Problems

Children with congenital anomalies share some general medical problems that can be anticipated and ameliorated by health-care providers. Many will have a turbulent early course complicated by feeding problems, frequent infections, and growth delay. Coordination of care by a generalist is thus essential, with frequent involvement of gastroenterology, otolaryngology, and ophthalmology specialists to optimize growth and neurosensory function. After early intervention for motor and speech delays, school placement becomes an important issue. There are still barriers to inclusive education and appropriate rehabilitation services in many public schools, and health professionals may need to advocate for their patients. Later there are issues of job readiness and training, with moderate independence and employment being important goals for all people with disabilities. Missed complications like crippling heart defects with pulmonary hypertension, hearing loss with poor speech skills, or poor vision can greatly compromise these goals of independence and employment. Providers also must be alert to earlier aging and dementia, as well as increased risks for certain cancers that accompany malformation syndromes. Improvements in management and survival are increasingly bringing individuals with syndromes to internists, general practitioners, and other adult specialists for care.

■ 11.6. CHROMOSOMAL SYNDROMES

The category of chromosomal syndromes was discussed extensively in Chapter 7, but is mentioned here because of its frequency in children with multiple congenital anomalies. Although the one hundred or so chromosomal syndromes are far outnumbered by the thousand-plus Mendelian syndromes and others of unknown etiology, their prevalence and easy diagnosis via the routine karyotype gives them disproportionate visibility. A karyotype is often the first consideration in children with an unusual appearance, developmental delay, and/or multiple congenital anomalies. Because of the variability of many syndromes, a karyotype should be considered even in children with presumptive diagnosis of nonchromosomal syndromes (e.g., those with Niikawa or Noonan syndrome as illustrated in Figures. 11.5 and 11.6.). Any child with unexplained developmental delay or multiple minor/major anomalies should probably have a karyotype; a karyotype is mandatory in the presence of both findings.

Genetic counseling also depends on the nature of the chromosome aberration. As stressed in Chapter 7, any rearrangement of chromosomal material (i.e., rings, microdeletions, translocations, deletions, duplications) mandates that parental chromosomes be examined. Normal parents may be carriers of balanced rearrangements that confer significant recurrence risks for future offspring. When simple aneuploidy is found, exemplified by trisomy 21 causing Down syndrome, then parental chromosome studies are unnecessary because balanced rearrangements will be rare. Because of their multiple anomalies and risks for medical complications, children with chromosomal disorders need early and aggressive preventive management. Medical complications implied by particular chromosomal syndromes can be found in references such as Schinzel (1984), and a sample program of preventive management is discussed in Chapter 15 using the example of Down syndrome.

■ 11.7. MALFORMATION SYNDROMES EXHIBITING MENDELIAN INHERITANCE INCLUDING METABOLIC DYSPLASIAS

The large Mendelian contribution to malformation syndromes is emphasized by more than 1040 syndromes in *Mendelian Inheritance in Man* (McKusick, 1994) compendium and the fact that about 80% of the disorders listed by Jones (1997) are Mendelian (Wilson, 1992). These disorders extend across every organ system and must be considered by every medical or surgical specialist when evaluating particular congenital anomalies. A few of these many disorders are discussed here to emphasize the importance of their diagnosis for genetic counseling.

Waardenburg Syndrome

Patients with Waardenburg syndrome (193500) have an abnormal gestalt because of increased distance between the eyes (hypertelorism), increased facial hair (hirsutism), and a white streak of hair in the midline (poliosis). The unusual gestalt can be analyzed by measuring the interpupillary distance. As discussed in Chapter 9, Waardenburg syndrome is caused by mutations in human *PAX* gene homologues to the *Drosophila paired* locus. It is thus possible to suspect the diagnosis based on the unusual facial gestalt, analyze the phenotype based on interpupillary measurements, and relate the syndrome to *PAX* gene mutations. True interpretation of the Waardenburg syndrome pattern will require future work showing how *PAX* genes influence midline facial development.

A major complication of Waardenburg syndrome is sensorineural deafness. Recognition of the syndrome thus allows early auditory assessment with treatment to promote hearing and speech. Genetic counseling also becomes possible, with unaffected parents having a minimal recurrence risk based on their child being a spontaneous mutation. Affected individuals have a 50% recurrence risk. Other disorders with hypertelorism must be distinguished from Waardenburg syndrome, illustrated by Greig syndrome with hypertelorism and polydactyly (145400), frontonasal dysplasia, and an X-linked disorder called Aarskog syndrome (100050). Frontonasal dysplasia is a sporadic disorder without a significant recurrence risk, emphasizing the importance of correct diagnosis in providing genetic counseling. The role of the primary care professional would be to recognize the unusual facial appearance with hypertelorism in these patients, then to obtain a specific diagnosis through specialty referral.

Metabolic Dysplasias—
Smith-Lemli-Opitz and
Zellweger Syndromes

Among the many syndromes exhibiting autosomal recessive inheritance are those associated with metabolic abnormalities. Although most inborn errors of metabolism like phenylketonuria (261600) are associated with normal morphology, some impact embryonic development and produce recognizable syndromes. In a sense, every genetic syndrome influences cellular and biochemical pathways and could be called metabolic. However, certain disorders impact development through alterations of intermediary metabolism and can be designated as metabolic dysplasias. The examples to be discussed here are two disorders of lipid metabolism, RSB or Smith-Lemli-Opitz (270400) and Zellweger (214100) syndromes. These disorders produce characteristic patterns of anomalies and can be suspected based on their unusual facial appearance.

As discussed in Chapter 9 and illustrated in Figure 9.10, the Smith-Lemli-Opitz syndrome of microcephaly, growth delay, facial and genital abnormalities is now known to be caused by a defect in cholesterol metabolism. The gestalt approach is useful for this condition, with hypertelorism, ptosis of the eyelids, and a broad nasal root being typical of the disorder. Descriptive examination often reveals extra fingers (polydactyly), fusion (syndactyly) of toes

2 and 3, and sex reversal to the degree that males may present with external female genitalia. The interpretation of mechanism can now be focused on elevated levels of 7-deoxycholesterol, with pathogenetic mechanisms including the need for cholesterol as part of the *sonic hedgehog* protein that influences brain development (see Fig. 9.10). The role of steroid hormones in sex differentiation may also be relevant (Opitz and De la Cruz, 1994).

In addition to severe growth delay and developmental disability, medical complications of Smith-Lemli-Opitz syndrome include eye misalignment (strabismus), seizures due to brain anomalies such as holoprosencephaly, agenesis of corpus callosum, and hypoplasia of the cerebellar vermis, undescended testes (cryptorchidism), congenital heart lesions such as tetralogy of Fallot, and renal anomalies. Pyloric stenosis and aganglionic megacolon (Hirschsprung disease with intestinal narrowing and constipation) can also occur. Early diagnosis allows preventive management including a comprehensive initial evaluation to screen for anomalies of brain, heart, skeleton, urinary tract, and internal genitalia. Some patients with Smith-Lemli-Opitz syndrome have a severe disorder that merits palliative management sufficient for diagnosis and genetic counseling. However, milder forms of the disorder have been described in which patients survive to adulthood. The diagnosis allows genetic counseling for autosomal recessive inheritance and a 25% recurrence risk, with options for prenatal diagnosis provided by elevated 7-dehydrocholesterol levels.

Zellweger syndrome (214100; Fig. 11.8) and related disorders are caused by dysfunction of a subcellular organelle, the peroxisome. Zellweger syndrome is an example of a generalized peroxisomal disorder in which peroxisome structure is severely deranged with multiple peroxisomal enzyme deficiencies. Another category of peroxisomal disease involves deficiencies of single enzymes, illustrated by the mild disorder acatalasemia (115500). Single peroxisomal enzyme deficiencies are more limited and specific in their

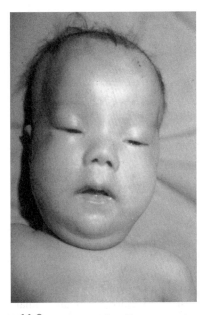

Figure 11.8. Patient with Zellweger syndrome illustrating a prominent forehead, broad nasal root, bitemporal hollowing and down-turned corners of the mouth. From Wilson et al. (1988).

manifestations and usually do not cause syndromes.

The approach to Zellweger syndrome and related generalized peroxisomal deficiency disorders is a good example of the approach to dysmorphology illustrated in Figure 11.2. There is often a characteristic face with bitemporal hollowing (shallow temples), shallow nasal bridge, anteverted nares (upturned nose), micrognathia (small jaw), single palmar creases, and bilateral clubfeet. Additional evaluation can disclose eye anomalies (retinitis pigmentosa), skeletal defects (punctate calcifications), and liver disease (periportal scarring, iron storage) through subspecialty examination, radiographic, or biopsy studies.

Once suspected by gestalt inspection and descriptive examination, the phenotype of Zellweger syndrome can be interpreted in terms of two major mechanisms—brain dysfunction with extreme hypotonia and abnormal bone growth. The hypotonia leads to bitemporal hollowing, single palmar creases, and clubfeet, while the abnormal bone growth leads to

the large fontanelle, short nose with anteverted nares, small jaw, and punctate calcifications. The hypotonia in turn is caused by brain dysfunction, as manifested by decreased myelination on head MRI scans and the pigmented retina. Analysis can be extended to the biochemical level where elevated metabolites such as very long chain fatty acids are diagnostic of peroxisomal dysfunction. Several genetic causes of Zellweger syndrome are now defined, each involving a protein that contributes to peroxisomal biogenesis in the cell. The chain from gestalt recognition to morphologic mechanism to biochemical and genetic cause is thus well defined for Zellweger syndrome, illustrating the steps of syndrome recognition and diagnosis that allow counseling and prenatal options for this autosomal recessive disorder (Fig. 11.2). Although palliative management is most appropriate for patients with Zellweger syndrome, preventive management anticipating vision, hearing, and developmental problems is useful in patients with milder peroxisomal disorders.

■ 11.8. MALFORMATION SYNDROMES WITH ABNORMAL GROWTH INCLUDING THE SKELETAL DYSPLASIAS

The importance of abnormal growth as a harbinger of syndrome risk was mentioned in Section 11.3. The presence of pre- or postnatal growth abnormality, coincident micro- or macrocephaly, or the presence of skeletal disproportion can be extremely helpful in assigning a syndrome category (Tables 11.4 and 11.5). Once the category is assigned, evaluation and referral can establish a specific syndrome diagnosis as illustrated by the following examples.

Cockayne Syndrome

Cockayne syndrome (216400) is now recognized as a group of disorders that share autosomal recessive inheritance, growth failure, and accelerated aging. The disorder can present as pre- or postnatal growth failure of unknown cause, and head measurements will disclose progressive microcephaly. Although difficult to recognize at birth, the face becomes characteristic during the first or second year with sunken eyes and a prominent nose. Once gestalt recognition and the characteristic growth pattern is apparent, other anomalies including red rashes due to photosensitivity of sun-exposed areas, pigment in the retina, uncoordinated movements and gait (ataxia), and decreased myelin appreciated on head MRI scan suggest the disease category. As the patient reaches mid- to later childhood, there are remarkable signs of aging including diabetes mellitus, hypertension, and osteoporosis. Death is inevitable in the severe form, but milder forms have been described. Skin fibroblasts from patients with Cockayne syndrome die more quickly when exposed to ultraviolet light, and one causative gene is a transcription factor involved in cell growth regulation.

The dividends of early diagnosis include genetic counseling for autosomal recessive inheritance and preventive management for vision or hearing problems. The anticipation of accelerated aging allows screening for abnormal glucose, blood pressure, or skeletal deformities which can greatly increase disability.

Niikawa-Kuroki (Kabuki) Syndrome

Patients with the Niikawa-Kuroki syndrome (147920) usually have normal birth weights and present with proportionate growth failure and developmental delay. The gestalt approach is useful in recognizing the characteristic face (Fig. 11.5), which can be described in terms of wide palpebral fissures, eversion of the lower eyelids, prominent ears, and down-turned corners of the mouth. There is often hypotonia, producing the open mouth shown by patients in Figure 11.5. Originally described in Japan, the syndrome has now been reported in more than 150 cases including many from the West. Japanese patients were noted to have a facial resemblance to Kabuki theatre masks, but Cau-

casian patients have an oriental appearance. Complications including postnatal growth retardation, mental disability, microcephaly, seizures, congenital hip dislocation, scoliosis (curved spine), chronic otitis with hearing loss, cardiac defects, and urogenital defects. Preventive management for Niikawa-Kuroki syndrome should thus include an early echocardiogram and renal sonogram, evaluation for chronic otitis (including periodic audiology screening), evaluation for skeletal anomalies (including dislocated hip in infancy and scoliosis in adolescence), and early intervention/speech therapy services for cognitive disabilty. The etiology is unknown, although some patients with X-chromosome anomalies and a few exhibiting autosomal dominant inheritance may point to a genetic cause.

Wiedemann-Beckwith Syndrome

Children with Wiedemann-Beckwith syndrome have a characteristic facial appearance with a hemangioma over the nasal root, malar flattening, and a large tongue. The birth weight is usually high (Table 11.5), followed by increased growth (pattern in Fig. 11.7E) in a majority of patients, some exhibiting asymmetry (hemihypertrophy). Once the large size and facial gestalt is appreciated, the descriptive examination often reveals characteristic pits behind the ears that can support the diagnosis. The large tongue (macroglossia) can be severe, causing respiratory obstruction, hypoxemia, apnea, feeding problems, and speech difficulties. Laboratory analysis may demonstrate neonatal hypoglycemia due to pancreatic islet cell hyperplasia. There are enlarged organs with increased risk for cardiac anomalies, hydrocephalus, umbilical or inguinal hernias, urinary tract anomalies, and abdominal tumors.

Diagnosis by appreciating the abnormal growth, unusual face, and hypoglycemia allows preventive management consisting of abdominal and renal imaging performed every 3–6 months until later childhood. The disorder is usually sporadic, but occasional familial transmission occurs due to autosomal dominant inheritance modified by incomplete penetrance and genomic imprinting as discussed in Chapter 10. Rare cases of Wiedemann-Beckwith syndrome resulted from a duplication of the chromosome 11p15 region, while others involved a deletion of this same region. It was soon demonstrated that the duplications always involved the paternally inherited chromosome 11, while deletions involved the maternally inherited chromosome. The implied alteration of parental imprinting has been confirmed by showing that the insulin-like growth factor-2 gene within the chromosome 11p15 region is expressed aberrantly in patients with Beckwith-Wiedemann syndrome. The number of genes involved and the pathogenesis by which altered gene expression produces the syndrome remain to be defined.

Achondroplasia

Achondroplasia (100800) and related conditions illustrate the value of recognizing syndrome categories, followed by referral to establish a precise diagnosis. The prominent forehead and shallow nasal bridge produce a characteristic facial appearance (see Fig. 9.9) that allows suspicion of skeletal dysplasia in the patient with short stature. The head often measures in the normal range, making it disproportionate for the short limbs and trunk (growth pattern C in Fig. 11.7). The descriptive approach consists of careful examination and skeletal radiography, which in achondroplasia should provide a definitive diagnosis. Often the child with short-limbed dwarfism can be categorized according to the limb segment (rhizo-, meso-, acromelic shortening) or skeletal structures (spondylo-, costo-, vertebral dysplasias) involved. Rhizomelic shortening is typical of achondroplasia and the related mutations in the fibroblast growth factor receptor-3 gene (thanatophoric dysplasia or hypochondroplasia, Table 11.4). In other disorders, specific findings such as absent clavicles (cleidocranial dysplasia), sparse hair (hair-cartilage hypoplasia), or multiple fractures (osteogenesis imperfecta) can lead to a diagnosis.

The diagnosis of achondroplasia implies substantial dwarfism with an adult height between $3^1/_2$ and $4^1/_2$ feet. Genetic counseling often addresses the minimal risk for normal parents to have another affected child, although achondroplast couples with a 50% recurrence risk for achondroplasia and a 25% risk for severe homozygous disease are sometimes encountered. Preventive management is discussed in Chapter 16.

■ 11.9. MALFORMATION SYNDROMES DUE TO TERATOGENS

Despite the fact that more than 50,000 drugs and chemicals are in common use, only 20 or so have been proven to be teratogenic to humans. Reproductive testing is mandated for drug development, and there are excellent references that summarize known exposures of animals or humans to particular drugs (Shardein, 1985; Shepard, 1992). Because some drugs and congenital infections are known to cause birth defects (Table 11.8), a gestational history is an important part of the morphologic evaluation as shown in Figure 11.2. Environmental exposures are frequently mentioned by parents when their child has a congenital anomaly, and it is reassuring that only one environmental chemical—methyl mercury—is a proven human teratogen.

Criteria for proving teratogenicity of an agent have been formulated, and these criteria have been met for agents such as alcohol or the notorious sedative thalidomide. Legal or scientific views are suspect when they claim that an agent increases the frequency of all types of congenital anomalies, rather than producing a specific anomaly or anomaly pattern. When unfounded parental concerns are encountered, it is important to emphasize the alternative diagnosis when present or to mention the background 3–5% risk for congenital anomalies to place the child in proper perspective. Counselors should allay parental guilt about exposures when appropriate, and avoid naive or deliberate support for unscientific claims.

■ **TABLE 11.8.** Syndromes Caused by Teratogens

Causal Agent	Syndrome	Complications
Ethanol	Fetal alcohol syndrome	Low BW, growth delay, strabismus, joint dislocations, heart defects, mild DD
Hydantoin	Fetal hydantoin syndrome	Low BW, coarse face, digital defects, small fingernails, cardiac defects, mild DD
Maternal diabetes	Infant of diabetic mother	Large BW, brain anomalies, cardiac defects, caudal regression, VATER association
Maternal PKU	Maternal PKU effects	Similar to fetal alcohol syndrome
Retinoic acid	Retinoic acid embryopathy	Craniofacial defects, heart defects, limb defects, severe DD
TORCH	Congenital infections	Low BW, microcephaly, hepatosplenomegaly, clotting defects
Trimethadione	Fetal trimethadione syndome	Low BW, unusual eyebrows, heart defects
Valproic acid	Fetal valproate syndrome	Neural tube defects, heart defects, mild DD
Varicella	Fetal varicella syndrome	Low BW, fetal scars, eye defects, limb defects, mild to severe DD
Warfarin	Warfarin embryopathy	Low BW, hypoplastic (fleur-de-lys) nose, punctate calcifications in bones

Notes: PKU, phenylketonuria with elevated phenylalanine levels; TORCH, *T*oxoplasmosis, *O*ther (e.g., syphilis), *R*ubella, *C*ytomegalovirus, *H*erpes; BW, birth weight; DD, developmental disability; VATER, *V*ertebral, *A*nal, *T*racheo-*E*sophageal, *R*adial, *R*enal defects.

Fetal Alcohol Syndrome (FAS)

Dangers of drinking during pregnancy were mentioned in biblical times and were emphasized during England's Gin Epidemic of 1720–1750. Despite this anecdotal evidence, specific patterns of physical anomalies in offspring of alcoholic women were not documented until the late 1960s. Children may be severely (fetal alcohol syndrome—FAS) or partially (fetal alcohol effects—FAE) affected, with an incidence of 1–2 per thousand that depends on socioeconomic conditions. Brain anomalies and small eyes produced by alcohol exposure of rodent or primate fetuses support the primary role of ethanol in FAS, and there is excellent correlation of syndrome severity with alcohol dosage and timing in humans or experimental animals.

A typical child with FAS has the growth pattern illustrated in profile B of Figure 11.7 and the facial appearance shown in Figure 11.9. Gestalt recognition is difficult, and the diagnosis is suggested by typical minor anomalies such as shallow nasal bridge, abnormal ears, thin upper lip, and an absent philtrum (crease between nose and upper lip—Fig. 11.9). Major anomalies include abnormal alignment (strabismus) of the eyes, orthopedic problems such as dislocated hips, and congenital heart defects. Ethanol teratogenesis may not produce an obvious phenotype at birth, and a positive maternal history is elicited in less than 50% of proven cases. Follow-up of children born to mothers with elevated blood alcohol levels show that few were diagnosed in the neonatal period and only half were identified by age 4. It is not yet possible to go beneath the surface anomalies of FAS to explain its pathogenesis, and no biochemical or molecular "footprint" of alcohol exposure is yet available to aid in diagnosis.

A major aspect of diagnosis is a good parental history. Blunt or judgmental questions often meet with denial or underestimates of drinking that are classic for alcoholic persons. Questioning of both parents (social customs are often congruent), initial focus on nonthreatening agents such as carbonated beverages and specific mention of beer and wine

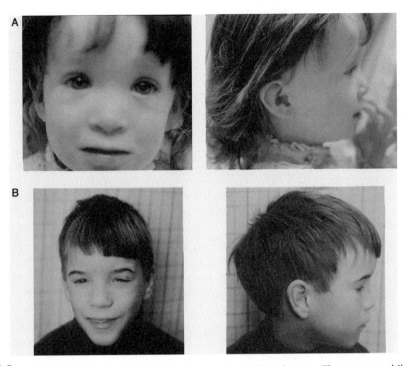

Figure 11.9. Individuals with fetal alcohol syndrome at ages 2 or 8 years. The younger child (A) has a broad nasal root, thin upper lip, shallow nasal bridge, and posteriorly rotated ears. The older child (B) has narrow palpebral fissures (eyes) and an absent philtrum (crease from nose to upper lip)

(sometimes not considered "drinks") are important strategies. Smoking histories are important, because cigarette smoking is a common correlate of alcoholism that also contributes to fetal growth restriction.

The impact of alcohol on the developing brain is evidenced by a high frequency of neurobehavioral problems including learning deficits (mean IQ of 40–65), hyperactivity, distractibility, and impulsivity. Neurosensory deficits include hearing loss and diminished vision in 50% of FAS patients. Recent debate concerns the reliability and specificity of a behavioral phenotype in FAS, and the use of soft neurologic signs or behavioral symptoms as diagnostic criteria in the absence of historical or morphologic evidence is inappropriate. Once the diagnosis of FAS or FAE is recognized, then preventive management in the form of early intervention, echocardiography, vision and hearing screening, and frequent developmental assessment is indicated.

Diabetic Embryopathy

Infants of diabetic mothers (IDM) have increased risk for congenital malformation that correlates with the degree of metabolic aberration during pregnancy. As the complications of stillbirth, neonatal hypoglycemia, and respiratory distress syndrome were ameliorated through better maternal management, increased risk for malformation in IDM was recognized. The common malformations in IDM all occur before 7 weeks of pregnancy, so that control of diabetes before conception must be emphasized to safeguard the embryo.

The etiology of anomalies resulting from maternal diabetes is still unclear. Maternal vasculopathy, hypo- and hyperglycemia, ketonemia, and somatomedin inhibitors have received experimental support as factors in diabetic embryopathy. Of great interest is a paradoxical growth *retardation* in some severely affected IDM (Pedersen and Mølsted-Pedersen, 1982);

delayed growth along with delayed maturation of lung and hematologic functions may be a unifying theme in the disorder.

Infants of diabetic mothers should be evaluated for major anomalies of the brain, heart, GI tract, urinary tract, and vertebrae. Caudal underdevelopment, ranging from sirenomelia (mermaid anomaly) to sacral agenesis, is the most characteristic anomaly, being present in about 1% of patients. Some children may require orthopedic, urologic, and neurosurgical follow-up when severe caudal regression produces limb hypoplasia, bladder, and spinal cord problems. Medical counseling should review the correlation of poor diabetic control with anomaly risk, particularly emphasizing the achievement of good control before attempting another pregnancy (see Chapter 15). Gestational diabetes is not associated with a higher risk for congenital anomalies, so these mothers can be reassured and their offspring evaluated for other causes of anomalies.

■ 11.10. MALFORMATION SYNDROMES AND ASSOCIATIONS OF UNKNOWN CAUSE

Many syndromes are recognized as patterns of anomalies for which no cause has been determined. Syndromes of unknown cause bring up a category that is even more frustrating for families and physicians—the child with an unrecognized syndrome. Some patients with multiple anomalies simply do not fit into described patterns, or else the disorder is so rare that it is not considered in the differential. Follow-up observation is particularly important for children with syndromes of unknown cause or with unnamed syndromes, because new findings can appear that change or discover the diagnosis. Despite the utility of the gestalt and descriptive approaches in defining syndrome categories, subjective impressions should always be reevaluated until imaging studies, specialty examinations, or laboratory analysis can provide objective confirmation. For syndromes that exhibit Mendelian inheritance,

and for many that are not yet recognized as such, the advances in molecular genetics and embryology discussed in Chapter 9 are providing DNA methods for objective diagnosis.

VATER Association

VATER association is an acronym that represents Vertebral defects, Anal atresia, Tracheo-Esophageal fistula, Radial limb and Renal defects. Synonyms include VACTERL association, where the "C" and "L" are added to emphasize cardiac and limb defects.

The etiology of VATER association is unknown, although infants of diabetic mothers show an increased incidence. As currently defined, the diagnosis is excluded if a recognizable chromosomal or genetic syndrome is found. The pathogenesis involves injury to developing mesoderm at 20–25 days after conception, resulting in abnormal development of vertebral, anorectal, cardiac, tracheosophageal, radial and renal derivatives. Dysmorphogenesis seems limited to major organ systems, with few minor anomalies of face, palate, or limbs.

Differential diagnosis is large because many genetic and chromosomal syndromes include one or more components of the VATER association. Most dangerous is the misdiagnosis of patients with trisomy 18 as VATER association, because the management of their cardiac, radial ray, and renal defects may be inappropriately aggressive and fraught with the operative instability manifested by patients with chromosomal disease. Appreciation of minor anomalies such as malformed ears, aberrant palmar creases, prominent heels, or rocker-bottom feet allows suspicion of trisomy 18 (see Fig. 7.14 and Fig. 11.3B).

Because there is no biological marker for VATER association, the diagnosis is made by documenting component anomalies. Severe anorectal, cardiac, tracheo-esophageal, and limb defects will present with obvious signs or symptoms, but milder anomalies of these systems plus vertebral or renal defects may require laboratory and imaging studies for diagnosis. VATER association should be considered after one cognate defect is recognized, but the degree of suspicion will depend on the presenting anomaly based on the epidemiologic data of Khoury et al. (1983) or the literature survey of Quan and Smith (1973).

A reasonable approach to the diagnostic evaluation is to screen for all of the cognate VATER anomalies once two of them have been documented. For example, in the absence of identified syndromes, children with limb and cardiac defects should have spinal X rays, renal sonogram, and surveillance for feeding/respiratory problems. Finding of a third cognate anomaly makes the diagnosis secure. When only one VATER cognate anomaly is present, screening for internal anomalies can be guided by the likelihood of association (Khoury et al. 1983; Quan and Smith, 1973). Patients with tracheo-esophageal fistula certainly deserve echocardiography and renal sonography, as do patients with imperforate anus (31.3% likelihood of renal defects once imperforate anus is documented; Khoury et al., 1983). Patients with renal defects or vertebral defects also deserve echocardiography (25.7% and 24.7% respective risks for cardiac defects according to Khoury et al., 1983). Patients with initial ascertainment of cardiac or limb anomalies have low risks for associated anomalies (Khoury et al., 1983).

Brachmann de Lange Syndrome

The facial appearance is usually sufficient for a diagnosis of Brachmann-de Lange syndrome. A remarkable gestalt can be described in terms of prominent eyebrows that meet in the midline (synophrys), arched eyebrows, upturned (anteverted) nose, down-turned corners of the mouth, and increased facial hair. (Fig. 11.10). Additional evaluation can disclose complications such as glaucoma, gastroesophageal reflux with risks for apnea or aspiration, chronic otitis, heart or renal defects, and severe cognitive disability in most cases. Diagnosis allows preventive management to screen for hearing and vision loss, urinary tract infection, and physical/occupational therapy to minimize the effects of contractures and hip malpositioning. The disorder is severe and often leads to early death because of apnea, aspiration, cardiac anomalies, intracranial bleeding, or postoperative events. A milder form of Brachmann-de Lange syndrome with reasonable self-help and communication skills is supported by observation of 8 individuals with IQ greater than 70.

Although a majority of cases with Brachmann de Lange syndrome have a normal karyotype, rare aberrations have highlighted two candidate regions for the hypothesized mutant gene. Rearrangements involving the distal long arm of chromosome 3 or of chro-

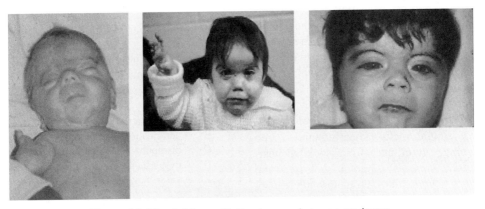

Figure 11.10. Children with Brackmann-de Lange syndrome.

mosome 9 produce a phenotype that is similar to the Brachmann-de Lange syndrome (Opitz, 1994).

Noonan Syndrome

Noonan syndrome (163950) involves short stature and unusual face with hypertelorism and anteverted ear lobes. The condition is usually sporadic, but families with apparent autosomal dominant inheritance account for the McKusick number. There are additional anomalies including webbed neck, cubitus valgus, characteristic pectus, and hypogonadism. Overlap of these features with those of women with a 45,X karyotype inspired the inaccurate term of "male Turner syndrome." However, both sexes are affected in Noonan syndrome and the karyotype is normal. Allanson (1989) has illustrated the changing facial appearance of Noonan syndrome patients over time, providing a challenge for gestalt diagnosis (Fig. 11.6).

Interpretation of defects in Noonan syndrome relates to an abnormality of fetal lymphatic circulation that produces a large neck mass (cystic hygroma) in the fetus. The fetal hygroma may cause the postnatal webbed neck, anteverted ear lobes, and chest deformities. Although it is expected to be normal, a karyotype should be performed in all but the most typical cases of Noonan syndrome. The heterogeneous Noonan phenotype can be mimicked by several chromosomal disorders including Turner syndrome. A normal life span with frequently normal intelligence warrants optimistic medical counseling for the parents of a child with Noonan syndrome. An echocardiogram is needed in early infancy to evaluate the degree of pulmonary valve dysplasia and cardiomyopathy in the 70–90% of patients with congenital heart anomalies.

Preventive management of Noonan syndrome should include hearing and vision screening, surveillance for associated heart (pulmonic stenosis), skeletal (scoliosis), and bleeding abnormalities. Problems with feeding can be severe, with one-quarter of patients requiring tube feedings. Although some patients experience motor and speech delays, the outlook for overall intelligence and learning is excellent, with 80–90% having normal intelligence and only 10% requiring special education. The etiology is unknown, but vertical transmission compatible with autosomal dominant inheritance occurs in some families. An affected individual will have about a 20% risk for affected offspring.

PROBLEM SET 11
Dysmorphology

Select the single most appropriate answer to the following questions:

11.1. Monozygotic twins with connected placental circulations can develop a pattern of vascular occlusions due to blood clots. A twin with a brain cyst, absent kidney, cleft palate, and absent digits has:
- (A) A malformation syndrome
- (B) A deformation syndrome
- (C) A disruption syndrome
- (D) A dysplasia syndrome
- (E) An association

11.2. A child has a small head, minor anomalies of the face including a thin upper lip, growth delay, and developmental disability. His mother becomes defensive when asked about her pregnancy. The child is likely to have:
- (A) A chromosomal syndrome
- (B) A teratogenic syndrome
- (C) A Mendelian syndrome
- (D) A polygenic syndrome
- (E) An association

11.3. A newborn has multiple blood vessel tumors (hemangiomas) over his trunk and legs, together with a large head and body asymmetry. He has:
- (A) A malformation syndrome
- (B) A deformation syndrome
- (C) A disruption syndrome
- (D) A dysplasia syndrome
- (E) An association

11.4. A child has congenital contractures (bent limbs) due to a large uterine fibroid that her mother developed during pregnancy. The child has:

- (A) A malformation syndrome
- (B) A deformation syndrome
- (C) A disruption syndrome
- (D) A dysplasia syndrome
- (E) An association

11.5. Several patients are described with similar congenital anomalies including defects of the sacral vertebrae, kidneys, anus, and trachea. The children do not have minor anomalies and their faces do not resemble one another. The child most likely has:

- (A) A malformation sequence
- (B) A deformation syndrome
- (C) A disruption syndrome
- (D) A dysplasia syndrome
- (E) An association

11.6–11.7. A family requests genetic counseling because the father has widely spaced eyes, increased facial hair, and deafness. One of their three children also has deafness with similar facial features. The mother is normal, but a paternal sister and the paternal grandfather are known to have deafness and increased facial hair.

11.6. The most likely pattern of inheritance of this disorder is

- (A) autosomal dominant
- (B) autosomal recessive
- (C) X-linked dominant
- (D) X-linked recessive
- (E) none of the above

11.7 The recurrence risk for this couple is

- (A) 100%
- (B) 67%
- (C) 50%
- (D) 25%
- (E) virtually 0

11.8–11.10. A man and woman have short stature, prominent forehead, shallow nasal bridge, short limbs, and other skeletal changes. Both have been told that they have achondroplasia (100800), and wish to know their recurrence risks for affected children. Match the recurrence risks with the questions below.

- (A) 100%
- (B) 75%
- (C) 50%
- (D) 25%
- (E) virtually 0

11.8. The probability for the first child of achondroplastic parents to be affected (heterozygous or homozygous)

11. 9. Following the birth of an affected child, the probability for the second child of achondroplastic parents to be affected

11.10. The probability for the first child to be affected if an achondroplast marries an unaffected person

PROBLEM SET 11
Answers

		11.4. B
11.10. C	11.7. C	11.3. D
11.9. B	11.6. A	11.2. B
11.8. B	11.5. E	11.1. C

PROBLEM SET 11
Solutions

11.1. The term syndrome, literally meaning "running together," refers to a pattern of several anomalies. Disruptions and deformations interrupt normal development, whereas malformations and dysplasias affect the primordium or anlage of a developing organ, causing development to be abnormal from the beginning. A blood clot interferes with the blood supply to a developing organ, interrupting normal development as a disruption. The multiple affected organs due to the same pathogenesis of vessel occlusion represent a disruption syndrome (answer C).

11.2. The small head (microcephaly), thin upper lip, and growth delay are typical of the fetal alcohol syndrome, which may explain the mother's defensiveness about the gestational history. Drugs that cause birth defects (teratogens) interrupt normal developmental processes and can be defined as disruptions. The multiple anomalies caused by alcohol cause a teratogenic syndrome (answer B).

11.3. Abnormal proliferation of blood vessels is an intrinsic abnormality of tissue (dysplasia) within a developing organ. The occurrence of vessel proliferation (hemangiomas) at several different sites in the body qualifies as a dysplasia syndrome (answer D). The benign vessel tumors, large head, and body asymmetry would also qualify as a hamartosis syndrome (see Table 11.5).

11.4. Extrinsic constraint on developing organs can interrupt normal development and cause deformations. Abnormal constraints such as uterine fibroid tumors or uterine anomalies can deform developing organs in otherwise normal fetuses, while normal uterine constraint can cause deformations in fetuses with low motor tone (hypotonia) and decreased movement. The multiple contractures described here can be classified as a deformation syndrome (answer B).

11.5. Multiple congenital anomalies can be described as a syndrome, but the presence of major anomalies without a pattern of minor anomalies is more precisely described as an association (answer E).

11.6–11.7. It is important to recognize the multiple components of a syndrome as an aggregate phenotype that can be produced by single mutant alleles. As stressed in Chapter 3, the vertical pattern of affected individuals in the family and the affliction of both men and women suggests autosomal dominant inheritance (answer 11.6A). The variable expression of syndrome features in several affected individuals is classic for autosomal dominant inheritance. Multifactorial determination would also be possible, but less likely with so many affected individuals. For autosomal dominant diseases, affected individuals have a 50% recurrence risk (answer 11.7C).

11.8–11.10. As indicated by the McKusick number, achondroplasia (100800) is an autosomal dominant condition. This implies a genotype of Aa for each parent, where A is the abnormal allele. The risk for affected children is then 75% (answer 11.8B), 50% for regular achondroplasia with an Aa genotype, and 25% for homozygous lethal achondroplasia with an AA genotype. Since chance has no memory, the same risk applies for each pregnancy re-

gardless of prior outcomes (answer 11.9B). If an achondroplast (Aa) and normal person (aa) marry, their risk is 50% to have a child with genotype Aa and regular achondroplastic dwarfism (11.10C).

BIBLIOGRAPHY

General References

Bankier A. 1998. *POSSUM Syndrome Database.* CD-ROM.

Jones KL. 1995. *Smith's Recognizable Patterns of Human Malformation.* Philadephia: W.B. Saunders.

Gorlin RJ, Cohen MM, Levin LS. 1999. *Syndromes of the Head and Neck,* 4th ed. New York: Oxford University.

Gould SJ. 1977. Ontogeny and Phylogeny. Cambridge MA: Belknap Press, p. 47.

McKusick VM. 1994. *Mendelian Inheritance in Man,* 11th ed. Baltimore: Johns Hopkins; on-line at http://www3.ncbi.nlm.nih.gov/omim.

Shepard T. 1992. *Catalogue of Teratogenic Agents,* 5th ed., Baltimore: Johns Hopkins.

Schardein JL. 1985. *Chemically Induced Birth Defects.* New York: Marcel Dekker.

Schinzel A. 1984. *Catalogue of Unbalanced Chromosome Aberrations in Man.* Berlin: de Gruyter.

Winter RM, Baraitser M. 1998. *London Dysmorphology Database.* Version 3.0. London: Oxford University. CD-ROM.

Examination and Classification of Anomalies

Friedman JM. 1990. A practical approach to dysmorphology. *Pediatr Ann* 19:95–101.

Gorlin RJ. 1980. Diagnosis of craniofacial anomalies: subjective evaluation—Gestalt. Birth Defects Original Articles Series 16:35–46, p. 46.

Kronick JB, Scriver CR, Goodyear PR, Kaplan PB. 1983. A perimortem protocol for suspected genetic disease. *Pediatrics* 71:960–962.

Leppig KA, Werler MW, Cann CI, Cook CA, Holmes LB. 1987. The predictive value of minor anomalies. I. Association with major malformations. *J Pediatr* 110: 531–537.

Little BB, Wilson GN, Jackson G. 1996. Is there a cocaine syndrome? Dysmorphic and anthropometric assessment of infants exposed to cocaine. *Teratology* 54:145–9.

Lubinsky M. 1986. VATER and other associations: Historical perspective and modern interpretations. *Am J Med Genet* 2 (suppl):9–16.

Opitz JM. 1982. The developmental field concept in genetics. *J Pediatr* 101:805–809.

Opitz JM, Wilson GN. 1997. Causes and pathogenesis of birth defects. In Gilbert-Barness E, ed. *Potter's Pathology of the Fetus and Infant,* St. Louis: Mosley, pp. 44–64.

Saul RA, Stevenson RE, Rogers RC, Skinner SA, Prouty LA, Flannery DB. 1988. *Growth References from Conception to Childhood.* Proc Greenwood Genet Center, Supplement 1.

Spranger J, Benirschke K, Hall JG, Lenz W, Lowry RB, Opitz JM, Pinsky L, Schwarzacher HG, Smith DW. 1982. Errors of morphogenesis: Concepts and terms. Recommendations of an international working group. *J Pediatr* 100:160–167.

Wilson GN. 1988. Heterochrony and human malformation. *Am J Med Genet* 29:311–321.

Wilson GN. 1990. Office approach to the genetics patient. *Pediatr Ann* 19:79–91.

Wilson GN. 1992. Genomics of human dysmorphogenesis. *Am J Med Genet* 42:187–196.

Management of Children with Syndromes and Disabilities

Committee on Genetics, American Academy of Pediatrics. 1994. Health supervision for children with Down syndrome. *Pediatrics* 93:855–859.

Cooley WC. 1994. The ecology of support for caregiving families. *J Behav Devel Pediatr* 15:117–119.

Gath A., Gumley D. 1984. Down syndrome and the family: follow-up of children first seen in infancy. *Developmental Medicine and Child Neurology* 26: 500–508.

Liptak GS, Revell GM. 1989. Community physician's role in the case management of children with chronic illness. *Pediatrics* 84:465–471.

Cassidy SB, Allanson J. 1999. *Preventive Management,* in press, New York: Wiley-Liss

Wilson GN, Cooley WC. 1999. *Preventive Management for Children With Congenital Anomalies and Syndromes,* in press. Cambridge: Cambridge University Press.

Specific Syndromes

Allanson JE. 1989. Time and natural history: The changing face. *J Craniofac Genet Devel Biol* 9:21–28.

Jones KL, Smith DW. 1975. The fetal alcohol syndrome. *Teratology* 12:1–10.

Khoury MJ, Cordero JF, Greenberg F, James LM, Erickson JD. 1983. A population study of the VACTERL association: evidence for its etiologic heterogeneity. *Pediatrics* 71:815–820.

Mills JL, Baker L, Goldman AS. 1979. Malformations in infants of diabetic mothers occur before the seventh gestational week. Implications for treatment. *Diabetes* 28:292–293.

Ohlsson R, Nystrom A, Pfeifer-Ohlsson S, Tohonen V, Hedborg F, Schofield P, Flam F, and Estrom TH. 1993. IGF2 is parentally imprinted during human embryogenesis and in the Beckwith-Wiedemann syndrome. *Nat Genet* 4:94–97.

Opitz JM. 1994. Brachmann-de Lange syndrome: A continuing enigma. *Arch Pediatr Adol Med* 148:1206–1207.

Opitz JM, de la Cruz F. 1995. Cholesterol metabolism in RSH/Smith-Lemli-Opitz syndrome. Summary of an NICHD conference. *Am J Med Genet* 50:326–38.

Pederson JF, Molsted-Pederson L. 1982. Early growth delay predisposes the fetus in diabetic pregnancy to congenital malformation. Lancet 1:737.

Quan L, Smith DW. 1973. The VATER association, Vertebral defects, Anal atresia, *T-E* fistula with esophageal atresia, Radial and Renal dysplasia; A spectrum of associated defects. *Journal of Pediatrics* 82:104–7.

Wilson GN. 1998. Thirteen cases of Niikawa-Kuroki syndrome: Report and review with emphasis on medical complications and preventive management. *Am J Med Genet* 79:112–120.

Wilson GN, Holmes RD, Hajra AK. 1988. Peroxisomal disorders: Clinical commentary and future prospects. *Am J Med Genet* 30:771–92.

12

PEDIATRIC GENETICS: INBORN ERRORS OF METABOLISM

■ LEARNING OBJECTIVES

1. Inborn errors of metabolism occur in about 1 in 600 births, presenting as acute or chronic illness.

2. Inborn errors are caused by enzyme deficiencies that exhibit autosomal or X-linked recessive inheritance.

3. Infants with catastrophic disease of the newborn present with lethargy, coma, acidosis, and/or increased jaundice after routine nursery feedings. Urea cycle disorders, galactosemia, and organic acidemias are common causes.

4. Acute metabolic diseases of early childhood commonly present with hypoglycemia, acidosis, and/or liver disease. Fatty acid oxidation, amino acid, and organic acid disorders are common causes.

5. Diagnostic categories for acute metabolic disease are deduced from a panel of initial tests including blood ammonia, amino acids, glucose, pH, and electrolytes; urine organic acids and reducing substances; and, in certain cases, blood carnitine and acylcarnitine profile.

6. Diagnostic categories for chronic metabolic (storage) diseases are recognized by organ histology and lysosomal enzyme assays that differentiate between glycogen, lipid, or mucopolysaccharide accumulation.

7. Disorders characteristic of carbohydrate, amino acid, urea cycle, organic acid, fatty acid oxidation, and organellar (peroxisomal, mitochondrial) exemplify characteristics of metabolic disease categories.

8. Criteria for genetic screening include high frequency of disease, potential for treatment, accurate testing, provision for counseling, and equal access.

9. Newborn metabolic screening best fulfills these criteria, while heterozygote, presymptomatic, and prenatal screening have significant disadvantages.

10. Therapies for metabolic disease include dietary avoidance, provision of cofactors, provision of deficient products, sparing of defective pathways, stimulation of alternative pathways,

enzyme replacement, transplantation, and (theoretically) gene therapy.

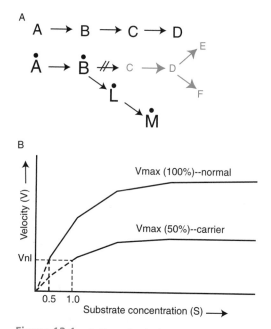

Case 12A: **The Lethargic Newborn**
A male infant does well for the first 12 hours of life and breast-feeds vigorously. The next morning the child appears lethargic and hypotonic (low muscle tone), and he exhibits rapid, shallow breathing. By 36 hours after birth, he is almost unresponsive and comatose but continues with rapid breathing. The gestational history and physical examination are unremarkable, but the family history reveals that the parents are second cousins. A neonatal blood spot is obtained and sent to the state metabolic screening laboratory.

■ 12.1. INTRODUCTION

Enzyme deficiencies are responsible for *inborn errors of metabolism,* explaining two major characteristics of these diseases. The first characteristic of inborn errors is diagrammed in Figure 12.1A: Metabolic diseases are caused by abnormal alleles that encode dysfunctional enzymes. In Figure 12.1A, the enzyme catalyzing conversion of substrate B to product C is deficient due to the presence of one (X-linked) or two (autosomal) mutant alleles. The block in substrate conversion due to enzyme deficiency causes build-up and increased concentrations of substances before the block (e.g., A and B in Fig. 12.1A) and deficiency of substances distal to the block (e.g., C and D in Fig. 12.1A). Cellular functions that depend on calibrated amounts of these metabolites then become deranged and lead to symptoms of metabolic disease. Because the multiple and interconnected metabolic pathways of cells are analogous to highway interchanges within cities, blocks in one pathway may impact conversions (traffic) and alter concentrations of metabolites in other pathways (e.g., substances L, M, E, F in Fig. 12.1A). Enzymes often require vitamins or other cofactors to facilitate their catalytic actions. Vitamin deficiencies may mimic certain metabolic disorders, and

Figure 12.1. *A,* Hypothetical metabolic pathway showing normal levels of metabolites (above) and alterations caused by deficiency of the enzyme converting substance B to substance C (below). Note the increased levels of substances (A, B, L, M—dots above symbol) and lower levels of substances C–F (shaded). The arrows (→) represent steps of enzyme catalysis; *B,* consequences of enzyme reserve showing a moderate increase in substrate concentration (S) to restore normal enzyme velocity (V_{nl}) in carriers with 50% of enzyme amount and 50% of maximal enzyme velocity (V_{max}).

the provision of specific vitamins in excess provides a means to assist dysfunctional enzymes in certain inborn errors.

A second general characteristic of inborn errors is diagrammed in Figure 12.1B. The standard saturation curve for enzyme catalysis is illustrated, demonstrating the attainment of maximal reaction velocity (Vmax) in the presence of excess substrate (S). A person with one-half the amount of enzyme in her cells (e.g., a heterozygous carrier with one normal allele) will attain half the maximum velocity with excess substrate concentration as compared to a normal individual with two functional alleles. Under physiologic conditions, however, substrates are present at low concentrations during their flux toward the next reaction and enzymes are present in great excess over the amounts needed to convert substrates. This excess of enzyme is known as *enzyme reserve*. The same normal reaction velocity (Vnl) can thus be obtained in heterozygotes by a twofold increase in substrate concentration (Fig. 12.1*B*). This small increase in substrate concentration required for normal reaction velocity does not influence the precursor or distal reactions diagrammed in Figure 12.1*A*, with the result that heterozygotes for alleles producing enzyme deficiency will be normal. Because of enzyme reserve, inborn errors of metabolism exhibit autosomal or X-linked *recessive* inheritance with few exceptions.

Inborn errors of metabolism are individually rare but collectively have an incidence of about 1 in 600 births. Although some diseases are detected automatically through governmentally mandated newborn screening, most must be recognized by generalists so that specialty referral and analysis can establish a specific diagnosis (Table 12.1). Dietary therapy is possible for many metabolic disorders, emphasizing the need for early clinical suspicion and diagnosis before abnormal metabolites produce lasting damage. Advances in analytical

chemistry and molecular biology now provide a formidable armamentarium for the diagnosis of metabolic disease, and it is essential to recognize suspect symptoms so that these methods can be applied (Table 12.2). The signs and symptoms listed in Table 12.1 should be borne in mind by all health professionals who care for young children.

The causation of metabolic disease by chemical alterations arising from enzyme deficiencies also implies that most patients will appear normal at birth. Since the fetus is a small part of the maternal tissue load, maternal metabolism can compensate for fetal alterations when they involve diffusible molecules. Central metabolic pathways also have an all-or-none feature that implies early death for embryos lacking key enzymes. As a result, those metabolic errors compatible with fetal survival rarely exhibit dysmorphology. Exceptions to this rule do occur, as illustrated by the discussion of metabolic dysplasias such as Zellweger syndrome (214400) in Chapter 11 and in Section 12.9.

The approach to inborn errors of metabolism must emphasize simple principles that guide the clinician toward a diagnostic category. Although the complexities of laboratory evaluation and treatment require the involve-

■ **TABLE 12.1.** Presentations and Investigations of Inborn Errors

Type	Signs and Symptoms	Laboratory Investigations
Acute metabolic disease	Lethargy, coma	Blood glucose, ammonia
	Coexisting infection	Blood pH, lactate
	Exaggerated jaundice	Blood amino acids
	Hypoglycemia with or without urinary ketones	Blood carnitine
	Acidosis with increased anion gap	Blood acylcarnitine profile
	Lactic acidosis	Urinary ketones
	Neutropenia, thrombocytopenia	Urinary reducing substances
	Unusual odors	Urinary organic acids
	Later developmental delay,	Enzyme assays
	hypotonia, seizures	DNA diagnosis
Chronic metabolic disease	Hypotonia, seizures	Skin, liver, or muscle biopsy
	Developmental delay, regression	Leucocyte preparations
	Retinal or corneal changes	Enzyme assays
	Visceromegaly	Skeletal radiographs
	Skeletal changes	DNA diagnosis

■TABLE 12.2. Laboratory Diagnosis of Inborn Errors

Disease Examples	Presenting Symptoms	Laboratory Abnormalities
Small molecule diseases		
Urea cycle disorder (e.g., OTC deficiency)	MD, lethargy, coma, mild alkalosis due to tachypnea	Blood—high ammonia, abnormal amino acids (high glutamine, asparagine)
Organic acidemias (e.g., propionic acidemia)	MD, hypoglycemia, lethargy, coma, acidosis	Blood—high anion gap, low pH, low glucose, abnormal amino acids (high glycine)
		Urine—abnormal organic acids (e.g., high propionic acid), abnormal metabolite (methylcitrate), absent ketones
Maple syrup urine disease	MD, hypoglycemia, lethargy, coma, acidosis	Blood—abnormal amino acids (leucine, isoleucine, valine)
		Urine—high organic acids (ketoacids)
Galactosemia	MD, cataracts, sepsis, hepatic disease if untreated	Blood—high galactose
		Urine—reducing substances
Tyrosinemia	MD, hypoglycemia, hepatic disease, hepatomegaly	Blood—high amino acids (tyrosine), abnormal metabolite (succinylacetone)
Fatty acid oxidation disorders (e.g., MCAD deficiency)	Hypoglycemia, hepatic disease, hepatomegaly, cardiomyopathy, sudden death	Blood—low glucose, low carnitine, abnormal acylcarnitine profile (e.g., MC acylcarnitines)
		Urine—abnormal organic acids (e.g., MC dicarboxylic acids), absent ketones
Phenylketonuria	MD, seizures if untreated	Blood—abnormal amino acid screen (phenylalanine)
Large molecule diseases		
Glycogenoses (e.g., GSD type Ia)	Hypoglycemia, hepatic disease, hepatomegaly	Blood—low glucose, high uric acid, lipids, lactic acid
		Liver biopsy—glycogen storage
Neurolipidoses (e.g., Tay-Sachs dis.)	Developmental regression, seizures ± hepatomegaly	Leukocytes or fibroblasts—deficient enzyme
MLS, MPS (e.g., Hurler syndrome)	Developmental regression, dysotosis, hepatomegaly	Leukocytes—granules in some disorders
		Leukocytes or fibroblasts—deficient enzyme
Organellar diseases		
Kearns-Sayre disease	MD, muscle weakness, ataxia	Blood—high lactic acid
		Leucocytes—mitochondrial DNA mutation
Pearson syndrome	MD, muscle weakness, ataxia, neutropenia	Blood—high lactic acid, low neutrophils
		Leucocytes—mitochondrial DNA mutation
Zellweger syndrome	MD, hypotonia, liver disease, bone disease	Blood—high very long chain fatty acids
		Liver biopsy—absent peroxisomes
		Fibroblasts—deficient enzymes

Notes: OTC, ornithine transcarbamylase; MCAD, medium chain coenzyme A dehydrogenase; MLS, mucolipidoses; MPS, mucopolysaccharidoses, MD, mental deficiency.

ment of metabolic disease specialists, it is the primary care provider that must recognize the initial symptoms listed in Table 12.1. There is some overlap between more physiologic diseases like diabetes mellitus or congenital adrenal hyperplasia that are treated by endocrinologists and the inborn errors of metabolism that comprise the specialty of biochemical genetics. Hypoglycemia, acidosis, and lactic acidemia can be symptoms of endocrine, gastrointestinal, or cardiac diseases, frequently necessitating cooperation between these specialists and biochemical geneticists in arriving at the correct diagnosis.

■ 12.2. RECOGNIZING METABOLIC DISEASES

In order to simplify the processes of symptom recognition and classification, inborn errors can be divided into acute disorders, involving smaller molecules with rapid turnover, and chronic disorders, involving larger molecules with slow turnover (e.g., *storage diseases*). This classification is of course oversimplified, and a more detailed summary of algorithms for metabolic disease can be found in the general references. Different laboratory evaluations are implied for acute versus chronic metabolic diseases (Table 12.2), emphasizing the importance of this distinction. Because these are recessive Mendelian diseases, a family history seeking evidence of consanguinity and genetic counseling following the diagnosis are important components in the approach to inborn errors of metabolism.

Acute Metabolic Disorders: The Newborn with Catastrophic Disease

The metabolic pathways responsible for the conversion of small molecules are crucial as sources of energy and building blocks for the organism. Amino acids, sugars, fatty acids, and nucleotides are examples of small molecules that are interconverted by enzyme action. Because of their rapid metabolism and turnover,

small-molecule diseases tend to be acute or episodic in presentation, with symptoms of lethargy, coma, seizures, or unusual odors as summarized in Table 12.1. A common and vivid presentation of small molecule diseases is the newborn with catastrophic illness. Once the fetus is removed from the protection of maternal metabolism, and after the newborn has ingested sufficient formula or breast milk to present substances for catabolism, an enzyme block can produce multiple chemical alterations as diagrammed in Fig. 12.1A. Symptoms such as lethargy, seizures, or exaggerated jaundice (hyperbilirubinemia) then appear that may be confused with infection. Sometimes the metabolic disease confers increased susceptibility to infection, causing the metabolic and infectious symptoms to coincide.

Common causes of newborn metabolic disease include urea cycle disorders with hyperammonemia, severe organic acidemias, or severe amino acid abnormalities as listed in Table 12.2. Specific screening tests are suggested by these possibilities, including blood amino acid and ammonia levels, urine organic acids, and reducing substances. Simultaneous monitoring of blood glucose, electrolytes, pH, hemogram (including red cells, white cells, and platelets), and bilirubin will assist in the decision between sepsis (high white blood cell counts, normal metabolic parameters), metabolic disease (normal or low white blood cell counts, low glucose, low pH, abnormal electrolytes), or both. Since neonatal sepsis must be suspected and treated immediately, sick newborns are always placed on broad spectrum antibiotic coverage until a diagnosis is made. Since metabolic disorders like galactosemia (230400) predispose to infection with *E. coli,* and others (e.g., propionic acidemia 232000) are associated with neutropenia, coexisting metabolic disease and sepsis are not unusual.

Case 12A Follow-up: The symptoms of acute presentation with progressive lethargy after feeding suggest catastrophic disease of the newborn, and the child should have specific metabolic testing directed at the most probable disease categories. These will include urea cycle disorders (blood ammonia), organic acidemias (blood pH, electrolytes, and urine organic acids), or severe amino acidopathies (blood amino acids, urine organic acids). The term *metabolic screen* is sometimes used to imply that a simple panel of urine screening tests can rule out the presence of inborn errors. This is never the case. A blood spot was sent to the state metabolic laboratory, but this also was not intended as a general screen. Each geographic region screens for specific metabolic diseases based on their frequency and severity in the regional population (see Section 12.8).

Acute Presentations of Later Infancy and Childhood

With slightly milder but still devastating inborn errors, the enzyme block may not cause disease until later infancy or childhood. The child may be entirely healthy until the time of acute illness, or there may be subtle abnormalities like mild growth delay, developmental delay, or increased susceptibility to infection that in retrospect were harbingers of disease. Often an environmental insult such as an infectious illness, dehydration, a prolonged fast, or a high-protein meal will provoke the acute metabolic episode. The child may present with vomiting, seizures, altered mental status, or with prolonged sleepiness and coma. Occasionally there is rapid progression with shock or sudden death prior to medical consultation. Such tragedies emphasize the importance of suspecting and defining metabolic diseases.

An important group of diseases that can present in later infancy or childhood are the glycogen storage diseases or disorders of fatty acid oxidation. Children with these diseases may appear normal until they stop feeding because of vomiting or loss of appetite due to infection. Interruption in the supply of carbohydrates and glucose prompts the liver to degrade glycogen and increase fatty acid oxidation in an attempt to maintain blood glucose for brain metabolism. In glycogen storage diseases, inability to release glucose from glycogen causes the blood glucose to fall, fatty acid metabolism and blood lipids to increase, and increases in blood lactic acid. In disorders of fatty acid oxidation, glycogen stores are consumed in several hours and the body becomes dependent on fatty acid breakdown with restoration of glucose levels by gluconeogenesis (manufacture of glucose from acids like pyruvate). In each disease category, the low blood glucose (hypoglycemia) may cause vomiting or seizures with progression toward severe neurologic disease and shock. As discussed in the following paragraphs, diagnosis allows dietary therapy by providing continuous carbohydrate infusions (glycogen storage diseases) or frequent feedings (fatty acid oxidation disorders).

Disorders of Insidious Onset: Storage Diseases

Storage diseases contrast with small-molecule diseases because of protein, carbohydrate, or lipid polymers that cannot be catabolized and slowly accumulate in the affected tissues. Acute metabolic disorders may be treated by dietary means, allowing true primary prevention by removing the disease. Large-molecule (storage) disorders often have a chronic onset with symptoms such as neurodegeneration and/or hepatosplenomegaly. The buildup of abnormal polymers within tissues is not curable by diet or cofactor administration, but new methods of enzyme replacement, gene therapy, and tissue transplantation are increasingly useful. It is also possible to minimize complications by anticipatory guidance in these disorders: Preventive management is important for chronic metabolic disorders.

In large-molecule disorders, the substrates that increase in concentration due to enzyme deficiency are polymers like glycogen (glucose chains), glycoproteins (carbohydrate and aminoacid chains), mucopolysaccharides or glycosaminoglycans (chains of various sugars modified by sulfate and amino groups), or complex lipids (glycerol and sphingolipid polymers). Most of the deficient enzymes are components of lysosomes, where their role is to degrade the large molecule polymers as they are replaced by new synthesis.

Accumulation of one polymer in lysosomes often interferes with the degradation of other polymers, causing accumulation or *storage* of several polymer types. Examples include the glycogen storage diseases, neurolipidoses, and mucopolysaccharidoses (Table 12.2). The overlap between small- and large-molecule disease categories is illustrated by glycogen storage diseases. These disorders may have acute or chronic presentations depending on the severity of hypoglycemic episodes that were mentioned previously.

Because levels of small molecules like amino acids, organic acids, or carbohydrates are generally normal in storage diseases, diagnosis depends on the effects of stored polymers within tissues. Sometimes undegraded polymer fragments may be detected in urine as with the mucopolysaccharidoses (Table 12.2). More often, the stored substances must be detected through unusual granules in white blood cells, abnormal histology on liver biopsy, unusual structures in the retina or skeleton, or increased size of organs like liver. Once a storage disease is suspected based on eye examination, tissue biopsy, radiography, or imaging studies, enzyme assays are necessary to establish a specific diagnosis. Although dietary therapy is rarely available (continuous starch feedings for glycogenoses being an exception), diagnosis of a storage disease often leads to important preventive measures such as screening for hydrocephalus in the mucopolysaccharidoses.

Disorders with Chronic Neurologic Presentation

Although many small molecule disorders present acutely, occasional children with urea cycle disorders or organic acidemias escape catastrophic episodes and present solely with neurologic impairments. The child with developmental delay must therefore be examined with the possibility of morphologic or metabolic causes in mind, with evidence from the history and physical used to decide on appropriate testing. Another group of metabolic disorders have elevations in molecules like uric acid (Lesch-Nyhan syndrome, 308000) or the amino acid glycine (hyperglycinemia, 238300) with symptoms of severe mental retardation with or without behavioral abnormalities. Finally, many large molecule diseases with storage of polymers in the brain exhibit early developmental progress with later leveling and degeneration. Early progress with later loss of developmental milestones is a strong indication for evaluation of storage disease even when there is no evidence of organ enlargement or other tissue changes. The many metabolic disorders that present with neurologic damage are beyond the scope of this chapter but should be not be forgotten despite the emphasis on acute illnesses and storage diseases.

The Laboratory Diagnosis of Metabolic Disease

Metabolic testing examines the protein product of a specific gene by enzyme/antibody assay or, less precisely, by measuring altered metabolite levels that are created by enzyme deficiency. The most accurate level of testing involves DNA diagnosis, since the isolation and characterization of mutant alleles avoids the requirement of enzyme expression in particular tissues. For example, deficiency of ornithine transcarbamylase (311250) that causes one form of hyperammonemia can only be detected in liver, making DNA diagnosis necessary for the analysis of amniotic or chorionic villus cells.

Although DNA testing is available for a growing number of metabolic disorders, the initial diagnosis usually requires measurement of abnormal metabolites that accumulate as a result of enzyme deficiency (Table 12.2). Acute metabolic disorders often present with alterations of blood electrolytes, pH, glucose, ammonia, or lactate levels. Important in the determination of electrolytes is the anion gap, roughly estimated by the sum of sodium (~145 mEq per L) and potassium (~4 mEq per L) minus the sum of chloride (~110 mEq per L) and bicarbonate (~20 mEq L). The resulting normal value of 19–20 for the anion gap is increased when high concentrations of organic acids like propionate or methylmalonate are present in the blood, because the negative charge of organic anions plus the chloride and bicarbonate anions must be equal to the positive charge of sodium and potassium cations. Low blood pH and a high anion gap, with or without low glucose or high ammonia, thus strongly suggests acute metabolic disease if hypoxia is not present.

Children with one or more of these blood abnormalities often need a quantitative determination of blood amino acids (amino acids are retained by the kidney and have highest concentrations in blood) and urine organic acids (organic acids are excreted by the kidney and attain highest levels in urine). Exceptions to this rule of testing are disorders of renal transport such as cystinuria (220100) where amino acids are normal in blood but abnormally excreted in urine. If a fatty acid oxidation disorder is suspected, then measurement of carnitine is indicated. Carnitine forms complexes with fatty acids (acylcarnitines) that enables transport across the mitochondrial membrane. A serious complication of elevated fatty acids or organic acids is to tie up carnitine and interfere with normal fatty acid transport. A blood acylcarnitine profile provides a way of detecting which fatty acids are bound to carnitine, suggesting the level at which fatty acid oxidation is blocked (Table 12.2).

The goal of initial metabolic testing is to characterize the abnormal metabolites in blood, urine, or affected tissues. These measurements define the category of abnormal metabolism and guide the evaluation toward definitive assays for enzyme deficiency or mutant DNA alleles. Children with storage diseases often have normal blood testing except for the possibility of storage granules in white blood cells. These diseases are often suspected from symptoms of organ enlargement (e.g., hepatomegaly), organ dysfunction (e.g., vision loss), and neurodegeneration as mentioned

previously. Preliminary testing for these diseases may involve the detection of accumulating substances in urine (e.g., mucopolysaccharides) or in tissues (e.g., liver glycogen) obtained through biopsy. The diagnosis is again established by the detection of specific enzyme deficiencies or mutant alleles.

Participation of a metabolic disease specialist is necessary for the performance and interpretation of complex laboratory results (e.g., urine organic acid profiles). After recognition, referral, and diagnosis, the primary physician assumes an important role by ensuring dietary compliance or coordinating a preventive management program.

Case 12A Follow-up: The neonate with lethargy had blood glucose, electrolytes, and ammonia that showed marked hyperammonemia. Subsequent blood amino acids showed elevations of glutamine and argininosuccinic acid consistent with one of the urea cycle disorders (see Fig. 12.4). The autosomal recessive disease correlates with the presence of consanguinity in the parents.

■ 12.3. DISORDERS OF CARBOHYDRATE METABOLISM

The structure of the simple sugars glucose, fructose, and galactose are shown in Figure 12.2. Note that they contain an aldehyde or ketone group that will register as a reducing substance in urine. Tests for urine reducing substances can thus be used to detect the excretion of increased amounts of glucose, galactose, or fructose. Simple sugars can be phosphorylated to provide high-energy precursors for metabolism or polymer formation. Glycogen is a polymer of glucose formed by linear 1–4 links and branches of 1–6 links (Fig. 12.2.). Some carbohydrate disorders arise from blocks in the conversion of carbohydrate substrates, while others interfere with the formation or degradation of carbohydrate polymers (Fig. 12.3). Glycogen is an example of a pure carbohydrate polymer, while mucopolysaccharides or oligosaccharides are polymers formed by mixtures

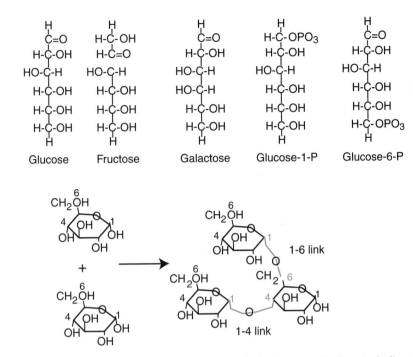

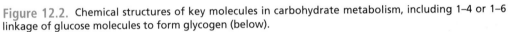

Figure 12.2. Chemical structures of key molecules in carbohydrate metabolism, including 1–4 or 1–6 linkage of glucose molecules to form glycogen (below).

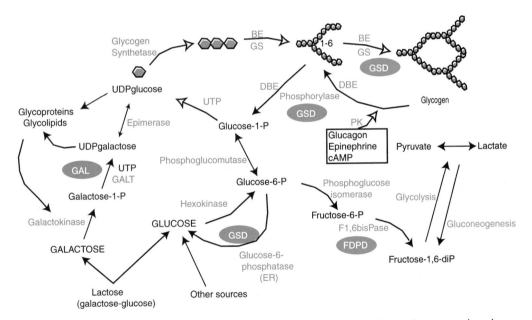

Figure 12.3. Clinically relevant pathways of carbohydrate metabolism. Galactose is converted to glucose via uridine diphosphate intermediates (left), while conversion of pyruvate and fructose-1–6-diphosphate is a key process of gluconeogenesis (right). Dietary glucose is activated to glucose-6-phosphate and used for energy metabolism or incorporated into glycogen (center). Hormones such as glucagon and epinephrine mediate the release of glucose from glycogen under conditions of hypoglycemia or stress (center). The sites of inborn errors involving this pathway are shown, includinge galactosemia (GAL), glycogen storage diseases (GSD), and fructose-1,6-diphosphatase deficiency (FDPD). P, phosphate; PK, phosphorylase kinase; GS, glycogen synthase; BE, branching enzyme; DBE, debranching enzyme; GALT, galactose-1-Pyridyl transferase; ER, endoplasmic reticulum.

■TABLE 12.3. Selected Disorders of Carbohydrate Metabolism

Disease or Syndrome	Incidence	Deficient Enzyme, Locus	Clinical Manifestations
Fructose-1,6-diphosphatase deficiency (229700)	Unknown	Fructose-1,6-diphosphatase	Hypoglycemia, lactic acidosis
Galactosemia, severe (230400)	1 in 50,000	GALT, 9p13, 4 kb gene, 11 exons, Q188R mutation in 70%	Neonatal liver disease, sepsis, later MR if untreated, ovarian failure with certain mutations
Galactosemia, mild (230200)	Unknown	Galactokinase 17q21	Cataracts
GSD type Ia (von Gierke) (232200)	1 in 100,000	G-6-Pase, 17p	Hypoglycemia, hyperuricemia, lactic acidemia, hepatomegaly
GSD type Ib (232220)	1 in 200,000	Abnormal microsomal transport G-6-Pase	Type Ia plus neutropenia
GSD type II (Pompe) (232300)	1 in 100,000	α-Glucosidase	Cardiac disease, early death
GSD types III and IV (232400, 232500)	1 in 100,000	Debrancher (1p21) or brancher (3p12) enzyme	Mild type Ia (III) or fatal cirrhosis (type IV)
GSD types VI and VIII (232700, 306000)	1 in 200,000	Phosphorylase kinase (unknown or Xp22)	Mild type Ia

Notes: GSD, glycogen storage disease; GALT, galactose-1-phosphate uridyl transferase; G-6-P, glucose-6-phosphate; 9p17, band 17 on the short arm of chromosome 9.

of sugars (e.g., glucose, galactose, mannose) with modified side chains (e.g., sulfate or amino groups).

The provision of glucose to cells is important for energy production in highly active tissues such as liver, skeletal muscle, and heart. Numerous steps in the provision of glucose to cells can be interrupted. These include dietary intake, digestion into small molecules, absorption into the blood stream, conversion of other carbohydrates like galactose into glucose, maintenance of serum glucose levels, intake of glucose into cells, and storage of materials for gluconeogenesis during fasting (Fig. 12.3). Hypoglycemia is the prototypic symptom of certain inborn errors of carbohydrate metabolism such as the hepatic glycogen storage diseases or fructose-1,6-diphosphate deficiency (FDPD—Table 12.3). Hypoglycemia may not be prominent in disorders like galactosemia, despite a block in the conversion of galactose to glucose (Fig. 12.3). Dietary deprivation, intestinal malabsorption, or inaccessibility of glucose to cells (e.g., in diabetes mellitus with

insulin deficiency) represent other alterations of carbohydrate metabolism that usually present to specialists in gastroenterology or endocrinology.

An overview of carbohydrate metabolism is shown in Figure 12.3. The conversion of galactose into glucose is shown at the left, of glucose to fructose at the right, and of glucose to glycogen at the center and top. When glucose is plentiful, glucagon and cyclic AMP levels are low, glycogen is made for future use, and glycolysis rather than gluconeogenesis is active. When glucose becomes scarce, as after a few hours of fasting, glucagon is increased, phosphorylase and phosphorylase kinases are activated, glycogen is broken down, and gluconeogenesis with its intermediate of fructose-1,6-diphosphate becomes active. When glycogen cannot be released, or when fructose-1,6-diphosphate cannot be cleaved and converted to glucose, then fatty acid oxidation is stimulated to provide alternative fuels for energy metabolism. These circumstances account for the hypoglycemia, increased lactate production, and increased blood lipids that occur in certain glycogen storage diseases and in FDPD deficiency. The conversion of galactose to glucose is less essential for metabolism, but the accumulation of toxic metabolites from elevated levels of galactose account for the liver and eye disease of galactosemia. These three disorders of carbohydrate metabolism thus illustrate how the pathogenesis of metabolic disorders can be understood based on the interconnections of metabolic pathways.

Acute Disorders of Carbohydrate Metabolism: Galactosemia

The most common cause of galactosemia is deficiency of the enzyme galactose-1-phosphate uridyl transferase (GALT—230400; Table 12.3). The diagnosis is often suspected from clinical manifestations of vomiting, diarrhea, and jaundice after breast or formula feeding in the newborn period, and a urine clinitest will be positive for reducing substances. Neonatal screening for galactosemia is conducted in 38 states, returning positive results within 1–2 weeks. With severe GALT deficiency, neonates usually manifest symptoms of enhanced jaundice, liver disease, and possible sepsis. Note that the block interferes with conversion of uridine diphosphate (UDP)-galactose to UDP-glucose (Fig. 12.3). The excess galactose that accumulates prior to this block is converted to intermediates such as galactitol that are thought to be toxic. A change to lactose-free formula should be instituted immediately once galactosemia is considered, pending referral to metabolic specialists and assay of blood for GALT enzyme deficiency (Table 12.3). Lactose is a disaccharide of glucose and galactose that is the main dietary source of galactose.

Acute Disorders of Carbohydrate Metabolism: Fructose 1,6-Bisphosphatase Deficiency

Fructose 1,6-bisphosphatase deficiency (FDPD—229700) is a severe disorder that presents during infancy and can be diagnosed by assaying the cognate enzyme in liver biopsy specimens. FDPD may present in the newborn period, with severe hypoglyemia, acidosis, hyperventilation, hypotonia, and coma. Unlike a milder disorder called hereditary fructose intolerance (229600), patients with FDPD do not have aversion to sweets or fruits containing fructose. They often have episodic attacks of inanition, vomiting, convulsions, hypoglycemia, and acidosis before the diagnosis is recognized. These attacks are provoked by febrile illnesses and fasting. The clinical course is benign once fructose and sucrose (a glucose-fructose disaccharide) are excluded from the diet. Other patients require frequent feeding to avert hypoglycemia and have numerous crises that must be treated with glucose and intravenous fluids. Preventive management consists of nutritional counseling, early treatment of infections, and surveillance for vomiting, diarrhea, and acidosis.

Glycogen Storage Diseases: Carbohydrate Disorders with Acute or Chronic Presentations

Glycogen storage diseases are a group of genetic disorders that produce alterations in the amount or structure of glycogen. Since storage of glycogen occurs mainly in liver and muscle, the diseases were first classified based on the spectrum of hepatic and muscular disease. Differential diagnosis for the hepatic disorders includes other causes of hypoglycemia and acidosis: FDPD, fatty acid oxidation disorders, or even infectious hepatitis. Glycogen storage diseases I–IV, VI and VIII are variations on a theme of hepatic disease, while types V and VII predominantly affect the muscles (Table 12.3). Pompe disease (type II) is very different, producing lethal cardiac disease with a characteristic shortening of the P-R interval by electrocardiography.

Although a variety of intravenous tolerance tests and associated imaging studies can be performed, the primary technique for diagnosis of glycogen storage diseases consists of liver or muscle biopsy followed by histologic analysis and enzyme assay. The key derangement in patients with hepatic glycogenosis is the inability to mobilize hepatic glycogen into circulating glucose. Abnormal amounts or structures of glycogen accumulate and produce hepatomegaly, while the block in glucose liberation causes hypoglycemia, lactic acidosis, hyperuricemia, and hyperlipidemia. Lipids also accumulate in the liver and contribute to the hepatomegaly. The types of hepatic glycogenoses present variations on this theme of glycogen accumulation and glucose scarcity. In type I, shunting of glucose-6-phosphate through glycolysis causes increased lactate and acidosis (Fig. 12.3). The lactate competes with renal urate excretion, and joins with increased nucleotide turnover to cause hyperuricemia. The exaggerated glycolysis also increases pools of NADH/NADPH and glycerol, favoring triglyceride synthesis and fatty liver. Types III and VI involve the same pathogenetic mechanisms as in type I, but to lesser degrees. Type IV is similar to galactosemia in that the accumulating glycogen is toxic and leads to early death from liver scarring (cirrhosis) and liver failure. The cause of toxicity is not known (Chen and Burchell, 1995).

Preventive management for children with hepatic glycogenosis is to restore glucose homeostasis and prevent hypoglycemic seizures, lactic acidosis, hyperuricemia, and hyperlipidemia. Nocturnal glucose drip feedings can be administered by nasogastric tube, or cornstarch can be given orally at frequent intervals to provide a slow-release source of glucose. Frequent monitoring of growth and development, glucose levels, liver size, and liver function tests is necessary for children with more severe disease, and those with Type Ib require periodic blood counts to monitor neutropenia. Surveillance for the occurrence of hepatomas should include periodic abdominal examinations and abdominal ultrasound studies. Many patients with long-term dietary treatment are now reaching adulthood, and the outlook for normal stature and regression of hepatic adenomas seems good (Chen and Burchell, 1995).

■ 12.4. DISORDERS OF AMINO ACID METABOLISM

Case 12B: **Developmental Delay with Unusual Odor**

A 2-year-old female with moderate developmental delay and a "mousy" odor is referred for genetic evaluation by Child Protective Services, who suspect fetal alcohol syndrome. The child was discharged less than 24 hours after birth, and she has had poor medical care with no immunizations. Family history is normal, as is the physical examination except for a mousy odor. The child has lighter pigmentation than her family background with strikingly pale eyes and hair.

Urea Cycle Disorders

The urea cycle illustrated in Figure 12.4 is the central pathway in humans for eliminating nitrogen wastes. Ammonia liberated from degraded protein and amino acids is complexed with bicarbonate and phosphate in the unique carbamyl phosphate synthase (CPS) reaction, then metabolized to urea with two ammonia equivalents for excretion (Fig. 12.4). The amino acid ornithine that results from the final step in urea synthesis is then recycled, accepting a molecule of carbamyl phosphate to form citrulline. N-acetyl-glutamate is a cofactor for CPS that exerts regulatory controls on the cycle that are outside the scope of this discussion (Fig. 12.4). Several of the enzymes are located within the mitochondrion, so alteration of N-terminal peptides that mediate mitochondrial uptake can cause enzyme misplacement rather than true deficiency. Each of the enzymes in the urea cycle has been associated with a specific inborn error of metabolism, as shown in Table 12.4.

As might be predicted, deficiencies of enzymes like CPS or ornithine transcarbamylase (OTC) that occur early in the cycle cause the most severe disease. These children (affected males in the X-linked OTC deficiency) present as catastrophic disease of the newborn that is nicely illustrated by Case 12A. Once the diges-

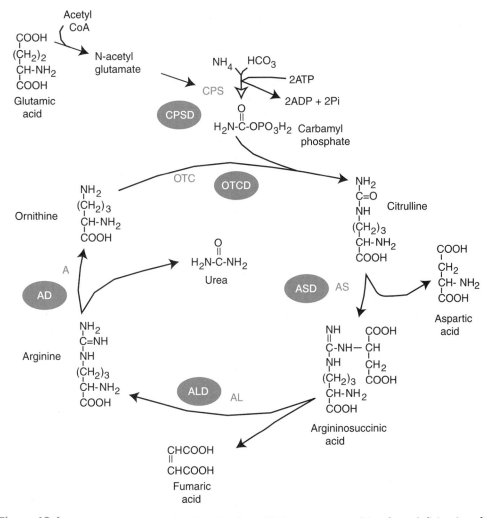

Figure 12.4. Urea cycle pathway showing the sites of inborn errors resulting from deficiencies of carbamyl phosphate synthase (CPSD), ornithine transcarbamylase (OTCD), argininosuccinate synthase (citrullinemia—ASD), argininosuccinase (lyase-ALD), and arginase (AD).

tion of protein provided in ingested maternal blood, formula, or breast milk begins, ammonia levels rise and cause progressive lethargy and coma. The ammonia also stimulates the respiratory center in the brain, producing rapid breathing with increased exhalation of carbon dioxide, increased blood bicarbonate, and mild increase in blood pH (alkalosis). Testing of blood ammonia will establish the diagnostic category, with simultaneous blood amino acids and urine organic acids needed to discriminate various causes of hyperammonemia. Organic

acidemias such as propionic or methylmalonic acidemia (Table 12.5) can cause moderate elevations in blood ammonia, but these will be associated with characteristic organic acid profiles in urine and severe acidosis in blood.

When the organic acids are normal, the blood amino acid profile gives clues as to the precise urea cycle block (Fig. 12.4). High levels of citrulline point to a block in argininosuccinic acid synthase (215700—Table 12.4), while high levels of argininosuccinate predict deficiency of argininosuccinase (207900—

■TABLE 12.4. Amino Acid and Urea Cycle Disorders

Disease or Syndrome	Incidence	Deficient Enzyme, Locus	Clinical Manifestations
Urea cycle disorders			
CPS deficiency (237300)	~1 in 100,000	As named, 2p, >100 kb gene with >40 exons	MD, hyperammonemia, seizures, death
Ornithine transcarb mylase (OTC) deficiency (311250)	~1 in 100,000	As named, Xp2185 kb gene with 10 exons, deletions and diverse point mutations	Same as CPS deficiency
Citrullinemia (215700)	~1 in 100,000	ASA synthetase, 9q34, 63 kb gene with 16 exons, diverse mutations	Same as CPS deficiency
Argininosuccinase (lyase) deficiency (207900)	~1 in 100,000	As named, 7cen-7p21, 1.3 kb gene, diverse mutations	Same as CPS deficiency
Arginase deficiency (207800)	~1 in 100,000	As named, 6q23, 11.5 kb gene with 8 exons, diverse mutations	MD, spasticity with less severe and frequent hyperammonemia
Other aminoacidopathies			
Phenylketonuria (261600)	1 in 10,000	< 1% PAH, 12q22, 90 kb gene with 13 exons, > 100 diverse mutations	MD, mousy odor, seizures if untreated
Hyperphenylalani-nemia (261630)	1 in 20,000	> 1% PAH, 12q22, subset of mutations	None—benign phenotype
Hyperphenylalani-nemia (233910)	1 in 1,000,000	Dihydropteridine reductase, 4p15, 730 bp open reading frame	Severe MD, seizures
Tyrosinemia type I (276700)	Unknown	Fumarylacetoacetate hydrolase, 15q23	Liver disease, cirrhosis
Oculocutaneous albinism (203100)	1 in 30,000	Tyrosinase, 11q14	Pale skin, eyes, sun sensitivity, nystagmus
Alkaptonuria (203500)	1 in 100,000	Homogentisic acid oxidase, 3q2	Dark urine, pigmented cartilage, arthritis
Homocystinuria (236200)	1 in 350,000	Cystathionine-β-synthase deficiency, 21q21	Marfanoid habitus, vascular thromboses
Maple syrup urine disease (248600)	1 in 180,000	Branched chain keto-acid dehydrogenase subunits, 1p31, 6p21, 7q31, 19q13	MD, ketoacidosis; lactic acidosis with E3 subunit deficiency

Notes: CPS, carbamyl phosphate synthetase; ASA, argininosuccinic acid; Xp21, band 21 on the short arm of the X chromosome. PAH, phenylalanine hydroxylase; MD, mental deficiency.

Table 12.4). Amino acids like arginine and glutamine (converted from glutamic acid in Fig. 12.4) are elevated in most of the urea cycle defects as expected when the pathway is blocked and arginine cannot be recycled. All of the intermediates shown in Figure 12.4 are in equilibrium with other metabolic pathways, and this ability to shunt into alternative pathways provided a new concept of therapy.

Management of children with urea cycle defects is directed toward the control of ammonia levels by minimizing dietary protein. Unfortunately, hyperammonemic episodes can be very damaging to the central nervous system, caus-

■ **TABLE 12.5.** Organic Acidemias and Fatty Acid Oxidation Disorders

Disease or Syndrome	Incidence	Deficient Enzyme, Locus	Clinical Manifestations
Propionic acidemia (232000)	Unknown	Propionyl-CoA carboxylase subunits, 3q13, 13q22	MD, acidosis, hypo glycemia, hyperammone mia, neutropenia
Methylmalonic acidemia (251000)	1 in 20,000	Methylmalonyl-CoA mutase, 6p12	Same as propionic
Methylmalonic acidemia plus homocystinuria (277410)	Unknown	Methylcobalamin (vit. B_{12}) synthesis	MD, milder acidosis, neutropenia
Multiple carboxylase deficiency (253260)	1 in 25,000	Biotinidase	Sparse hair, rashes, acidosis, anion gap
Multiple carboxylase deficiency (253270)	Unknown	Holocarboxylase synthetase deficiency	Sparse hair, rashes, acidosis, anion gap
LCHAD deficiency	Unknown	Long chain hydroxyacyl CoA dehydrogenase	Liver disease, cardiomyopathy
MCAD deficiency (201450)	1 in 20,000	Medium chain acyl-CoA dehydrogenase, 1p31	Nonketotic hypoglycemia, acidosis, sudden death
SCAD deficiency (201470)	Unknown	Short chain acyl-CoA dehydrogenase	MD, lethargy, vomiting, hypotonia

Notes: LCHAD, long chain hydroxyacyl CoA dehydrogenase; MCAD, medium chain acyl-CoA dehydrogenase; SCAD, short chain acyl-CoA dehydrogease; CoA, coenzyme A; MD, mental deficiency; 3q13, band 13 on the long arm of chromosome 3.

ing severe disabilities before transplantation can be accomplished. Therapy by stimulating alternative pathways for ammonia excretion is effective and is often combined with dietary protein restriction. Children with argininosuccinase deficiency (207900) respond rapidly to arginine infusions and have excellent outcomes when treated with this drug alone. The urea cycle disorders provide an elegant example of genetic heterogeneity (one phenotype of hyperammonemia, multiple genetic causes) that has been definitively explained by biochemical and molecular techniques.

Phenylketonuria

The pathways illustrated in Figure 12.5 illustrate another group of inborn errors that can be understood based on chemical interconversions. Phenylalanine, like several others, is an essential amino acid that cannot be synthesized by the body. Although necessary for protein synthesis, phenylalanine must be catabolized when present in excess and is first hydroxy-

lated by the enzyme phenylalanine hydroxylase (Table 12.4). Hydroxylated phenylalanine is tyrosine, an example of a nonessential amino acid that can be synthesized by the body. Tyrosine has several metabolic fates, including conversion to homogentisic and fumaric acids or conversion to the neurotransmitter DOPA and melanin pigments. These reactions are the basis for a group of metabolic disorders.

Elevated blood levels of phenylalanine are associated with three categories of disease (Scriver et al., 1995). The most frequent is classical phenylketonuria (PKU) due to deficiency of phenylalanine hydroxylase enzyme (261630, Table 12.4). Patients with PKU require diets low in phenylalanine to have normal mental development. Milder deficiencies of phenylalanine hydroxylase produce hyperphenylalaninemia (261630), a benign variant that rarely requires dietary treatment. A third and fortunately rare cause of high phenylalanine levels are errors affecting biopterin (e.g., 233910—Table 12.4), a cofactor for phenylalanine hydroxylase. This group of disorders

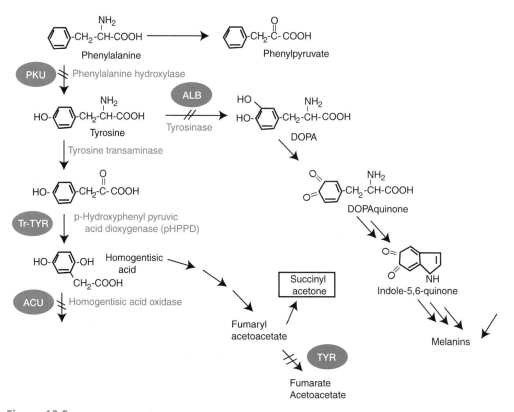

Figure 12.5. Conversions of aromatic amino acids with the inborn errors phenylketonuria (PKU), albinism (ALB), transient tyrosinemia of the newborn (Tr-TYR), tyrosinemia type I (TYR), and alkaptonuria (ACU).

is more refractory to dietary management. Another disease results from exposure of fetuses to high phenylalanine levels in their mothers with PKU. These infants have the maternal PKU syndrome of congenital anomalies and developmental delay that resembles fetal alcohol syndrome.

The incidence of PKU is 1 in 10,000 births in Caucasian populations, while hyperphenylalaninemia is four- or fivefold lower and the biopterin deficiences 100-fold lower (Table 12.4). Children with PKU are often lightly pigmented, presumably because of tyrosine deficiency after the phenylalanine hydroxylase block and decreased melanin synthesis (Fig.12.5). Developmental delay, seizures, scleroderma-like changes, and skin rashes may occur. Children with elevated blood phenylalanine should be referred to a metabolic disease center for diagnosis of PKU, followed by treatment with a diet low in phenylalanine. As would be predicted from the pathways in Figure 12.5, tyrosine must be supplemented when protein is restricted. Parents should also be cautioned about aspartame, the artifical sweetener that contains phenylalanine.

Case 12B Follow-up: The light pigmentation and mousy odor are classic signs of untreated PKU. As shown in Figure 12.5, deficiency of tyrosine and decreased melanin synthesis due to deficiency of phenylalanine hydroxylase causes the lighter pigmentation. Early discharge has complicated neonatal screening because increased levels of metabolites may not be evident by 12–24 hours after birth. Follow-up screening of early discharge patients is therefore necessary. The child has undoubtedly sustained mental damage because the diagnosis of PKU was not made and the protective low-phenylalanine diet was not instituted. Although the child does not have fetal alcohol syndrome, the involvement of Child Protective Services may be appropriate to ensure dietary compliance. Even at age 2 years, initiation of the low-protein diet would be beneficial for subsequent intellectual outcome.

Albinism, Tyrosinemia, and Alkaptonuria

Other diseases associated with defects in the pathways shown in Figure 12.5 include oculocutaneous albinism (several types including tyrosinase deficiency—203100, Table 12.4). The block in tyrosine catabolism interferes with melanin production and causes lightening of pigment in the eyes and skin. Albinos are particularly sensitive to the carcinogenic effects of sunlight, so prevention of exposure with sunscreens is vital. The lack of eye pigment is associated with complex changes in ocular nervous control that result in nystagmus (jerking eye movements). Regular ophthalmology evaluations are thus needed for patients with severe forms of albinism. Albinism is a complex and heterogenous category of disease that extends beyond the simple defect in tyrosine deaminase mentioned here. Associations with deafness, immune defects, and other medical complications in the various forms of albinism mandate that these patients have appropriate specialty evaluation.

Tyrosinemia type I (276700, Table 12.4) is a rare disorder except in certain regions of Quebec, where a founder effect has led to exaggerated frequency. The chief manifestation is severe neonatal liver disease, and most patients with this presentation excrete the unusual metabolite succinyl acetone (Fig. 12.5). Dietary protein restriction to lower phenylalanine and tyrosine is of benefit, and the disease is sufficiently frequent in parts of Quebec to justify neonatal screening. There is a transient form of tyrosinemia that reflects immaturity of the liver (Fig. 12.5).

Alkaptonuria (203500, Table 12.4) is a rare inborn error that achieved fame as the first inborn error to be recognized. The disorder leads to excess levels of homogentisic acid (Fig. 12.5), which oxidizes in light to produce a black color. Children were recognized by their black diapers, and adults can be recognized by darkly pigmented cartilage (ochronosis). Some of the increased pigmentation may derive from diversion of elevated homogentisic acid into melanin metabolites (Fig. 12.5). The chief complication of the disease is adult arthritis.

Maple Syrup Urine Disease

Maple syrup urine disease (248600, Table 12.4) involves the accumulation of branched chain amino and organic acids, producing acidosis and neurologic symptoms (Chuang and Shih, 1995). The primary defects affect the branched chain α-keto acid dehydrogenase, a complex of at least five proteins and a thiamine (vitamin B1) cofactor. In the most severe variety, neonates become lethargic by age 1 week and progress to hypotonia with unusual posturing, ketosis, and acidosis. Figure 12.6A illustrates the subtle dysmorphology that may accompany acidosis in patients with maple syrup urine disease. Seizures, coma, a bulging fontanelle, and a maple syrup odor may be noted. The diagnosis is made by blood amino acid and urine organic acid profiles, which show elevated branched-chain amino acids in blood (valine, leucine, isoleucine; Fig. 12.6B) and elevated levels of their corresponding ketoacids in urine (Fig. 12.6B). Several milder forms of the disease have been described and discriminated by molecular analysis; one of these responds to dietary supplementation of excess thiamine.

The management of maple syrup urine disease relies on a sufficiently early diagnosis to avoid severe neurologic lesions. The initial diagnosis and dietary counseling is best made at a metabolic center, where specialized testing and dietary management is available. Once the diagnosis is suspected, thiamine is adminis-

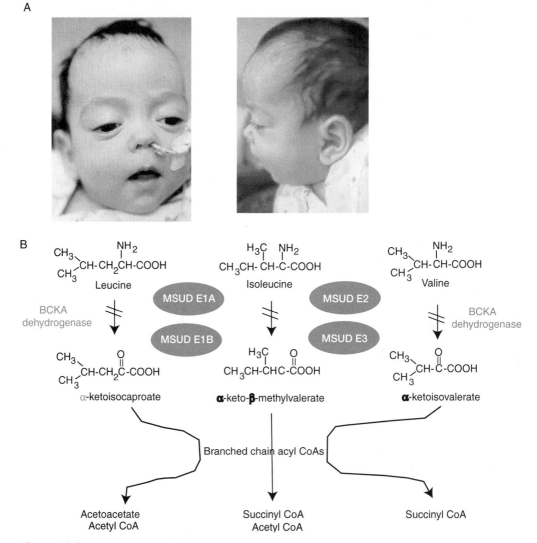

Figure 12.6. *A*, Patient with maple syrup urine disease (MSUD) showing subtle dysmorphology including shallow orbits and malar flattening; *B*, pathways for the degradation of branched chain amino acids into branched chain keto-acids (BCKA) and four inborn errors affecting subunits (E1A, E1B, E2, E3) of the BCKA dehydrogenase.

tered for at least 3 weeks to see if it produces decreased levels of amino and ketoacids (Chuang and Shih, 1995). Special formulas lacking in branched chain amino acids are administered, and blood branched chain amino acid levels are monitored. Intercurrent infections and/or dehydration can be lethal to these patients, and parents should be encouraged to seek early evalution for symptoms of illness, loss of appetite, or behavioral changes. Exchange transfusion and parenteral nutrition may be required during acute episodes (Chuang and Shih, 1995). Many patients sustain some neurologic damage, so early intervention and other services appropriate for children with disabilities are needed.

Homocystinuria

Homocystinuria (236300, Table 12.4) is named for its increased levels of homocystine in blood and urine, and is one of the metabolic disorders that produces altered morphology. Homocystinuria is a finding that can arise in conjunction with several metabolic defects including those with deficiencies of folic acid, pyridoxine (vitamin B_6), or one form of cobalamin (vitamin B_{12}—see Fig. 12.7). Children with severe starvation may thus have homocystinuria due to vitamin deficiencies. The most common form of homocystinuria is caused by inherited deficiency of cystathionine-β-synthase (236200—Table 12.4). Other causes include alterations in folic acid and vitamin B_{12} metabolism; these disorders are not associated with a Marfanoid phenotype and connective tissue abnormality.

Tall stature and body build (Marfanoid habitus), lens dislocation, arachnodactyly (long fingers), scoliosis (curved spine), and flat feet are frequent findings in patients with homocystinuria. Similarity of the phenotype to that of Marfan syndrome (154700) requires that some patients suspected of the latter, more common syndrome have urine tests for sulfhydryl (SH) groups to rule out homocystinuria. Differences from Marfan syndrome in-

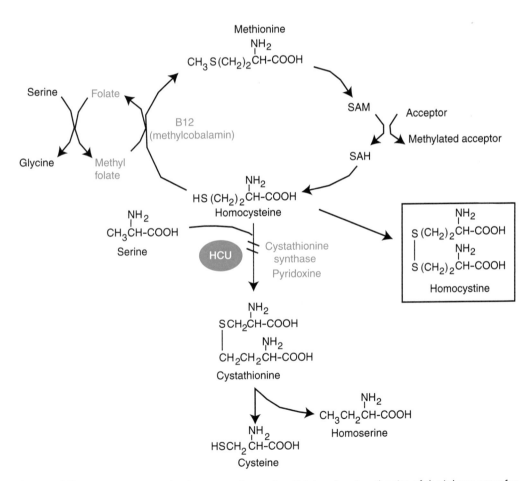

Figure 12.7. Pathways converting homocysteine and methinine showing the site of the inborn error for homocystinuria (HCU). Note the involvement of three vitamins—folate, B_{12}, and pyridoxine (B_6), a cofactor for cystathionine synthase.

clude downward rather than upward dislocation of the lens, and neurologic manifestations including mental deficiency (median IQ of 64 for patients with homocystinuria who do not respond to vitamin supplementation). Seizures and psychiatric disorders can occur in up to 50% of patients, but these may be complications of thromboembolic (vaso-occlusive) episodes. Preventive management can include dietary treatment with pyridoxine to lower homocysteine levels, with ophthalmology, cardiology, and skeletal evaluations. Patients undergoing surgery should have preoperative hydration and anticoagulation with careful anesthesia to lower the risks for thromboembolism.

Cystinuria

Many metabolic abnormalities arise from dysfunction of the kidney as graphically illustrated by renal osteodystrophy, a pattern of skeletal changes and fractures due to renal phosphate loss and hypocalcemia. These disorders are more properly discussed under renal diseases, but cystinuria (220100) is mentioned here to emphasize the one use of urinary amino acids. Despite the frequent listing of urinary amino acids as options for hospital laboratories, quantitative blood amino acids are most useful for evaluating children with potential inborn errors. Diseases that affect renal amino acid excretion are an exception to this rule of testing, as illustrated by cystinuria. Individuals with the disorder are predisposed to the development of kidney stones due to excess excretion of the basic amino acids ornithine, lysine, arginine, and cystine. Characterization of cystinuria and related disorders has led to the identification of specific renal transporters that are specific for families of amino acids. The major management strategy for cystinuria is frequent drinking to dilute the urine and prevent kidney stone formation. Cystinosis (219800), a more serious disorder with accumulation of cystine in multiple tissues, should be distinguished from cystinuria.

◼ 12.5. FATTY ACID OXIDATION DISORDERS AND ORGANIC ACIDEMIAS

Case 12C: *Febrile Illness, Hypoglycemia, and a Deceased Sibling*

A 2-year-old boy presents with fever, lethargy, decreased appetite, and signs of dehydration (decreased skin turgor, dry lips, no tears). Infection is suspected because of a high white blood cell count, and broad spectrum antibiotics are begun after appropriate fluids are sent for culture. The initial laboratory studies are somewhat unusual, showing hypoglycemia, slightly increased anion gap, and a decreased blood pH. The urinalysis is normal, but there are no ketones despite the dehydration and low blood sugar. Family history reveals that a sister died at age 14 months from the sudden infant death syndrome (SIDS).

Metabolic acidosis with an increased anion gap is a characteristic presentation for children with organic acidemias (Table 12.5). These disorders involve enzyme deficiencies that result in elevated levels of organic acids—that is, organic molecules with carboxyl groups such as uric acid, lactic acid, propionic acid, or methylmalonic acid (Fig. 12.8). In order to maintain the total anions (negative charges) equal to the cations (positive charges) in blood, deep breaths (Kussmaul respirations) are initiated to blow off carbon dioxide and increase blood. Bicarbonate is lost as the kidney attempts to excrete the excess organic acids, and the blood pH drops despite attempts to raise bicarbonate and lower carbon dioxide. The organic acid is hidden among the cations and ions recorded as electolytes, producing an elevated ion gap (sodium plus potassium ion minus bicarbonate plus chloride ions) as discussed previously. The diagnosis of organic acidemias requires mass spectrometry to characterize the organic molecules appearing in the urine. Once the abnormal molecule(s) are characterized, a disease category can be suspected and the diagnosis confirmed by enzyme assay or DNA studies.

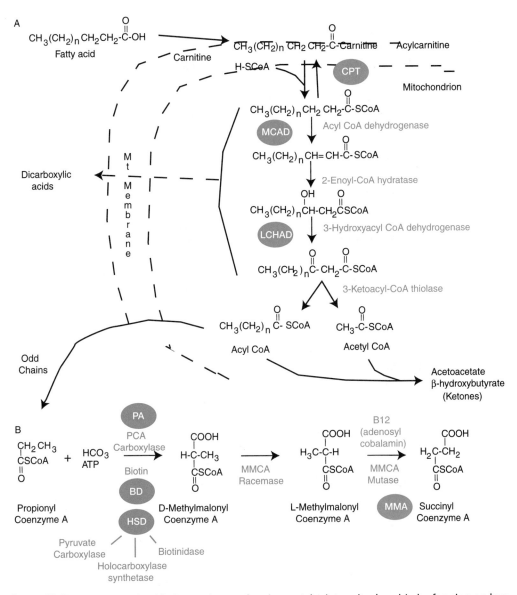

Figure 12.8. A, Fatty acid oxidation pathways showing uptake into mitochondria by forming acylcarnitines and a cycle that removes two carbon units with each passage of a fatty acid. The site of the inborn errors carnitine-palmitoyl transferase (CPT), medium chain acyl-CoA dehydrogenase (MCAD), and long chain acyl-CoA hydroxyacyl dehydrogenase (LCHAD) are shown, although these disorders would involve enzymes of different chain-length specificity (see text). B, Pathway converting odd chain fatty acids and certain amino acids to propionic acid, methylmalonic acid, and ketones. Sites of the inborn errors propionic acidemia (PA), biotinidase deficiency (BD), holocarboxylase synthase deficiency (HSD), and methylmalonic acidemia (MMA) are shown.

Fatty acids are also organic anions, but they do not reach sufficient concentrations to cause a significant anion gap. Disorders of fatty acid oxidation (Table 12.5) can cause mild acidosis through buildup of smaller molecules like propionate or pyruvate (Fig. 12.8), but their major effect is to increase lactate by interfering with gluconeogenesis. A lethal complication is depletion of carnitine, the molecule that complexes with fatty acids to form acylcarnitines that can be transported across the mitochondrial membrane. When carnitine is depleted or tied up by excess fatty acid, the inability of fatty acids to penetrate the mitochondria for oxidation results in energy depletion, cardiac and liver failure, and death. There is also a severe disorder caused by deficiency of the enzyme that transfers acyl groups between carnitine and coenzyme A (carnitine palmitoyl transferase deficiency, 255122, see Fig. 12.8).

Less commonly with organic acidemias, but more commonly with fatty acid oxidation disorders, acute decompensation may occur after a normal early childhood. These severe episodes are often precipitated by intercurrent infections, often exacerbated by decreased food intake. Because the flow from pyruvate to glucose (gluconeogenesis) is disrupted by several organic acidemias and fatty acid oxidation disorders, hypoglycemia is a common presenting symptom. In certain organic acidemias and fatty acid oxidation disorders, the generation of ketones such as acetoacetate or β-hydroxybutyrate is blocked because of the oxidation defect (Fig. 12.8). The result is nonketotic hypoglycemia, a distinctive laboratory finding that alerts the clinician to this disease category.

Propionic and Methylmalonic Acidemias

Propionic (232000) and methylmalonic acidemia (251000) are heterogenous genetic disorders that usually present as catastrophic disease of the newborn. Hypoglycemia, acidosis with an increased anion gap, hyperammonemia, and absent ketones are typical. Certain patients with these disorders have bone marrow suppression with neutropenia and thrombocy-

topenia. The blood amino acids show elevated glycine, while the urine organic acids reveal large amounts of the cognate organic acid. Methylmalonic acidemia is particularly heterogenous because the mutase enzyme (Fig. 12.8) employs adenosyl cobalamin (one form of vitamin B_{12}) as a cofactor. This heterogeneity was initially demonstrated by cocultivation of fibroblasts from different patients. If sharing of substances among the fibroblasts could correct the metabolic defects, then these defects must involve different genes (different complementation groups). The several complementation groups were then matched with particular steps in cobalamin metabolism. One of these (277410, Table 12.5), producing deficiency of methylcobalamin, affects the pathways involved in both homocystine (Fig. 12.7) and methymalonate (Fig. 12.8) metabolism.

Treatment of the organic acidemias involves intravenous infusion to correct acidosis and hypoglycemia, protein and fat restriction to lower organic acid and ammonia levels, and maintenance on a moderate protein and fat diet. Vitamin B_{12} therapy is attempted in patients with methylmalonic acidemia, and biotin may be therapeutic in certain patients with propionic acidemia. Many patients are so severely affected that they incur brain injury and demonstrate scarring or demyelination on head MRI. Anticipation of developmental delays, seizures, and other neurologic problems is included in the preventive management of these disorders.

Multiple Carboxylase Deficiency

Propionic acidemia may also occur as part of multiple carboxylase deficiency, since propionyl coenzyme A carboxylase, pyruvate carboxylase, and β-methylcrotonyl CoA carboxylase all share biotin as a cofactor. These mitochondrial carboxylases are important for fatty acid synthesis and amino acid catabolism, and their combined absence in multiple carboxylase deficiency produces elevations of lactate, propionate, ammonia, alanine, and ketone bodies. Biotin is chemically attached to these carboxylases (biotinylation), and must be recycled through action of the enzyme biotinidase. Defective biotinylation (holocarboxylase synthetase deficiency, 253270) or defective biotin recycling (biotinidase deficiency, 253260) are two causes of multiple carboxylase deficiency that produce similar clinical results: organic aciduria with propionate, pyruvate, and lactate acidosis, variable neurologic problems, skin rashes, and alopecia. These disorders are important to recognize because they can be partially or completely cured by administration of biotin (Wolf, 1995).

Fatty Acid Oxidation Disorders Including MCAD Ddeficiency

Nine disorders of human fatty acid oxidation have been described, epitomized by medium chain coenzyme A dehydrogenase (MCAD) deficiency (201450). As shown in Figure 12.8, fatty acids must complex with carnitine to form acylcarnitines that allow transport into the mitochondrion. Transfer of the fatty acid from carnitine to acetyl coenzyme A then allows a cycle of oxidation steps that remove two carbons at a time from the fatty acid. Four enzymes are involved in each 2-carbon removal, and these have overlapping specificity for long chain (C12-C18), medium chain (C4-C12), and short chain (C4-C6) fatty acids. When one of these enzymes is deficient, oxidation of fatty acids below its chain length specificity is blocked. The accumulated fatty acid CoA molecules form increased amounts of acylcarnitines of similar chain length, and are excreted as dicarboxylic acids of similar chain length. In the example of MCAD deficiency, acyl carnitines of C6-C12 length will accumulate in blood and dicarboxylic acids of C6-C10 chain length will accumulate in urine. Detection of these intermediates by a blood acylcarnitine profile or urine organic acids supports the diagnosis of MCAD deficiency.

Although the different fatty acid oxidation defects listed in Table 12.5 exhibit somewhat different metabolic symptoms and severity, their common effects will be episodic hypoglycemia and acidosis without ketones (Fig. 12.8). Some disorders, like long chain CoA hydroxyacyl dehydrogenase (LCHAD) deficiency, present with severe heart failure due to cardiac muscle disease and liver disease. Biopsy of liver or autopsy of liver, heart, and skeletal muscle may show fat accumulation in these disorders, but this can be a nonspecific finding that must be supported by specific enzyme assays in fibroblasts. Disorders of fatty acid oxidation are important to recognize since acylcarnitine accumulation may deplete carnitine and lead to death from heart and liver failure. Treatment is relatively simple, consisting of low fat diets, frequent feeding to prevent the need for fat oxidation, and carnitine supplementation to avoid the possibility of depletion. There has been emphasis on fatty acid oxidation disorders as a potential cause for sudden infant death syndrome (SIDS, "cot deaths" in Britain). However, most children with true SIDS are younger than age 6 months and die from accidental suffocation or apnea due to immaturity of the respiratory center. Children may die suddenly from unrecognized disorders of fatty acid oxidation, but they are usually older than age 6 months.

Case 12C Follow-up: The presence of unusually marked acidosis and nonketotic hypoglycemia in this child with an infection should raise suspicion of a metabolic disease. Biotinidase deficiency would be one possibility, although sparse hair and rashes were not described. Presentation at age 2 years would be unusual but not unheard of for propionic or methylmalonic acidemia, and would be very possible for milder forms of the latter disease. The history of a sibling whose death was attributed to sudden infant death syndrome would be applicable to any of these autosomal recessive disorders. The acute illness after an apparently normal childhood history is most typical of a fatty acid oxidation disorder, of which MCAD deficiency is the most common (Table 12.5). Analysis of urine organic acids did show typical C6-C8 dicarboxylic acids, and the blood carnitine level was low.

MCAD deficiency is associated with a prevalent K328E mutation that is homozygous in up to 80% and compound in 17% of patients with this disease. DNA testing for this predominant allele is thus particularly useful for confirming the metabolic findings.

▪ 12.6. STORAGE DISEASES: LIPIDOSES AND MUCOLIPIDOSES (OLIGOSACCHARIDOSES)

The degradation of lipid, glycoprotein, and carbohydrate polymers is an important function of lysosomes. Lysosomal enzyme deficiencies are thus common causes of storage disease, with the type of storage material leading to disease categories based on common clinical symptoms (Fig. 12.9). Many are cruel diseases, causing severe degeneration and death in children who initially thrive and appear healthy. The metabolic consequences of lysosomal enzyme deficiencies are illustrated by the steps in degradation of dermatan sulfate as shown in Figure 12.10. The mucopolysaccharide polymer is successively degraded by

different enzymes with appropriate specificity for sulfate, glucosamine, or glycoside bonds. Absence of any particular enzyme in the sequence will block degradation at that point and lead to accumulation of the truncated mucopolysaccharide. The resulting clinical symptoms depend on the biological effects of the accumulating polymer and its tissue distribution.

Neurolipidoses

The storage of lipid polymers seems particularly damaging to brain function as reflected by the disease category of neurolipidosis (Table 12.6). Neurolipidoses have similar insidious presentations that vary by age of onset and the types of neurologic symptoms (e.g., seizures, spasticity, blindness, deafness, ataxias, startle reactions). The type of neurolipidosis may be difficult to assign clinically unless there are distinctive findings like the cherry red spot and startle reactions of Tay-Sachs disease (272800, Table 12.6). The diagnosis rests on the demonstration of particular deficient enzymes or mutant alleles and is usually accomplished by sending blood leucocyte samples

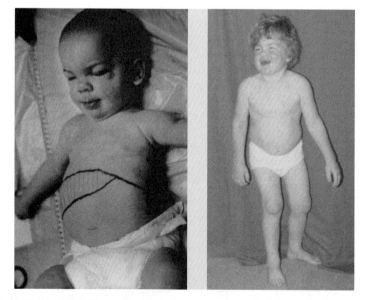

Figure 12.9. *Left*, Child with GM1 gangliosidosis showing a coarse facial appearance and hepatomegaly; *Right*, boy with Hunter syndrome illlustrating a coarse facial appearance, finger contractures, and spinal curvature (gibbus) accounting for the unusual posture.

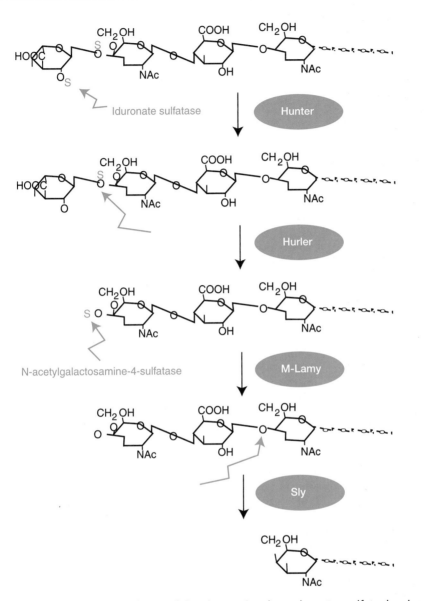

Figure 12.10. Successive degradation of the glycosaminoglycan dermatan sulfate showing the sites of the inborn errors Hunter, Hurler, Maroteaux-Lamy (M-Lamy), and Sly syndromes. Modified from Neufeld and Meunzer (1995).

for panels of assays that include the relevant enzymes (Table 12.6).

Some lipidoses involve the storage of both lipids and oligosaccharides (mucopolysaccharides with smaller chain length). These oligosaccharides may not register on standard urine tests for mucopolysaccharides, but they may cause symptoms of both lipidosis and mu-copolysaccharidosis. One example, GM1 gangliosidosis (252400—Fig. 12.9, Table 12.6) has cherry red spots in the eyes with the skeletal and facial changes suggestive of the mucopolysaccharidoses. These disorders have been called mucolipidoses, but oligosaccharidosis is now preferred because there is no "mucolipid" substance. Disorders of glycoprotein

■TABLE 12.6. Selected Diseases with Accumulation (Storage) of Large Molecules

Disease or Syndrome	Incidence	Deficient Enzyme, Locus	Clinical Manifestations
Neurolipidoses			
Metachromatic leukodystrophy (250100)	1 in 50,000	Arylsulfatase A, 22q13, 3.2 kb gene with 8 exons, P426L common in adults	ND, altered gait, incontinence, seizures, quadriparesis
Tay-Sachs G_{M2} gangliosidosis (272800)	1 in 4000 (J) 1 in 100,000	Hexaminidase A, 15q23, 35 kb gene with 14 exons, 4 bp insertion common in Jews	ND, hypotonia, startle response, cherry red spot
Sandhoff G_{M2} gangliosidosis (268800)	1 in 100,000	Hexaminidase B, 5q13, 45 kb gene with 14 exons, diverse mutations	ND, hypotonia, startle response, cherry red spot
Other Lipidoses			
Fabry disease (301500)	1 in 40,000	β-galactosidase, Xq22, 12 kb gene with 7 exons, diverse mutations	Angiokeratoma, band cataract, vascular disease, nerve pain, renal failure, hypohidrosis
Gaucher disease (230800)	1 in 1000 (J) 1 in 100,000	Glucocerebrosidase, 1q21, 7 kb gene with 11 exons, N379S mutation common in Jews	ND (types 2,3), visceromegaly, bleeding, bone crises, joint disease, pulmonary disease
Oligosaccharidoses			
G_{M1} gangliosidosis (230500)	Unknown	β-Galactosidase, 3p21, 60 kb gene with 16 exons, diverse mutations	ND, Hurler-like, cherry red spots
I-cell disease (252500)	Unknown	Phosphotransferase	ND, Hurler-like
Mannosidosis (248500) cataracts	Unknown	α-Mannosidase, 19p13	ND, Hurler-like, seizures,
Fucosidosis (230000)	Unknown	α-Fucosidase, 1p34, 23 kb gene with 8 exons, diverse mutations	ND, Hurler-like, angiokeratomas, hypohidrosis
Mucopolysaccharidoses			
Hurler (type IH—252800)	1 in 100,000	α-Iduronidase, 4p16	ND, coarse face and skin, viscous mucous, pectus, gibbus, dysostosis, visceromegaly
Scheie (type IS—252800)	1 in 500,000	α-Iduronidase, 4p16	Mild or no features
Hunter (type II—309900)	1 in 65,000	Iduronate sulfatase, Xq27	ND, Hurler-like
San Filippo (type III—252900)	1 in 24,000	Heparan sulfatase, 12q14	ND, Hurler-like (later onset)
Morquio (type IV—253000)	1 in 40,000	β-Galactosidase, 3p21	Dysostosis, short neck and trunk
Maroteaux-Lamy (type VI—253200)	1 in 100,000	Arylsulfatase B, 5q13	Hurler-like
Sly (type VII—253220)	Unknown	β-Glucuronidase, 7q21	ND, Hurler-like

Notes: (J), Jewish population; ND, neurodegeneration; 22q13, band 13 of the long arm of chromosome 22.

degradation, including mannosidosis (248500) or fucosidosis (230000), can also be classified as oligosaccharidoses (Table 12.6).

Other Lipidoses—Fabry Disease

Fabry disease (301500, Table 12.6) is a rather unique lipidosis where most symptoms are due to the progressive deposition of glycolipids into blood vessel endothelium. The skin is particularly distinctive with dark-red to blue spots (telangiectasias) that cluster over the umbilicus, thorax, thighs, buttocks, and knees. There is also ectodermal dysplasia with sparse body and facial hair together with decreased ability to sweat. Blood vessel changes in other organs can produce cloudy corneas, white bands in the lens called "Fabry cataract," renal disease with proteinuria and eventual failure, myocardial infarction, and cerebrovascular disease due to vessel occlusion. Chronic pain from peripheral nerve damage and vaso-occlusion begins in childhood, and crises of burning pain may drive patients to attempt suicide.

Other Lipidoses—Gaucher Disease

Gaucher disease (230800, Table 12.6) involves the accumulation of glucocerebroside due to deficiency of β-glucosidase. Clinical manifestions of type 1 Gaucher disease include neurologic (spinal cord compression due to collapse of vertebrae), pulmonary (infiltrative disease with clubbing), gastoenterologic (hepatomegaly and occasional liver failure), hematologic (thrombocytopenia, splenic infarction, or rupture), and skeletal (painful "bone crises," fractures) abnormalities (Beutler and Grabowski, 1995). The diagnostic evaluation may include a bone marrow to demonstrate the foam-laden Gaucher cells, but should rest on the demonstration of β-glucosidase deficiency in leucocytes. DNA analysis for β-glucosidase gene mutations is also available and is preferred when a mutation has been demonstrated in affected relatives.

As with Fabry disease, the ability to target exogenous enzymes to lysosomes has prompted trials of enzyme therapy in Gaucher disease.

Modified enzyme from human placenta Ceredase (alglucerase) has been produced in quantity and administered with improvement of hematologic and skeletal abnormalities. Although the amounts of enzyme needed decline during the course of therapy, initial costs can be as high as $400,000 per year for an adult male (Figueroa et al., 1992). Furthermore, some manifestations (e.g., pulmonary disease) appear unaffected by enzyme therapy. A recombinant enzyme produced in bacteria (Cerezyme) has recently become available and may decrease these expenses. Bone marrow transplant is also effective and expensive, but has the usual disadvantage of a 10–15% mortality rate.

The Mucopolysaccharidoses

The mucopolysaccharidoses are a group of neurodegenerative disorders that exhibit somatic changes of the face and skeleton (Table 12.6). They are lysosomal storage diseases, caused by a deficiency of enzymes that sculpt complex chains of carbohydrate and protein (glycosaminoglycans or mucopolysaccharides, Fig. 12.10). Glycosaminoglycans are a prominent component of the extracellular matrix, explaining the thickened secretions and subcutaneous tissues in children with mucopolysaccharidosis. Most categories of mucopolysaccharidosis produce a coarse appearance with visceromegaly as illustrated in Figure 12.9; these disorders are distinguished from similar lipidoses or oligosaccharidoses by high levels of urinary glycosaminoglycans. As with other lysosomal enzyme deficiencies mentioned previously, the mucopolysaccharide storage disorders offer a compelling strategy for enzyme or gene therapy that is derived from the classic experiments of Neufeld and colleagues (Neufeld and Muenzer, 1995). The deficient enzymes often contain a mannose-6-phosphate "tag" that targets them to lysosomes of the appropriate cells and allows a restoration of degradative function.

Complications of the mucopolysaccharidoses include hydrocephalus with enlarged head, neurodegeneration, and behavioral changes of poor attention span, aggression or temper tantrums, chronic rhinorrhea and otitis, and potential sleep apnea due to a large tongue with thick mucous. Corneal clouding is prominent in the Hurter and Maroteaux-Lamy syndromes, but absent in Hunter syndrome. Skeletal changes include progressive contractures of the extremities, deformities of the chest that combine with thickened alveolar secretions to cause lung disease, and spinal deformities (gibbus, scoliosis). Preventive management should include regular vision and hearing assessments, early intervention and behavioral therapy, cardiac, orthopedic, ear, nose, and throat (ENT), and dental involvement.

■ 12.7. ORGANELLAR DISORDERS

Case 12D: **Anemia and Ataxia**
An 11-year old boy had been followed for years with a bizarre combination of symptoms. He had ataxia (unbalanced gait and dyscoordination), pancreatic insufficiency with malabsorption of nutrients, chronic lactic acidosis, and bone marrow failure with anemia and neutropenia. He had mild developmental delay with muscle atrophy and an otherwise normal physical examination. The family history was unremarkable.

A select group of metabolic disorders involves organelles within the cell—the mitochondria or peroxisomes. Peroxisomal disorders are discussed in Chapter 11 as an example of a metabolic disorder that causes morphologic changes.

Mitochondrial Disorders Encoded by Mitochondrial DNA

The mitochondrial genome (Fig. 12.11) comprises a 24th chromosome in human cells that can be the site of gene mutations. The entire mitochondrial chromosome is only 16 kb in length, but it is present in about two copies per mitochondrion with >500 mitochondria per

cell in most tissues. The circular mitochondrial genome encodes a minority of the proteins present in the mitochondrial organelle, with the rest being encoded by genes in the nuclear genome. Mitochondrial disorders are diseases caused by abnormal mitochondrial structure and/or function, and they can be produced by mutations in either the nuclear or mitochondrial chromosomes. Although well recognized for their role in energy metabolism, the characterization of mitochondrial diseases shows that mitochondria have important roles in development as well as in functions such as hematopoiesis or glucose homeostasis.

When a mitochondrial disease is caused by mutations in the mitochondrial genome, the disease may exhibit maternal inheritance. Because sperm contribute little but DNA to the fertilized egg, the mitochondria of offspring are inherited from the mother. Mitochondrial genomic mutations therefore exhibit maternal transmission. In theory, this means that all offspring of affected mothers are affected, but that no offspring of affected fathers are affected. In practice, the maternal cytoplasm may contain mixtures of normal and mutant mitochondrial genomes such that unaffected mothers can have variably affected offspring. A mixture of mutant and normal mitochondria genomes is termed *heteroplasmy,* and it is known that the proportion of mutant mitochondria can change during development or during aging in the same individual, producing variable timing of disease. Heteroplasmy may allow some offspring of affected mothers to be normal and obscure the pattern of maternal inheritance.

Some mitochondrial disorders are caused mainly by point mutations in the mitochondrial genome (Figure 12.11, Table 12.7). An example is Leber hereditary optic neuropathy (LHON) with its phenotype limited to optic nerve development. Other mitochondrial disorders have extensive deletions that remove multiple genes from mitochondrial genomes. Disorders such as Pearson syndrome (bone marrow failure, ataxia, pancreatic dysfunction) often have more extensive abnormalities due to large mitochondrial DNA deletions. Once a deletion

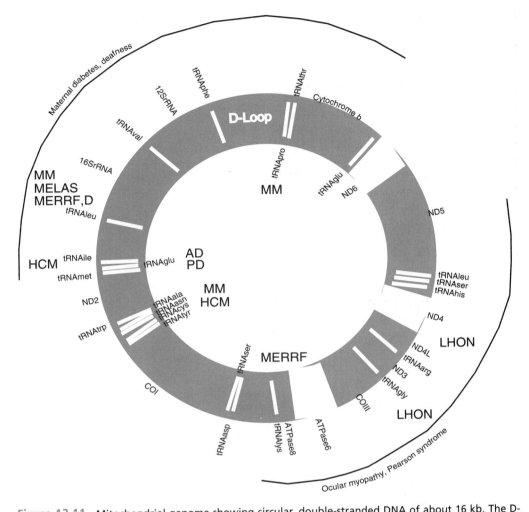

Figure 12.11. Mitochondrial genome showing circular, double-stranded DNA of about 16 kb. The D-loop is important for genome replication. Genes transcribed from the heavy (outer) strand are shown outside the circle and those transcribed from the inner strand are shown inside the circle. The positions of mutations causing certain diseases are illustrated, including MM, mitochondrial myopathy; MELAS, mitochondrial encephalopathy with lactic acidosis and strokes; MERRF, D, mitochondrial encephalopathy with ragged red fibers and deafness; AD, Alzheimer disease; PD, Parkinson disease; HCM, hypertrophic cardiomyopathy; LHON, Leber hereditary optic neuropathy. The large duplication causing maternal diabetes with deafness, and the large deletion causing ocular myopathy and Pearson syndrome are shown.

has occurred, mitochondrial DNA replication may be altered to produce additional abnormalities. Progressive alterations of mitochondrial DNA may produce worsening of disease with age, just as heteroplasmy may produce fewer abnormal cells and produce improvement. The spectrum of mitochondrial genomic diseases is quite broad as listed in Table 12.7, encompassing unusual findings such as predis-

position to diabetes mellitus or strokes. Many mutations of the mitochondrial genome have common symptoms such as lactic acidosis or muscles that show ragged red fibers on biopsy.

Case 12D Follow-up: Studies of mitochondrial DNA revealed that the young man had a large deletion as shown in Figure 12.11 that is typical of Pearson syndrome. His mother was

■ TABLE 12.7. Organellar Metabolic Diseases

Disease or Syndrome	Incidence	Deficient Gene, Locus	Clinical Manifestations
Mitochondrial Diseases Caused by Nuclear Genes			
Glutaric aciduria II (231670)	Unknown	ETF, 15q23	ND, acidosis, hypotonia, abnormal facies, demyelination, renal cysts, genital anomalies.
Leigh (266150)	Unknown	Complex IV, oxidative phosphorylation	ND, lactic acidemia, hypotonia, brain anomalies, optic atrophy
Pyruvate dehydrogenase deficiency (246900, 312170)	Unknown	Pyruvate dehydrogenase, multiple subunits	ND, lactic acidemia, labored respirations, optic atrophy
Mitochondrial Diseases Caused by Mitochondrial Genes			
Kearns-Sayre (165100)	Unknown	Mt DNA deletions of tRNA, rRNA genes	Ptosis, retinital changes, hearing loss, diabetes, lactic acidosis
Pearson syndrome (260560)	Unknown	Mt DNA deletions and duplications	Pancytopenia, similar to Kearns-Sayre syndrome
Leber hereditary optic neuropathy (308900)	Unknown	Mt DNA mutations in complex I, III, IV subunits	Vision loss and optic atrophy
Peroxisomal Diseases			
Acatalasemia (115500)	1 in 25,000	Catalase, 11p13	Gum disease
ALD (300100)	1 in 100,000	ALD PMP, Xq28	ND, visual loss, adrenal insufficiency
Generalized disorders: ZS (214100) IRD (266510) Neonatal ALD (202370)	1 in 50,000	Several different PMPs	ND, hypotonia, unusual face, liver disease, hearing loss, retinitis with vision loss, scaly skin (ichthyosis)

Notes: ETF, electron transport flavoprotein; Mt, mitochondrial; ZS, Zellweger syndrome; IRD, infantile Refsum disease; ALD, adrenoleukodystrophy; PMP, peroxisomal membrane protein; ND, neurodegeneration; 15q23, band 23 on the long arm of chromosome 15.

heteroplasmic with low levels of mitochondria with the deletion. The deletion in Pearson syndrome encompasses the D-loop, causing mitochondrial DNA replication to be very unstable. This may account for the rapid proliferation of deleted mitochondria in the affected boy.

Mitochondrial Disorders Caused by Nuclear Genes—Glutaric Acidemia Type II

Type II glutaric acidemia is caused by an abnormality of the electron transfer flavoprotein (ETF) that is part of the mitochondrial respiratory chain (Frerman and Goodman, 1995). Similar disorders are caused by deficiencies of ETF or its dehydrogenase, and both exhibit autosomal recessive inheritance consistent with their encoding by the nuclear genome.

Clinical manifestations of glutaric acidemia type II include macrocephaly (large head), large anterior fontanelle (soft spot), high forehead, broad nasal root, rocker bottom feet, renal cysts, and genital anomalies (hypospadias or chordee). The neonatal presentation usually includes hypotonia and hepatomegaly associated with severe hypoglycemia and metabolic acidosis. Most patients with neonatal onset die in early infancy, often with enlargements and dysfunction of the heart muscle (hypertrophic cardiomyopathy). Attempted therapy of glutaric acidemia II, like that for other disorders impacting the mitochondrial respiratory chain, has included oral riboflavin (to boost flavin intermediates), vitamin K (a quinone related to electron transport quinones), ascorbic acid (to boost cytochrome activity), and oral carnitine (to improve import and offset carnitine depletion by glutarylcarnitine). These medicines have had some benefit in later-onset patients but not with neonates (Frerman and Goodman, 1995). A low fat and protein diet may also be helpful.

Mitochondrial Disorders Caused by Nuclear Genes—Leigh Disease and Lactic Acidemias

Leigh disease, also known as subacute necrotizing encephalomyelopathy, is a phenotype that is produced by a variety of defects in the mitochondrial respiratory chain. The presentation has onset from early infancy to middle childhood, and includes hypotonia, developmental delay with regression, optic atrophy, strabismus (deviated eyes), nystagmus (jerking eye movements), irregularities in breathing, muscle weakness, and lactic acidosis. Later neurologic symptoms may include ataxia (altered gait) and spasticity (increased muscle tone). The cranial MRI scan shows demyelination and/or hyperintense areas near the thalamus and basal ganglia. The diagnosis of Leigh disease involves an analysis of respiratory chain components in muscle or leucocytes. Alterations in cytochrome c (respiratory complex IV) are most common, but abnormalities of NADH dehydrogenase (respiratory complex I) or pyruvate dehydrogenase have also been reported. While most mutations causing Leigh disease have been in nuclear-encoded genes, a few examples with maternal inheritance have been demonstrated. It is important to realize that the phenotype is extremely variable and heterogeneous, overlapping with other mitochondrial diseases such as pigmentary retinopathy with degeneration or mitochondrial myopathy.

■ 12.8. GENETIC SCREENING

The ability to detect abnormal metabolites in the blood and urine of patients with inborn errors, together with the availability of dietary

■ TABLE 12.8. Considerations in Genetic Screening

Criteria for disease	High frequency in target population
	Serious morbidity for affecteds or relatives
	Benefits of early diagnosis (treatment, genetic counseling, life planning)
Criteria for disease test	Inconvenience and cost small compared to disease
	High sensitivity (few false negatives and high specificity (few false positives)
Criteria for screening program	Voluntary with informed consent
	Access to education and counseling regarding significance of positive or negative results
	Equal access to testing regardless of geography or insurance funding
	Quality control of screening laboratories with review of false positive and negative result
Advantages of screening	Early diagnosis with treatment or amelioration
	Awareness of genetic risk with informed reproductive decisions
	Improved awareness and understanding of disease
Disadvantages of screening	Discrimination against affecteds or carriers by society, health insurance, employment
	Governmental, societal, family pressures to participate in screening
	Anxiety with positive results, survivor guilt or inappropriate behaviors with negative results

therapy, brought up the possibility of detection and treatment before symptoms appeared. The detection of individuals with genetic disease by testing of a general or defined population is known as genetic screening. Table 12.8 summarizes important considerations and criteria for genetic screening.

Genetic screening is usually directed at individuals with no signs or symptoms of disease, exemplified by newborn screening for phenylketonuria (Table 12.9). It sometimes involves testing a subgroup of individuals with particular characteristics or symptoms, such as amniocentesis offered to women over age 35

■ TABLE 12.9. Examples of Genetic Screening

Disease	Frequency	Type of Test	Potential Problems
Newborn screening			
Phenylketonuria	1 in 12,000	Bacterial (Guthrie)	False positives
Galactosemia	1 in 50,000	Bacterial, enzyme	False positives
Maple syrup urine disease	1 in 100,000	Bacterial	False positives
Hypothyroidism	1 in 5000	RIA	False positives
Congenital adrenal hyperplasia	1 in 10,000	RIA	False positives
Duchenne muscular dystrophy	1 in 3000 males	Enzyme	No treatment
Carrier screening			
Sickle cell anemia	1/12 in Blacks	Hgb electrophoresis	Stigmatization
Cystic fibrosis	1/23 in Whites	DNA test, many mutations	Many mutations, false negatives
Tay-Sachs	1/30 in Jews	Enzyme assay	Stigmatization
α-Thalassemia	1/30 in Greeks, Italians	Red cell indices Hgb electrophoresis	Stigmatization
β-Thalassemia	1/25 in Chinese	Red cell indices Hgb electrophoresis	Stigmatization
Presymptomatic screening			
Huntington chorea	1 in 20,000 1 in 2 if parent affected	DNA test for expanding tri- nucleotide repeats	No treatment Anxiety Behavior changes
BRCA1 gene mutation	1 in 10 with family history[a]	DNA test, many mutations	False negatives Survivor guilt Lax behavior
Prenatal screening			
Down syndrome	1 in 1000	Maternal serum AFP	False positives Absent or biased counseling
Congenital anomalies	1 in 200 (MA > 35) 1 in 20	Amniocentesis Fetal ultrasound	Biased counseling False negatives False positives

[a]breast and ovarian cancer.

Notes: BRCA, breast cancer; MA, maternal age; Hgb, hemoglobin; RIA, radioimmunoassay.

or cystic fibrosis testing of individuals with failure to thrive. Although applied appropriately or inappropriately to other types of genetic disorders, genetic screening first achieved widespread use and attention with metabolic diseases. This chapter is thus the natural place to address genetic screening with additional mention in Chapters 5 (genetic risk factors), 14 (adult disorders), and 15 (reproductive genetics).

Criteria for genetic screening can be considered according to the nature of disease, disease test, and the screening program (Table 12.9). Because screening programs involve populations and therefore institutions, cost is always an important consideration. Cost-effectiveness dictates that the disease in question be of reasonable frequency in the targeted population (minimize the number of negative tests), that it be of import for affected individuals or their relatives, and that there be some amelioration or treatment possible to decrease costs of disease care (Table 12.9). Tests must also be cost-effective with minimal cost compared to the disease and high specificity (few false positives that must be tracked down). Ethical criteria also require individual benefits from early disease detection, provision for adequate counseling and education after results are reported, and equal access to the screening program regardless of location or socioeconomic status (Table 12.8). Note how the eugenics programs mentioned in Chapter 1 violated these principles of genetic screening. The test (mental retardation) was not at all specific for genetic disease, there was no benefit to the affected individuals or their relatives, and the "therapeutic" action following a positive test (sterilization) did not reduce care costs.

Experience with genetic screening using these modern criteria, as gathered from several disease examples summarized in Table 12.9, discloses several advantages and disadvantages. There is no question that newborn screening for phenylketonuria (PKU) or galactosemia has allowed early diagnosis and treatment of individuals with improved intellectual and medical outcomes. Relatives of these individuals receive education regarding the nature and treatment of the disease, and they become aware of genetic risks with options such as artificial insemination or prenatal diagnosis. Disadvantages of screening have occurred, including discrimination against diagnosed individuals for employment or health insurance. Governmental pressures are less likely now in the United States, but were very detrimental in the early history of screening for sickle cell anemia (Markel, 1992). Laws mandating screening of blacks for sickle cell anemia were racially insensitive and led to negative perceptions of screening programs that persist today. Also dramatic was the fate of thalassemia carriers in Greece, some of whom became social outcasts with regard to dating and marriage (Modell, 1992).

Various strategies for genetic screening are summarized according to sample diseases in Table 12.9. General newborn screening targets a very large population (about three million births annually in the United States) with laudable goals of preventing mental impairment (e.g., in PKU or hypothyroidism) or severe disease (e.g., in galactosemia or congenital adrenal hyperplasia). The feasibility of screening for a relatively common disease (PKU, frequency 1 in 12,000) versus a relatively rare disease (maple syrup urine disease, MSUD, frequency 1 in 100,000) is shown in Figure 12.12.

The calculation of sensitivity, specificity, and positive predictive value for tests was illustrated in Chapter 5 and is revisited here. If a specificity of 99.99% is postulated for neonatal screening, then the false positive rate (1-specificity) for annual testing in a state such as Texas (300,000 newborns) will be 0.0001% or 30 out of 300,000. The positive predictive value for PKU screening is 45%, while that for MSUD screening is only 6% (Fig. 12.12). The cost of such testing, made feasible by the Guthrie bacterial inhibition assay, is about $1 per test. This converts to a cost of $12,000 per patient with PKU detected (true positive), but more than $150,000 per patient with MSUD detected. Since treatment of PKU is much

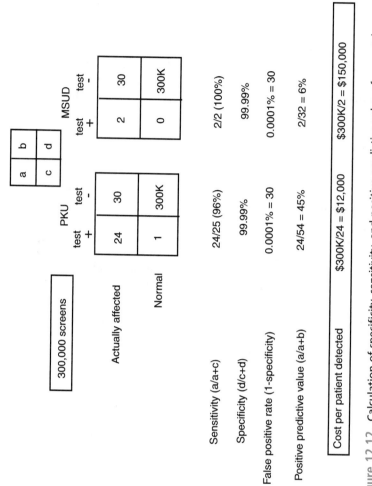

Figure 12.12. Calculation of specificity, sensitivity, and positive predictive value of neonatal screening for phenylketonuria (PKU) or maple syrup urine disease (MSUD—see text).

more effective than that for MSUD (see prior discussions), these calculations explain why PKU but not MSUD screening is performed in most states (including Texas).

As illustrated in Figure 12.12, higher disease frequencies in targeted populations will yield higher positive predictive values for testing and greater cost-effectiveness. Rare diseases such as MSUD are usually not candidates for neonatal screening, but founder effects in some populations produce higher frequencies of disease and regional variations in policy (e.g., tyrosinemia in Quebec). States (and countries) also vary in their political emphasis on public health, accounting for the large menu for neonatal screening in states like Massachusetts that gave early emphasis to screening programs. The ability to do multiple screening tests on single samples can influence screening policies, because tests for rare diseases can be piggy-backed onto tests for more common diseases with little increase in cost.

Carrier screening, presymptomatic screening, and prenatal screening examples cited in Table 12.9 raise more controversial issues due to their lesser benefits for individuals with positive results. Carriers are certainly given better awareness and understanding of disease if the educational criteria are fulfilled, but the benefits of reproductive decisions are not quite in the league with the prevention of mental retardation. Stigmatization of individuals with positive results has occurred as mentioned previously, and efforts to avoid negative self-image or family/social bias may not be successful. Because most carrier screening is targeted toward specific ethnic groups with higher frequencies of disease, cultural awareness is second only to test accuracy as important attributes of the screening program.

Presymptomatic screening for severe diseases like Huntington chorea (143100, Table 12.9) brings up other disadvantages of screening such as survivor guilt (my sister will develop disease but I will not). Individuals testing negative for the BRCA1 gene may become lax about routine mammography or breast exams, despite their continued risk for multifac-

torial breast cancer. The lack of treatment for Huntington chorea, and the extreme treatment (mastectomy) for breast cancer risk detracts from the advantages of these screening programs and is considered in more detail in Chapter 14. Prenatal screening has potential benefits for at-risk couples, but usually enforces difficult choices that require thorough counseling. Disadvantages include the lack of real treatment for affected fetuses, the need for ethically and socially controversial abortions, the low positive predictive value of many prenatal tests, and the lack of counseling for many positive tests due to their high volume in busy obstetric practices. These concerns are discussed in Chapter 15.

■ 12.9. TREATMENT OF METABOLIC DISORDERS: REVIEW AND SUMMARY

Metabolic diseases provide an important rebuttal to the assumption that genetic diseases cannot be treated. Approaches to treatment have been discussed under individual diseases in this chapter, and they are summarized here for review and emphasis (Table 12.10). The presence of an enzyme deficiency with a block in metabolic conversion can be supervened by several strategies. Deficient products can be supplied as illustrated by carnitine supplementation in the fatty acid oxidation disorders. Excess cofactors (usually vitamins) can be supplied to stimulate partially active enzymes that have been incapacitated by mutation. Vitamin supplementation is most effective when the metabolic defect lies in vitamin synthesis, illustrated by biotinidase deficiency (Table 12.5). Dietary avoidance of substances that impact the blocked pathway is effective in many disorders such as PKU, and often ameliorate diseases where no true therapy is available. Sparing of the pathway by providing alternative routes of metabolism is illustrated by glucose infusion in glycogen storage diseases or frequent feeding in the disorders of fatty acid oxidation. Substances can also be administered

■TABLE 12.10. Therapies for Inborn Errors of Metabolism

Strategy	Disease Example	Rationale
Provision of deficient product	Carnitine	Poor carnitine absorption
	Cortisone, mineralocorticoids	Congenital adrenal hyperplasia
	Vitamin D	Rickets due to breast feeding
Provision of excess cofactor	Thiamine (vitamin B_1)	Maple syrup urine disease
		Mitochondrial Complex I–IV defects
	Biotin	Biotinidase deficiency
		Multiple carboxylase deficiency
	Pyridoxine (vitamin B_6)	Homocystinuria
	Methylcobalamin (vitamin B_{12})	Homocystinuria, methylmalonic acidemia
	Adenosylcobalamin (vitamin B_{12})	Methylmalonic aciduria
	Carnitine	Fatty acid oxidation disorders, organic acidemias
Dietary avoidance	Low phenylalanine diet	Phenylketonuria
	Low lactose diet	Galactosemia
	Low protein diet	Urea cycle, organic acidemias
	Low fat diet	Fatty acid oxidation disorders
Sparing of pathway	Carbohydrate infusion	Glycogen storage disease
	Frequent feeding	Fatty acid oxidation disorders
Alternative pathway	Urea cycle disorders	Sodium benzoate, phenyl acetate to divert nitrogen from cycle
Enzyme replacement	Gaucher disease	Infusion of glucocerebrosidase
Transplantation	Storage diseases, small molecule diseases refractory to treatment	Bone marrow, liver transplants
Gene therapy	Adenosine deaminase deficiency	Replace defective gene in key tissues

to divert intermediates in a blocked pathway to another metabolic route, illustrated by the provision of phenylacetate to divert ammonia from the urea cycle to an excretable substance (hippuric acid).

More direct therapies have also been pioneered in biochemical genetic disorders through provision of deficient enzymes or replacement genes. Enzyme infusions have been successful in some disorders, particularly for lysosomal enzyme deficiencies where a mannose-6-phosphate targeting signal directs the foreign enzyme to host lysosomes. Transplantation offers a way to replace enzymes and defective genes, but is limited by the ability of larger molecules such as enzyme proteins to cross the blood–brain barrier.

Gene therapy has replaced a deficient enzyme in bone marrow (adenosine deaminase), and is being tried for other enzyme deficiencies including that of phenylalanine hydroxylase (see Chapter 10). Vectors that can target genes to brain are particularly needed to impact severe neurolipidoses and mucopolysaccharidoses that cause neurodegeneration. Some improvements have been noted in patients receiving bone marrow or enzyme infusions for these disorders, despite the presence of the blood–brain barrier. It may also be feasible to target macrophages and other cells that can cross this barrier, allowing sources of corrective enzyme to enter the central nervous system. Multiple strategies for early screening, metabolite and enzyme therapy, and gene replacements predict a bright future for therapy of metabolic diseases, particularly for those many diseases in which affected individuals are normal at birth.

PROBLEM SET 12
Inborn Errors of Metabolism

Select the one most appropriate answer to the following questions:

12.1–12.5. A 3-day-old infant is the fourth child of immigrant parents. She stops feeding, becomes lethargic, and appears more noticeably jaundiced. In addition to cultures of blood, cerebrospinal fluid, and urine, a blood pH of 7.1 is found. The electrolytes show a sodium of 135, potassium 4, chloride 99, and bicarbonate 15 mEq per L. A family history reveals that the parents are first cousins, and that a prior child died in the nursery because of infection.

12.1. The blood pH and electrolyte values suggest:
- (A) Alkalosis with high bicarbonate
- (B) Increased anion gap with acidosis
- (C) Increased anion gap with alkalosis
- (D) Acidosis with high bicarbonate
- (E) Alkalosis with low bicarbonate

12.2. The most important metabolic test in this setting is:
- (A) Blood glucose
- (B) Blood amino acids
- (C) Blood organic acids
- (D) Urine amino acids
- (E) Urine organic acids

12.3. Other initial metabolic tests to consider would be:
- (A) Blood glucose
- (B) Blood carnitine
- (C) Blood amino acids
- (D) Blood ammonia
- (E) All of the above

12.4. The disease category that best describes this child is:
- (A) Catastrophic disease of the newborn
- (B) Sudden infant death syndrome (SIDS)
- (C) Large molecule storage disease
- (D) Urea cycle disorder
- (E) Amino acid disorder

12.5. The finding most suggestive of metabolic disease is:
- (A) A prior child dying from infection
- (B) Abnormal blood pH
- (C) Increased amount of jaundice

- (D) Consanguinity in the parents
- (E) Absence of documented infection in the baby

12.6–12.10. A 2-year-old child presents with lethargy and decreased appetite. On physical examination, she appears dehydrated with an enlarged liver. Initial testing reveals a low blood glucose of 55 mg per dl, a pH of 7.3, and a slightly low bicarbonate of 15 mEq per L. The prior childhood and family history are normal. A urine test was run and was negative.

12.6. The urine test is most likely:
- (A) Urine pH
- (B) Urine reducing substances
- (C) Urine organic acids
- (D) Urine glucose
- (E) Urine ketones

12.7. The negative ketone test is suggestive of the category of:
- (A) Amino acid disorders
- (B) Carbohydrate disorders
- (C) Nonketotic hypoglycemia
- (D) Nonketotic hyperglycinemia
- (E) Organic acidemias

12.8. The most likely diagnosis in this child is:
- (A) Organic acidemia
- (B) Fatty acid oxidation disorder
- (C) Urea cycle disorder
- (D) Amino acid disorder
- (E) Glycogen storage disease

12.9. Additional tests that should be considered are:
- (A) Urine organic acids, urine reducing substances
- (B) Blood amino acids, blood carnitine
- (C) Urine organic acids, blood carnitine and acylcarnitine profile
- (D) Blood ammonia, liver biopsy for enzyme assay
- (E) Blood amino acids, urine reducing substances

12.10. After the preliminary tests were completed, a specific mutation was demonstrated using the polymerase chain reaction and allele-specific oligonucleotide hybridization. The most likely diagnosis is:
- (A) Maple syrup urine disease

(B) Galactosemia
(C) Long chain hydroxyacyl-CoA dehydrogenase (LCHAD) deficiency
(D) Short chain acyl-CoA dehydrogenase (SCAD) deficiency
(E) Medium chain acyl-CoA dehydrogenase (MCAD) deficiency

PROBLEM SET 12
Answers

		12.4. A
12.10. E	12.7. C	12.3. E
12.9. C	12.6. E	12.2. E
12.8. B	12.5. D	12.1. B

PROBLEM SET 12
Solutions

12.1–12.5. The child suggests catastrophic disease of the newborn (answer 12.3A) because of sudden disease with lethargy and acidosis. The low pH and increased anion gap (139 − 114 = 25, answer 12.1B) suggest the possibility of an organic acidemia, which is best diagnosed by urine organic acids (answer 12.2E). Recall that amino acids are retained by the kidney and best tested in blood (except for disorders of renal transport like cystinuria) and that organic acids are excreted by the kidney and best screened in urine. Organic acidemias can cause hypoglycemia, elevated amino acids like glycine, elevated blood ammonia, and depleted carnitine (answer 12.3E). The prior death in the family was probably due to unrecognized metabolic disease rather than sepsis, but the undisputed fact in the history that suggests metabolic disease is parental relatedness (Answer 12.5D).

12.6–12.10. Hypoglycemia with the absence of ketones in the urine (answer 12.6E) was initially described as nonketotic hypoglycemia (answer 12.7C) to discriminate these patients from those with diabetes mellitus or glycogen storage disease with hypoglycemia and ketosis. Nonketotic hyperglycinemia is a disorder of glycine metabolism. The mild acidosis in this child is most suggestive of a fatty acid oxidation disorder (answer 12.8B), because or-

ganic acidemias usually have more severe acidosis. A block in fatty acid or organic acid degradation (see Fig. 12.8) will interfere with the formation of ketones like acetoacetate and β-hydroxybutyrate, although more sophisticated analyses can demonstrate ketones of higher chain length. Elevated fatty or organic acid intermediates can tie up carnitine as acylcarnitine, providing a useful test (answer 12.9C) and a danger for blocking access of fatty acids to mitochondria with energy failure and death. MCAD deficiency (answer 12.10E) is unusual because a single mutant allele accounts for 80% of homozygotes and another 17% of heterozygotes with the disease. PCR/ASO methods to detect this mutant allele are thus very sensitive for diagnosis of MCAD deficiency.

BIBLIOGRAPHY

General Texts and References

Berry GT, Bennett MJ. 1998. A focused approach to diagnosing inborn errors of metabolism. *Contemp Pediatr* 15:79–102.

Gorlin RJ, Cohen MM Jr, Levin LS. 1990. *Syndromes of the Head and Neck.* New York: Oxford.

Saudubray JM, Carpentier C. 1995. Clinical phenotypes: diagnosis/algorithms. In Scriver CR, Beaudet AL, Sly WS, Valle D, eds. *The Metabolic and Molecular Bases of Inherited Disease,* 7th ed. New York: McGraw-Hill, pp. 327–400.

Scriver CR, Beaudet AL, Sly WS, Valle D. 1995. *The Metabolic and Molecular Bases of Inherited Disease,* 7th ed. New York: McGraw-Hill.

Waber L. 1990. Inborn errors of metabolism. *Pediatr Ann* 19:105–118.

Disorders of Carbohydrate Metabolism

Chen YT, Burchell A. 1995. Glycogen storage diseases. In Scriver CR, Beaudet AL, Sly WS, Valle D, eds. *The Metabolic and Molecular Bases of Inherited Disease.* 7th ed. New York: McGraw-Hill, pp. 935–965.

Kaufman FR, Donnell GN, Roe TF, Kogut MD. 1986. Hypergonadotropic hypogonadism in female patients with galactosemia. *N Engl J Med* 305:464–467.

Levy HL, Sepe SJ, Shih VE, Vawter FG, Klein JO. 1977. Sepsis due to *Escherichia coli* in neonates with galactosemia. *N Engl J Med* 297:823–825.

Pagliara AS, Karl IE, Hammond M, Kipnis DM. 1973. Hypoglycemia in infancy and childhood. *J Pediatr* 82:365–379; 558–577.

Parker PH, Ballew M, Greene HL. 1993. Nutritional management of glycogen storage disease. *Ann Rev Nutr* 13:83–109.

Rallison ML, Meikle AW, Zigrang ZD. 1979. Hypoglycemia and lactic acidosis associated with fructose-1,6-diphosphatase deficiency. *J Pediatr* 94:933–936.

Segal S, Berry GT. 1995. Disorders of galactose metabolism. In Scriver CR, Beaudet AL, Sly WS, Valle D, eds. *The Metabolic and Molecular Bases of Inherited Disease,* 7th ed. New York: McGraw-Hill, pp. 967–1000.

Waggoner DD, Buist NR, Donnell GN. 1990. Long-term prognosis in galactosemia: results of a survey of 350 cases. *J Inborn Errors Metab* 13: 802–808.

Wendel U, Schroten H, Burdach S, Wahn V. 1993. Glycogen storage disease type Ib: infectious complications and measures for prevention. *Eur J Pediatr* 152 (Suppl. 1):S49–S51.

Disorders of Amino Acid Metabolism and the Urea Cycle

Chuang DT, Shih VE. 1995. Disorders of branched chain amino acid and keto acid metabolism. In Scriver CR, Beaudet AL, Sly WS, Valle D, eds. *The Metabolic and Molecular Bases of Inherited Disease,* 7th ed. New York: McGraw-Hill, pp. 1239–1277.

Goodman SI, Pollak S, Miles B, O'Brien D. 1969. The treatment of maple syrup urine disease. *J Pediatr* 75:485–488.

Kaplan P, Mazur A, Field M, Berlin JA, Berry GT, Heidenreich R, Yudkoff M, Segal S. 1991. Intellectual outcome in children with maple syrup urine disease. *J Pediatr* 119:46–50.

Koch R, Azen CG, Friedman EG, Williamson ML. 1982. Preliminary report on the effects of diet discontinuation in PKU. *J Pediatr* 100: 870–875.

Scriver CR, Kaufman S, Eisensmith RC, Woo SLC. 1995. The hyperphenylalaninemias. In Scriver CR, Beaudet AL, Sly WS, Valle D, eds. *The Metabolic and Molecular Bases of Inherited Disease,* 7th ed. New York: McGraw-Hill, pp. 1015–1076.

Williamson ML, Koch R, Azen C, Chang C. 1981. Correlates of intelligence test results in treated phenylketonuria children. *Pediatrics* 68: 161–167.

Organic Acidemias and Disorders of Fatty Acid Oxidation

Fenton WA, Rosenberg LE. 1995. Disorders of propionate and methylmalonate metabolism. In Scriver CR, Beaudet AL, Sly WS, Valle D, eds. *The Metabolic and Molecular Bases of Inherited Disease,* 7th ed. New York: McGraw-Hill, pp. 1423–1450.

Roe CR, Coates PM. 1995. Mitochondrial fatty acid oxidation disorders. In Scriver CR, Beaudet AL, Sly WS, Valle D, eds. *The Metabolic and Molecular Bases of Inherited Disease,* 7th ed. New York: McGraw-Hill, pp. 1501–1534.

Wolf B. 1995. Disorders of biotin metabolism. In Scriver CR, Beaudet AL, Sly WS, Valle D, eds. *The Metabolic and Molecular Bases of Inherited Disease,* 7th ed. New York: McGraw-Hill, pp. 3151–3177.

Wolf B, Heard GS. 1991. Biotinidase deficiency. *Adv Pediatr* 38:1–22.

Storage Disorders

Beutler E, Grabowski GA. 1995. Gaucher disease. In Scriver CR, Beaudet AL, Sly WS, Valle D, eds. *The Metabolic and Molecular Bases of Inherited Disease,* 7th ed, New York: McGraw-Hill, pp. 2641–2670.

Desnick RJ, Ioannou YA, Eng CM. 1995. α-galactosidase A deficiency: Fabry disease. In Scriver CR, Beaudet AL, Sly WS, Valle D, eds. *The Metabolic and Molecular Bases of Inherited Disease,* 7th ed, New York: McGraw-Hill, pp. 2741–2784.

Figueroa ML, Rosenbloom BE, Kay AC, Garver P, Thuerston DW, Koziol JA, Gelbart T, Beutler E. 1992. A less costly regimen of alglucerase to treat Gaucher's disease. *N Engl J Med* 327:1632.

Kolodny EH, Fluharty AL. 1995. Metachromatic leukodystrophy and multiple sulfatase deficiency: Sulfatide lipidosis. In Scriver CR, Beaudet AL, Sly WS, Valle D, eds. *The Metabolic and Molecular Bases of Inherited Disease,* 7th ed, New York: McGraw-Hill, pp. 2693–2739.

Lockman LA, Hunninghake DB, Krivit W, Desnick RJ. 1973. Relief of pain of Fabry's disease by diphenylhydantoin. *Neurology* 23:871–875.

Neufeld EF, Meunzer J. 1995. The Mucopolysac-
charidoses. In Scriver CR, Beaudet AL, Sly WS,
Valle D, eds. *The Metabolic and Molecular
Bases of Inherited Disease,* 7th ed. New York:
McGraw-Hill, pp. 2465–2494.

Spranger J. 1987. Mini review: Inborn errors of
complex carbohydrate metabolism. *Am J Med
Genet* 28:489–499.

Organellar Disorders

Frerman FE, Goodman SI. 1995. Nuclear-encoded
defects of the mitochondrial respiratory chain,
including glutaric acidemia type II. In Scriver
CR, Beaudet AL, Sly WS, Valle D, eds. *The
Metabolic and Molecular Bases of Inherited
Disease,* 7th ed. New York: McGraw-Hill,
pp. 1611–1630.

Robinson BH. 1995. Mitochondrial defects: An
overview of inborn errors associated with lactic
acidemia. *Int Pediatr* 10:82–87.

Robinson BH. 1995. Lactic acidemia (disorders of
pyruvate carboxylase, pyruvate dehydrogenase).
In Scriver CR, Beaudet AL, Sly WS, Valle D,

eds. *The Metabolic and Molecular Bases of Inherited Disease,* 7th ed. New York: McGraw-
Hill, pp. 1479–1499.

Shofner JM, Wallace DC. 1995. In Scriver CR,
Beaudet AL, Sly WS, Valle D, eds. *The Metabolic
and Molecular Bases of Inherited Disease,* 7th ed.
New York: McGraw-Hill, pp. 1535–1609.

Suomalainen A. 1997. Mitochondrial DNA and disease. *Ann Med* 29:235–246.

Wallace DC. 1995. Mitochondrial DNA variation in
human evolution, degenerative disease, and aging. *Am J Hum Genet* 57:201–223.

Warner TT, Schapira AH. 1997. Genetic counselling
in mitochondrial diseases. *Curr Opin Neurol* 10:
408–412.

Genetic Screening

Markel H. 1992. The stigma of disease: Implications
of genetic screening. *Am J Med* 93: 209–215.

Modell B. 1992. Ethical aspects of genetic screening. *Ann Med* 24:549–555.

Rowley PT. 1984. Genetic screening: Marvel or
menace. *Science* 225:138–142.

13

GENETICS IN THE SURGICAL SPECIALITIES

■ LEARNING OBJECTIVES

1. Anomaly associations may complicate the surgical treatment of congenital anomalies.
2. Minor anomalies and disease patterns are important to recognize before surgical management and genetic counseling is provided.
3. Each common anomaly presenting to surgical specialists can be present in malformation syndromes with higher complication and recurrence risks.
4. Recognition of genetic factors in multifactorial anomalies or syndromes is essential for pre- and postoperative management.

*Case 13: **Anal Atresia in a Newborn***
A newborn requires surgical evaluation because of absent (imperforate) anus. The family and gestation histories are normal, but the birth weight is low.

■ 13.1. INTRODUCTION: EVALUATION AND RISKS OF SURGICALLY CORRECTIBLE CONGENITAL ANOMALIES

Congenital anomalies make a large contribution to the work of pediatric surgeons and other surgical specialists who operate on children. A decision central to surgical management was discussed in Chapter 11: Does the patient have an isolated congenital anomaly or are there associated anomalies that might constitute a syndrome? The presence of unsuspected anomalies may lead to unanticipated complications in the operating room or change the prognosis towards palliative rather than aggressive management. For this reason, common associations and syndromes are presented for each anomaly discussed in this chapter.

As reviewed in Chapter 11, anomaly associations often have a low genetic risk with an excellent prognosis for intellectual development if the anomalies can be corrected surgically. Syndromes, on the other hand, exhibit a pattern of major and minor anomalies that often cause an abnormal facial appearance, growth failure without obvious medical causes, and developmental delay. In the neonatal nursery where many congenital anomalies present for surgical treatment, developmental and growth potential will not be evident to help in the decision between anomaly associations and syndrome. Minor anomalies such as epicanthal folds, broad nasal root, malformed ears, high palate, single palmar crease, redundant neck skin, or abnormally placed toes are therefore critical to recognize for consideration of a syndrome diagnosis. Once the possibility of a syndrome is raised, then evaluation by genetic specialists and tests such as chromosome studies and/or skeletal radiographic survey are indicated. Rapid karyotyping methods using bone marrow cells or fluorescent in situ hybridization techniques can provide important information in a time frame (12–24 h) that allows for urgent surgical decisions.

The suspicion of syndromes rather than anomaly associations is important because of their higher risk for medical complications and recurrence in the family. Children with syndromes, particularly those caused by chromosomal aberrations, often have abnormal homeostatic regulation that renders them more vulnerable to stress. Such children may not tolerate the acute stress of operation, and their healing and resistance to infection in the postoperative period is also decreased. The importance of the decision between isolated anomalies or anomaly associations and syndromes is illustrated in subsequent sections by showing genetic risk as a shark lurking under the water's surface. Thorough surface examination and internal imaging studies are often needed to recognize the syndrome beneath the obvious congenital anomaly, but forewarning of malformation or genetic pattern is forearming for operative and postoperative management. Although the many different syndromes that may include anomalies such as anal atresia cannot be listed in detail, examples and referral to the

appropriate texts serve as reminders to their presence.

When no other major or minor anomalies are found besides the one presenting for surgical evaluation, then the genetic recurrence risk is often low (Table 13.1). Most isolated anomalies are either sporadic, meaning that they exhibit minimal recurrence in families (less than 1%), or they are multifactorial. The model for multifactorial determination with threshold was discussed in Chapter 3 and predicts a recurrence risk of 2–5% for parents having a child with a major birth defect. Multifactorial determination (i.e., several genes plus the environment) rather than sporadic occurrence is suggested by a sex predilection or an increase in empiric recurrence risk when additional relatives are defined with the anomaly. For an anomaly such as pyloric stenosis, males are more often affected than females and two affected children raises the parents' recurrence risk from 3 to 6% (Table 13.1; see Chapter 3). A corollary is that an affected female, requiring genetic predisposition in her parents to have crossed the threshold, will predict a higher recurrence risk (5–6%) than an affected male. In most cases, the general risk of 2–3% for one affected child, raised to 4–6% for a second affected child, are adequate figures for genetic counseling. References are available for more exact numbers (see Bibliography), but small differences are usually not significant for families. The risk for a sporadically occurring (< 1%) or multifactorially determined (~3%) anomaly can be favorably compared to the general risk of 2–3% for major birth defects in the average pregnancy.

It should be mentioned also that surgical management has an important role in lessening handicap and morbidity even when it is not curative. The rehabilitative aspects of surgery are too vast to cover here, but are exemplified by gastostomy placement in the child who cannot feed, tracheostomy insertion in the child with respiratory obstruction, or release of tendons in children whose joints are contracted with restricted movement. Although the surgeon's role may be secondary rather than pri-

■ **TABLE 13.1. Risks for Relatives to Have a Multifactorial Anomaly**

Anomaly (favored sex)	If index case M Risk %	If index case F Risk %	Incidence Increase Risk (%)
Pyloric stenosis (M)			3 per 1000
Sibling (1°)	3.2	6.5	× 25 (7.5) [b]
Son (1°)	5.5	19	
Daughter (1°)	2.4	7.0	
Nephew or niece (2°)	1.4	4.7[b]	× 9 (2.7) [b]
First cousin (3°)	0.65	0.5	× 1.5 (0.45) [b]
Cleft lip/palate (M)			1 per 1000
Two affected sibs	11	21	
Sibling (1°)	4.1[a]		× 40 (4.0) [a]
Child (1°)	5.3[a]		
Nephew or niece (2°)	0.9[a]		× 7 (0.7) [a]
First cousin (3°)	0.33[a]		× 3 (0.3) [a]
Cardiac tissue (M)			1 per 1000
Sibling (1°)	1.5–3.0[a]		× 25 (2.5) [a]
Child (1°)	1.9	2.9	
Cardiac flow (M)			1 per 2000
Sibling (1°)	0.6–3.6[a]		× 40 (2.0) [a]
Child (1°)	2.0	8.5	
Cardiac ECM (M)			1 in 6500
Sibling (1°)	1.5–8.7[a]		× 325 (5.0) [a]
Child (1°)	7.0	10.5	
Spina bifida (F)			2 per 1000
Two affected sibs	10.0[a]		
Sibling (1°)	5.0[a]		× 15 (3.0) [a]
Child (1°)	4.0[a]		
Nephew or niece (2°)	2.0[a]		
First cousin (3°)	1.0[a]		× 2 (0.4) [a]

Sources: Riopel (1993), Lettieri (1993), Laurence (1990), Carter (1974), Dennis and Warren (1981), Pierpont and Moller (1986).

[a]sex of index case unspecified.

[b]for males only.

Notes: M, male; F, female; 1°, primary relative (1/2 related); 2°, secondary relative (1/4 related); 3°, tertiary relative (1/8 related); Cardiac tissue, mesenchymal tissue defects like tetralogy of Fallot; Cardiac flow, flow defects like coarctation of the aorta; Cardiac ECM, extracellular matrix defects like atrioventricular septal defect.

mary in such circumstances, the resulting improvements in patient outcome and in patient care can be enormous. It is thus important for surgeons to be familiar with genetic diseases and syndromes as a category and to recognize the benefits of being involved with these patients and their families.

■ **13.2. GENERAL PEDIATRIC SURGERY**

Congenital Diaphragmatic Hernia

The diaphragm derives chiefly from the septum transversum of the early anterior region of the embryo, and divides the thoracic and abdominal cavities by 6–7 weeks of gestation. When this dividing septum is delayed or interfered with, an opening (hernia) between the cavities persists. Diaphragmatic hernias present dramatically in the newborn with cyanosis and breathing difficulties. Examination may reveal bowel sounds in the chest with deviation of the heartbeat, and radiography shows the presence of intestines in the thorax where lungs should be. Surgical outlook is chiefly determined by the degree of fetal lung growth; smaller or later herniation interferes less with the fetal breathing that is essential for lung development.

Diaphragmatic defects can include complete absence of the diaphragm (complete hernia), posterolateral absence (Bochdalek hernia), anterior absence (Morgagni hernia), hernia surrounding the esophagus (hiatus hernia), and eventration or upfolding of the diagragm. The incidence of diaphragmatic hernia is about 1 in 2000 births, with the majority of cases presenting as stillbirths or severely compromised infants that do not survive to undergo surgery. Associated malformations occur in about 20% of infants with diaphragmatic hernia, including particularly midline defects of the heart (~10%), central nervous system (~5–10%), and palate (~5%). Infants with multiple anomalies predominate in the stillborn group, some having associations and some having genetic syndromes. The surgeon must be alert to the presence of other anomalies both in planning corrective surgery and in ensuring correct genetic diagnosis and counseling.

As an isolated defect, diaphragmatic hernias have a recurrence risk of less than 1% (Fig. 13.1). Very rarely, isolated diaphragmatic hernias exhibit autosomal or X-linked recessive inheritance (306950) with recurrence rates of 25%. Two large studies have examined 181 sibs of 127 cases, and 559 sibs of 333 cases, respectively (Winter and Baraitser, 1998). Recurrences were observed in less than 1% of cases.

Additional anomalies have been reported in about one-half of children with diaphragmatic hernia, most commonly congenital heart defects that occur in 18% of children with multiple anomalies. Another common association has been described as the schisis association of midline defects like spina bifida, oral cleft, omphalocele, and diaphragmatic hernia (Fig. 13.1). Upper limb anomalies are also reported: Martinez-Frias (1996) described 9 infants out of a registry of 21,000 with congenital malformations who had diaphragmatic hernia and upper limb anomalies. Sometimes these associations are caused by teratogens, with vitamin A, coumadin, and influenza exposure being linked with congenital diaphragmatic hernia.

When multiple major and minor anomalies are noted in conjunction with diaphragmatic hernia, a syndrome must be suspected as illustrated in Figure 13.1. The many syndromes and associations that include diaphragmatic hernia mandate careful examination of infants to facilitate operative and postoperative management.

Large diaphragmatic hernias constitute an indication for emergency surgery, which has a high success rate when lung growth has been adequate. Fetal correction of diaphragmatic hernias detected prenatally has been tried using the rationale of relieving pressure on the developing lung. Unfortunately, most cases detected early by ultrasound have had associated anomalies with the risks for syndromes exemplified in Figure 13.1. Postnatal surgery is an extensive procedure that requires return of large thoracic structures to the abdomen. High levels of cardiorespiratory support are necessary to maintain oxygenation until the heart and lungs can function normally, and extracorporeal membrane oxygenation (a heart-lung machine) is frequently used for postoperative recovery.

Omphalocele and Gastroschisis

Omphalocele consists of an opening through the umbilicus with protrusion of the abdominal contents. This is a normal stage of the early embryo that may persist into postnatal life. The incidence is 2.5 cases per 10,000 births, with

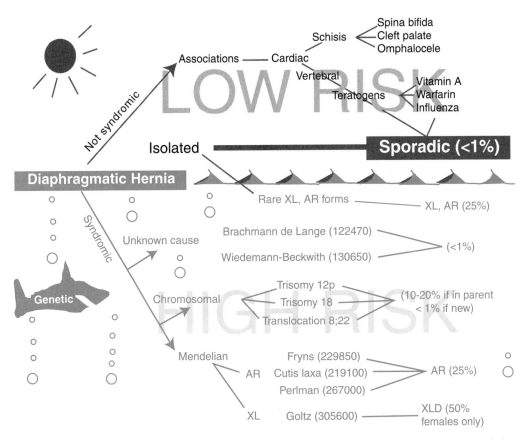

Figure 13.1. Causes of congenital diaphragmatic hernia. Conditions with lower recurrence risk (sequence leading to small lungs, other anomaly and teratogenic associations) are shown above, with rare but important genetic forms shown below. AR, autosomal recessive; XL, X-linked; XLD, X-linked dominant.

about 25% presenting as stillbirths associated with multiple anomalies. Gastroschisis is a rent in the abdominal wall that occurs to the side (usually the right side) of the umbilicus and does not mimic a normal embryologic stage. The intestines and abdominal organs may sustain damage in gastroschisis, which does not protect these organs with the umbilical sac that is present in omphalocele. The incidence of gastroschisis is 1 case per 10,000 births with a much different maternal age distribution than omphalocele. Omphalocele is much more likely to be associated with syndromes and chromosomal aberrations. Omphalocele is thus more common in offspring of older mothers, due to their increased risk for chromosomal

anomalies, while gastroschisis is much more common younger mothers. Because of its increased rate (approaching 9 per 10,000 in very young mothers), the overall frequency of gastroschisis is increasing compared to a stable rate for omphalocele.

Depending on the study sample, between 40 and 88% of infants with omphalocele have associated anomalies compared to 20% for those with gastroschisis. As a result, more than 90% of children with gastroschisis have corrective surgery compared to less than 40% with omphalocele. Anomalies associated with gastroschisis are typically vascular disruptions like porencephaly (cavity in the brain due to vessel disruption and lysis), Poland anomaly of digital defects and absent pectoral muscle, and renal agenesis (interruption of kidney development by vessel disruption). Anomalies associated with omphalocele include the pentalogy of Cantrell (omphalocele, lower sternal defect, absent lower pericardium, anterior diaphragmatic hernia, cardiac anomaly), cardiac defects (in 50%), and spina bifida/anencephaly (40%). Teratogens such as cocaine have been associated with both anomalies, while vitamin A and valproic acid exposure have been associated with omphalocele only. The main syndrome associated with gastroschisis is amyoplasia (108100), a generalized hypoplasia of muscles that produces decreased fetal limb movements and arthrogryposis (congenital contractures).

Gastroschisis and even omphalocele, when isolated, are usually sporadic anomalies with recurrence risks of less than 1%. However, several families in which multiple individuals have omphalocele have been reported, including one with four affected males that suggested X-linked recessive inheritance of isolated omphalocele and one in which five affected boys and girls were born to one mother. The presence of additional anomalies with the omphalocele increases the chances for a syndrome with genetic etiology, and these infants often require chromosome studies.

Prenatal diagnosis of gastroschisis and omphalocele by ultrasound is increasingly common, and between 20 and 50% of prenatally diagnosed infants with omphalocele have chromosome aberrations (trisomy 13/18 and others). As discussed in Chapter 15, these infants often merit percutaneous umblical blood sampling (PUBS) for rapid karyotyping. Gastroschisis may be confused with more severe disruptions of the abdominal wall as occurs in the lethal limb-body wall complex, so a search for severe anomalies is also needed when ultrasound diagnosis is made. For isolated anomalies, postnatal surgical treatment has improved dramatically since the mid-sixties with greater than 85% survival for repair of gastroschisis and almost 100% for repair of omphalocele. The latter anomaly may required a staged closure, since the extrusion of abdominal contents may produce a small cavity that will not accommodate the return of liver, spleen, and intestines in one procedure. A cylinder ("silo") of plastic material may be used to enclose the extruded contents until the infant grows sufficiently to allow a final replacement and closure.

Anal Atresia

The developing gut has foregut (pharynx, esophagus, stomach and duodenum), midgut (intestines from duodenum through cecum), and hindgut (cecum through anus) regions that can be altered to produce anomalies. Anal atresia is a spectrum of defects that impact variable extents of the anus and rectum. In high and intermediate anal atresias, the rectum ends above or within the levator muscles that must contract to allow fecal continence. In low anal atresias, the rectum ends beneath the levator muscles, allowing a more straightforward surgical repair. In higher lesions, the fecal contents (fetal meconium) dissect through the tissues to exit through a passage known as a fistula. High lesions are more likely to be associated with the anomalies listed in Figure 13.2.

All types of anal atresias have an incidence of 1 in 5000 live births. Males outnumber females about 1.5 to 1, suggesting that some cases involve multifactorial determination. Nevertheless, recurrences are rare with an overall risk for isolated anal atresia of less than 1% (Figure 13.2).

Associations with anal atresia are dominated by the VATER association of vertebral, anorectal, tracheoesophageal, radial (thumb ray), and renal defects. This association was discussed in Chapter 11, and may include cardiac defects as well. Urogenital (20%), skeletal (13%), and other gastrointestinal (10%) defects are the most common associated anomalies, sometimes caused by teratogens such as alcohol, thalidomide, and the thyroid inhibitor propylthiouracil (Figure 13.2).

Winter and Baraitser (1998) list more than 100 syndromes including anal atresia and sev-

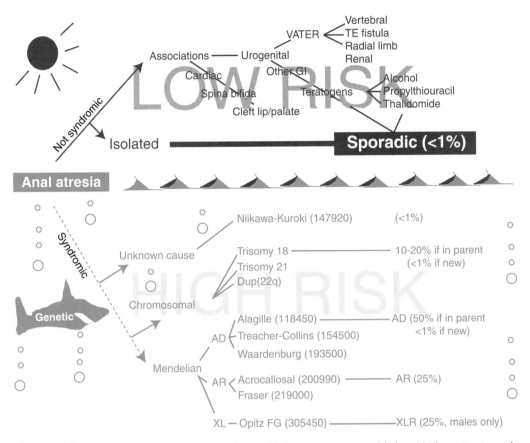

Figure 13.2. Causes of anal atresia. Conditions with lower recurrence risk (associations, teratogenic problems) are shown above, while rare but important genetic forms are shown below. AD, autosomal dominant; AR, autosomal recessive; XL, X-linked; XLR, X-linked recessive.

eral shown in Figure 13.2. Isolated anal atresia of the low type has an excellent surgical outcome, usually corrected in one stage in the newborn period with complete attainment of fecal continence. High or intermediate lesions often require a staged repair with interim use of a colostomy. These procedures often cause additional complications such as fistulas or infections, and one large study cited a mortality of 20%. Some of this mortality is probably caused by other anomalies that tend to occur with high anal atresias. The lower survival and higher syndrome risk portended by associated anomalies emphasize the importance of thorough examination and internal imaging studies in assessing children with anal atresia.

Case 13 Follow-up: Additional investigations showed the presence of vertebral and cardiac anomalies that led to a diagnosis of VATER association. The cardiac anomaly was a septal defect that was sufficiently stable to allow one-stage closure of the anal atresia. Although the presence of multiple anomalies in VATER association may cause a 1-year survival less than 50%, those children amenable to surgical correction have a normal prognosis for growth and development. Aggressive surgical management with genetic counseling for a minimal recurrence risk was therefore provided, and awareness of the risk for associated anomalies allowed the recognition and appropriate evaluation of a congenital heart defect.

Pyloric Stenosis

The pylorus is the lower valve of the stomach that connects it to the duodenum, and narrowing (stenosis) of this valve occurs due to muscular hypertrophy in 3 per 1000 births. There is a striking male to female predominance that fits with multifactorial determination. The risks for pyloric stenosis were covered in Chapter 3, ranging from a 6% recurrence risk if a daughter is affected to a 3% recurrence risk if a son is affected. Some cases have been proven to develop after birth, but many occur early in embryogenesis as indicated by a 6–12% incidence of associated anomalies.

As with other anomalies discussed in this section, isolated pyloric stenosis rarely exhibits Mendelian inheritance with an autosomal dominant pattern. Exposures to teratogens such thalidomide and hydantoin (Dilantin) have caused pyloric stenosis. Chromosomal syndromes with pyloric stenosis as one component include Down syndrome (trisomy 21), trisomy 18, and the partial trisomies dup(1q), dup(9q), and del(11q). Mendelian syndromes with this anomaly include the Smith-Lemli-Opitz syndrome (270400) with broad nasal root, ambiguous genitalia, and fusion of the toes due to abnormal cholesterol metabolism; Marden-Walker syndrome (248700) with immobility of facial muscles, small head, congenital contractures, and growth failure; Zellweger syndrome (214100) with severe hypotonia and liver disease due to abnormal peroxisome biogenesis; and the Opitz FG syndrome (305450) with frontal cowlick and constipation are other examples.

The prognosis for pyloric stenosis is excellent if the typical hypochloremic alkalosis (low blood chloride, high blood pH) is anticipated. The condition will resolve spontaneously after several months, so careful restoration of fluid balance and optimization of surgical risks are important. The anomaly may be detected as an olive shape that is palpated during careful abdominal examination. The optimal examination occurs after the child has vomited to empty the stomach contents, with palpation for

30 minutes needed to exclude the lesion. Modern detection is more rapid using radiography after barium ingestion or abdominal ultrasound.

■ 13.3. CRANIOFACIAL AND PLASTIC SURGERY

Advances in surgical technique and medical support have produced dramatic improvements in the ability to rectify abnormal skull shape and facial deformities. Portions of the skull can literally be ground up (morcellation) and reshaped, while skull and facial regions can be mobilized and rearranged like the continental plates were moved to reshape the earth. The multidisciplinary approaches required for operations involving the brain, skull, ears, eyes and mouth have fostered the development of a craniofacial team at many medical centers that includes plastic surgeons, neurosurgeons, ophthalmologists, otolaryngologists, dentists, and experts in prosthetic or reconstructive devices. Candidates for craniofacial surgery would include individuals such as those with Treacher-Collins syndrome (154500) as illustrated in Figure 11.4. The ability to remold an abnormal facial appearance is truly remarkable. Many of the children with craniofacial anomalies have underlying syndromes that must be identified to ensure proper surgical and medical management.

Craniosynostoses

Craniosynostosis refers to premature fusion of the cranial sutures. The pressure of infantile brain growth usually forces expansion of the skull around the fused suture, causing abnormal head shape. Fusion of the coronal sutures restricts anteroposterior skull growth to produce brachycephaly (flattened skull) and force compensatory growth in the vertical direction. Fusion of the sagittal suture restricts outward growth (narrow skull or dolichocephaly) with compensation in the anteroposterior direction (elongated head or scaphocephaly). Other unusual head shapes produced by craniosynostosis include trigonocephaly (triangular shape as viewed from above with pointed forehead) caused by fusion of the metopic suture, plagiocephaly (asymmetrical head shape) produced by unilateral craniosynostoses, and clover leaf skull anomaly caused by fusion of multiple sutures. Fusion of multiple sutures may also occur with severe undergrowth of the brain (microcephaly), but the absence of brain pressure leads to a relatively normal or pointed shape (acrocephaly or oxycephaly). When brain growth is normal, early recognition of craniosynostosis is critical because increased intracranial pressure can compress the brain and cranial nerves to produce mental retardation, deafness, and blindness.

The frequency of craniosynostosis is variably reported between 1 and 3 cases per thousand live births. Sagittal synostosis is present in over half the cases, with coronal (22%), metopic (6%), and multiple synostoses (23%) accounting for the rest (Toriello, 1993). Plagiocephaly (lop-sided skull shape) and brachycephaly (flattened occiput) can be deformations caused by abnormal pre- or postnatal positioning of the baby rather than true craniosynostoses. Cranial radiographs or ultrasound may be required to demonstrate patency of the sutures, with the conclusion that immobility of the fetus or child has led to abnormal head shape. Brachycephaly occurs in infants that are bedridden for long periods, and may be a sign of neurologic disability or child neglect. The distinction between craniosynostosis and positional deformations is critical because the latter can be treated by restoring activity or by molding the head with a helmet.

If true craniosynostosis is present, there is a 20–25% risk for accessory anomalies. Once a careful physical examination and, if necessary, imaging studies exclude other anomalies, the recurrence risk for isolated craniosynostosis is less than 1%. Rare autosomal dominant inheritance of isolated craniosynostosis has been reported, illustrated by one family who traced their "breadhead" shape back several generations. Associated anomalies may indicate exposure to teratogens such as valproic acid, hydantoin, folate inhibitors such as methotrexate, or vitamin A. Many syndromes include craniosynostosis, with some specificity for the sutures involved. The Apert (101200) and Crouzon (123500) syndromes usually produce coronal synostosis, although multiple synostoses with cloverleaf skull anomaly can occur in Crouzon syndrome. Since these disorders have now been traced to mutations in different regions of the fibroblast growth factor receptor-2 gene, it is evident that variations in synostosis pattern may reflect the timing or degree of abnormal gene expression rather than causation by different syndromes.

Additional examples of syndromes with craniosynostosis include the Pfeiffer syndrome (101600) with frequent clover-leaf anomaly and broad thumbs/great toes, the Carpenter syndrome (201000) with coronal or multiple synostoses and postaxial polydactyly, and the Saethre-Chotzen syndrome (101400) with milder synostosis, prominent eyes, and cleft palate. Among the more common craniosynostosis syndromes, most are autosomal dominant with the exception of the autosomal recessive Carpenter syndrome. The diversity of other syndromes emphasizes the need to consider all modes of inheritance, exemplified by the Say-Meyer syndrome (314320) with metopic synostosis and growth delay. Altered head shape without synostosis can also occur in numerous syndromes as listed in detail by Toriello (1993), mandating again that skull imaging be performed when the presence of craniosynostosis is not clear.

Early surgical correction is usually indicated when craniosynostosis is recognized, and the outcome for children without other anomalies is excellent. Variable frequencies of mental disability reported in certain case series (10–25%) most likely reflect underlying syndromes or brain anomalies, particularly when the disability persists despite early recognition and treatment. The presence of mental retardation should thus promote a careful reevaluation to search for subtle signs of syndrome involvement.

Cleft Lip/Cleft Palate

During embryogenesis, a primary palate forms at the anterior roof of the mouth and contributes to the lip and anterior palate. Somewhat later, the secondary palate closes posteriorly completed by fusion of the uvula. Failure of the primary palate to produce cleft lip and cleft palate varies by ethnic origin from about 0.5 per 1000 live births in blacks to 2.1 per 1000 live births in Asians (Lettieri, 1993). Failure of the secondary palate to close produces cleft palate alone in 0.5 per 1000 live births and bifid uvula in 20 per 1000 live births with little ethnic variation. As discussed in Chapter 11 and illustrated in Figure 11.1D, interference with palatal closure by maldescent of the tongue due to a small jaw produces the U-shaped cleft of Robin sequence. V-shaped clefts are primary malformations that disrupt palatal closure. Most oral clefts are obvious at birth, but mild defects interfere with soft palate motility (velopalatine incompetence) or occur as bony defects beneath a skin-covered palate (submucous clefts).

As with other more common congenital anomalies, the distinction between isolated cleft lip/palate and cleft palate is essential for management and counseling. Isolated cleft lip/palate and cleft palate usually imply multifactorial determination with a 3–5% recurrence risk. Since clefts occur more often in males, affliction of a female infant and more severe, bilateral clefts are predictive of higher recurrence risks.

Cleft lip/palate and cleft palate are associated with additional anomalies in 50–60% of cases in some series (Lettieri, 1993). Although the presence of cleft lip/palate tends to predict recurrence of cleft lip/palate when the cleft is isolated (Table 13.1), particular associations or syndromes often have either anomaly. Associations include other midline anomalies such as heart defects, spina bifida, or omphalocele, illustrated by the schisis or CHARGE associations (Fig. 13.3). Teratogens such as hydantoin, vitamin A, alcohol, and valproate are associated with oral clefts, as are more than 370 syndromes and associations listed by Winter and Baraitser (1996). The many Mendelian causes of cleft lip/palate provide potential examples of extreme mutations that in milder form can interact to produce multifactorial cleft lip/palate.

The prognosis for isolated cleft lip/palate is excellent, with nasal speech being the major residual complication after surgery. Severe clefts cause feeding problems that require special nipples and nutritional counseling. Regurgitation of feedings causes chronic otitis with risks for hearing problems if not aggressively treated. Early closure of cleft lip is often performed for cosmetic reasons, and early closure of the soft palate is recommended by some to facilitate feeding and speech development. Closure of the hard palate is often postponed until later childhood. About 25% of children have residual speech defects that are severe enough to require a second operation to ensure adequate coverage and motion of the soft palate (velum).

Eye Anomalies

Ophthalmologists have a unique opportunity to witness evidence of genetic disease through their repertoire of special instruments. The slit lamp allows detailed visualization of the cornea, lens, and anterior chamber, revealing subtle abnormalities like the corneal crystals seen in cystinosis (219800), the lax ciliary ligament that suspends the optic lens in Marfan syndrome (154700), or the changes in the optic cup (the insertion point of the optic nerve in the retina) that occur in neurofibromatosis-1 (162200). Eye complications caused by many craniofacial malformations also make ophthalmologists important members of the craniofacial surgery team.

Table 13.2 lists several types of ocular anomalies and provides examples of disorders presenting as isolated eye problems or as syndromes. The theme of isolated versus multiple anomalies as a guide to management is again emphasized for ocular disease, because the aggressiveness of surgical management must be

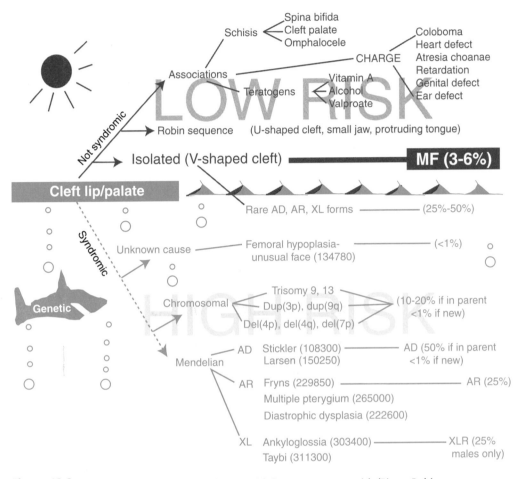

Figure 13.3. Causes of cleft palate. Conditions with lower recurrence risk (Pierre Robin sequence, associations, teratogenic problems) are shown above, while rare but important genetic forms are shown below. AD, autosomal dominant; AR, autosomal recessive; XL, X-linked; XLR, X-linked recessive; MF, multifactorial determination.

matched with patient prognosis. Many, if not most, malformation syndromes have an increased risk for glaucoma (increased pressure within the eye), cataracts, strabismus, or refractive errors, emphasizing the importance of ophthalmology for preventive management.

Complete or partial absence of the eye (anophthalmia) is a rare defect that can be associated with abnormal forebrain development (holoprosencephaly—Table 13.2). The optic cup arises from the neural tube and forebrain during early embryonic development, perhaps accounting for this association. Isolated cases may be sporadic or autosomal recessive (206900), and the presence of anophthalmia in Goldenhar syndrome (164210) is predictive of developmental disability. The Waardenberg syndrome (206920) of anophthalmia and limb anomalies (different from other Waardenberg syndromes) and trisomy 13 illustrate the possibilities for syndrome involvement.

Clefts in the eyelids, iris, and/or retinae (colobomas) arise from persistence of a normal fissure in the optic cup that allows mesoderm and blood vessels to invest the eye. It may be difficult to distinguish small, underdeveloped eyes (microphthalmia) from iris colobomas.

■**TABLE 13.2.** Optic Anomalies: Isolated, Associated, and Syndromic

Isolated Anomaly	Associations	Syndromes
Anophthalmia (MF) AR form (206900)	Holoprosencephaly (S, C, M)	Waardenberg (206920) Lenz (309800) Sjogren-Larssen (270200) Trisomy 13 (C)

Small iris, coloboma (MF)
  AD form (120200, 120430)
  AR form (216820)
	CHARGE (S, 214800)
	Frontonasal dysplasia (S)
	Rubella (T)
	Cytomegalovirus (T)
	Toxoplasmosis (T)
	Alcohol (T)
	Vitamin A (T)
		Rieger (180500)
		Cohen (216550)
		Goldenhar (MF;164210)
		Goltz (305600)
		Trisomy 13 (C)
		Triploidy (C)
		Del(4p), dup(22q)—C

Congenital cataract (MF)
  AD form (116100)
  AR form (212540)
  XL form (302200)
	Various ocular anomalies
	Rubella (T)
	Toxoplasmosis (T)
	Thalidomide (T)
	Varicella (T)
		Larsen (150250)
		Cerebrooculofacial (214150)
		Cockayne (216400)
		Galactosemia (230400)
		Gyrate atrophy (258870)
		Homocystinuria (236200)
		Nance-Horan (302350)
		Trisomy 13 (C)
		Del(11p13)—C

Retinal dysplasia XL form (312350)	Ocular microphthalmia Ocular cyclopia Ocular PHPV Aprosencephaly (S or AR) ?LSD ?Agent orange	PXE (177850, 264800) Gyrate atrophy (258870) Warburg (236670) Aicardi syndrome (304050) Trisomy 13, 18 (C) Triploidy (C) Del(4p)—C
Blephariphimosis AD form (110100)	Ocular ptosis Alcohol (T)	Saethre-Chotzen (101400) Dubowitz (223370) Ohdo (249620) Schwartz-Jampel (255800)

Notes: MF, multifactorial; AD, autosomal dominant; AR, autosomal recessive; XL, X-linked; T, teratogenic; S, sporadic; PXE, pseudoxanthoma elasticum; CHARGE, coloboma, heart defects, atresia choanae, retardation, genital defects, ear defects; PHPV, persistent hyperplastic primary vitreous; LSD, lysergic acid diamide.

Taken together, these eye anomalies occur in about 0.5 per 1000 live births and are listed in more than 150 syndromes by Winter and Baraitser (1998). Isolated forms are usually sporadic, but rarely can exhibit autosomal dominant (120200, 120430) or autosomal recessive (216820) inheritance. Teratogens such as alcohol or congenital infectious agents, Mendelian syndromes such as Rieger syndrome (180500) with absent facial fat and abnormal teeth, and many chromosomal syndromes including tri-somy 13 can include eye colobomas (Table 13.2). Colobomas that extend through the retina can cause significant vision loss.

Congenital cataracts are opacities of the optic lens that occur in even more associations and syndromes than colobomas, with more than 350 listed by Winter and Baraitser (1998). Cataracts can be classified according to their type and location in the lens, and they often occur secondarily to other types of eye anomalies and injuries. Although some forms of isolated congenital cataract are sporadic with a low recurrence, the presence of cataracts should alert the examiner to suspect a genetic disease. In addition to many teratogens such as the congenital infections rubella or varicella, inherited malformation syndromes, metabolic diseases, or chromosomal syndromes can all present with cataract (Table 13.2). Homocystinuria (236200) and galactosemia (230400) were discussed in Chapter 12, and gyrate atrophy of the choroid and retina (258870) is another enzyme deficiency that affects metabolism of the amino acid ornithine.

Retinal dysplasia is a congenital anomaly that is different from the retinal or macular degenerations of later life. The organized retinal layers are disrupted in this anomaly, producing a thickened region that may be mistaken for tumors such as retinoblastoma or detachments that occur with retinopathy of prematurity. Retinal organization is not well developed until 8 months of gestation, and the macula (most sensitive part of the retina) does not attain optimal vision until age 1–2 years (Traboulsi, 1993). Accordingly, certain suspected teratogens and many chromosomal disorders such as trisomy 13 can cause retinal dysplasia (Table 13.2). A later-onset disorder called pseudoxanthoma elasticum can present with retinal dysplasia and "orange-peel" skin that is caused by abnormal blood vessels. The disease occurs in both autosomal dominant (177850) and autosomal recessive (264800) forms. The neural origin of retina correlates with the presence of retinal dysplasia in two severe neurologic disorders: the Warburg syndrome (236670) with encephalocele or other brain anomalies and the Aicardi syndrome (304050) with myoclonic (jerking) seizures and vertebral anomalies. Aicardi syndrome manifests only in females, suggesting that it is an X-linked dominant disorder with lethality in males.

Anomalies outside the ocular globes are common and constitute some of the most common minor anomalies noted in syndromes. Minor anomalies such as telecanthus (wide space between the canthi or corners of the eyes), epicanthal folds, ptosis (drooping eyelids), altered slant to the palpebral fissures, double rows of eyelashes (distichiasis), outfolding of the lower palpebral fissure (ectropion), and altered width of the palpebral fissures occur in numerous syndromes. More severe examples of anomalies such as ptosis can be classified as major anomalies because they may require surgical correction. Blepharophimosis or narrowing of the palpebral fissures is such an anomaly, with most cases being minor aids to syndrome diagnosis rather than needing correction. The anomaly is common in fetal alcohol syndrome (see Fig. 11.9) and often associated with ptosis. Several Mendelian syndromes include blepharophimosis (Table 13.2), and it is listed in more than 50 syndromes or associations by Winter and Baraitser (1998).

Ear Anomalies

Origin of the external ears from the branchial arches of the neck region makes them extremely vulnerable to developmental aberrations. Ear anomalies occur in about 1 in 1000 births, although different terms such as lop ear or dysplastic ear complicate such estimates. Interference with ascent of the ears can produce common minor anomalies (low-set ears, posteriorly rotated ears) and interruptions of branchial arch fusions can produce absent or aberrant external ears associated with facial and jaw anomalies. A pit located anterior to the external ear (ear pit) is a helpful minor anomaly that can raise suspicion of Mendelian disorders like the branchio-oto-renal syndrome (113650) or chromosomal disorders like the Wolf-Hirshhorn (4p deletion) or *cri-du-chat* (5p deletion) syndromes (see Chapter 7).

Isolated external ear anomalies can occur sporadically or by Mendelian inheritance (128600). Most syndromes involve incomplete formation of the external ear with microtia or small ears. External ear anomalies are common in teratogenic syndromes caused by vitamin A, alcohol, or thalidomide exposure, and in a variety of Mendelian syndromes. Most characteristic are branchial arch syndromes like Treacher-Collins (154500—Fig. 11.1*C*), Nager (154400—Fig. 11.1*B*), Miller (263750) or Goldenhar (164210) syndromes that present for craniofacial surgery. These syndromes often involve hypoplasia of the pharyngeal muscles and jaw with airway and feeding problems, and the middle and/or internal ears are often malformed to cause hearing loss.

Anomalies of the middle and internal ears often accompany external ear anomalies, particularly if the ear canal (meatus) is absent. Abnormalities of the middle ear ossicles produce conductive or bone deafness, while abnormalities of the inner ear and otic nerve produce sensorineural or nerve deafness. Middle ear anomalies occur as sporadic or Mendelian disorders, illustrated by the X-linked form of stapes fixation (304400). Skeletal dysplasias such as achondroplasia (100800) or chromosomal disorders such as trisomy 13/18 can have fusions or malformations of the ear ossicles, and these anomalies are probably present but undocumented in many other syndromes. Sensorineural deafness due to anomalies of the cochlear apparatus (Michel and Mondini types) can also occur as isolated or syndromic forms. Thalidomide and rubella teratogenesis is notable for affecting the inner ear, and common Mendelian causes syndromes include the Waardenburg syndrome with white forelock and hypertelorism (193510) and the Wildervanck syndrome (314600) with abnormal cervical vertebrae and eye anomalies. Many other genetic forms of sensorineural deafness occur in the absence of notable congenital anomalies, and these are discussed in Chapter 14.

Dental Anomalies

Like the ophthalmologists, dentists have made enormous contributions to clinical genetics by utilizing their unique view of tooth morphology. The dentists Robert Gorlin and Michael Cohen Jr. have written the most comprehensive reference for syndromes (Gorlin et al., 1990) that provides a useful supplement to the pictorial atlas of Jones (1997) and the database

of Winter and Baraitser (1998). Conically shaped teeth are helpful in appreciating the large category of ectodermal dysplasias that present with sparse hair, hypoplastic nails, and decreased sweating. Malposition of the teeth is common in chromosomal syndromes, and dental care is an important preventive strategy in disorders like Down syndrome. Absence of one or more teeth can be a normal variant (absence of the third molar), an inherited trait (absence of the central incisors or canines), or a component of numerous malformation syndromes including the Johanson-Blizzard syndrome (243800) with pancreatic insufficiency and facial abnormalities (Jorgenson, 1993). Dysplasias of the enamel (outer) or dentin (inner) tooth substance occurs in numerous syndromes, highlighted by dentinogenesis imperfecta (125490). The impact of facial or jaw misalignment on teeth, and the value of tooth malformations in syndrome diagnosis makes the dentist and oral surgeon an important component of the craniofacial surgical team.

■ 13.4. CARDIOTHORACIC SURGERY

Cardiac anomalies are second only to hypospadias as the most common birth defects, with an overall frequency of 1 in 170 live births. More than 50% of cardiac defects occur with associated anomalies, and they are a component of most chromosomal syndromes. Teratogens such as rubella virus, chromosomal aneuploidies such as Down syndrome, and microdeletions on chromosomes 7 (Williams syndrome) or 22 (Shprintzen/DiGeorge syndrome) are well known for their high frequencies of congenital heart defects. Although most isolated heart defects exhibit multifactorial determination (Table 13.1), there are 36 Mendelian forms of isolated heart anomalies and 166 Mendelian syndromes that include congenital heart defects (Wilson, 1998).

Clark (1996) has integrated a large amount of epidemiologic, genetic, and embryologic data to postulate six major categories of congenital heart disease (Table 13.3). The first

■**TABLE 13.3.** Cardiac Anomalies: Isolated, Associated, and Syndromic

Isolated Anomaly	Associations	Syndromes

Tetralogy of Fallot (MF)
  AD form (187500)
  XL form (304750)
	Asternia (S, 313850)
	CHARGE (S, 214800)
	Alcohol (T), Vit. A (T) Primadione (T)
		Adams-Oliver (100300)
		Nager (154400)
		Hallerman-Streif (234100)
		Shprintzen (C, 192430)

Coarctation of aorta (MF) AD form (120000)	Sternal clefts (140850) Propylthiouracil (T) Vitamin A (T)	Robinow (180700) Majewski dysplasia (263530) Perlman (267000) Shprintzen (C, 192430)

Ebstein anomaly (MF)
  AR form (224700)
  XL form (314400)
	Lithium (T)	

AVSD (MF) AR form (208530, 270100)	Dandy-Walker cyst (220200) CHARGE (S, 214800)	Hypochondrogenesis (200600) Ritscher-Schinzel (220210) Jarcho-Levin (277300) Ohdo (249620) Trisomy 21 (C)
TAPVR (MF) AD form (106100)		Holt-Oram (142900) Baller-Gerold (218600) Fryns (229850) Marden-Walker (248700) Robin sequence plus (311900)

Heterotaxy (MF)
  AR form (208530, 270100)
  XL form (304750)
	Agnathia-holoprosencephaly (202650)
	Poland sequence (173800)
	MURCS
		Goldenhar (164210)
		Ellis van Crevald (225500)
		Meckel-Gruber (249000)
		Mosaic trisomy 16 (C)

Notes: MF, multifactorial; AD, autosomal dominant; AR, autosomal recessive; XL, X-linked; T, teratogenic; S, sporadic; C, chromosomal; PXE, pseudoxanthoma elasticum; CHARGE, coloboma, heart defects, atresia choanae, retardation, genital defects, ear defects; MURCS, mullerian (uterine) derivatives, renal, cervical somite anomalies.

group involves aberrant migration of neural crest and mesenchymal tissue into the conotruncal region of the heart, producing outflow tract anomalies such as double-outlet right ventricle, tetralogy of Fallot, and pulmonary valve stenosis (narrowing), and aortic valve stenosis. The second group involves alterations of intracardiac blood flow to produce anomalies like hypoplastic left heart or coarctation of the aorta. The third group involves increased programmed cell death, leading to anomalies like Ebstein malformation of the tricuspid valve. The fourth affects the extracellular matrix to produce anomalies like atrioventricular septal defect (atrioventricular canal, single ventricle), and the fifth involves abnormal cell growth to produce anomalous pulmonary venous return. Finally, the category of abnormal laterality (situs defects) produces changes in cardiac orientation with or without changes in overall situs (liver on right, spleen on left).

Cardiac malformations within each category tend to cluster together in families and occur within particular syndromes. Relatives of individuals with double-outlet right ventricle have higher risks for defects in the outflow tract category (Table 13.1), and particular syndromes like trisomy 21 exhibit high rates of defects in one category (atrioventricular, atrial, or ventricular septal defects (Table 13.3). The type of cardiac anomaly is not only important for surgical management, but is a preliminary indicator of the likelihood and type of associated defects. Table 13.3 emphasizes these correlations with a few examples from the many syndromes involving cardiac anomalies.

Mesenchymal Defects (e.g., Tetralogy of Fallot)

These anomalies affect the separation of the major pulmonary and aortic arteries to form the outflow tract of the heart. If either major artery is severely compromised, there must be a coexisting septal defect to allow mixing of blood from the pulmonary and systemic circulation. The four features of tetralogy of Fallot are pulmonary stenosis, ventricular septal defect, pulmonic outflow tract displaced anteriorly to overide the left ventricle, and, because of pulmonary narrowing, right ventricular enlargement. Most patients present with cyanosis in the newborn period, with tetralogy of Fallot patients having characteristic "squatting" episodes reflecting intermittent cyanosis. The incidences of tetralogy of Fallot, transposition of the great arteries, and truncus arteriosus are 5, 3, and 0.8 cases per 10,000 live births, respectively (Riopel, 1993).

Tetralogy of Fallot and other mesenchymal defects exhibit multifactorial determination (Table 13.1) with rare autosomal or X-linked forms (Table 13.3). Most congenital heart defects predominate in males, with slightly higher recurrence risks for relatives of female index cases (Table 13.1). The increased risk for offspring of affected females is particularly striking for several types of heart defects, suggesting a maternal affect (Table 13.1). Recalling the effects of maternal genes on early patterning discussed in Chapter 9, this maternal effect could represent gene products expressed in the egg cytoplasm, teratogenic factors, or effects of major loci on the X chromosome. There is an X-linked form (304750) of tetralogy of Fallot that includes abnormal laterality (heterotaxy).

More than 150 associations or syndromes with congenital heart defects are listed by Winter and Baraitser (1996), and nearly all of the 100+ chromosomal syndromes can include

cardiac anomalies. Although there is some specificity for types of cardiac defects within particular syndromes, it should be realized that a particular syndrome may include cardiac anomalies of various types and even of different mechanistic categories. This variability is illustrated by X-linked heterotaxy (304750) listed under two categories in Table 13.3, and is particularly true of chromosomal syndromes.

There are 55 associations or syndromes that include tetralogy of Fallot (Winter and Baraitser, 1996), including associations with asternia, the CHARGE group, and exposure to teratogens such as alcohol and the antiepileptic drug primadione (Table 13.3). Several Mendelian syndromes include tetralogy of Fallot, exemplified by the Adams-Oliver syndrome of scalp and limb defects (100300), the Nager syndrome (154400) of branchial arch and limb defects (see Fig. 11.1B), and the Hallerman-Streif syndrome (234100) with unusual facial appearance, sparse hair, accelerated aging, and growth delay.

The key to management for most cardiac defects is early detection before damage occurs due to hypoxia or pulmonary hypertension. The latter complication occurs when circulation through the pulmonary arteries and veins is increased in infancy because of anomalous circulation. Over time, the pulmonary arteries become thickened, causing increased resistance to pulmonary flow and forcing underoxygenated blood into the systemic circulation. Children with disorders that have high frequencies of cardiac anomalies like Down syndrome must be rigorously examined using techniques like echocardiography to image the cardiopulmonary anatomy. Physical examination alone is not enough in high-risk situations, because large septal defects may be present that do not produce audible cardiac murmurs. The early left-to-right flow of blood from the high-pressure systemic circulation to the low pressure pulmonary circulation is reversed once pulmonary hypertension develops. A previously asymptomatic child may thus develop cyanosis indicative of an undetected ventricular septal defect with pulmonary hypertension: This scenario is tragic because the pulmonary hypertension cannot be corrected by surgery.

Most congenital heart diseases are surgically correctable if recognized promptly. Often the lesions are corrected in two stages, as exemplified by tetralogy of Fallot. Palliative procedures are done during early infancy to alleviate severe cyanosis; these involve several types of shunts to circumvent the blocked (stenosed) pulmonary artery in the case of tetralogy of Fallot. Once sufficient growth has occurred to decrease risks of major surgery with heart-lung bypass, a definitive correction is performed. Corrected patients still need follow-up for risks of infection to the operated heart, and antibiotic prophylaxis is provided. Certain operations also confer risks in later life because regions of the heart (e.g., the right ventricle) must carry a inappropriate circulatory load dictated by the corrected anatomy. Nevertheless, the excellent outcomes for most patients with congenital heart lesions is a dramatic success story in the field of birth defects.

Cardiac Anomalies in Other Mechanistic Categories

As shown in Table 13.1, most isolated cases of cardiac anomalies in all mechanistic categories fit the model for multifactorial determination. Recurrence risks for primary relatives of patients with congenital heart disease will be in the range of 1–4%, adjusted upward when the affected person is female. Each mechanistic category occasionally exhibits Mendelian inheritance when isolated, and each is associated with particular anomalies and syndromes (Table 13.3).

Rare malformations such as the Ebstein tricuspid valve stenosis (1 in 30,000 live births) show a specific association with maternal lithium ingestion (a drug for manic-depressive illness). Flow defects such as coarctation of the aorta (1 in 2500 live births) are included in more than 50 syndromes listed by Winter and Baraitser (1998) and are seen in the sternal disruption-hemangioma sequence (140850)

that is usually sporadic. Absence of the entire atrial and ventricular septa (endocardial cushion defect, atrioventricular septal defect, atrioventricular canal) occurs in 1 in 6500 live births. Atrioventricular septal defect is associated with 21 different syndromes by Winter and Baraitser (1998), and can be associated with Dandy-Walker cyst (enlargement of the fourth ventricle within the brain) as an isolated defect (220200) or as part of the Ritscher-Schinzel syndrome (220210). Anomalous pulmonary venous return (1 in 2000 live births with more cases probably unrecognized) is rarely diagnosed in teratogenic syndromes but is listed in 33 associations and syndromes by Winter and Baraitser (1998). This anomaly, along with cardiac septal defects, occurs in the Holt-Oram syndrome (142900) of heart and limb defects and an X-linked pattern of Robin sequence with congenital dislocated hip (311900).

Cardiac defects of different mechanistic categories can occur in syndromes with altered situs (heterotaxy), including outflow tract and atrioventricular septal defects. When the cardiac situs (i.e., right superior vena cava and pulmonary artery, left pulmonary veins and aorta) matches the body situs (i.e., right liver, right appendix, and right three-lobed lung, left spleen, left colon, and left two-lobed lung), the person is normal and has situs inversus. When the cardiac situs is mismatched with the body situs (*heterotaxy* or different positions), then severe cyanosis and heart disease can ensue. X-linked recessive forms of heterotaxy (304750) have been documented where some individuals have heart defects only (e.g., tetralogy of Fallot) and others in the same family have heart defects plus midline liver and absent or multiple spleens (*polyasplenia*).

Study of inherited congenital heart defects has led to the definition of numerous genes involved in cardiac morphogenesis. A Mendelian form of supravalvular aortic stenosis (185500) was explained by mutations in the elastin gene on chromosome 7. Based on the high frequency of supravalvular aortic stenosis in the sporadic Williams syndrome (194050) of unknown etiology, a specific microdeletion of chromosome 7 that encompasses the elastin gene was defined (see Chapter 7). Current research is examining the role of elastin and other genes within the deletion on the pathogenesis of Williams syndrome, which includes interesting behavioral characteristics such as a happy affect, musical ability, and intense hearing (hyperacusis). Other genes such as the WT-1 tumor suppressor associated with Wilms tumor (194070) and the neurofibromin tumor suppressor associated with neurofibromatosis-1 (162200) have been associated with cardiac morphogenesis by finding anomalies in knock-out mice (Strauss and Johnson, 1996). As with coronary artery disease, the polygenic determination of most congenital heart anomalies has, through clinical phenotypes and molecular analysis, been related to specific genes of major effect. Such genes provide new diagnostic methods for patients with cardiac anomalies and syndromes and predict a better understanding of abnormal cardiac morphogenesis and its prevention.

Tracheoesophageal Fistula

Tracheoesophageal (TE) fistula represents a connection between the trachea and esophagus that is usually associated with respiratory and swallowing problems. The overall frequency is about 1 in 3000 live births. Several types of TE fistula occur, with 90% involving a blind esophageal pouch and distal connection of the esophagus and stomach to the trachea. Inspired air thus goes directly from trachea to gastrointestinal tract, and neonatal radiographs show a prominent, air-filled stomach. Affected infants drool copious saliva because of the blind esophageal ending, and a small amount of dye may be administered to visualize the esophageal pouch. Modern surgical techniques have changed TE fistula from a universally lethal anomaly to one with excellent survival when present in isolated form. More than one-half of cases are associated with other anomalies, accounting for a 10–15% mortality after surgical correction.

Common associations with TE fistula include cardiac anomalies (~30%), anal atresia (10–15%), vertebral defects (20–50%), and genitourinary defects (10–30%). Many of these are components of the VATER association (192350), which almost always occurs sporadically with minimal recurrence risk. TE fistula also occurs as a component of CHARGE association (214800) and the teratogenic syndrome produced when fetuses are exposed to high phenylalanine concentrations from their mothers with phenylketonuria (261600). Chromosomal syndromes such as trisomy 18 can include TE fistula, and tracheal or laryngeal defects are listed as components in more than 70 syndromes by Winter and Baraitser (1998). Those syndromes with TE fistula include Goldenhar (164210—usually sporadic), dyskeratosis congenita with hyperpigmented skin, bony changes, and mental deficiency (224230, 305000), and the Opitz BBB/G syndrome (145410) with laryngeal clefts, severe swallowing problems, and facial changes including hypertelorism. TE fistula also occurs in the Shprintzen/DiGeorge spectrum that can include patients with Opitz BBB/G syndrome, so testing for the characteristic microdeletion on chromosome 22 should be considered in some patients with TE fistula and multiple anomalies. The many syndromes associated with TE fistula emphasize the need for careful evaluation before proceeding with a fairly demanding operation.

▪ 13.5. NEUROSURGERY

Hydrocephalus

Hydrocephalus refers to an increase in size of the cerebral ventricular system compared to that of the surrounding brain substance. The incidence depends on how hydrocephalus is reported, because it often occurs as a secondary phenomenon after congenital or postnatal infections, intracranial bleeding as occurs frequently during prematurity, or congenital anomalies of the spinal cord like spina bifida. The overall frequency of about 3.5 per 1000 live births is thus reduced to 0.5 to 0.8 per 1000 when primary congenital forms of hydrocephalus are included. Hydrocephalus can also be separated into communicating forms with decreased absorption of cerebrospinal fluid (CSF) and noncommunicating forms with obstruction of fluid flow. Most congenital defects fall into the latter category.

As shown in Figure 13.4, isolated primary hydrocephalus is usually multifactorial with occasional Mendelian forms. X-linked aqueductal stenosis (307000) is often an alternative phenotype to the MASA syndrome (303350) of mental deficiency, aphasia, spasticity, and adducted thumbs caused by mutations in the L1CAM gene at chromosome band Xq28 (see Chapter 9). Abnormal expression of this cell adhesion molecule provides a framework for understanding the pathogenesis of hydrocephalus due to aqueductal stenosis (the aqueduct is a narrow opening between the third and fourth ventricles). Many anomaly associations can include hydrocephalus, and it is a common accessory finding in VATER association. Amniotic band disruptions may intefere with CSF circulation and produce hydrocephalus. Other associations include spina bifida, Goldenhar syndrome (164210) together with caudal defects called axial mesodermal dysplasia spectrum (Russell et al., 1981), and caudal regres-

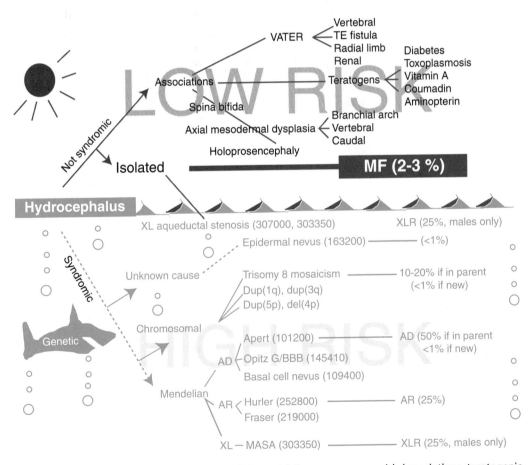

Figure 13.4. Causes of hydrocephalus. Conditions with lower recurrence risk (associations, teratogenic problems) are shown above, while rare but important genetic forms are shown below. AD, autosomal dominant; AR, autosomal recessive; XL, X-linked; XLR, X-linked recessive; MF, multifactorial determination.

sion (hypoplasia of the sacrum and lower limbs) together with brain anomalies such as holoprosencephaly.

Teratogenic syndromes include maternal diabetes, influenza, toxoplasmosis, vitamin A, Coumadin, and folic acid inhibitors (aminopterin, methotrexate), and many chromosomal disorders can include the anomaly (Fig. 13.4). Mendelian syndromes include many skeletal dysplasias exemplified by achondroplasia (100800), craniosynostosis syndromes exemplified by Apert syndrome (101200), metabolic disorders exemplified by Hurler syndrome (252800), and syndromes with midline defects exemplified by the Opitz G/BBB (145410) syndrome with laryngotracheal defects and hypertelorism. Winter and Baraitser (1998) list more than 250 syndromes with hydrocephalus.

The treatment of hydrocephalus is surgical and is aimed at preventing increased intracranial pressure due to the accumulation of cerebrospinal fluid. Shunts are placed between the ventricles and right atrium of the heart or the perioneum to allow for fluid drainage. Early recognition of hydrocephalus before pressure causes damage to cerebral structures, optic, or otic nerves is critical, but even early shunting is associated with significant disabilities at later ages. If children with spina bifida are excluded, those with hydrocephalus treated before age 3 months had decrements in IQ below 80 in about 30% and below 60 in 45–50%. Significant complications of some series have included spasticity typical of cerebral palsy in 30% and seizures in 50–60%. As with other anomalies discussed in this chapter, the prognosis of hydrocephalus is significantly changed when it is associated with other anomalies. Prenatal detection of hydrocephalus by ultrasound is increasingly frequent, and fetal surgery has been performed on more than 40 cases with improved postnatal survival. Complications such as seizures or spasticity have not been reduced by fetal surgery, perhaps because prenatal detection is biased toward more severe cases. As was the case for omphalocele, most cases detected prenatally are associated with additional anomalies and are not good candidates for surgery.

Spina Bifida

Spina bifida presents as a mass on the dorsal midline that represents extrusion of spinal cord tissue through a defect in the vertebral arches. Extrusion of the lining (meninges) alone is called meningocele, while extrusion of spinal cord with the meninges is called myelomeningocele and accounts for more than 90% of the anomalies. Spina bifida is one of several defects that occur along the neural tube present in the embryo at 3–5 weeks of gestation. Defects at the anterior end cause anencephaly and certain types of encephalocele, while defects along the middle and posterior end cause spina bifida at the level of the cervical (~4%), thoracic (~7.5%), thoracolumbar (~10%), lumbar (~40%), lumbosacral (~30%), or sacral (~8%) vertebrae. There are occult forms of spina bifida with absence of the vertebrae but without skin penetration above the skin, and there are rare anterior spina bifidas (~0.5%) that extrude into the abdominal cavity.

Most cases of spina bifida are isolated and exhibit multifactorial determination with female predominance (Table 13.1). The increased risk to relatives is not only for spina bifida, but also for other types of neural tube defects. The incidence of neural tube defects varies widely among ethnic groups. There are higher rates in certain areas of Britain and Ireland (6 per 1000 live births) and lower rates in the United States (1–2 per 1000 live births). Environmental factors such as socioeconomic status and nutrition are clearly important for the causation of neural tube defects, as emphasized by the lowered rates after perinatal vitamin supplementation. The spectrum of associated anomalies suggests that most neural tube defects are disruptions. Associations with amniotic bands, ectrodactylies (absent fingers), bladder exstrophy and gut atresias in the OIES association (*O*mphaloceles, bladder *E*xstrophy, *I*mperforate anus, *S*pina bifida, abnormal genitalia, renal anomalies, gut atresias; 258040,

Carey et al., 1978) and hemangiomas imply vascular disruptions as a cause. Spina bifida is also associated with omphalocele, cleft palate, and diaphragmatic hernia in the schisis association (Czeizel, 1981), and with teratogenic disorders such as the maternal diabetes, maternal hyperthermia, and maternal valproate syndromes.

Rare cases of isolated neural tube defects exhibit X-linked recessive inheritance (301410) rather than multifactorial determination. Relatively few syndromes include spina bifida, although it is occasionally present in the triploidy, trisomy 18, dup(3q), ring(22), and dup(11q) chromosomal syndromes (Schinzel, 1995). Mendelian disorders include the Lehman syndrome (166720) with a Marfanoid habitus and increased bone density; CHILD syndrome (308050) with asymmetric undergrowth, scaly skin, and skeletal anomalies; Goltz syndrome (305600) with skin, nail, and dental anomalies; and some cases of abnormal situs (heart, liver, spleen anomalies—see Table 13.3) that can exhibit X-linked inheritance (304570). Several mutant mouse strains with higher incidence of spina bifida have been defined, including the *splotch* phenotype that is caused by *Pax* gene mutations (see Chapter 9). One type of human Waardenburg syndrome (193500) also involves *PAX* gene mutations, and this condition can exhibit spina bifida.

Anencephaly is a lethal malformation and merits palliative care. The treatment of spina bifida is surgical, but the selection of patients and timing of surgery is controversial. When the defect is low (toward the sacrum), small, and not associated with other anomalies, the outcome is excellent. Higher and larger degrees of spina bifida will cause complications after surgery, including urinary incontinence and chronic bladder infections due to paralysis, lower limb dysfunction without ambulation, secondary hydrocephalus with need for shunting, and developmental disability. Some authors recommend selection of patients with reasonable prognosis for operation while others suggest this is unnecessary or unethical.

Representative figures for children with moderate severity of spina bifida show that 86% survive, 87% achieve urinary continence, 54% can walk, and 73% have normal development (McLone, 1983). Longer periods of follow-up may give less optimistic figures with 41% dying by age 16 years, 32% having mental disability, 51% confined to a wheelchair, and 12% having no handicap (Hunt, 1990). Although nonneural anomalies are not commonly associated with spina bifida, brain imaging in these patients has revealed brain anomalies such as migration defects, cerebellar hypoplasia, and agenesis of the corpus callosum in addition to the usual hydrocephalus. Such anomalies may be additional factors influencing outcome that can be predicted by brain imaging prior to surgery (Hunter, 1993).

Patients with spina bifida should be managed by a multidisciplinary team that includes developmental pediatricians, neurosurgeons, rehabilitative medicine specialists, urologists, and allied care providers (occupational, physical, and speech therapists). Genetic counseling for the 3–5% recurrence risks in isolated cases is important because the defect can be truly prevented and detected by various means of prenatal diagnosis. Prevention requires preconceptional supplementation with folic acid, usually as a mixture of other multivitamins. Supplements should be begun before attempting pregnancy because of the early gestational timing of neural tube defects. Prenatal detection is by maternal serum or amniotic fluid alpha-fetoprotein as discussed in Chapter 15.

■ 13.6. ORTHOPEDIC SURGERY

Clubfoot

Talipes equinovarus or clubfoot can be an intrinsic malformation or a deformation produced by intrauterine constraint or fetal immobility. The anomaly is obvious at birth, with the foot being deviated inwards (varus position) and extended downwards so that the toes are beneath the heel (equinus like the horse). The frequency is 1–2 per 1000 live births, with a 2:1 preponderance of males over females. Associated malformations occur in 10–20% of cases, with spina bifida being the most common association. Isolated clubfoot malformation exhibits multifactorial determination with a 2–3% recurrence risk for primary relatives.

Syndromes include trisomy 13/18, *cri-du-chat*, and Mendelian conditions that produce severe in utero hypotonia such as Zellweger syndrome (214100). More than 250 associations and syndromes that include clubfoot are listed by Winter and Baraitser (1996), including those associated with exposure to folic acid inhibitors (methotrexate), valproic acid, and thalidomide. Syndromes with joint laxity (e.g., Larsen syndrome, 150250, 245600), skeletal dysplasia (e.g., dyssegmental dysplasia, 224400) or multiple joint contractures (e.g., Pena-Shokeir syndrome, 208150) can include clubfoot in addition to those with severe hypotonia or spina bifida as mentioned previously.

Early treatment is important for clubfoot, as deformations can become more rigid and painful to manipulate. True malformations require surgery, with laceration and realignment of the connective tissue structures. Splints and special shoes can be used for milder deformations, as well as during the rehabilitation after corrective surgery. Therapy of clubfoot secondary to nerve paralysis, as with spina bifida, is more difficult and protracted. As for most other anomalies discussed in this chapter, isolated clubfoot has an excellent outcome and low recurrence risk. Exclusion or documentation of associated anomalies is thus crucial for proper management.

Congenital Hip Dislocation

Dislocation exists when the femoral heads can be manipulated outside of the acetabulum (the hip cavity articulating with the femoral head). Congenital hip dislocation can be mild, detected by manipulation in the newborn period, or severe with subluxation of the femoral head outside and behind the acetabulum. Severe cases often involve some degree of acetabular deformity (acetabular dysplasia). Congenital hip dislocation with subluxation implies prenatal dislocation and is much more difficult to treat.

The incidence of congenital dislocation of the hip depends on the thoroughness of neonatal examinations, but is generally estimated to be 1 in 1000. Multifactorial determination is suspected in most isolated cases, consistent with the 3:1 preponderance in females. The recurrence risk for isolated congenital dislocated hip is between 2–5%, with relatives of affected males being at the higher range.

Syndromes that interfere with fetal movement are common causes of congenital dislocated hip, just as they are for clubfoot. Autosomal dominant conditions with congenital dislocated hip include Larsen syndrome (150250) with cleft palate and joint laxity; Marfan syndrome (154700) with severe childhood presentation; and Freeman-Sheldon (whistling face—193700) with arthrogyposis and puckered lips. Autosomal recessive conditions include Antley-Bixler syndrome (207410) with craniosynostosis; Cohen syndrome (216550) with pleasant personality, obesity, and prominent incisors; and familial dysautonomia (223900) with sensory nerve dysfunction and pain insensitivity. Many metabolic disorders with neural or skeletal dysfunction can include congenital dislocated hip, as illustrated by Hurler syndrome (252800). X-linked disorders include Taybi syndrome (311300) with prominent forehead, broad thumbs, and digital anomalies. Associations include clubfoot and exposures to teratogens such as Dilantin or thalidomide. There is also a strong association with breech delivery (25% versus 0.7% for cephalic births in similar case series), and with infant swaddling in appropriate cultures.

Early detection is useful in dislocated hip but neonatal screening programs have not been effective. Experience of the examiner is crucial, because the Ortolani and Barlow signs require subjective interpretation. The Ortalani maneuver extends the hips outward while palpating for a "click" at the acetabular joint. The Barlow maneuver stabilizes one hip while the other is pulled toward the examiner to assess its freedom to move out of the acetabulum. Infants with hypotonia, arthrogryposis, or skeletal dysplasia should be examined carefully for congenital dislocation of the hip. An abnormal hip examination can be followed by orthopedic specialists, with more obvious dislocations requiring bracing (e.g., triple diapers) or immobilization in the flexed and reduced position with casts. Prenatal dislocations with subluxation usually require surgical reduction and prolonged therapy.

Limb Deficiencies

Orthopedic surgeons have an extremely important role in the recognition and treatment of children with limb deficiencies. Many of these children have short limbs caused by teratogenic drugs such as thalidomide or more than 100 genetic types of skeletal dysplasia. Others have absent or missing parts of limbs, a group of anomalies sometimes called limb reduction defects. Limb deficiency is a more accurate term that incorporates both absence and size reduction of the 120 human limb bones, and this group of anomalies is discussed here. Descriptive terms such as amelia (absence of limbs), hemimelia (medial or lateral limb rays), acheiria or apodia (absences of hands or feet), adactyly (absence of fingers), or phocomelia (absence of middle limb segments with retention of distal segments) are often encountered with limb deficiencies. Meromelia is a more inclusive term that contrasts with amelia and refers to any partial absence of a limb.

The incidence of limb deficiencies has been particularly well documented by a large study of over 1 million live births in British Columbia over 18 years (Froster-Iskenius and Baird, 1989). Recognizable syndromes or cases with relevant teratogenic exposures were excluded from this study. Among the 659 cases with limb deficiencies (6.0 per 10,000 live births), 3.4 per 1000 only affected the upper limbs and 1.1 per 10,000 the lower limbs. A comparison of this epidemiologic survey of limb deficiencies to Mendelian syndromes including limb

deficiencies allows some interesting conclusions to be drawn regarding skeletal birth defects. Data on Mendelian syndromes that include limb deficiencies (Wilson, 1998) were drawn from a survey of Mendelian Inheritance of Man (McKusick, 1994).

There are 80 autosomal dominant, 85 autosomal recessive, and 7 X-linked limb deficiency disorders listed by McKusick (1994), with an additional 32 being of uncertain inheritance. Upper limb deficiencies are more predominant in the epidemiologic survey (57%) as opposed to the genetic database (32%), with 61% of the genetic disorders involving upper and lower limbs as opposed to 16% of the birth registry cases. This correlates with the rarity of unilateral involvement in genetic disorders (2%) as opposed to 86% of the birth registry cases. One would expect mutant genes to act equally on the four limb buds. The proportionate involvement of limb segments is very similar between the birth registry and genetic cases (e.g., humerus 1.5, radius-ulna 16.5, hand 39% of birth registry cases; humerus 2.9, radius-ulna 19.3, hand 33% of genetic disorders). Absence of the hands was rarely included in Mendelian syndromes, while complete amelias were more common (5.4% of Mendelian syndromes versus 2.5% of survey cases.

When excluded syndromic cases of limb deficiencies in the epidemiologic survey were reviewed, more than 50% of the limb deficiencies observed over the 18-year period were associated with anomalies outside of the skeletal system. Deficiencies involving the radius and humerus were most likely to be syndromic in the epidemiologic survey, and these bones were more often deficient in Mendelian syndromes. Aplasia or hypoplasia of the radius with inward deviation (club hand) is particularly worrisome for syndromic involvement. Radial aplasia is present in the VATER association; Baller-Gerold syndrome (218600) with craniosynostosis; Okihiro syndrome (126800) with eye anomalies; Goldenhar syndrome (164210) with branchial arch, heart, and vertebral defects; Holt-Oram syndrome (142900) with heart defects; Juberg-Hayward syndrome (216100) with cleft palate and microcephaly; Nager syndrome (154400) with branchial arch and heart defects; and thrombocytopenia-absent radius syndrome (274000). It is also present in teratogenic syndromes caused by co-caine, valproate, thalidomide, and vitamin A (Winter and Baraitser, 1998).

Other Mendelian syndromes causing limb deficiencies include the Roberts syndrome (268300) with amelia, phocomelia, or radial aplasia plus microcephaly and cleft lip/palate; the Antley-Bixler syndrome (207410) with hypoplastic humeri, radiohumeral synostosis, craniosynostosis, and choanal atresia; Adams-Oliver syndrome (100300) with limb deficiencies of the lower legs, feet, hands or digits combined with cutis aplasia of the scalp, eye, and renal anomalies; Fanconi syndrome (227650) with radial aplasia or thumb anomalies combined with congenital hip dislocation, pancytopenia, cardiac anomalies, urogenital anomalies, and predisposition to leukemia.

This comparison of epidemiologic and genetic syndrome data should illustrate how the distribution and location of certain birth defects can be utilized to estimate the likelihood of associated anomalies. Once the type of limb deficiency is defined by physical examination and radiographic skeletal survey, potential associations and syndromes can be ascertained in textbooks or databases to allow appropriate evaluation and preventive management. Orthopedic management of limb deficiencies can include braces, prostheses, and bone lengthening procedures that ameliorate or correct the deficiency in many children (Herring and Birch, 1998). Genetic limb deficiencies are being investigated with knowledge of molecules involved in limb bud development (see Chapter 9), and disorders such as Holt-Oram syndrome have now been matched with the responsible genes. The ability to fracture limbs and stretch them to grow new bone via the Alizaroff procedure, coupled with molecular knowledge of limb growth regulators, points toward a future therapy of limb deficiencies where regeneration exceeds replacement.

■ 13.7. UROLOGY

Hypospadias/Ambiguous Genitalia

Hypospadias refers to displacement of the urethral opening toward the ventral surface or base of the penis (Fig. 13.5). Hypospadias varies in severity, reaching the glans (first degree), penile base (second degree), or the scrotum and perineum (third degree). The incidence is 4–5 per 1000 live births, with the majority being mild or first degree cases. Glandular hypospadias may be missed at birth and detected because of a deviated urinary stream (McGillivray, 1993). Isolated hypospadias is usually multifactorially determined with a rather high 9–10% recurrence risk. The high recurrence risk reflects the high frequency of the anomaly as well as genetic disorders of sex differentiation that are discussed in the following paragraphs (Fig. 13.5, Table 13.4). Associated anomalies are detected in about 10% of isolated hypospadias, including particularly those of the genitourinary system.

More than 150 associations and syndromes that include hypospadias are listed by Winter and Baraitser (1998), including those caused by teratogens such as thalidomide, valproate, trimethadione, and propylthiouracil (Table 13.4). The Smith-Lemli-Opitz syndrome (270400) includes hypospadias or complete sex reversal due to a defect in cholesterol metabolism (see Chapter 9). More isolated defects of sex differentiation also derive from defects in the conversion of cholesterol to sex steroid hormones (Fig. 13.5).

Hypospadias together with chordee (bending of the penis) and/or cryptorchidism (undescended testes) is most often a sign of incomplete genital development in a genetic (46,XY) male. Occasionally, however, it is an important sign of ambiguous genitalia as in genetic (46,XX) females exposed in utero to elevated steroid hormone intermediates. Figure 13.5 illustrates the major pathways for sex steroid synthesis from cholesterol. Five enzymes convert cholesterol to feminizing hormones (estrogens) such as progesterone and estrogen

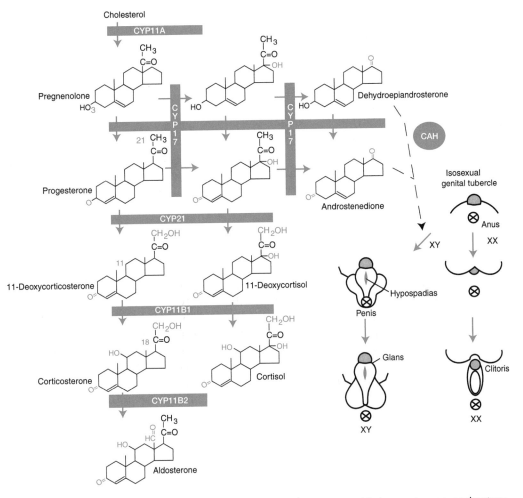

Figure 13.5. Major steps in the conversion of cholesterol to sex steroids (progesterone, androstene-dione) and mineralocorticoids (aldosterone) in the adrenal gland. Blocks in the 3βHSD (3-β-hydroxys-teroid dehydrogenase), CYP 21 (21-hydroxylase), or CYP11 (11-β- or 18-hydroxylase) can cause congenital adrenal hyperplasia (CAH) with diversion of steroid synthesis to produce excess androgens (e.g., androstenedione). Androgens such as dihydrotestosterone or testosterone convert the isosexual fetal gonad to male external genitalia (right side). Androgen synthesis is normally directed by the SRY transcription factor on the Y chromosome.

or virilizing hormones (androgens) such as androstenedione and testosterone. These same pathways produce cortisol that acts to maintain glucose levels among many other functions, and aldosterone that regulates salt retention by the kidney for maintenance of normal serum electrolytes and blood pressure. Blocks in various parts of this steroidogenesis pathway can produce deficiencies and elevations in various sex or corticoid hormones. Several defects can

■TABLE 13.4. Syndromes with Hypospadias and Ambiguous Genitalia

Anomaly or Enzyme Defect	Phenotype	Syndromes or Disease
Hypospadias (MF) 　AD form (146450) 　AR form (241750)	First degree (glans) Second degree (shaft) Third degree (perineum)	Opitz (145110) WAGR (194070) Acrocallosal (200990) McKusick-Kaufman (226700) Smith-Lemli-Opitz (270400) Shprintzen (C, 192430) Dup(1p), dup(3q), del(4q)—C X/XY mosaicism, Y aberrations—C
CYP11A 20,22-desmolase 　15q23-q24	Female internal and external 　genitalia	Lipoid CAH (201710)
3β-HSB (hydroxysteroid de 　hydrogenase) 1p13.1	Male or female pseudoH	Salt-losing CAH (210810)
CYP17 17α-hydroxylase 10q24-q25	Male pseudoH	Hypertensive CAH (202110)
CYP21 21-hydroxylase 6p21	Female pseudoH	Virilizing and salt-losing CAH 　(201910)
CYP11B1, CYP11B2 11β-hydroxylase 18-hydroxylase 8q22	Female pseudoH	Hypertensive, virilizing CAH 　(202010)
5α-reductase-2 5p15	Female external genitalia 　(third degree hypospadias) Male internal genitalia	Steroid 5α-reductase deficiency 　(264600)
Androgen receptor Xq1.1	Female external and internal 　genitalia	Testicular feminization (313700)
Androgen receptor Xq1.1	Female external genitalia 　(third degree hypospadias) Male internal genitalia	Reifenstein syndrome (312300)
Androgen receptor Xq1.1	Male internal and external 　genitalia Decreased spermatogenesis	Infertile male syndrome (308370)
SRY mutations Yp	Female genitalia	Pure gonadal dysgenesis 　(XY sex reversal)
Y/X translocations	Male genitalia	XX sex reversal 　(SRY translocated to X)

Sources: Donahue et al. (1995); Griffin et al. (1995).

Notes: MF, multifactorial; AD, autosomal dominant; AR, autosomal recessive; 8q22, chromosome 8 band q22; pseudoH, pseudohermaphrotidism; WAGR, Wilms tumor, aniridia, genital defect, retardation; CAH, congenital adenal hyperplasia.

result in congenital adrenal hyperplasias with mild or severe hypospadias with accessory changes.

The right side of Figure 13.5 illustrates the external genitalia of an isosexual embryo like that found in embryos up to 6–7 weeks of gestation. After this time, female sexual differentiation is the default pathway unless testes form under the direction of the SRY (sex-determining region on Y) transcription factor that is en-coded by a locus on the Y chromosome short arm (Table 13.4). Testis formation produces testosterone and dihydrotestosterone that are responsible for external conversion of the genital tubercle into penis and testes, and internal conversion of urogenital ducts into the vas deferens. Several events must occur before default female genital development is diverted to that of a male—inheritance of a normal Y chromosome containing SRY, steroidogenesis with production of testosterone, synthesis of dihydrotestosterone by 5α-reductase enzyme, and action of these hormones on the X chromosome-encoded androgen receptor. The resulting normal female appearance in a genetic male is called complete sex reversal. Apparent sex reversal can occur in females who carry a small piece of the Y-chromosome (including the SRY region) on their X chromosome due to translocation (Table 13.4).

Sex reversal should not be confused with hermaphroditism, a rare disorder associated with XX/XY mosaicism and other causes that produces combinations of ovarian and testicular tissue in the same individual.

In addition to complete sex reversal, partial defects in androgen synthesis or androgen receptors can produce males with incomplete genital development that present with hypospadias or infertility (Table 13.4). Blocks in adrenal steroid synthesis cause partial defects in male development because of their resulting excesses or deficiencies of steroid hormones (Fig. 13.5). Blocks in steroid synthesis can also lead to masculinization of females due to excesses of androgens. These disorders are called congenital adrenal hyperplasias because they produce enlarged adrenal glands due to feedback stimulation from the pituitary. Depending on the particular enzyme deficiency and the sex of the individual, congenital adrenal hyperplasias have several presentations. These can include virilization of a female (female pseudohermaphroditism), inadequate genital development in a male (male pseudohermaphroditism), deficiencies of cortisol with hypoglycemia, deficiency of aldosterone to cause salt wasting with depletion of electolytes and dehydration, or increased blood pressure (Fig. 13.5; Table 13.4). Although most types of congenital adrenal hyperplasia present in the newborn period, milder forms can present as hypertension or abnormal genitalia recognized later in life. Precocious puberty often occurs in these milder forms, facilitating the examination and recognition of abnormal genitalia.

Surgical correction of hypospadias is effective and associated with little morbidity. However, the associated sexual disorders make the preoperative evaluation of hypospadias even more important than that for other congenital anomalies discussed in this chapter. If hypoglycemia and salt wasting are not recognized and treated, the child will expire from hypotensive shock. When second or third degree hypospadias is present, particularly when associated with chordee or undescended testes, the genitalia may be sufficiently ambiguous to prevent sex assignment. Because recognition of sex is a pivotal birth event, the child with ambiguous genitalia is as much of a medical emergency as the child with salt wasting and hypoglycemia. Both types of children require a thorough diagnostic evaluation for the disorders listed in Table 13.4. Initial laboratory data may include glucose and electrolyte levels, a karyotype to determine genetic sex, levels of estrogen and androgen hormones, and imaging studies of the internal genitalia.

Once recognized, the treatment of hormone and electrolyte abnormalities in children with congenital adrenal hyperplasia is straightforward. As discussed in Chapter 12, neonatal screening for congenital adrenal hyperplasia is performed in many states to ensure prompt diagnosis and treatment. However, the charged decision of sex assignment makes the management of ambiguous genitalia more complex. In many medical centers, a multidisciplinary team of urologists, endocrinologists, and geneticists are convened to make this decision. Sex assignment should be as early as possible to foster parental identification and bonding, but should never be made cavalierly or without necessary studies. Sexually neutral names such as Lynn may be suggested to anxious families, and supportive counseling by nursing, social work, genetic counseling, and pastoral staff is important. Often the nexus is the size of the phallus or clitoris. Hypospadias repair or vaginoplasty is more technically feasible than creating an erectile penis. (See the problem set for new information on this ethical dilemma).

Because many disorders of sex differentiation are autosomal or X-linked recessive, genetic counseling is extremely important for these families. A novel aspect of this counseling is prenatal treatment to prevent virilization in certain forms of congenital adrenal hyperplasia. For women at risk for a second child with 21-hydroxylase deficiency (Table 13.4), early prenatal treatment with dexamethasone can suppress steroidogenesis and prevent the secretion of excess androgens like androstenedione (Fig. 13.5). Prenatal diagnosis is then performed at 14–16 weeks of gestation to determine fetal sex. Treatment is stopped for male fetuses, but continued for female fetuses to prevent virilization of their external genitalia (see Chapter 15).

Urinary Tract Anomalies

Anomalies of the urethra, bladder, ureters, and kidney are estimated to occur in 10% of the population, and in 2–6% of children under age 12 (Van Allen, 1993). The obstruction of urinary flow is associated with dilation of the ureters (hydronephrosis) and is damaging to the kidney when it occurs prenatally or postnatally. More than 70% of urinary tract anomalies occur in associations or syndromes. Alertness for urologic anomalies is important because of their subtle presentations, their amelioration by timely management, and their predictive value for associations or syndromes. Table 13.5 lists some physical findings that indicate a higher risk for urinary tract anomalies.

Atresia or agenesis of the ureter can produce a grotesquely abnormal fetus due to engorgement of the bladder (megacystis). If a fistula forms around the urethral obstruction, the bladder may decompress and cause the prune belly anomaly with loose abdominal musculature and redundant skin. Because pressure from urinary retention will damage and destroy the fetal kidneys, all neonates with megacystis and at least one-third with prune belly die. The anomaly is rare, slightly more common in males, and associated with a low recurrence risk appropriate for sporadic occurrence (Table 13.5). The Meckel-Gruber syndrome (249100) with encephalocele, polydactyly, and cystic liver and kidneys can include urethral atresia.

■**TABLE 13.5. Physical Findings Suggestive of Urinary Tract Anomalies**

Fetal and neonatal

Oligohydramnios
Anuria, oliguria
High anal atresia
Ambiguous genitalia
Exstrophy of the bladder
Prune belly
Supernumerary nipples

Later childhood

Aniridia, hemihypertrophy
Poor urinary stream
Persistent wetness
Polydipsia, polyuria

Childhood and adult

Polydipsia, polyuria
Recurrent urinary tract infection
Hypertension

Source: Van Allen (1993).

Posterior urethral valves are folds of tissue that obstruct the outflow of urine from the bladder. They almost always occur in males where they have an incidence of 1.5–2 per 10,000 male births. Posterior urethral valves may present during fetal life with oligohydramnios, or in the first year of life with failure to thrive, abdominal mass, weak urinary stream, or recurrent urinary tract infections (Allen, 1993). They have similar associations as documented for urethral agenesis (Table 13.6), but can also occur in the VATER association. Posterior urethal valves occur in several syndromes, including the McKusick-Kaufman syndrome (236700) of uterine anomalies, polydactyly, and cardiac disease. The success of surgical treatment depends on the presence of associated anomalies and the degree of renal damage. When the anomaly is isolated and recognized early, simple instrumentation of the urethra to remove the valves is curative. Later recognized or more severe obstructions may be associated with significant frequencies of renal failure when the children

■ **TABLE 13.6.** Urinary Tract Anomalies: Isolated, Associated, and Syndromic

Isolated Anomaly	Associations	Syndromes
Urethral atresia (S)	Potter sequence (S) Urorectal septum defects (S) Caudal regression (S) Cocaine (T)	Meckel-Gruber (249100)
Posterior urethral valves (S)	Potter sequence (S) Urorectal septum defects (S) Caudal regression (S) VATER association (S)	Townes-Brocks (107480) Neurofibromatosis (162200) Rubinstein-Taybi (C, 268600)
Renal agenesis (MF)	Maternal diabetes (T) Cocaine (T) CHARGE, MURCS, VATER associations (S) Klippel-Feil (S, 148680)	Brachmann-de Lange (S) Fanconi (227650) Kallman (147950, 308700) Kouseff (245210) Roberts (268300) Del(4p), trisomy 21 (C)
Renal dysplasia (MF)	Neural tube defects (MF) Sirenomelia (S) Prune belly anomaly (S) MURCS, VATER(S) Maternal diabetes (T) Alcohol, rubella (T)	Perlman (267000) Simpson-Golabi-Behmel (312870) McKusick-Kaufman (236700) Fanconi (227650) Kallman (147950, 308700) Trisomy 7, trisomy 13 (C)

Notes: MF, multifactorial; T, teratogenic; S, sporadic; C, chromosomal; CHARGE, coloboma, heart defects, atresia choanae, retardation, genital defects, ear defects; MURCS, mullerian (uterine) derivatives, renal, cervical somite anomalies; VATER, vertebral, anorectal, tracheoesophageal, radial, and renal defects.

reach adulthood. Fetuses with lung hypoplasia may require extensive respiratory support and repeated surgeries with multiple complications. Fetal surgery has been attempted in select cases (see Chapter 15).

Renal agenesis has been discussed with regard to the Potter sequence in Chapter 11. When bilateral, renal agenesis is lethal due to its effects on lung development in utero. When unilateral, it is usually detected as a chance finding on surgery or autopsy. The incidence of unilateral renal agenesis is 1–2 per 1000 live births based on autopsy series (Van Allen, 1993). The incidence of bilateral disease is harder to estimate, but it does occur in about 1 in 250 fetal or early infantile autopsies. Isolated renal agenesis seems to obey the multifactorial model with a recurrence risk of 4–5% for a renal anomaly. This risk was obtained by performing renal ultrasounds on relatives, and suggests similar management be considered for new cases with asymptomatic parents or siblings. The overall risk for urogenital anomalies in these patients was even higher at 9–10%.

Renal agenesis may occur in infants of diabetic mothers or in offspring of those exposed to cocaine or thalidomide. The sequence of decreased fetal urine, oligohydramnios, pulmonary hypoplasia, and compression anomalies of the face, skin, and feet (clubfeet) is well recognized (Potter sequence). Renal agenesis can be part of the CHARGE, MURCS, and VATER associations, and occurs in the sirenomelia (mermaid) anomaly as well as the early body wall disruptions that lead to severe fetal anomalies. Syndromic disorders with renal agenesis are many and include the Brachmann-de Lange syndrome with unusual face, growth delay, and limb anomalies; the Fanconi syndrome (227650) with pancytopenia and thumb anomalies; and the Roberts syndrome (268300) of severe limb anomalies.

Renal dysplasias result from abnormalities of the primitive embryonic kidney, the metanephros. Histology of the abnormal kidney shows disorganized primitive ducts and cartilage. The irregular nature of the differentiation distinguishes renal dysplasias from renal cystic diseases that are discussed in Chapter 14. The cysts in dysplastic kidneys are often irregular (multicystic kidneys) in contrast to the fine honeycombing pattern in cystic kidneys.

The incidence of renal dysplasia is about 0.7 per 10,000, and the anomaly exhibits multifactorial determination with a 3–4% recurrence risk. As with renal agenesis, the risk for all types of urinary tract anomalies is also increased to 9% in relatives of affected individuals. Teratogens causing renal dysplasia include alcohol, maternal diabetes, and thalidomide. The MURCS and VATER associations also include renal dysplasias, as do neural tube defects, anomalies of the urorectal septum, prune belly anomaly, and sirenomelia. Involved syndromes include overgrowth disorders such as the Perlman (267000) or Simpson-Golabi-Behmel (312870) syndromes. The risks for urinary tract anomalies mentioned previously for Smith-Lemli-Opitz, Fanconi, and McKusick-Kaufman syndromes also include renal dysplasia (Table 13.6). Surgical considerations for renal dysplasia, like those for posterior urethal valves, depend on the extent of renal damage and presence of associated anomalies. Unilateral renal dysplasias do not require surgery in the absence of recurrent urinary tract infections.

■ 13.8. CANCER SURGERY

Cancer surgery is another large contribution to the work of surgeons, extending much more into adult medicine than does the typical correction of congenital anomalies. Chapter 9 discussed the radical change in perception of cancer as a genetic disease that has accompanied

the revolution in molecular technology. Although every cancer involves genetic changes, hereditable aspects of cancer are relatively small compared to the vast impact of environment and aging. Nevertheless, specific cancers must be evaluated for the possibility of genetic causation in the same way that congenital anomalies are evaluated for associated malformations that may indicate genetic syndromes.

As with a congenital anomaly, the management of a tumor mass may be changed by its presence in a genetic syndrome. Tumors in neurofibromatosis (162200), for example, are almost always benign. Resection is rarely required unless they cause dysfunction by impinging on neighboring tissues (malignant by position). An example is the pheochromocytoma that occurs in this condition, causing severe hypertension unless it is resected.

Tumors in adenomatous polyposis coli (175100), on the other hand, are almost always malignant. The transformation of polyps into colon cancer is so frequent in this syndrome that prophylatic colectomy is usually required. While rare, the cancer syndromes listed in Table 9.6 are important to bear in mind when evaluating tumors in various body regions. Recognition of the cancer syndrome is essential for planning operative management and for genetic counseling. Because many of these disorders present during adulthood, and because surgeons often function as part of a multidisciplinary cancer team, more detailed discussion and additional examples of cancer-prone disease are provided in Chapter 14.

PROBLEM SET 13
Genetics in the Surgical Specialties

Respond to the following questions with short answers, consulting Tables 13.1–13.6 or Figs. 13.1–13.5. For each clinical presentation, discuss the genetic evaluation, possible diagnoses, and potential recurrence risks for the family:

13.1. A newborn presents with anal atresia and cyanosis (bluish lips and face). The physical examination and radiographic studies suggest the presence of high anal atresia and a congenital heart defect.

13.2. A 1-month-old child presents to the ophthalmology clinic with bilateral cataracts. The parents are new immigrants and the pregnancy and neonatal histories are not documented.

13.3. A newborn presents with severe respiratory distress and is thought to have a diaphragmatic hernia. Physical examination reveals no other major or minor anomalies.

13.4. A 12-year-old female is noted to have short stature and hypertension. A cardiac evaluation reveals coarctation of the aorta.

13.5. A 1-year-old male presents with a dribbling urinary stream and is found to have severe hypospadias.

13.6. A 3-year-old female is hospitalized because of high fever and urinary tract infection. She is noted to have extra nipples on examination, but no other anomalies.

13.7. A newborn is noted to have anophthalmia and digital anomalies consisting of syndactyly (fused fingers) and oligodactyly (missing fingers).

13.8. A newborn is noted to have an omphalocele with a large birth weight, hypoglycemia, large organs, and unusual creases behind the ears.

13.9. A newborn presents with bilateral cleft lip and palate. There are numerous other anomalies including microphthalmia (small eyes), polydactyly (extra fingers), and micropenis with chordee.

13.10. One of presumed monozygotic twin boys begins projectile vomiting after each feeding when he is two weeks old. No major or minor anomalies are noted on physical examination.

PROBLEM SET 13
Answers

13.1–13.10. See Solutions

PROBLEM SET 13
Solutions

13.1. The two major anomalies of anal atresia and a congenital heart defect suggest an association or a syndrome. The VATER or VACTERL association with vertebral, anorectal, cardiac, tracheoesophageal (TE) fistula, renal, and limb defects is a possibility, and evaluation for the other characteristic defects is necessary. If minor anomalies like single palmar crease were also noted, a karyotype would be mandatory. Possible etiologies include VATER association (sporadic with < 1% recurrence risk), trisomy 18 or partial trisomy 22 (1 % recurrence risk if trisomy, higher 5–15% if parental translocation), or a Mendelian disorder such as FG syndrome with a possible 25% recurrence risk (Fig. 13.2).

13.2. Bilateral cataracts may be caused by teratogens such as rubella virus, metabolic disorders such as galactosemia, or syndromes with eye anomalies such as Nance-Horan syndrome (302350). The lack of neonatal history mandates that galactosemia be excluded by looking for reducing substances in the urine (see Chapter 12). The presence of deafness and skeletal anomalies might suggest teratogenesis by rubella virus, while other anomalies would require a karytype to exclude chromosome disorders (Table 13.2). Even when isolated, bilateral cataracts can exhibit Mendelian inheritance with a maximal 25% recurrence risk.

13.3. Isolated diaphragmatic hernia is a sporadic event with a < 1% recurrence risk. The anomaly can be associated with hypoplastic lungs, which will be critical in assessing the newborn's prognosis for surgical correction (Fig. 13.1).

13.4. Short stature and coarctation of the aorta in a female suggest the presence of Turner syndrome. A chromosome study looking for the characteristic 45,X karyotype should be documented. The recurrence risk for the parents would be < 1%, and the child would be infertile.

13.5. Isolated hypospadias exhibits multifactorial determination with a 9–10% recurrence risk. Careful evaluation of the infant for other genital anomalies (e.g., cryptorchidism or undescended testes) is needed to rule out incomplete masculinization due to congenital adrenal hyperplasia or other disorder of sex differentiation (Fig. 13.5).

13.6. Extra or supernumerary nipples are associated with urinary tract anomalies, as are urinary tract infections. Radiographic studies of the urinary tract are indicated in this child, since undetected anomalies with recurrent infection may lead to renal failure. Isolated renal tract anomalies may result from multifactorial etiology with significant (5–10%) recurrence risks (Tables 13.5, 13.6).

13.7. Two unusual anomalies such as anophthalmia and syndactyly suggest a syndrome, and chromosome studies will be needed. A likely diagnosis is the Waardenburg anophthalmia syndrome (206920) that predicts a 25% recurrence risk (Table 13.2). This Waardenburg syndrome is different than that associated with *PAX* gene defects (see Chapter 9).

13.8. The omphalocele together with other anomalies suggests a syndrome, and the findings are typical of Wiedemann-Beckwith syndrome (130650). Although its McKusick number implies autosomal dominant inheritance, Wiedemann-Beckwith syndrome is probably a disorder of imprinting resulting from aneuploidy or uniparental disomy for a region of chromosome 11 (see Chapter 10).

13.9. The findings suggest trisomy 13 and mandate a karyotype (Fig. 13.3).

13.10. Projectile vomiting in a male infant suggests a diagnosis of pyloric stenosis with a 2.4–5.5% recurrence risk for the next child to be affected depending on whether it is a boy or girl. The twin will be at even higher risk for concordance (30–40%) and requires careful monitoring for symptoms. Examination to exclude other anomalies is important, because several chromosomal or malformation syndromes can include pyloric stenosis.

BIBLIOGRAPHY

General References

Gorlin RJ, Cohen MM Jr, Levin LS. 1990. *Syndromes of the Head and Neck.* New York: Oxford.

Jones KL. 1997. *Smith's Recognizable Patterns of Human Malformation.* Philadelphia: WB Saunders.

McKusick VA. 1994. *Mendelian Inheritance in Man,* 11th ed. Baltimore: Johns Hopkins; online at http://www3.ncbi.nlm.nih.gov/omim.

Rimoin DL, Emery AEH, Pyeritz R. 1995. *Principles and Practice of Medical Genetics.* Edinburgh: Churchill Livingstone.

Schinzel A. 1995. *Catalogue of Unbalanced Chromosome Aberrations in Man,* 2nd ed. Berlin: de Gruyter.

Stevenson RE, Hall JG, Goodman RM. 1993. *Human Malformations and Related Anomalies.* New York: Oxford University Press.

Winter RM, Baraitser M. 1998. *London Dysmorphology Database,* Vers. 3.0. Oxford: Oxford University Press.

General Pediatric Surgery

Cantrell JR, Haller JA, Ravitsch MA. 1958. A syndrome of congenital defects involving the abdominal wall, sternum, diaphragm, pericardium and heart. *Surg Gynecol Obstet* 28:602–614.

Cunniff C, Jones KL, Jones MC. 1990. Patterns of malformation in children with congenital diaphragmatic defects. *J Pediatr* 116:258–261.

Czeizel A. 1981. Schisis-association. *Am J Med Genet* 10:25–35.

Donahue PA, Parker K, Migeon CJ. 1995. Congenital adrenal hyperplasia. In Scriver CR, Beaudet AL, Sly WS, Valle D, eds. *The Metabolic and Molecular Bases of Inherited Disease.* 7th ed, New York: McGraw-Hill, pp. 2929–66.

Gordon H, Davies D, Berman MM. 1969. Camptodactyly, cleft palate and club foot. A syndrome showing autosomal dominant pattern of inheritance. *J Med Genet* 6:266–274.

Griffin JE, McPhaul MJ, Russell DW, Wilson JD. 1995. The androgen resistance syndromes: steroid 5α-reductase 2 deficiency, testicular feminization, and related disorders. In Scriver CR, Beaudet AL, Sly WS, Valle D, eds. *The Metabolic and Molecular Bases of Inherited Disease.* 7th ed, New York: McGraw-Hill, pp. 2929–66.

Martinez-Frias ML. 1996. Epidemiological analysis of the association of congenital diaphragmatic hernia with upper-limb deficiencies: a primary polytopic developmental field defect. *Am J Med Genet* 62:68–70.

McGillivray BC. 1993. Male genital system. In Stevenson RE, Hall JG, Goodman RM, eds. *Human Malformations and Related Anomalies.* New York: Oxford University Press, pp. 551–52.

Opitz JM, Kaveggia EG, Adkins WN. 1982. Studies of malformation syndromes of humans XXXIIIC. The FG syndrome—further studies on three affected individuals from the FG family. *Am J Med Genet* 12:147–154.

Russell LJ, Weaver DD, Bull MJ. 1981. The axial mesodermal dysplasia spectrum. J Pediatr 67: 176–82.

Schinzel A. 1968. The acrocallosal syndrome in first cousins: widening of the spectrum of clinical features and further support for autosomal recessive inheritance. *J Med Genet* 25:332–336.

Soltan HC, Holmes LB. 1986. Familial occurrence of malformations possibly attributable to vascular abnormalities. *J Pediatr* 108:112–114.

Sweed Y, Puri P. 1993. Congenital diaphragmatic hernia: influence of associated malformations on survival. *Arch Dis Child* 69:68–70.

Van Allen MI. 1993. Urinary tract. In Stevenson RE, Hall JG, Goodman RM, eds. *Human Malformations and Related Anomalies.* New York: Oxford University Press, pp. 501–50.

Craniofacial and Plastic Surgery

Carey JC. 1993. External ear, middle ear, inner ear. In Stevenson RE, Hall JG, Goodman RM, eds. *Human Malformations and Related Anomalies.* New York: Oxford University Press, pp. 193–236.

Cohen MM Jr, Fraser FC, Gorlin RJ. 1990. Craniofacial disorders. In Rimoin DL, Emery AEH, Pyeritz R, eds. *Principles and Practice of Medical Genetics,* 2nd ed. Edinburgh: Churchill Livingstone, pp 749–798.

Jorgenson RJ. 1993. Teeth. In Stevenson RE, Hall JG, Goodman RM, eds. *Human Malformations and Related Anomalies.* New York: Oxford University Press, pp. 383–396.

Lettieri J. 1993. Lips and oral cavity. In Stevenson RE, Hall JG, Goodman RM, eds. *Human Malformations and Related Anomalies.* New York: Oxford University Press, pp. 367–382.

Toriello H. 1993. Cranium. In Stevenson RE, Hall JG, Goodman RM, eds. *Human Malformations and Related Anomalies.* New York: Oxford University Press, pp. 589–628.

Traboulsi E. 1993. The eye. In Stevenson RE, Hall JG, Goodman RM, eds. *Human Malformations and Related Anomalies.* New York: Oxford University Press.

Warkany J. 1971. *Congenital Malformations: Notes and Comments.* Chicago: Year Book Medical Publishers.

Cardiac Surgery

Carter CO. 1974. Clues to the aetiology of neural tube malformations. *Dev Med Child Neurol* 16:Suppl 32:3–15.

Clark EB. 1996. Pathogenetic mechanisms of congenital cardiovascular malformations revisited. *Sem Perinatol* 20:465–472.

Dennis NR, Warren J. 1981. Risks to the offspring of patients with some common congenital heart defects. *J Med Genet* 18:8–16.

Pierpont MEM, Moller JH. 1986. Congenital cardiac malformations. In Pierpont ME, Moller JH, eds. *Genetics of Cardiovascular Disease.* New York: Marinus Nijhoff, pp. 1–24.

Riopel DA. 1993. The heart. In Stevenson RE, Hall JG, Goodman RM, eds. *Human Malformations and Related Anomalies.* New York: Oxford University Press, pp. 237–254.

Strauss AW, Johnson MC. 1996. The genetic basis of pediatric cardiovascular disease. *Sem Perinatol* 20:564–576.

Neurosurgery

Carey JC, Greenbaum B, Hall BD. 1978. The OEIS Complex (omphalocele, exstrophy, imperforate anus, spinal defects). *Birth Defects Original Article Series* 14(6B):253–263.

Hunt GM. 1990. Open spina bifida; outcome for a complete cohort treated unselectively and followed into adulthood. *Dev Med Child Neurol* 32:108–112.

Hunter AGW. 1993. Brain and spinal cord. In Stevenson RE, Hall JG, Goodman RM, eds. *Human Malformations and Related Anomalies.* New York: Oxford University Press, pp. 109–138.

Laurence KM. 1990. The genetics and prevention of neural tube defects and 'uncomplicated' hydrocephalus. In Emery AEH, Rimoin DL, eds.,

Principles and Practice of Medical Genetics. New York: Churchill Livingstone.

McLone DG. 1983. Results of treatment of children born with a myelomeningocele. *Clin Neurosurg* 30:407–415.

Orthopedics

Froster-Iskenius UG, Baird PA. 1989. Limb reduction defects in over one million consecutive live-births. *Teratology* 39:127–135.

Herring JA, Birch JG. 1998. *The Child with a Limb Deficiency.* Rosemont, IL: American Academy of Orthopedic Surgeons.

Stevenson RE and Meyer LC. 1993. The limbs. In Stevenson RE, Hall JG, and Goodman RM, eds., *Human Malformations and Related Anomalies.* New York: Oxford University Press, pp. 699–804.

Wilson GN. 1998. Heritable limb deficiencies. In Herring JA, Birch JG, eds., *The Child with a Limb Deficiency.* Rosemont, IL: American Academy of Orthopedic Surgeons, pp. 39–50.

14

GENETICS AND ADULT MEDICINE

■ LEARNING OBJECTIVES

1. Common adult diseases like coronary artery disease, manic depressive illness, or colon cancer often have genetic predisposition.

2. Accessory or extreme symptoms should prompt suspicion of unusual Mendelian forms of these common adult diseases.

3. Study of Mendelian extremes like familial hypercholesterolemia can provide biological markers for risk assessment in common diseases like coronary atherosclerosis.

4. Risk factors and mutant alleles can be used for presymptomatic diagnosis of adult-onset diseases.

5. Risk factors have been defined for most common diseases in medicine, illustrated by disorders such as cardiomyopathy, anemia, rheumatoid arthritis, inflammatory bowel disease, dementias, psychoses, colon cancer, breast cancer, and prostate cancer.

6. Huntington chorea is a model of predictive testing that emphasizes the importance of counseling prior to rather than after the report of test results.

7. Recognition of genetic factors in common diseases through a positive family history and early or atypical onset has vastly important implications for family risk and disease management.

*Case 14: **A Female with Myocardial Infarction***
A 40-year-old woman presents for genetic counseling after a myocardial infarction and coronary artery bypass. She has three sons and is concerned about their risk for premature heart disease. Her husband and her parents are healthy with no history of cardiovascular disease.

■ 14.1. INTRODUCTION

A medical catastrophe that remains to be solved is the tragedy of sudden cardiac death. Whether because of unrecognized apnea during infancy, of cardiac collapse during sporting events in young adults, or of unrecognized coronary artery disease in older adults, sudden death is the antithesis of prevention that has become so important in modern medicine. Except for trauma, most cases of sudden death in adolescence and adulthood are cardiovascular. Several categories of genetic disease that can cause sudden cardiac decompensation and death are presented as a reminder to suspect genetic causes when confronted with an extreme or unusual phenotype.

The large toll of morphologic and metabolic disease on children (Chapters 11–13) emphasizes the importance of pediatric genetics. An equally important fraction of genetic disease presents to general practitioners or internists, often masquerading as genetic forms of common diseases. The appearance of genetic disease in older patients partly reflects a relaxation of negative selective pressure—mutations beneficial for earlier reproduction and fertility are free to extract costs during the less fertile periods of middle and older age. Another factor is increased survival of individuals with genetic disorders because of improvements in public health and medical treatment. Adult genetic disorders can be mentioned for every organ system, and the genetic predisposition to coronary atherosclerosis and diabetes mellitus has already been discussed in Chapter 3. Recognition of these genetic factors is important in guiding effective evaluation, management, and counseling.

As with pediatric diseases, recognition of a genetic possibility rather than specific diagnoses is the most important goal for health providers. As emphasized in Chapter 3, genetic diseases often present as extreme or unusual forms of common diseases. The patient with a severe form of emphysema may thus have α-1-antitrypsin deficiency, and the individual with congestive heart failure in middle age may have a genetic cardiomyopathy. Once the possibility of genetic causation is entertained, consultation of the appropriate references and specialists can establish the precise diagnosis essential for prognostic and genetic counseling.

Awareness that Mendelian forms can lurk behind routine disorders should be complemented by an appreciation of genetic risk factors. Rare genetic diseases have value beyond their frequency through their insights into dis-

ease pathogenesis. The characterization of familial hypercholesterolemia thus explained why elevated cholesterol conferred higher risks for coronary artery disease and supported the use of cholesterol and blood lipid levels for assessing risks for cardiovascular disease. As later onset diseases are traced to particular mutant alleles or associated with polymorphisms, predictive testing is becoming a more common strategy in medicine. Testing to divine future risks for Alzheimer disease or Huntington has enormous implications for individuals and families that must be anticipated by medical practitioners. As predictive testing is coupled with therapy, illustrated by current treatment of hypercholesterolemia with lipid-lowering agents, then predictive testing and early or presymptomatic diagnosis becomes a central theme of adult medical care and prevention. Every area of adult medicine involves common diseases with genetic predisposition as well as Mendelian disorders. A small sample of diseases concerning the heart, blood, immune, gastrointestinal, and nervous systems are discussed here. Certain common cancers are also mentioned. Important for each disease category is the identification of genetic risk factors as keys to early diagnosis and preventive management (Table 14.1).

■ 14.2. CARDIOLOGY

Premature Atherosclerosis and Coronary Artery Disease

The multifactorial determination of coronary artery disease, suggested by its male predominance and ethnic variability, was discussed in Chapter 3. The role of diet was shown by low rates of coronary artery disease in populations with diets low in animal fat. The role of genes was demonstrated by familial clustering of heart attack victims and correlated lipid levels in twins. One of these genetic risk factors was discovered in a classic paradigm for defining genetic risk factors that should be remembered for all multifactorial diseases. Individuals with

■**TABLE 14.1.** Genetics of Selected Adult Diseases

Disease	Risk for Disease (%)				Mendelian Forms of Disease
	Gen	*Sib*	*DZ*	*MZ*	
Coronary artery disease[a]	5	15	20	40	FH (143890), others
Rheumatoid arthritis	0.1	3–5	10	32	Stickler syndrome (108300)
Crohn's disease	0.4	7.5	18[b]	84[b]	Hermansky-Pudlak syndrome (203300)
Anemias	?2–3				Many
Alcoholism	3	6	12	26	
Liver cirrhosis	0.02		5.4[c]	14[c]	Hemachromatosis (235200)
Renal disease	1–2				Many—Adult PKD (173900) Infantile PKD (263200)
Presenile dementia[a]	2–3	8	40[b]	41[b]	Huntington chorea (143100)
Deafness	0.1				Many
Schizophrenia	0.1	10.5		50	Acute intermittent
Unipolar depression	4		11	40	porphyria (176000)
Bipolar depression	0.7	16	14	72	Wilson disease (277900)
Colon cancer[a]	0.04	0.13			Adenomatous polyposis coli (175100) Lynch syndrome (114500)
Breast cancer[a]	0.03	0.1	17	13	Li-Fraumeni syndrome (114480) Cowden disease (158350)
Prostate cancer[a]	0.03	0.15			Rare AD form

[a]Risks highly dependent on age of affected individual;

[b]Small numbers studied;

[c]For alcoholic cirrhosis;

Notes: Gen, general population, DZ, dizygotic twins, MZ, monozygotic twins, AD, autosomal dominant.

the extreme phenotype (heart attacks at an early age) were studied to separate a Mendelian disease (hypercholesterolemia, 143890) from other risk factors for heart attacks (Goldstein et al., 1995). Characterization of this locus of major effect (low density lipoprotein receptor locus—see Chapter 8) defined a relatively common predisposition for heart attacks and provided insight as to why elevated cholesterol is associated with heart attack risk. To the general risk of diets high in animal fat was added the genetic risk of inherited mutations in a receptor protein necessary for cholesterol metabolism.

The pathogenesis of hyperlipidemia in causing coronary atherosclerosis (hardening of the arteries) was illustrated in Figure 5.2. Although ways in which high blood lipids lead to

the formation of plaques on artery walls (atheromata) are still under investigation, the management of individuals with signs of coronary artery occlusion (e.g., angina pectoris) or overt heart attacks includes the measurement of blood lipid profiles. The amounts and types of blood lipids, together with the clinical presentation and family history, are helpful in recognizing genetic disorders that predispose individuals to coronary artery disease (Table 14.2).

Lipoproteins are complexes of lipid and apoprotein molecules that are present as partially solubilized droplets (microemulsions) in blood. Lipoproteins with higher amounts of certain types of lipidlike cholesterol have a lower density in aqueous solutions and float to the top of stored blood or exhibit characteristic

■**TABLE 14.2.** Genetic Disorders of the Heart That May Present with Sudden Death

Disease	Clinical Signs and Symptoms	Cause or Risk Factors
Dyslipidemias		
Familial hypercholesterolemia, heterozygous and severe homozygous (143890)	Xanthomas on tendons, white arc around the cornea (corneal arcus), atherosclerosis	LDL receptor mutations with impaired degradation of LDL, high LDL, cholesterol
Familial combined hypercholesterolemia (144250)	Pancreatitis if hyper-triglyceridemia; atherosclerosis	?autosomal dominant or multifactorial trait, high VLDL
Lecithin-cholesterol acyltransferase (LCAT) deficiency (245900)	Corneal opacities, anemia, renal disease, sea-blue histiocytes, atherosclerosis	LCAT deficiency with structurally abnormal LDL, HDL
Hyperchylomicronemia (238600)[a]	Skin xanthomas, pancreatitis, no atherosclerosis	High triglycerides, low cholesterol and LDL levels
Apolipoprotein E4/E4 genotype	Higher risk for atherosclerosis	Apo E polymorphism, higher cholesterol levels
High apolipoprotein (a) levels	Higher risk for atherosclerosis	Lp(a) polymorphism, higher cholesterol levels
Cardiomyopathies and arrythmias		
Hypertrophic cardiomyopathy (192600)	Syncope, dyspnea, chest pain on exertion; thickened myocardium, sudden death	β-Cardiac myosin gene mutation, α-tropomyosin gene mutation, troponin T gene mutation
Familial idiopathic cardiomyopathy (115200)	Heterogenous families with dilated hearts or congestive heart failure	Unknown
Dilated cardiomyopathy (212110)	Heterogenous families with dilated hearts or congestive heart failure	Unknown
Jervell and Lange-Nielsen syndrome (220400)	Long Q-T interval, deafness, sudden death from arrythmia	Unknown
Wolf-Parkinson-White syndrome (194200)	Short P-R interval, long QRS, paroxysmal tachycardia with sudden death, occasional cardiomyopathy	Unknown
Connective tissue diseases		
Marfan syndrome (154700)	Tall stature, arachnodactyly, joint laxity, lens dislocation, pectus, aortic aneurysm with rupture and sudden death	Fibrillin gene mutations
Homocystinuria (236200)	Tall stature, arachnodactyly, milder or no joint laxity, lens dislocation, blood clots, myocardial infarction	Cystathionine synthase gene mutations

[a]Example of a dyslipidemia not associated with heart disease.

bands after ultracentrifugation. Three large categories of blood lipoproteins that can be demonstrated after centrifugation include high-density lipoproteins (HDL), low-density lipoproteins (LDL), and very-low-density lipoproteins (VLDL). Abnormalities in the amounts of these lipoprotein fractions were first described generally as Types I–V, then specifically according to the particular apoprotein that was involved. The genes for many apoproteins have now been cloned, including those for Apo A–I (locus at chromosome region 11q), Apo A–II (1p), Apo B (2p), Apo C-I (19q), and Apo E (19q). The apoproteins and their associated lipids are involved in a complex interchange of lipids absorbed from the intestine and those synthesized or stored by the liver and other tissues. Proteins that degrade, transport, or mediate the cellular uptake of lipoproteins have also been defined, including lipoprotein lipase that cleaves lipids in chylomicrons or the LDL receptor that binds Apo B and Apo E in LDL to bring these molecules into the cell for degradation. Genetic alterations in the apoproteins themselves, or in the proteins involved in lipoprotein transport or uptake, alter this lipid interchange and change the blood lipid profile.

Interesting sequence variations have been defined in several of the apoproteins, including several that are relevant to genetic disease. One is an example of general mechanism called RNA editing. A large apoprotein called B-100 is a prominent component of blood that is in LDL and VLDL synthesized by liver. Chylomicrons that transport dietary lipids from intestinal cells contain a smaller version of this apoprotein called B-48 that is due to replacement of a cytosine with a uracil at position 6666 of the messenger RNA. This replacement changes a glutamine codon to a stop codon, terminating translation and producing the smaller B-48 apoprotein rather than B-100 in intestinal cells. Two different mRNAs thus arise from the same apo B gene, causing differently sized apoproteins to be produced in liver versus intestine.

Other apoprotein polymorphisms have been recognized at the DNA sequence level, with particular attention to those involving apoproteins E and Lp(a). Four major polymorphisms have been defined for the apo E gene, and the apo E genotypes are associated with different levels of plasma cholesterol. This effect means that apo E alleles confer different risks for coronary atherosclerosis, perhaps because apo E is a recognition site (ligand) by which LDL binds to the LDL receptor. Lp(a) is a lipoprotein that was first detected as an antigen, then studied when its blood levels were found to vary over a thousandfold range in various individuals and ethnic groups. Higher Lp(a) levels are an independent risk factor for coronary artery disease and stroke. The mechanism for this risk is not yet defined, but Lp(a) levels correlate with variation in the number of tandem repeats of a 90 amino acid unit within its apoprotein, apo(a). Different apo(a) alleles contain between 11 and 60 of these repeats, producing variably sized apo(a) proteins and different amounts of Lp(a) lipoprotein in serum.

The overlapping types and polymorphism of apoproteins within various lipoprotein fractions produce a continuous spectrum of blood lipid concentrations that varies by diet, age, sex, and population. Blood lipid values are thus relative rather than absolute measures that must be related to population norms. With this caveat in mind, the measurement of plasma triglycerides, chylomicrons, and cholesterol (including its LDL and HDL fraction) is often sufficient to define risks for coronary artery disease and possibilities for inborn errors in lipoprotein metabolism. Table 14.2 lists several abnormalities of lipoproteins and their metabolic conversions that cause specific clinical phenotypes including coronary artery disease. Most of these disorders are rare compared to dietary elevations of lipoproteins and cholesterol. Fatty skin deposits called xanthomas are striking symptoms for several dyslipoproteinemias. When xanthomas occur on the tendons and the LDL cholesterol is high, a diagnosis of hypercholesterolemia is suggested. Other dyslipoproteinemias are suggested by the presence of corneal clouding or pancreatitis (Table 14.2), and additional apoprotein or enzyme assays are often required for a precise diagnosis. Once an abnormal lipid profile has been defined, family studies may be indicated to discern other individuals at risk for cardiovascular disease.

The management of overt or suspected coronary artery disease begins with cardiac studies to define the extent of coronary artery occlusion. An electrocardiogram during rest or stress is useful for recognizing myocardial ischemia by changes in the S and T waves. For acute coronary artery disease (heart attacks), visualization of the blockage by cardiac catheterization and dissolution of any clots with thrombolytic agents may be indicated. After the acute phase, or after stress testing to demonstrate chronic coronary occlusion with atherosclerosis, dietary therapy is important. Rare forms of hyperlipidemia or coronary thrombosis such as those listed in Table 14.2 should also be borne in mind, because agents like pyridoxine are helpful in disorders like homocystinuria. For hyperlipidemias, low-fat diets can lower blood lipids and cholesterol by 10–15% but is inadequate for genetic disorders like hypercholesterolemia. Inhibitors of hydroxymethylglutaryl (HMG)-CoA reductase such as lovastatin are much more useful for higher elevations of cholesterol, and newer derivatives can produce a 50% lowering of blood cholesterol at costs of about one dollar per day. Surgical treatments are needed for some patients with severe coronary artery obstruction, including coronary artery bypass achieved by grafting veins from elsewhere in the body to circumvent the blocked coronary vessel.

Case 14 Follow-up: A blood lipid profile on the woman with early onset coronary artery disease showed elevated cholesterol that prompted additional studies. Clinical findings included corneal opacities, mild anemia, and elevated protein in her urine. Enzyme assay confirmed the diagnosis of lecithin-cholesterol

acyltransferase deficiency (245900) and explained why her parents were not affected by this autosomal recessive disease. Because her husband was unlikely to be a carrier for this rare disease, the risk for coronary artery disease in her sons would be no greater than for others with their ethnicity and dietary habits.

Cardiomyopathies

Although coronary artery disease is the most common cause of sudden death, diseases of the cardiac muscle (cardiomyopathies) also produce this phenotype. Certain heart muscle diseases produce a large, dilated heart wall with thinning of the muscles (dilated cardiomyopathies). The dilated cardiomyopathies often present in early childhood because of metabolic diseases like the carnitine deficiencies or glycogen storage diseases discussed in Chapter 12. Hypertrophic cardiomyopathies produce increased thickness of the cardiac muscle with smaller cardiac chambers; these often present during adolescence or adulthood with the tragedy of sudden death.

Hypertrophic cardiomyopathies are a heterogenous group of genetic diseases that can present with symptoms at any age. There may be a history of breathlessness (dyspnea), fainting, or chest pain during physical exertion. About 50% of patients present with such symptoms, while the other half are diagnosed after family screening due to an affected relative. Since 15–20% of individuals with no cardiac disease experience fainting spells, selection of patients who require cardiac evaluation may be difficult (McKenna and Watkins, 1995). A diagnostic evaluation should include an electrocardiogram to detect arrhythmias because of thickened cardiac muscle and an echocardiogram to visualize heart wall thickness. Hypertrophic cardiomyopathy can be viewed as an extreme Mendelian cause of the common multifactorial phenotype of fainting spells (syncope).

Molecular analysis has demonstrated that various forms of hypertrophic cardiomyopathy are due to mutations affecting cardiac muscle proteins. The availability of large families exhibiting autosomal dominant inheritance allowed linkage studies that defined a locus for HCM on chromosome 14. Candidates in this region included two genes encoding the cardiac muscle protein myosin that were tandemly arranged within a 4-kb region in chromosome band 14q11. Since the α-myosin gene was expressed mainly in the cardiac atrium, the β-myosin gene that was expressed in the cardiac ventricles was screened for mutations in affected patients. Many different point mutations and a few deletions affecting this gene have now been characterized in affected families and in individuals with sporadic disease (Table 14.2). Mutations at the α-tropomyosin T locus on 15q2 and the troponin T locus at chromosome band 1q have also been defined in families with HCM. DNA diagnosis is now available to assist in defining patients with risk for sudden death due to HCM, and certain mutant alleles are being associated with higher risks.

Medical and surgical therapy is available for patients recognized to have HCM. The presence of ventricular tachycardia is a predictive marker for sudden death in adults with HCM, having a sensitivity of 0.7, a specificity of 0.8, and a positive predictive value of 0.2. The low positive predictive value reflects a low but substantial risk of 4–6% for sudden death once the diagnosis is made. Positive findings such as fainting symptoms or thickness of the heart wall cannot be used to refine these risks. Medical therapy involves reduction of the force of cardiac contraction using drugs such as propranolol. In patients unresponsive to medical therapy, heart muscle thickness is reduced by removing a portion of the cardiac septum. Surgery is effective at reducing long-term risks and symptoms but is associated with an operative mortality of 5–10% (McKenna and Watkins, 1995).

Disorders with Abnormal Connective Tissue

Genetic disorders that alter connective tissue strength often affect the skin, eyes, heart, blood vessels, gut, and skeleton. Examples include the supravalvular aortic stenosis (185500) that occurs in Williams syndrome (194050, see Chapter 7) and the abnormal skin in cutis laxa (123700, 219100). As emphasized in Chapter 11, connective tissue laxity can be a nonspecific feature of many syndromes or a more defining characteristic of specific diseases. Among these disorders that can present in adolescence or adulthood are the Marfan (154700), Ehlers-Danlos (130000), and cutis laxa syndromes. The books by Royce and Steinmann (1993) and Beighton (1993) provide excellent guides to this category of disorders.

Marfan syndrome is an example of a connective tissue disease that can cause cardiac complications and sudden death in adults. As illustrated in Figure 2.2, the disorder exhibits variable expressivity that can cause severe symptoms in infants or children. Mapping of the causative locus to chromosome 15 allowed mutations in the fibrillin gene to be identified that are now pathognomonic for the disorder. Unfortunately, the large size of the fibrillin gene and the diversity of mutations in Marfan syndrome have restricted DNA diagnosis to research laboratories.

Clinical features of Marfan syndrome include a tall, thin body build (Marfanoid habitus) with several major or minor findings. Major diagnostic criteria for Marfan syndrome include dislocation of the optic lens, dilatation of the ascending aorta, aortic dissection (tearing of the wall), and dural ectasia (stretching of the meningeal lining of the brain and spinal cord, with widening of the spinal canal or meningocele). Minor criteria for diagnosis include skeletal changes like high palate, pectus excavatum (concave chest), scoliosis, arachnodactyly (thin fingers), flat feet, hernias of the diaphragm or inguinal region; pneumothorax (rupture of the lung to allow air into the chest cavity), stretch marks, or an aged appearance of the skin. Stretching of the mitral valve may also occur, producing an extra click sound on auschultation that is characteristic of mitral valve prolapse. The latter anomaly can be inherited as an isolated defect and is relatively common in the general population. However, unlike its benign phenotype in the isolated form, mitral valve prolapse often progresses to mitral insufficiency with heart problems in people with Marfan syndrome.

The diagnosis of Marfan syndrome is often suspected by minor skeletal criteria of the Marfanoid habitus, arachnodactyly, pectus, and flat feet. The joint laxity plus arachnodactyly allows patients to wrap their hands around their wrists. The major diagnostic criteria of lens dislocation or aortic dilation can then be sought by specialty referral with appropriate studies. The skilled ophthalmologist may detect ciliary ligament weakening by iridodonesis (lens fluttering), the cardiologist may employ echocardiography to demonstrate that the aortic valve or aortic diameters are above age-appropriate norms, and MRI or computerized tomography (CT) imaging can detect widening of the spinal canal. If minor criteria involving more than one organ system and at least one major criterion are present, then the diagnosis of Marfan syndrome is likely (Pyeritz, 1993). This likelihood is of course increased if a first-degree relative is known to have Marfan syndrome.

The differential diagnosis of Marfan syndrome includes homocystinuria (236200) with a similar Marfanoid habitus and lens dislocation but without aortic dissection (Table 14.1). Homocystinuria is due to cystathionine synthase deficiency, and has the potential for therapy with the pyridoxine cofactor of that enzyme (see Chapter 12). Beals congenital contractural arachnodactyly (121050) is due to mutation of another fibrillin gene on chromosome 5, but has unusual "crumpled" ears with joint contractures in addition to a Marfanoid habitus. Stickler syndrome (108300) also can present with a Marfanoid habitus and mitral valve prolapse, but other findings such as neonatal Pierre Robin sequence, retinal detachments, and skeletal dysplasias distinguish the disorder. Adults with certain forms of Ehlers-Danlos syndrome also have a lanky build, but those with blood vessel fragility rarely have cardiac valve dilatation.

In individuals suspected of having Marfan syndrome, echocardiography to measure the diameter of the aortic valve provides a diagnostic and therapeutic guide. Drugs that block the myocardial β-andrenergic receptors are helpful in delaying the progression of aortic and mitral valve dissection. Other preventive management includes surveillance for skeletal problems such as scoliosis or flat feet, eye examinations to detect lens dislocation or myopia, and restriction of participation in highly competitive or traumatic sports. Patients with marked dilations of the aorta valve or with early signs of aortic dissection will need surgical repairs of both valve and aorta. Mitral valve insufficiencies also may need surgical repair or replacements (Pyeritz, 1993).

■ 14.3. AUTOIMMUNE DISORDERS

Certain diseases of immune function involve a breakdown of tolerance that is built in to the immune system during fetal life. Diffuse alterations of the immune system in these "autoimmune" diseases provoke reactions to normal host tissues rather than to invading foreign tissues. Several autoimmune disorders are common in adults, often involving genetic predisposition in association with particular alleles of the human leucocyte antigen (HLA) region on chromosome 6. Individual susceptibility may thus be predicted based on the number and degrees of affected relatives and the presence of associated HLA alleles. The use of associated HLA alleles as risk factors for disease was discussed for diabetes mellitus in Chapter 5.

Rheumatoid Arthritis

Arthritis refers to inflammation of the joints that occurs in a huge number of medical conditions. Rheumatoid arthritis refers particularly to inflammation that occurs in joints with a synovial membrane, often associated with small inflammatory nodules (rheumatoid nodules). Altered immune function as a causative factor in rheumatoid arthritis is indicated by the presence of abnormal antibodies to the heavy chain of host immunoglobulins. These abnormal antibodies were initially detected by their ability to agglutinate (complex) immunoglobulin-coated sheep red blood cells. Now radioimmunoassay methods are available for sensitive detection of this rheumatoid factor.

Although the heterogenous causation of arthritis complicates estimates of frequency, it affects between 0.1 and 10% of people older than age 15 in all regions of the world. These frequencies vary greatly according to ethnic origin, being high in areas like Finland and very low in Japan. There is a 1.5- to 3-fold preponderance of females and a great increase in frequency with age. Discrimination of rheumatoid arthritis from other diseases with arthritis may be difficult, since only 10–30% of individuals who meet the diagnostic criteria test positive for rheumatoid factor.

With these difficulties of diagnosis in mind, a significant familial component to rheumatoid arthritis has been demonstrated by multiple studies. Most surveys document a 3–5% risk for siblings of patients with rheumatoid arthritis to be affected, with concordance (both affected) rates of 32–33% in monozygotic (identical) twins and 7–13% in dizygotic (fraternal) twins. These risks and the sex predilection fit with the model of multifactorial determination and show even greater correlation between risk and relationship when only patients testing positive for rheumatoid factor are studied. Stickler syndrome (108300) represents a Mendelian form of arthritis that occurs in patients with tall or short stature, retinal detachments, and midface or jaw hypoplasia due to type II collagen deficiency (Table 14.1).

The examination of HLA types in patients with rheumatoid arthritis revealed that certain alleles of the HLA-D locus (see Fig. 5.3) were 4–5 times more common. Alleles associated with rheumatoid arthritis include the HLA-DR4 allele together with a DQw3 allele in the neighboring HLA-DQ locus. Molecular analysis determining particular versions of HLA-DR and HLA-DQ alleles have increased these associations somewhat, but there is no correla-

tion of disease severity in patients with DR4 and DQw3 alleles and those without. These associated alleles probably do not have a direct role in causing rheumatoid arthritis because most affected patients have other HLA alleles. Since there is no preventive treatment for rheumatoid arthritis, and since a minority of patients have DR4/DQw3 alleles, screening of individuals to determine their predisposition for rheumatoid arthritis is not indicated. A positive family history, the presence of rheumatoid factor, and the presence of associated HLA-DR4/DQ3 alleles does increase the precision of diagnosis of rheumatoid arthritis in symptomatic patients. Therapy consists of drugs like gold or penicillamine that induce symptom-free remissions or anti-inflammatory drugs like aspirin and steroids that suppress symptoms during flares. HLA typing does have some value in predicting which patients will have toxic reactions to gold or penicillamine, with individuals positive for HLA-B8 having higher frequencies of reactions and those positive for HLA-DR3 having lower frequencies of reactions (King, 1992).

Inflammatory Bowel Disease

Ulcerative colitis and Crohn's disease exhibit chronic, episodic inflammation of the bowel that manifests as abdominal pain and hematochezia (bloody stools). Ulcerative colitis typically affects the colon and Crohn's disease the small intestine, but each has characteristic pathology that has been defined at various regions of the gastrointestinal tract. Given that 20% of cases cannot be specifically classified, ulcerative colitis has a prevalence of 4–8 per thousand and Crohn's disease a frequency of 3–5 per thousand. The higher prevalence of inflammatory bowel disease in whites indicate possible genetic factors in causation, while the increase in prevalence of the disease in black immigrants emphasizes environmental factors such as diet. Definite familial aggregations are more prominent for Crohn's disease, with recurrence risks as high as 7.5% in siblings of patients with Crohn's disease compared to 6%

for siblings of patients with ulcerative colitis. Higher concordance rates for monozygotic twins in Crohn's disease (84%) versus those with ulcerative colitis (36%) have also been documented.

Despite these suggestions of multifactorial determination with considerable heritability, HLA association studies have not been revealing for risks of inflammatory bowel disease. Some evidence associating HLA-DR2 alleles with ulcerative colitis has been reported. Despite these studies, the autoimmune disease ankylosing spondylitis has 10–50-fold increased frequency in patients with Crohn's disease or ulcerative colitis. The well-known association of ankylosing spondylitis (an inflammation of vertebral joints in the lower back) with the HLA-B27 allele does hold when ankylosing spondylitis and inflammatory bowel disease are present together—80% of these patients are HLA-B27 positive. Nonetheless, the frequency of HLA-B27 in patients with inflammatory bowel disease alone is no greater than that of the general population.

Perhaps more revealing than the HLA locus in discerning genes responsible for familial clustering of inflammatory bowel disease will be associated diseases like Turner syndrome or Hermansky-Pudlak syndrome (203300). The higher frequency of inflammatory bowel disease in Turner syndrome correlates with increased incidence of other autoimmune diseases (e.g., thyroiditis) and is particularly striking in patients with structural rearrangements of the X chromosome (i.e., patients with 46,Xi(Xq) karyotypes—see Chapter 7). The Hermansky-Pudlak syndrome involves albinism and low platelets with high frequencies of inflammatory bowel disease that is particularly resistant to therapy.

Genetic studies do not assist in the diagnosis of inflammatory bowel disease unless its combination with ankylosing spondylitis leads to positive testing for HLA-B27 alleles. Management includes a low fiber diet with anti-inflammatory drugs such as steroidal or nonsteroidal agents. Surgical resection of bowel

segments or of the entire colon is required in refractory cases. Genetic counseling may be provided, with an average 2–3% risk for siblings and 1–2% risk for offspring of affected patients (McConnell and Vadheim, 1992). Some studies suggest earlier onset and greater severity for familial cases, but no methods for screening and prevention are available.

■ 14.4. MEDICAL SUBSPECIALTY DISEASES

As emphasized in Chapter 1, multifactorial and Mendelian diseases occur in every organ system and medical specialty. Common diseases with multifactorial determination have been emphasized in the preceding discussions, with emphasis on early onset, more severe disease, and unusual or extreme presentations as indicators of Mendelian loci hidden within this multifactorial causation. Here, additional examples of Mendelian disorders are presented to emphasize the ubiquity of genetic causation (Table 14.3).

Hematology—Anemias

Anemia refers to a decreased percentage of hemoglobin in blood, and it is a common phenotype produced by many environmental and genetic factors (see Table 6.5). When genes or the environment affect the bone marrow and stem cells producing erythrocytes, then anemia is due to inadequate red blood cell production. Anemias due to inadequate red cell production have decreased numbers of reticulocytes, the immature precursor of erythrocytes that can be identified on blood smears by its residual nuclear material. Anemias due to accelerated red blood cell destruction or blood loss will have increased numbers of reticulocytes as the marrow attempts to replace destroyed red cells, and the increased load of degraded hemoglobin may produce jaundice (yellow color due to increased bilirubin).

Nutritional deprivations like iron, folic acid, or vitamin B12 deficiencies, bleeding

■ TABLE 14.3. Genetics of Selected Medical Specialty Diseases

Disease Category	Signs and Symptoms	Cause or Risk Factors
Anemias, decreased RBC production (low reticulocyte count)		
Iron deficiency	Smaller (microcytic) RBCs	Environmental
Folic acid deficiency	Larger (macrocytic) RBCs	Environmental
Aase syndrome (205600)	Normal RBCs, thumb anomalies	AR
Blackfan-Diamond anemia (205900)	Normal RBCs	AR
Fanconi anemia (227650)	Normal RBCs, WBCs, platelets, thumb anomalies, growth delay	AR
Anemias, increased RBC destruction, abnormal hemoglobins		
Sickle cell anemia (141900)	Sickled RBCs	AR
α-Thalassemia (273500)	Targeted RBCs	AR
β-Thalassemia (273500)	Targeted RBCs	AR
Anemias, increased RBC destruction, red cell membrane defects		
Hereditary spherocytosis (182900, others)	Spherical RBCs	AD, AR, spectrin, ankyrin mutations
Heriditary elliptocytosis (130450, others)	Elliptical RBCs	AD, AR, spectrin, protein 4.1 mutations
Anemias, red cell enzyme deficiencies		
Pyruvate dehydrogenase deficiency (266200)	Hemolyzed RBCs (chronic)	AR
Glutathione reductase deficiency (138300)	Hemolyzed RBCs (chronic)	AR
Glucose-6-P dehydrogenase deficiency (350900)	Hemolyzed RBCs (acute)	XLR
Chronic liver disease		
Alcoholic cirrhosis	Alcoholism, fatty liver, liver scarring (cirrhosis)	Multifactorial
Primary biliary cirrhosis	Liver disease, cholestasis	Multifactorial, mitochondrial antibodies
Chronic active hepatitis	Liver disease, ankylosing spondylitis	Multifactorial, HLA-B8 and HLA-B27 alleles
Hemachromatosis (235200)	Increased iron storage, liver cirrhosis	HFE gene mutations
Polycystic renal disease		
Multicystic kidneys	Renal cysts, renal failure	Urinary tract obstruction, certain drugs (environmental)
Adult polycystic kidney disease (173900)	Renal cysts, renal failure, liver, pancreas, lung cysts, mostly adults	PKD1 gene on chrom. 16 PKD2 gene on chrom. 4
Infantile polycystic kidney disease (263200)	Renal cysts, renal failure, liver fibrosis, mostly infants	Gene on chromosome 6

Notes: RBCs, red blood cells; WBCs, white blood cells; P, phosphate: AD, autosomal dominant inheritance, AR, autosomal recessive inheritance; XLR, X-linked recessive inheritance; PKD, polycystic kidney.

from trauma or occult sites like gastric ulcers, numerous chronic illnesses like kidney failure, and various infections like infectious mononucleosis are associated with anemia. Genetic anemias therefore affect an important minority of cases that will require a different style of management and counseling.

The initial evaluation of anemia includes a gestation and family history to rule out congenital infections like toxoplasmosis that cause anemia, and to ascertain the likelihood of a familial disease. The physical examination will discern associated malformations like absent thumb in Aase syndrome (205600) and search for jaundice, splenomegaly (due to trapping of abnormal cells), or signs of disease in other organs. Preliminary laboratory analyses include blood cell counts to determine if the anemia is isolated or part of general bone marrow failure, and red cell studies to determine the shape, fragility, and volume of erythrocytes. The preliminary evaluation should determine whether the anemia is isolated or part of systemic disease, whether the defect concerns synthesis or survival, and whether the red cell shape or volume is abnormal. Smaller red cells (iron deficiency) or larger red cells (folic acid, vitamin B_{12} deficiency) often suggest the presence of a nutritional anemia that can be cured by dietary supplementation. When the anemia is chronic and persists regardless of nutritional or chronic disease therapy, a genetic disease must be considered.

One category of anemias involves decreased red cell synthesis. The anemia may be isolated as in Blackfan-Diamond anemia (205900) or combined with deficiency of other blood cell types like Fanconi anemia (227650). Deficiency of red blood cell synthesis may be acquired in skeletal disorders that encroach on the bone marrow space or in leukemias where the bone marrow is replaced with cancer cells. Genetic disorders comprise a small portion of anemias with decreased red cell synthesis and are often signaled by associated anomalies such as the abnormal thumbs in Aase (205600) or Fanconi (227650) syndromes (Table 14.3).

Many genetic anemias like sickle cell anemia in blacks, β-thalassemia in Mediterraneans, and α-thalassemias in Orientals often exhibit higher frequencies in certain ethnic groups. Although most patients with sickle cell anemia or thalassemia present during childhood, many require treatment or present as adults. Red cell destruction by hemolysis, jaundice, and scarred or dysfunctional spleens often accompany these forms of anemia, and characteristic cell shapes (sickle cell, target cell) aid their recognition. Sickle cell exhibits remarkable variability, with some infants having severe disease and some adults having few symptoms. The molecular basis of sickle cell disease and certain thalassemias was discussed in Chapter 6 and illustrated in Figure 6.7. Hemoglobin electrophoresis to define the presence of globin proteins with abnormal mobility and DNA diagnosis to define mutations that decrease α- or β-globin expression allow the definitive diagnosis of these and related anemias.

A second class of anemias with accelerated red cell destruction affect the red cell membrane rather than the protein components of hemoglobin. Defective membrane proteins alter the red cell shape, producing several types of spherocytosis (182900, 182870, 183010, 270970) or elliptocytosis (130500, 130450, 130600, 182860, 225450). The altered membrane also exhibits decreased stability in solutions of low ionic strength, allowing red cell hemolysis testing as an aid to diagnosis. A growing number of mutations have been characterized in these structural alterations of red cell membranes, including those affecting the spectin, ankyrin, and band 3 proteins in hereditary spherocytosis, and those affecting the spectin and protein 4.1 molecules in elliptocytosis (Becker and Lux, 1995). The more severe derangements of membrane structure produce spherocytosis rather than elliptocytosis, and mutations interfering with regions of the spectrin molecule that bind to other membrane proteins produce the more severe phenotype.

A third group of anemias that exhibit accelerated red cell destruction involve red cell enzyme deficiencies that impair energy supplies in the red cell (Tanaka and Pagila, 1995). The red cell is highly evolved to carry a viscous hemoglobin solution for delivery of oxygen to tissues, and its metabolic flexibility is limited. Energy is required to maintain membrane components and to protect enzymes and hemoglobin from denaturation by oxidizing agents. Figure 14.1 illustrates the energy-producing glycolytic pathway (left) and the oxidation-protecting glutathione pathway (right) that depends on NADPH generated by glucose-6-phosphate dehydrogenase (center).

Enzymes that may be deficient in patients with hemolytic anemia are illustrated, and produce two broad phenotypes. The first, illustrated by enzyme deficiencies in the glycolytic pathway, produce decreased amounts of ATP and chronic hemolyis. The second, illustrated by deficiencies of glucose-6-phosphate dehydrogenase and certain enzymes of glutathione metabolism, exhibit increased susceptibility to oxidative agents with sudden and episodic hemolytic crises. Glucose-6-phosphate dehydrogenase deficiency (305900) and the susceptibility of affected males to dietary or pharma-

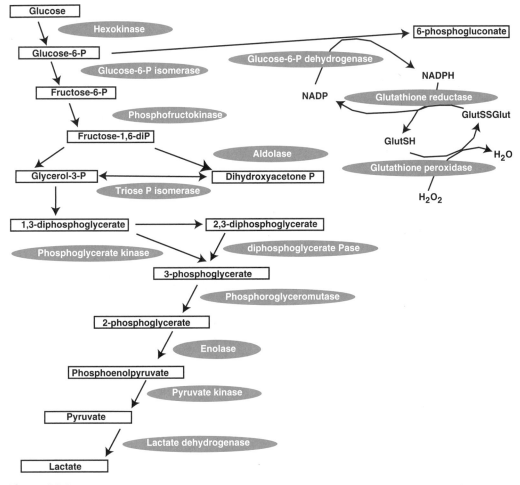

Figure 14.1. Enzyme defects (shaded) that can cause increased red blood cell hemolysis and anemia. P, phosphate; NADP, NADPH, nicotinamide adenosine dinucleotide phosphate and its reduced form; glutSH, glutSSglut, glutathione and its disulfide form.

ceutical substances was discussed in Chapter 5. The most common glycolytic enzyme deficiency is that of pyruvate kinase (266200). The anemia may be severe enough to require neonatal transfusions or mild enough to escape detection until adulthood. Jaundice, enlargment of the spleen, and gall stones due to hyperbilirubinemia may be seen in patients with chronic anemias such as that due to pyruvate kinase deficiency.

The spectrum of anemia provides another illustration of the genetic contribution to disease. Although nutritional deficiencies and chronic diseases are responsible for anemia in most patients, numerous genetic defects at various stages of hemoglobin synthesis, red cell development, and red cell function can produce inherited disease. A simple history, physical, and laboratory examination will quickly identify those more chronic or recurrent anemias that are likely to be genetic, and a considerable array of specialized tests are available to provide an exact diagnosis. Therapies for anemias range from nutritional supplements to chronic transfusion, and the prognosis is usually good. The anemias are also a model for molecular analysis, since sickle cell anemia was the first mutation to be defined and most genetic anemias have been characterized at the molecular level. Within the large pulp of anemias was the seed of genetic disease that has provided a fruitful synthesis of clinical and laboratory methods.

Gastroenterology— Chronic Liver Disease

Chronic liver disease with inflammation (hepatitis) and scarring (cirrhosis) is another example of a common medical problem with genetic predisposition. The multifactorial determination of most common diseases is again illustrated, with alcohol and hepatitis viruses representing environmental factors and hemachromatosis or HLA alleles representing genetic factors. Alcoholism is in turn a multifactorial disorder where a toxin causes the disease and genes promote ingestion of the toxin.

Chronic liver diseases often present with jaundice, hepatomegaly, and elevated activities of liver-based enzymes in serum. The liver inflammation destroys hepatic cells, releasing enzymes and producing scarring (cirrhosis) that blocks the routing of bilirubin to the gall bladder. The presenting symptoms and course of chronic disease is often the same, with laboratory evidence of infections, toxins, or genetic causation plus occasional liver biopsy required for a precise diagnosis. Some cases of chronic liver disease and cirrhosis are idiopathic—that is, they do not have defined causes.

Alcoholic liver disease is a continuum from fatty liver to alcoholic hepatitis to scarring and cirrhosis. All three processes correlate with the amount and duration of alcohol intake, and only the first two are reversible by abstinence. The frequency of alcoholism is estimated at 3–5% of males and 1–2% of females, with deaths from alcoholic cirrhosis estimated at 1.1–1.3 per 10,000 (Kang et al., 1992). Formulae have been derived to estimate the amount of intake needed to produce cirrhosis—one version suggests that 10% of 70 kg males drinking 90 gram of ethanol daily (about 5 beers) for 10 years will develop cirrhosis (Lelbach, 1976). Such formulae ignore individual differences in susceptibility, with females requiring less intake for damage.

The prevalence of alcoholism is of course highly dependent on the diagnostic criterion, and this imprecision complicates studies of heritability. One study of almost 16,000 male twin pairs revealed a concordance of 26% (monozygotic) and 12% (dizygotic) for alcoholism and 15% (monozygotic) and 5.4% (dizygotic) for cirrhosis (Kang et al., 1992). Since at least 50% of alcoholics have a parent who is alcoholic, the importance of social factors in addition to genetic influences must be considered.

Causes for this apparent genetic predisposition have been sought in the pathways for alcohol metabolism. Genetic polymorphism has been demonstrated in alcohol dehydrogenase and in acetaldehyde dehydrogenase, the initial enzymes in alcohol metabolism. A variant acetaldehyde dehydrogenase is present in many

Orientals, causing slower metabolism and a flush after drinking due to high leves of acetaldehyde. The flush is part of an adrenalin response that is unpleasant, and it is thought that this reaction may explain the lower frequency of alcoholism in Orientals. However, different frequencies of the polymorphic forms of either enzyme have not been observed in alcoholics of any ethnic group.

Despite increased sensitivity in females, 67% of those with alcoholic cirrhosis and 80% of those with chronic liver disease from hepatitis B are males. These factors probably reflect higher frequencies of alcoholism and high-risk sex or drug behaviors in males. Two chronic liver diseases with abnormal antibodies suggestive of autoimmune dysfunction—biliary cirrhosis and chronic active hepatitis—have the opposite sex predilection with 80–90 percent of affected individuals being female.

In primary biliary cirrhosis, antibodies develop to mitochondria in 80% of affected persons. Genetic predisposition is suggested by elevation of these antibodies in asymptomatic family members, and there are occasional families with multiple affected individuals. In chronic active hepatitis, fewer (< 20%) individuals have mitochondrial antibodies but other indicators of autoimmune disease like rheumatoid factor may be present. Evidence of familial clustering is more striking in chronic active hepatitis, and particular HLA alleles are more frequent in the disease. When discerning diagnostic criteria are used, more than 80% of patients with chronic active hepatitis will have the HLA-B8 allele (Kang et al., 1992). Individuals with HLA-B8 thus have an 11–15-fold higher risk to develop chronic active hepatitis that contrasts with their lower risk for toxic reactions to rheumatoid arthritis therapies mentioned previously. These associations emphasize the complex relationship between alleles of the HLA system and disease causation.

Many Mendelian disorders can cause chronic liver disease as exemplified by the few listed in Table 14.3. One of the most common is hereditary hemochromatosis (235200), reaching a frequency of 3 per thousand in Caucasian populations. The disease involves increased deposition of iron in various tissues, with particularly damage caused by iron deposition in liver. Since chronic transfusions or red cell hemolysis also release iron for deposition, chronic anemias and other disorders lead to hemochromatosis that is different from the hereditary form.

Of the 3–4 grams of iron in a representative adult male, some 2–3 grams is present in hemoglobin and other heme-containing proteins. From 0–1 gram is present as soluble (ferritin) or insoluble (hemosiderin) storage material, constituting the iron reserve. Transferrins are involved in the transport of iron between tissues, and specific receptors are available for uptake of transferring into cells. These aspects of iron use as cofactors for enzymes, iron transport, and iron storage are usually regulated by the amount of dietary iron intake. In individuals with hemochromatosis, excess iron is absorbed by the gastric mucosa than is needed for protein use or storage. Over time that usually extends into adulthood, the storage produces chronic liver disease and cirrhosis (Bothwell et al., 1995).

The hemochromatosis gene was linked to the HLA locus on chromosome 6, exhibiting less than 1% recombination with the HLA-A locus. Not expected from the linkage data was a strong association with particular HLA-A alleles. In Europeans, about 30% of normal and more than 70% of hemochromatosis individuals are positive for the HLA-A3 allele. This association may indicate a role of immune or at least cell surface molecules in the development of iron overload and cirrhosis. Candidate genes were isolated near the HLA-A locus and mutations were found in an *HFE* gene. This gene is homologous to genes in the HLA complex that attach to the cell surface via β2-microglobulin. Individuals with mutant *HFE* alleles do not express the coupled *HFE*-β2-microglobulin complex on their cell surfaces, providing a first step in understanding the pathogenesis of hemochromatosis. Surface expression of *HFE* must be necessary to signal cellular iron sufficiency, and this signal must be transmitted to or expressed in the mucosal cells that mediate iron absorption.

Although the causes of chronic liver disease are extremely varied, the final common pathway of cirrhosis is often difficult to treat. Prevention of liver injury is the best form of therapy, illustrated by alcoholic recovery, avoidance of dietary lactose in galactosemia, or the avoidance of unnecessary transfusions in chronic anemias. Treatment of hemochromatosis has an option not available with most chronic anemias: that of removing blood and its high iron content. Weekly withdrawal of 500 ml of blood is usually well tolerated, and is effective in preventing the lethal complications of liver and heart disease. Desferoxamine or other iron chelators that must be used in patients with hemachromatosis due to chronic anemias are much less effective. Many patients with hemochromatosis never develop toxic levels that require therapy, while others present with liver and heart toxicity. Once these complications develop, they are inadequately reversed by venipuncture and portend decreased survival. The preliminary suggestion that certain mutations in the *HFE* gene seem to cause more severe hemochromatosis, coupled with the high frequency and treatable nature of the disease, make this disorder a superb candidate for carrier and homozygote screening. DNA diagnostic testing is already commercially available.

Nephrology—Renal Cystic Disease

Urinary tract anomalies that often present for surgical care in the pediatric age group were discussed in Chapter 13. Another group of renal disorders that may exhibit genetic predisposition are the renal cystic diseases. These disorders account for about 10% of patients with renal failure who require chronic dialysis (Jordan and Kangarloo, 1990). The impact of renal cysts thus falls upon adult care providers.

Environmental causes of cystic kidneys include many drugs such as the chemotherapeutic agent cis platinum. Renal cysts may also form as a secondary phenomenon from urinary tract obstructions or chronic dialysis. Some types of renal cysts like multicystic kidney and medullary cysts are developmental anomalies related to the renal dysplasias discussed in Chapter 13. These forms of renal cystic disease have minimal genetic predisposition and are not considered here.

More than 90 different malformation syndromes include renal cysts as listed by Winter and Baraitser (1998), including the Bardet-Biedl syndrome (209900) with obesity and polydactyly, the metabolic disorder glutaric acidemia type II (231680) with acidosis and defective electron transport, or the Perlman syndrome (267000) with overgrowth and renal tumors. Renal cystic disease occurs without obvious additional anomalies in two important disorders—the autosomal recessive (infantile) polycystic kidney disease (PKD—263200) and the autosomal dominant (adult) polycystic kidney disease (173900). Both diseases can present in infancy or adulthood, but are more frequent in their cognate age period (Table 14.3).

Infantile PKD often presents at birth with large abdominal masses. If renal function is severely impaired during fetal life, the fatal Potter sequence of oligohydramnios, clubfeet, facial compression, and lung hypoplasia can occur. These severe presentations and early renal failure in many patients promoted a view of infantile PKD as a lethal disease. However, many patients can survive into adulthood. Hepatic fibrosis (scarring) is associated with infantile PKD, but most patients do not have severe liver disease. The disorder can be detected during fetal life by early ultrasound studies, so recognition and counseling for the 25% recurrence risk is important.

Adult PKD has exhibited the reverse trend with most cases being recognized in the fourth or fifth decades until better methods of detection led to diagnosis during childhood. The series of Cole et al. (1987) found 12.5% of infants with PKD had the adult dominant form, while 35% had the infantile recessive form. The renal cysts are larger in adult PKD and can be distinguished pathologically from the infantile form with its medullary tubular dilation. Additional cysts can occur in the liver, pancreas, or lung, and some patients have cardiovascular anomalies such as cerebral aneurysms or mitral valve prolapse. These two forms of polycystic disease can cause dilemmas in genetic counseling, particularly when distinguishing between a new mutation for the dominant form and an inherited recessive case. Variable expressivity in adult PKD mandates abdominal ultrasound studies in parents of affected children before assigning a recurrence risk. DNA testing should soon supplant these imaging strategies, since two genes responsible for adult PKD have been localized to chromosomes 16 (*PKD1*) and 4 (*PKD2*).

The gene for adult PKD1 is responsible for 80–85% of cases and encodes a membrane protein that is part of a signal transduction pathway. Interaction of the protein with protein kinases and transcription factors may indicate a role for stimulating growth of embryonic renal tubules. Excess expression of the gene may thus lead to tubular expansion and cysts. An interesting aspect of the *PKD1* gene is the presence of several homologous copies (pseudogenes) that can recombine to cause mutations. The gene for one form of tuberous sclerosis (191100) is also located nearby, and unusual infants presenting with the white spots and seizures of tuberous sclerosis together with polycystic kidneys are now explained by chromosome microdeletions that inactivate these contiguous genes. The gene for infantile PKD has been localized to chromosome 6, and candidate genes are being evaluated to determine the cause of this recessive disease.

■ 14.5. NEUROLOGIC AND PSYCHIATRIC DISEASES

Two large contributors to adult neurologic and psychiatric practice are disease with neurodegeneration or mental illness. As with the other medical fields discussed here, relatively common neurologic diseases like early onset senility (presenile dementia) are multifactorial with occasional Mendelian causes. As with the other common illnesses, study of rare Mendelian phenotypes has yielded insights that illuminate the entire spectrum of neurodegenerative and psychiatric disease. Several examples of these Mendelian diseases are listed in Table 14.4

Adult Degenerative Diseases Including Alzheimer Disease

Dementia refers to the deterioration of mental function. Although mental illnesses such as schizophrenia were once known as dementia praecox, the term dementia now denotes loss of previously acquired memory or mental skills. Confusion and memory loss rather than psychosis (loss of touch with reality) are prominent parts of dementia. Dementia can occur in many chronic illnesses, including vascular occlusions that compromise blood supply to the brain. Cases where dementia is secondary to defined medical problems are often described as organic brain syndromes. Dementia accompanied by particular neuropathologic changes, often with earlier onset than expected, is characteristic of Alzheimer disease.

The characteristic pathology of Alzheimer disease includes coils of protein filaments surrounding neurons (neurofibrillary tangles) and deposits of cell debris and amyloid in the brain substance (senile plaques). The incidence of dementia is about 1% at age 70, rising to about 50% at age 90. When strict neuropathologic criteria are used for diagnosis of the dementia, Alzheimer disease accounts for 45% of dementia in persons in their forties and over 90% of dementia in persons over age 80. The prevalence of Alzheimer disease thus rises markedly with age over 70, with substantial causation of presenile dementia—that is, 1–3% of people in their sixties and seventies who lose mental function while remaining healthy in other areas.

Although the high prevalence and age-dependence of dementia complicate genetic studies, numerous investigators agree that the phenotype exhibits significant heritability. When first degree relatives over age 60 are compared with controls having no history of

■**TABLE 14.4.** Genetics of Selected Common Neurologic Diseases

Disease Category	Signs and Symptoms	Cause or Risk Factors
Dementias		
Alzheimer disease—later onset	Loss of cognitive functions, memory loss, confusion, ages 65 plus	Associated with apolipoprotein E A4 alleles
Alzheimer disease—early onset (104300, 104310)	Loss of cognitive functions, memory loss, confusion, age < 60	Amyloid β-protein (*APP*) gene, chromosome 21
Alzheimer disease—early onset (104300, 104310)	Loss of cognitive functions, memory loss, confusion, age < 60	*Presenilin*-1 locus on chromosome 14
Alzheimer disease—early onset (104300, 104310)	Loss of cognitive functions, memory loss, confusion, age < 60	*Presenilin*-2 locus on chromosome 1
Huntington disease (143100)	Early clumsiness, restlessness, dysarthria, later chorea, dystonia, dementia, depression	AD, Huntington gene on chromosome 4, CAG triplet repeat expansion above 37 repeats
Neurosensory		
Adult open angle glaucoma	Mild headaches, halos	MF—four- to fivefold increased risk in primary relatives
Secondary glaucomas	Variable	More than 50 Mendelian syndromes
Infantile glaucoma (231300)	Enlarged eye (buphthalmos), tearing, photophobia	AR
Deafness	Hearing loss	More than 100 Mendelian syndromes
Deafness, low frequency (124910)	Hearing loss	AD
Deafness, neural (221600)	Hearing loss	AR
Deafness with stapes fixation (304400)	Hearing loss	XLR
Mental illness		
Schizophrenia	Loose associations, flat affect, ambivalence	MF
Manic depressive illness	Depression, mania	MF
Acute intermittent porphyria (176000)	Abdominal pain, vomiting, neuropathy, anxiety, depression	AD, porphobilinogen reductase, heme deficiency
Wilson disease (277900)	Hepatitis, cirrhosis, chorea, schizophrenia, depression	AR, copper transporter

Notes: AD, autosomal dominant; AR, autosomal recessive; XLR, X-linked recessive; MF, multifactorial.

dementia, their prevalence of dementia was 6–10% compared to 2–3% for controls (Heston, 1992). Another way of looking at the data is to estimate that the steep rise in prevalence of dementia occurs at about age 70 for the general population.

For those with first-degree relatives having dementia (usually siblings), the steep rise begins ten years earlier at age 60. Another consequence of this multifactorial predisposition to dementia is the younger age of affected individuals who have affected relatives. As illustrated by hypercholesterolemia, heart attacks or dementia at a younger age is predictive of greater genetic contribution and higher recurrence risks for relatives. Unlike other multifactorial diseases, dementia does not exhibit a sex predilection if longer survival of females is accounted for.

Because most family studies have not employed neuropathologic criteria for diagnosis, it can only be presumed that the measured cases are truly Alzheimer disease. Two types of genetic data support a genetic predisposition for Alzheimer disease rather than other types of dementia. One is the high incidence of Alzheimer pathology in adults with Down syndrome. Based on autopsy studies, the characteristic neurofibrillary tangles and senile plaques begin appearing at age 20 and are universal at age 40 for patients with Down syndrome. The mental disability in this disorder makes assessment of dementia more difficult, but it is estimated that at least 25% of patients in their middle decades will show signs of dementia. Additional evidence comes from rare families who exhibit autosomal dominant inheritance of Alzheimer disease. Genetic linkage studies have linked disease in these families to the amyloid β-protein (APP) locus on chromosome 21. The *APP* gene can also be overexpressed in transgenic mice, and its amyloid protein product accumulates in plaques similar to those in Alzheimer disease. Other rare families have identified a *presenilin*-1 locus on chromosome 14 and a *presenilin*-2 locus on chromosome 1 that can cause autosomal dominant Alzheimer disease. Altogether, these rare Mendelian mutations account for about one-half of patients with early onset (age < 60) Alzheimer disease.

For the more prevalent cases of Alzheimer disease with later onset, an association with particular alleles of the polymorphic apolipoprotein E locus has been demonstrated. The *apo* (E) locus was discussed in Section 14.1 and Table 14.1 as an independent risk factor for atherosclerosis. The E4 allele with higher risk for atherosclerosis also exhibits a higher frequency in patients with late-onset Alzheimer disease (Blacker and Tanzi, 1998). These patients exhibit a 10-fold higher incidence of homozygosity for the E4 allele than does the normal population. This association is strong enough to be used for confirmatory diagnostic testing, with a positive predictive value of 97% in patients already suspected of having Alzheimer disease (in other words, most patients with later onset dementia who later have autopsy-proven Alzheimer disease will test positive for the E4 allele). The use of E4 apolipoprotein E alleles as a screening test for Alzheimer predisposition in the general population is not recommended, however, because the majority of E4 homozygotes will not be affected (the lack of preventive measures also mitigates against screening).

Identification of the E4 allele association has led to the recognition that this locus has an important role in brain lipoprotein metabolism, and that apoprotein E is deposited in Alzheimer lesions. Homozygous E4 patients with Alzheimer disease do have increased levels of atherosclerosis as expected (Table 14.1), but they do not have evidence for cerebral artery atherosclerosis as a cause for their Alzheimer disease. The E4 allele is also more common in adult patients with Down syndrome who develop early onset Alzheimer disease. The E4 allele is associated with increased levels of apolipoprotein E in blood, but its role in Alzheimer disease remains to be defined. The occurrence of disease in patients without trisomy 21, without any of the Mendelian mutations described, and without E4 alleles emphasizes that other environmental and genetic factors predisposing to Alzheimer disease remain to be defined.

Huntington Disease

Huntington disease (HD-143100) is a single locus disorder associated with chorea (jerking movements), neurodegeneration, and dementia. The prevalence of HD varies from 7 per 1000 in certain isolated populations like that of Maracaibo, Venezuela, to 3–7 per 100,000 in Northern American populations, to 0.5 per 100,000 in low prevalence areas such as Finland. The onset of HD is insidious with abnormal eye movements, clumsiness, restlessness, dysarthria (inarticulate speech), and inappropriate hand and finger movements with stress. Involuntary jerking movements (chorea) and rigidity (dystonia) signal the obvious phase of disease that may occur several years after the subtle symptoms. The decline of cognitive function (dementia) and memory loss then follow, with psychosis, depression and suicidal tendencies in some patients. The average age of diagnosis is at about 40 years, with the average age of death some 15 years later.

Genetic linkage studies assigned the locus for Huntington chorea to the short arm of chromosome 4. The successful linkage study was one of the first to employ restriction fragment length polymorphisms (RFLP), finding coinheritance of the HD mutant allele with alternative forms of a DNA marker called G8. Subsequent cloning of DNA fragments from this region allowed a contig to be assembled, and recombinations between DNA markers flanking the region and HD mutations allowed a candidate gene region to be identified. Among nine different genes identified in this region, a Huntington gene was identified adjacent to an unstable region containing CAG trinucleotide repeats that were amplified in patients with HD. The gene or its deduced protein (Huntingtin) has no homology to other characterized genes and has not provided insight into pathogenesis.

The fact that repeat numbers exceeding 37 on one of the two HD alleles correlated with the presence of HD symptoms provided a diagnostic and predictive test. Higher numbers of CAG repeats (e.g., 55–65) do correlate with younger ages of onset (e.g., ages 15–35 years), but not with particular symptoms or severity. Males with amplified repeats can transmit even higher numbers (e.g., 65–75) to their offspring and producing juvenile HD (onset at ages 5–15 years). The reason for this predilection for repeat instability during male meiosis is unknown, but it conforms to selective instability in female meiosis for the triplet repeats in fragile X syndrome (309550) or myotonic dystrophy (160900).

Predictive testing for HD became available when the G8 marker exhibited close linkage to the causative locus in 1983. Considerable effort has been expended in designing protocols for testing, since it has long been known that there is a high rate of depression and suicide that can accompany the diagnosis. With the advent of accurate testing by measurement of triplet repeat number, predictive testing for HD has been offered by many centers worldwide under a consensus protocol. At-risk patients must have psychiatric evaluations and extensive counseling prior to testing and agree to participate in counseling sessions for the divulgence of test results.

Although there has been less participation in predictive testing than was predicted by surveys before its availability, the outcomes for both reassured and diagnosed patients have been encouraging (Hayden and Kremer, 1995). There have been few problems with depression in those individuals found to be at high risk, but many exhibit inordinate attention to symptoms and require frequent evaluation and reassurance. There is understandable relief on the part of individuals found to be at low risk, but about 10% have had problems adjusting. Reasons have included "survivor" guilt (discomfort at being normal while sibs are not) and sudden confrontation of an unplanned future. Interestingly, fewer than 20% of individuals who received a positive test result chose to have prenatal diagnosis after becoming pregnant. A predominant reason was the anticipation of new treatment methods by the time the fetus would reach middle age.

As with other dementias and neurodegenerative diseases, no current therapies can prevent or delay the loss of cognitive functions. Family and social supports should encourage normal routines for as long as possible, and neuroleptics that compete at dopamine receptors like phenothiazines may suppress the chorea. Antidepressive agents for psychiatric problems and anticonvulsants for seizures may also be indicated. Despite its rarity, HD has become an important model for predictive testing, with pretesting evaluations and counseling assuming great importance. The current hypothesis for disease pathogenesis involves excess of excitatory neurotransmitters, and it is hoped that blocking agents may be found to delay, diminish, or eliminate the neurologic progression of HD.

Neurosensory Disorders: Vision and Hearing Loss

A huge number of multifactorial and Mendelian disorders affect the senses. Many of these are congenital syndromes that impact eye or ear development, while others involve risks for compression of cranial nerves or damage through infection. Table 14.4 lists several among many multifactorial or Mendelian disorders that cause vision or hearing loss. Although most cases with neurosensory impairment present during childhood, several can have progressive or delayed onset with presentation during adulthood. The key to managing these disorders is to appreciate the numerous Mendelian diseases that present with neurosensory problems and to ensure that appropriate diagnostic studies are performed. Patients without family histories of neurosensory problems often assume that their problem is caused by toxins or injury. Genetic counseling, together with many DNA diagnostic tests that are available for neurosensory diseases, offers important information and options to affected individuals and their families. Two examples of many neurosensory disorders are discussed— glaucoma and sensorineural deafness. Similar constellations of multifactorial and Mendelian diseases occur for retinitis pigmentosa, optic atrophy, cataracts, and conductive hearing loss (e.g., otosclerosis).

Increased pressure in the eye (glaucoma) usually occurs when the outflow of intraocular fluid is blocked. The normal flow of intraocular fluid proceeds from the ciliary body in the posterior chamber through the pupil into the anterior chamber and out through a meshwork of vessels at the circumferential angle where the iris and cornea meet. Glaucoma occurs in many congenital anomalies and syndromes as a secondary phenomenon and can present as an autosomal recessive disorder (231300) during infancy. Infantile glaucoma occurs when the eye is expandible and produces enlargement of the eye and iris (buphthalmos). Once common association with early onset glaucoma is the Sturge-Weber syndrome with facial hemangiomas and seizures.

Later-onset glaucoma occurs as an open angle type and a closed angle type where the anterior chamber between the iris and cornea is narrowed (Isenberg and Heckenlively, 1990). The presence of glaucoma at any age requires immediate treatment to alleviate pressure on the optic disc that destroys vision. The open angle glaucoma exhibits multifactorial causation (Table 14.4). Onset is usually in middle to late adult life with a prevalence of about 1%. Affected relatives are found in about 50% of cases with chronic open angle glaucoma, and the reverse situation of a person with a known affected relative implies a four- to fivefold increase in that person's risk for glaucoma. No genetic markers of risk have been defined, but screening relatives of affected individuals for increases in intraocular pressure is recommended. The presentation in chronic glaucoma is subtle, with mild headaches or halos around lights due to corneal swelling. Acute glaucoma presents with more intense pain and decreased vision. Simple dilation or constriction of the pupil may relieve the obstruction in closed angle glaucoma, while open angle patients usually respond to topic medications or laser surgery.

Deafness occurs in more than 100 congenital or inherited syndromes, including some with ear anomalies that were discussed in Chapter 13. Beighton (1990) estimated from experience in South Africa that 30% of deafness was genetic, including 10% as syndromes, with 40% being acquired and 30% of unknown cause. Isolated deafness includes autosomal dominant, autosomal recessive, and X-linked forms, most of which are sensorineural (abnormal otic nerve) rather than conductive (abnormal ossicles or blockage due to middle ear fluid). Conductive deafness is particularly common in syndromes with ear anomalies (e.g., Treacher-Collins syndrome, 154500) or with predisposition to ear infections (e.g., Down syndrome). Deafness is frequently associated with skeletal, renal, or dental anomalies, and occurs as a secondary complication of certain craniofacial syndromes that lead to progressive compression of the otic nerve.

Early detection of deafness is of obvious importance for speech development and for genetic counseling. Evaluation of hearing can be performed during infancy by measuring brain signals evoked by sounds broadcast to the ear. Routine audiology screening can be initiated by age two in cooperative children, and any hearing loss quantified for particular frequencies or transmission (e.g., bone versus nerve). The large number of Mendelian conditions that cause nonsyndromic hearing loss means that many deaf couples who both have autosomal recessive disorders may have hearing children because of complementation (each transmits a normal allele from the locus that is homozygous abnormal in the opposite parent). Rapid progress is being made in the delineation of these many genes that cause isolated hearing loss, with implications for early detection and prenatal diagnosis. Based on the negative emotions provoked by cochlear implants and oral speech training in certain members of the deaf community, it behooves health providers to become culturally aware before discussing recurrence risks and prenatal options with deaf individuals.

Unlike glaucoma but like other causes for vision loss like retinitis pigmentosa, more than 20 genes for nonsyndromic deafness have now been mapped or characterized. Many more are characterized for syndromic forms of deafness, illustrated by the type IV collagen gene responsible for certain types of Alport syndrome (104200) with hearing loss and renal disease. The Jervell and Lange-Nielsen syndrome (220400) that includes cardiomyopathy has been associated with mutations in a gene that encodes a potassium channel in the cell membrane. Mutations responsible for isolated deafness include those impacting a gap junction molecule called connexin 26 and a gene encoding an atypical myosin. Such genes should provide insights into the mechanisms of inner ear development and of progressive hearing loss in adults.

Mental Illness Including Schizophrenia and Mood Disorders

Schizophrenia is a major contributor to the economic burden of disease, with prevalences between 0.1 and 1% and high costs due to chronic treatment and lost productivity. Diagnosis is subjective and variable, with symptoms such as loose or illogical associations, flat or inappropriate emotional responses, ambivalence, and autistic withdrawal from society with internal fantasies. Deviations from reality with hallucinations (imaginary occurrences) or delusions (altered perception of real occurrences) are common but not integral to the diagnosis. The Diagnostic and Statistical Manual (DSM)-IV criteria are most utilized for diagnosis and reveal an earlier onset in males. Genetic predisposition to schizophrenia is indicated by a 9–12% risk for primary relatives and a 50% rate in monozygotic twins compared to 0.8 percent in a control population (Kinney, 1990). Risk factors including particular HLA alleles have not been discovered for schizophrenia, although there is an association with gluten enteropathy (celiac disease). The higher recurrence risk for relatives has important clinical implications, because mortality is higher in schizophrenics and pharmacologic therapy is extensive and effective. Given the high prevalence, morbidity, and benefits of treatment, predictive testing for schizophrenia would be desirable if suitable genetic markers could be found. An international consortium has been formed to search for genetic markers, with preliminary associations between markers on chromosome regions 6p, 8p, and 10p (Cloninger et al., 1998; Straub et al., 1998). Environmental influences are likely to be important in this multifactorial group of disorders, because low socioeconomic status exhibits high correlation with the disease in urban areas.

Mood disorders can be divided into unipolar illness dominated by depression and bipolar illness wherein individuals exhibit manic episodes with or without depression. The latter bipolar or manic-depressive illness exhibits the greater genetic predisposition in most studies. Diagnosis is again subjective with criteria provided by the DSM-IV consensus guidelines. Depression is diagnosed in individuals with four of seven symptoms including: 1) increase or decrease in weight; 2) insomnia or hypersomnia; 3) psychomotor retardation or agitation; 4) lack of energy; 5) inappropriate guilt or self-reproach; 6) difficulty in concentrating or thinking; 7) recurring thoughts of death or suicide (Kinney, 1990). Manic behavior is diagnosed if three to four of the following seven symptoms are present: 1) increased activity or restlessness; 2) pressured speech or talkativeness; 3) racing thoughts or flight of ideas; 4) grandiosity; 5) decreased need for sleep; 6) distractibility; and 7) buying sprees, reckless driving, or other high risk behaviors (Kinney, 1990). Based on these criteria, the frequency of unipolar depression is about 3% for men and 5% for women with 0.8% of individuals having manic episodes and 0.6% having manic depressive illness.

The higher prevalence of unipolar illness in women is paralleled by higher risks for women (7–32%) than men (6–18%) to have a depressive illness when a first degree relative is affected (Gershon et al., 1976). Monozygotic (MZ) and dizygotic (DZ) twin concordant rates are correspondingly high, with 40/11 percent for MZ/DZ twins for unipolar cases and 72/14 MZ/DZ twins for bipolar cases (Kinney, 1990). Despite the clear genetic predisposition in bipolar illness, no HLA or DNA marker alleles have been associated with the phenotype.

Mendelian Causes of Psychiatric Disease—Acute Intermittent Porphyria and Wilson Disease

Although both disorders have additional symptoms that should separate them from other psychiatric disorders, patients with acute intermittent porphyria (AIP—176000) and Wilson disease (277900) may be misdiagnosed unless the underlying metabolic abnormality is pursued. AIP is one of several defects in the metabolism of porphyrin, the molecular precursor to heme. A block in the enzyme porphobilinogen deaminase causes the accumulation of porphobilinogen, heme deficiency, and a wide spectrum of intermittent symptoms in the estimated 1 per 10,000 people with AIP. Acute episodes of abdominal pain, vomiting, and diarrhea may lead to inappropriate surgical exploration, and concurrent adrenergic stimulation can produce fever, sweating, restlessness, tremors and even lethal cardiac arrhythmias. Toxicity to nervous tissue is indicated by muscle weakness due to involvement of the peripheral nerves and psychiatric symptoms such as anxiety, insomnia, depression, and hallucinations. The diagnosis of AIP can be made using the Watson-Schwartz test that detects urinary porphobilinogen as a purple complex, followed by the appropriate enzyme assays. The availability of effective therapy by averting crises with oral carbohydrates, by alleviating pain, and by administering of heme solutions makes it particularly important to recognize this rare cause of psychiatric symptoms.

Wilson disease manifests with hepatic and/or neurologic symptoms, with about half of patients presenting in adulthood. The prevalence is 1 in 30,000 with little ethnic variation. Increased copper levels are present in the blood,

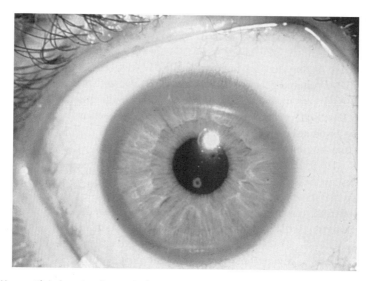

Figure 14.2. Kayser-Fleischer ring (green halo around edge of iris) in a patient with Wilson disease. Photograph courtesy of Dr. Harold Falls.

tissues, and urine of patients with Wilson disease due to a defect in cellular copper uptake. The responsible gene has been isolated and is a membrane-bound copper transporter at chromosome band 13q14 (Payne et al., 1998). Symptoms of liver disease occur in about half the patients and include hepatitis, chronic active hepatitis, and cirrhosis. A characteristic diagnostic sign that is usually present by adolescence is a greenish Kayser-Fleischer ring around the iris (Fig. 14. 2). Older patients with neurologic presentations thus always have a Kayser-Fleischer ring, and the absence of this sign upon examination by an experienced ophthalmologist can rule out the diagnosis in patients with psychiatric symptoms. Most patients with neurologic symptoms have a movement disorder with tremors, chorea, spasticity, and drooling. Psychiatric symptoms can mimic those of schizophrenia or manic depressive illness and fulfill many of the diagnostic criteria discussed previously. Because treatment with chelating agents such as penicillamine is effective, and interruption or delay in treatment can cause irreversible deterioration and death, Wilson disease is a Mendelian extreme that must be considered in patients with chronic liver or psychiatric disease.

■ 14.6 GENETICS OF COMMON CANCERS

The approach to cancer is similar to that of other multifactorial diseases described in this chapter. Most cancer cases occur sporadically with multifactorial determination. Attention to the family history and to accessory findings on physical examination will alert the practitioner to unusual cancer cases with strong genetic predisposition. The recognition of familial cancers allows genetic counseling and the possibility of predictive diagnosis, surveillance and intervention for at-risk relatives, and design of medical or surgical therapy appropriate for the underlying genetic diagnosis. As discussed in Chapter 9, the recognition of adenomatous polyposis coli (175100) in a parent with colon cancer allows evaluation of offspring at 50% risk; presence of a mutant *APC* gene would mandate colectomy rather than local tumor resection to prevent recurrence.

In Chapter 9, common changes in signal transduction pathways that lead to immune, developmental, or neoplastic disorders were emphasized. Although each cancer arises from a cascade of genetic events within certain somatic cells, the primary switch initiating this cascade is activated by a combination of environmental and genetic factors. All cancers are thus multifactorial diseases, with genes being more important in some than in others. Bishop and Skolnick (1984) evaluated the familial clustering of common cancers in a database of 1.5 million people. The likelihood of relatedness between individuals with particular types of cancer was compared to that of random individuals, yielding an estimate of genetic predisposition for each cancer. Individuals with skin cancers (2.5-fold), prostate cancers (2-fold), gastrointestinal cancers (1.7–2-fold), and breast cancers (1.7-fold) exhibited higher likelihood of relatedness, while those with lung cancers (1.3-fold) and lymphomas (equal) exhibited little increased likelihood. The data forecast the possibility of finding genes of major effect that initiate the pathway toward an isolated, common cancer. Such genes would be very useful as risk factors for isolated cancers, complementing those that have been defined in characteristic cancer syndromes such as adenomatous polyposis coli (see Table 9.6).

Leukemias

Just as anemia is a common phenotype with occasional genetic cause, leukemia (white blood) is a common cancer of white blood cells with higher frequency in particular Mendelian or chromosomal syndromes (Table 14.5). Because of access to dividing cells in peripheral blood or bone marrow, leukemias have led the way in defining characteristic chromosomal rearrangements that are unique to leukemic cells. An early example was the Philadelphia chromosome found in chronic myeloid leukemia—a chromosome 22 with a deleted long arm that was later revealed to be present on chromosome 9 as a balanced translocation. Molecular analysis has revealed that the translocation moves the c-*abl* proto-oncogene on chromosome 9 adjacent to the *bcr* proto-oncogene on chromosome 22, activiting *bcr* expression as a cause for white blood cell proliferation. Many other typical chromosome rearrangements (Table 14.5) have been

defined in lymphatic leukemias (cancers of lymphocytes) or myeloid leukemias (cancers from granulocytes). These changes en route to cancer provide useful diagnostic and prognostic markers, but the primary initiating event for leukemia is still unknown.

Abundant evidence for familial predisposition to leukemia has been garnered, exemplified by a study showing that relatives with leukemia are 16 times more likely in families with an affected individual. Consanguinity is also increased in such families, and there is a 17–25% concordance rate in monozygotic twins that must be viewed from the perspective of shared fetal circulations (Rowley, 1990). Despite the chromosomal or genetic changes that can be documented in almost every leukemia, the heritability of incidence is lower than that for many other cancers (e.g., colon cancer). The high frequency of leukemia in certain syndromes with altered DNA repair or chromosome structure (Table 14.5) may indicate that the inherited factor is DNA or chromosome instability, with leukemia being one of several possible outcomes that reflects the normal demand for white cell proliferation. Certain genetic disorders like deficiency of adenosine deaminase (102700—see Chapter 9) impose constraints on DNA replication and are manifest in cell types that must proliferate in the course of normal function (e.g., immune stem cells in the bone marrow and skeletal chondrocytes).

Two chronic leukemias and a disease with proliferation of red blood cells (polycythemia vera) are common problems in adult patients. Chronic leukemias present insidiously with fatigue, bone pain, or prolonged/unusual infections signaling malfunction of the blood elements. Chronic lymphocytic leukemia is the most common of all leukemias and accounts for 30% of affected patients (Rowley, 1990). The proliferating cells are usually B cells (see Chapter 9) that are harder to karyotype than T-cell leukemias. Characteristic translocations with a common breakpoint at chromosome band 14q32 are often observed in those patients with successful karyotypes (Table 14.5).

■**TABLE 14.5.** Genetics of Selected Common Cancers

Cancer	Associated Factors	Genetic Risk	Mendelian Disorders
Leukemias			
Chronic lymphocytic	Translocations with 14q32 breakpoints		Bloom syndrome (210900)
Chronic myelogenous	Philadelphia t(9;22) translocation	Slight increase	Fanconi anemia (227650, 227660)
Polycythemia vera	Translocations of 1, 20		Down syndrome (trisomy 21) Trisomy 8, 9
Gastrointestinal			
Colon	Ulcerative colitis Adenomatous polyps Dietary fat	3–3.5 fold (primary)	Adenomatous polyposis coli (175100), Lynch colon cancer (114500)
Stomach	Chronic gastritis Pernicious anemia Immune deficiency	1.5–7 fold (primary)	
Esophageal Small bowel	Alcohol, tobacco		Peutz-Jeghers syndrome (175200)
Liver	Hepatitis virus Alcoholic cirrhosis		α-1-antitrypsin deficiency (107400) Wilson disease (277900)
Hormone-responsive			
Breast	Ovarian cancer Estrogen production *Her2/Neu* oncogenes	2–3 fold (primary)	*BRCA*1, *BRCA*2 Cowden disease (158350) Li-Fraumeni syndrome (114480)
Prostate	Androgen production Prostate-specific antigen (PSA) Trisomy 7, 8 *BCL-2* oncogene expression	2–3 fold (primary)	Rare autosomal dominant forms

Note: Primary-primary or first-degree relatives.

Chronic myelogenous leukemia is associated with the Philadelphia chromosome in 80–90% of cases, and cells with this abnormality persist in the bone marrow after remission is induced by chemotherapeutic agents such as hydroxyurea. Patients with chronic myelogenous leukemia may develop an acute "blast crisis" after variable periods of remission, and these new proliferative white cells have new chromosome rearrangements in addition to the Philadelphia translocation. Adult disorders related to chronic myelogenous leukemia are myelofibrosis with myeloid metaplasia (bone marrow atrophic and replaced with altered myeloid cells) and myelodysplasia syndromes (alterations of hematopoetic stem cells with deficiencies of peripheral blood elements and numerous, immature cells in the bone marrow). These latter disorders also may enter an acute leukemic phase signaled by the appearance of new cells with new chromosome arrangements. The appearance of cells with new chromosome re-arrangements in chronic myeloid disorders is thus an ominous sign. New therapies are becoming available for these disorders using antibodies directed against the particular type of B- or T-cell that has proliferated to cause leukemia and/or bone marrow dysfunction.

Polycythemia vera is a proliferative disorder of red cell precursors and other marrow elements that usually present in late middle age. As with other chronic leukemias, occasional cases in relatives or monozygotic twins indicate a genetic predisposition. The increased production of red cells and other blood elements causes plethora (flushed appearance) with headaches, dizziness, and splenomegaly due to expanded blood volume. Cytogenetic changes are diverse with aneuploidy for chromosomes 8 or 9 and rearrangements involving chromosomes 1 and 20. As with other chronic myeloproliferative disorders, karyotype evolution with acute leukemia may occur with lethal implications. The acute transformation occurs more often in patients whose polycythemia vera is treated with chemotherapeutic agents, so chronic bleeding is used to lower blood volume as done in hemochromatosis to lower iron stores. Unlike patients with hemochromatosis, patients with polycythemia vera are at risk for iron deficiency anemia unless placed on iron supplements.

Advances in the treatment of leukemias has led to prolonged survival in most forms and remarkable cures in certain types of acute lymphocytic leukemias. Favorable types of childhood lymphocytic leukemias now have cure rates of greater than 50% due to aggressive use of chemotherapy and improved antibiotics for treating infections during the period of marrow suppression. Improvements in therapy have mainly resulted from better chemotherapeutic agents and registry approaches to study large patient groups; aside from antibodies to particular leukocyte surface molecules, the genetic associations with particular chromosomal rearrangements and oncogenes have been more useful as prognostic signs than as insights for new therapies. These insights are still needed

because successfully treated cases may mimic the acute transition in chronic myeloid diseases and develop secondary leukemias in later life. As in the Mendelian or chromosomal syndromes with higher risks for leukemia listed in Table 14.5, these secondary leukemias may reflect DNA and chromosomal damage inflicted on residual cells by chemotherapeutic agents.

Gastrointestinal Cancers

Gastrointestinal cancers that involve the lips and mouth are mainly caused by tobacco use and of a different type than those of the stomach and intestines. Cancer of the large bowel (colon and rectum) is the most common with an incidence of about 40 per year per 100,000 people over age 35 (about 150,000 total each year in the United States). Pancreatic (7), stomach (7), liver (3.5), esophagus (2.6), and small bowel (0.6) cancers have lower incidences with proportionately lower numbers of cases. Esophageal (2.5-fold) and gastric (1.5-fold) cancers exhibit higher frequencies in males, while the others exhibit equal sex predilection. Striking ethnic and geographic differences in incidence of gastrointestinal cancers have been documented, with colon cancer being 10-fold lower in certain African countries and gastric cancer being 7-fold higher in Japan. Several studies have documented a 3–3.5-fold increased risk for colon cancer in first degree relatives of affected persons, and a 1.5–7-fold increased risk for gastric cancer (Table 14.5). Twin studies revealing increased concordance for these cancers have been documented, but the number of cases was extremely small. Little familial data has been accumulated for other types of gastrointestinal cancer.

Epidemiologic studies have defined associated or predisposing factors for several types of gastrointestinal cancer (Table 14.5). Often these factors relate to chronic injury and regeneration of the organ tissue, as with ulcerative colitis in colon cancer, alcohol and gastritis from pernicious anemia in stomach cancer, alcohol and tobacco in esophageal cancer, and hepatitis virus or alcoholic cirrhosis in liver cancer. Colonic polyps are a risk factor for colon cancer whether they are inherited or not, and the finding of a polyp predicts the presence of others in the colon and a higher risk for colon cancer (Burt and Lipkin, 1992). Genetic disorders that favor polyp formation are associated with high rates of colon cancer. These include the Lynch syndrome of colon cancers (114500), adenomatous polyposis coli (175100) that can also have bony tumors and eye changes defined as Gardner syndrome, and Peutz-Jeghers syndrome (175200) with freckles on the lips and polyps of the small intestine (Table 14.5). Damage from chronic hepatitis and cirrhosis probably accounts for the increased risk for liver cancer in α-1-antitrypsin deficiency (107400) and Wilson disease (277900).

As with most cancers, successful management of gastrointestinal cancer relies on early detection. Although genetic tests are becoming available to predict risk for Mendelian syndromes that exhibit higher risks for gastrointestinal cancer (Table 14.5), there are no genetic markers that allow predictive testing for isolated gastrointestinal cancers. Individuals of appropriate age or with environmental exposure should be educated regarding symptoms and screening strategies (detection of occult blood) for colon cancer.

Hormone-Responsive Cancers— Breast and Prostate

Two common cancers with prevalence in older individuals almost equivalent to that of gastrointestinal cancer are those of the breast and prostate (Table 14.1). Each cancer is almost sex-specific (male breast cancer rarely occurs), with most forms exhibiting sensitivity to the appropriate sex hormone for their incidence and progression. The risk of breast cancer in women, for example, correlates with the lifetime exposure to higher estrogens as indicated by earlier menarche or later menopause. Each cancer has a two- to threefold higher prevalence in like-sex siblings of affected individu-

als. For breast cancer as with coronary heart disease, the risk to relatives increases greatly for individuals with early-onset disease.

The lifetime risks for breast or prostate cancers are about 10%, and it has been estimated that all individuals would develop cancers with sufficient longevity. Specific chromosomal abnormalities and the alterations of specific oncogenes have been defined in both types of cancer (Table 14.5), and the variety of these changes suggests greater heterogeneity in the type or progressions of these hormone-responsive cancers as opposed to the leukemias.

Rare families exhibiting autosomal dominant inheritance have been identified for breast and prostate cancer: Such families have led to the identification of the *BRCA1* (chromosome band 17q21) and *BRCA2* (13q12) genes predisposing to breast cancer with ongoing studies in prostate cancer. Identification of the *BRCA* breast cancer genes brought forward the possibility of predictive testing or screening to identify women with high risks of breast cancer. However, even those women from breast cancer families or with early onset have a 7% frequency of *BRCA* mutant alleles. Since the *BRCA* genes are large and most patients have different mutations, predictive testing is not routine. For prostate cancer, a prostate-specific antigen (PSA) is secreted into serum that allows mass screening of older men. The many alterations of oncogene expression in both types of cancer may offer future hope for predictive testing. Additional hope for understanding and predictive testing of patients with breast cancer is offered by its associated Mendelian syndromes that document the involvement of other specific genes like the *p53* (Li-Fraumeni) and *PTEN* (Cowden) protooncogenes in breast cancer causation (Table 14.5).

Prostate cancer is highly associated with androgen production and benign prostatic hypertrophy that occurs in 90% of men by age 80. Its presentation is usually asymptomatic or congruent with the slow, frequent voiding and urgency of urination that occurs with benign hypertrophy. Yearly rectal examination to palpate the prostate for men over age 50 is the best method for early detection, with blood PSA levels being a helpful adjunct that lacks sufficient sensitivity and specificity for mass screening. For women, self-examination of the breast after age 20, yearly physical examinations after age 40, and yearly radiographic mammography after age 50 are recommended to all women. High-risk women with strong family histories will need more aggressive and frequent monitoring, and DNA testing for *BRCA* or other hereditary factors can aid the difficult decision for prophylactic mastectomy. Treatment for breast or prostate cancer is best for smaller tumors using surgical excision, and withdrawal of hormone stimulus by oophorectomy or orchiectomy can stabilize tumor progression and improve pain from bony metastases. Chemotherapy and radiation therapy are available for both types of cancer, but the serious prognosis for metastatic cases emphasizes the importance of family history, routine screening, and early detection.

PROBLEM SET 14
Genetics and Adult Medicine

Respond to the following questions with short answers, consulting Tables 14.1–14.5 or Figs. 14.1–14.2. For each clinical presentation, discuss the genetic evaluation, possible diagnoses, and potential recurrence risks for the family:

14.1. A woman has a cardiac arrhythmia and deafness, while her younger sister has only deafness.

14.2. A 29-year-old male has a heart attack. His father and grandfather died of heart attacks in their early 40s.

14.3. A woman is diagnosed with Crohn's disease, and wishes to know the risk that her daughter will develop the disease. She is otherwise normal with an unremarkable family history.

14.4. A 24-year-old woman develops bilateral breast cancer. Her mother died of ovarian cancer, as did a maternal aunt. She has two daughters aged 12 and 16.

14.5. A male teenager presents for a school physical with tall stature, thin body build, concave chest (pectus), long fingers, flat feet, and increased joint laxity. His father died at age 35 with a heart attack. He wants approval to play basketball.

14.6. A 30-year-old man has hypertension controlled by diet and medication. His father died of kidney failure, and one of his three sons has been diagnosed with cystic kidneys.

14.7. A middle-aged man presents for his annual physical and admits to being a heavy drinker. His liver is small and firm on examination and blood tests reveal elevated levels of liver enzymes. His two brothers and one of three sisters also have liver disease but do not talk about it with him. They too are heavy drinkers.

14.8. A newborn is evaluated for increased jaundice, and a family history reveals chronic anemia in his mother and several maternal relatives.

14.9. A deaf couple present for genetic counseling. The husband has a white forelock in his hair and differently colored eyes. The wife has a normal physical examination.

14.10. A 20-year-old man presents to the emergency room with hallucinations and abusive behavior. A urine drug screen is normal, and blood testing reveals elevated liver enzymes.

PROBLEM SET 14
Answers

14.1–14.10. See Solutions

PROBLEM SET 14
Solutions

14.1. The cardiac arrhythmia and deafness are suggestive of a Mendelian disorder such as the Jervell and Lange-Nielsen syndrome (220400,

Table 14.2). This autosomal recessive disease implies a 25% risk that other siblings will be affected, but a minimal risk for the affected women to transmit the disease (their spouses are unlikely to be carriers unless they are related).

14.2. The early onset and family history of heart attacks suggests a genetic disorder. Familial hypercholesterolemia (143890, Table 14.2) would be most likely, with blood lipid levels, Lp(a), and Apo E marker studies being indicated if this diagnosis was excluded. In the case of familial hypercholesterolemia, offspring of the 29-year-old male would have 50% risk to inherit the LDL receptor mutation.

14.3. Crohn's disease is a multifactorial disorder with a 7.5% risk for siblings of affected individuals to develop the disease (Table 14.1). Approximately the same risk would apply to other primary relatives such as the woman's daughter.

14.4. The family history is suggestive of autosomal dominant breast cancer due to BRCA gene mutations or Li-Fraumeni syndrome (114480, Table 14.5). The daughters would be at 50% risk for breast cancer, and DNA testing on the mother could determine if a particular BRCA1, BRCA2, or p53 (Li-Fraumeni) tumor suppressor gene were present. Such testing is useful for women with early onset, familial breast cancer but has a low yield in isolated cases. Testing of the minor daughters raises the ethical issues of informed consent and autonomy (parent versus child), but would probably pursued because of the advantages of early screening or prophylactic mastectomy.

14.5. The physical findings in the teenager and sudden death in his father support a diagnosis of Marfan syndrome (154700). These individuals are at risk for aortic dissection and sudden death in collision or high intensity sports and should not participate. Note that the history of "heart attack" in the father was probably an aortic dissection, stressing the need for medical and autopsy information to discriminate among cardiac causes of sudden death (Table 14.2).

14.6. The family history and presence of hypertension is suggestive of autosomal dominant polycystic kidney disease (173900, Table 14.3). This disease may not manifest until adulthood, and renal imaging may be required for diagnosis. The 30-year-old man has imaging studies to confirm the diagnosis, followed by imaging studies of his two apparently normal sons and any siblings.

14.7. The history suggests alcoholic cirrhosis, which can be familial due to the multifactorial determination of both alcoholism and predisposition to cirrhosis in alcoholics. However, the possibility of autosomal recessive inheritance should prompt consideration of a Mendelian disorder exacerbated by drinking, and iron studies revealed the presence of hemochromatosis (235200).

14.8. Although increased jaundice in a newborn can have many different causes, the family history of chronic anemia suggests an inherited disorder of red cell, enzyme, or hemoglobin structure (Table 14.3). The family history sounds most compatible with an autosomal dominant anemia such as spherocytosis (182900). If confirmed, this diagnosis implies a 50% recurrence risk for the infant and his affected maternal relatives.

14.9. Deafness with a white forelock (poliosis) and differently colored eyes (heterochromia) are suggestive of autosomal dominant Waardenburg syndrome (193500) in the husband. The wife could also have a Mendelian form of deafness despite her normal physical examination (Table 14.4). If her form of deafness also followed autosomal dominant inheritance, the risk for deafness in their offspring would be 75%.

14.10. The combination of liver disease with possible psychotic behavior could represent acute alcoholism alone or mental illness with alcoholism. Rare diseases such as Wilson disease (277900) should also be considered, and the diagnosis could be made by eye examination (Fig. 14.2). A diagnosis of Wilson disease would imply a 25% risk for each sibling to be affected with a low recurrence risk for the patient's offspring.

BIBLIOGRAPHY

General References

Beighton P, ed. 1993. *McKusick's Heritable Disorders of Connective Tissue,* 5th ed. St. Louis: Mosby.

Gorlin RJ, Cohen MM Jr, Levin LS. 1990. *Syndromes of the Head and Neck.* New York: Oxford.

King RA, Rotter JI, Motulsky AG. 1992. *The Genetic Basis of Common Diseases.* New York: Oxford University Press.

McKusick VA. 1994. *Mendelian Inheritance in Man,* 11th ed. Baltimore: Johns Hopkins; online at http://www3.ncbi.nlm.nih.gov/omim.

Rimoin DL, Emery AEH, Pyeritz R. 1995. *Principles and Practice of Medical Genetics.* Edinburgh: Churchill Livingstone.

Royce PM, Steinmann B. 1993. *Connective Tissue and its Heritable Disorders.* New York: Wiley-Liss.

Scriver CR, Beaudet AL, Sly WS, Valle D, eds. 1995. *The Metabolic and Molecular Bases of Inherited Disease,* 7th ed. New York: McGraw-Hill, pp. 1015–1076.

Winter RM, Baraitser M. 1998. *London Dysmorphology Database.* Ver. 3.0. Oxford: Oxford University Press.

Cardiology

Boerwinkle E. 1996. Coronary artery disease. A contemporary paradigm for the genetic analysis of a common chronic disease. *Ann Med* 28: 451–457.

Boerwinkle E, Ellsworth DL, Hallman DM, Biddinger A. 1996. Genetic analysis of atherosclerosis: a research paradigm for the common chronic diseases. *Hum Mol Genet* 5:1405–1410.

Goldstein JL, Hobbs HH, Brown MS. 1995. Familial hypercholesterolemia. In Scriver CR, Beaudet AL, Sly WS, Valle D, eds. *The Metabolic and Molecular Bases of Inherited Disease,* 7th ed. New York: McGraw-Hill, pp. 1981–2030.

McKenna WJ, Watkins HC. 1995. Hypertrophic cardiomyopathy. In Scriver CR, Beaudet AL, Sly WS, Valle D, eds. *The Metabolic and Molecular*

Bases of Inherited Disease. 7th ed, New York: McGraw-Hill, pp. 4253–74.

Motulsky AG, Brunzell JD. 1992. The genetics of coronary atherosclerosis. In King RA, Rotter JI, Motulsky AG, eds. *The Genetic Basis of Common Diseases.* New York: Oxford University Press, pp. 150–169.

Pyeritz RE., 1993. The Marfan syndrome. In Royce PM, Steinmann B, eds. *Connective Tissue and its Heritable Disorders: Molecular, Genetic, and Medical Aspects.* New York: Wiley-Liss, pp. 437–506.

Autoimmune Diseases

Cole B, Conley S, Stapleton FB. 1987. Polycystic kidney disease in the first year of life. *J Pediatr* 111:693–9.

Goronzy JJ, Weyland CM. 1995. T cells in rheumatoid arthritis. Paradigms and facts. *Rheum Dis Clin North Am* 21:655–674.

Heyward J, Gough SC. 1997. Genetic susceptibility to the development of autoimmune disease. *Clin Sci* 93:479–491.

King RA. 1992. Rheumatoid arthritis. In King RA, Rotter JI, Motulsky AG, eds. *The Genetic Basis of Common Diseases.* New York: Oxford University Press, pp. 596–624.

McConnell RB, Vadheim CM. 1992. Inflammatory bowel disease. In King RA, Rotter JI, Motulsky AG, eds. *The Genetic Basis of Common Diseases.* New York: Oxford University Press, pp. 326–348.

Penn AS, Crusius JB. 1998. Genetics of inflammatory bowel disease: implications for the future. *World J Surg* 22:390–393.

Satsangi J, Parks M, Jewell DP, Bell JI. 1998. Genetics of inflammatory bowel disease. *Clin Sci* 94:473–478.

Wordsworth P. 1995. Genes and arthritis. *Br Med Bull* 51:249–266.

Selected Subspecialty Diseases

Becker PS, Lux SE. 1995. Hereditary spherocytosis and hereditary elliptocytosis. In Scriver CR, Beaudet AL, Sly WS, Valle D, eds. *The Metabolic and Molecular Bases of Inherited Disease,* 7th ed. New York: McGraw-Hill, pp. 3513–3562.

Bothwell TH, Charlton RW, Motulsky AG. 1995. Hemochromatosis. In Scriver CR, Beaudet AL, Sly WS, Valle D, eds. *The Metabolic and Molecular Bases of Inherited Disease,* 7th ed. New York: McGraw-Hill, pp. 2237–2270.

Jazwinska EC. 1998. Hemochromatosis: a genetic defect in iron metabolism. *Bioessays* 20: 562–568.

Jordan SC, Kangarloo H. 1990. Renal cystic diseases. In Rimoin DL, Emery AEH, Pyeritz R, eds. *Principles and Practice of Medical Genetics,* Edinburgh: Churchill Livingstone, pp. 1291–1313.

Kang K, Schwarzenberg SJ, Bloomer JR. 1992. Genetic basis of chronic liver disease. In King RA, Rotter JI, Motulsky AG, eds. *The Genetic Basis of Common Diseases.* New York: Oxford University Press, pp. 349–374.

Lelbach WK. 1976. Epidemiology of chronic alcoholic liver disease. *Progr Liver Dis* 5:494–515.

Ramrakhiani S, Bacon BR. 1998. Hemochromatosis: Advances in molecular genetics and clinical diagnosis. *J Clin Gastroenterol* 27:41–46.

Tanaka KR, Pagila DE. 1995. Pyruvate kinase and other enzymopathies of the erythrocyte. In Scriver CR, Beaudet AL, Sly WS, Valle D, eds. *The Metabolic and Molecular Bases of Inherited Disease,* 7th ed. New York: McGraw-Hill, pp. 3485–3512.

Torra R, Badenas C, Darnell A, Camacho JA, Aspinwall R, Harris PC, Estivill X. 1998. Facilitated diagnosis of the contiguous gene syndrome: tuberous sclerosis and polycystic kidneys by means of haplotype studies. *Am J Kidney Dis* 31:1038–1043.

Watnick TJ, Gandolph MA, Weber H, Neumann HP, Germino GG. 1998. Gene conversion is a likely cause of mutation in PKD1. *Hum Mol Genet* 7:1239–1243.

Zerres K, Rudnik-Schoneborn S, Steinkamm C, Becker J, Mucher G. 1998. Autosomal recessive polycystic kidney disease. *J Mol Med* 76: 303–309.

Neurologic Diseases

Beighton P. 1990. Hereditary deafness. In Emery AEH, Rimoin DL, eds. *Principles and Practice of Medical Genetics.* Edinburgh: Churchill Livingstone, pp. 1291–1304.

Blacker D, Tanzi RE. 1998. The genetics of Alzheimer disease: current status and future prospects. *Arch Neurol* 55:294–296.

Cloninger CR, Kaufmann CA, Faraone SV, Malaspina D, Svrakic DM, Harkavy-Friedman J, Suarez BK, Matise TC, Shore D, Lee H, Hampe CL, Wynne D, Drain C, Markel PD, Zambuto CT, Schmitt K , Tsuang MT. 1998. Genome-wide search for schizophrenia susceptibility loci:

the NIMH Genetics Initiative and Millenium Consortium. *Am J Med Genet* 81:275–281.

Danks DM. 1995. Disorders of copper transport. In Scriver CR, Beaudet AL, Sly WS, Valle D, eds. *The Metabolic and Molecular Bases of Inherited Disease,* 7th ed. New York: McGraw-Hill, pp. 2211–2236.

Gershon ES, Bunney WE, Leckman J, van Eerdewegh M, DeBauche B. 1976. The inheritance of affective disorders: a review of data and of hypotheses. *Behav Genet* 6:227–261.

Hayden MR, Kremer B. 1995. Huntington disease. In Scriver CR, Beaudet AL, Sly WS, Valle D, eds. *The Metabolic and Molecular Bases of Inherited Disease,* 7th ed. New York: McGraw-Hill, pp. 4483–4510.

Heston LL. 1992. Alzheimer's disease. In King RA, Rotter JI, Motulsky AG, eds. *The Genetic Basis of Common Diseases.* New York: Oxford University Press, pp. 792–800.

Isenberg SJ, Heckenlively JR. 1990. Glaucoma: congenital and later onset. In Rimoin DL, Emery AEH, Pyeritz R, eds. *Principles and Practice of Medical Genetics,* 2nd ed. Edinburgh: Churchill Livingstone, pp. 645–667.

Jarvik GP. 1997. Genetic predictors of common diseases: apolipoprotein E genotype as a paradigm. *Ann Epidemiol* 7:357–362.

Kinney DK. 1990. Schizophrenia and major mood disorders. In Rimoin DL, Emery AEH, Pyeritz R, eds. *Principles and Practice of Medical Genetics,* 2nd ed. Edinburgh: Churchill Livingstone, pp. 457–472.

Martini A, Mazzoli M, Kimberling W. 1997. An introduction to the genetics of normal and defective hearing. *Ann N Y Acad Sci* 830:361–374.

Payne AS, Kelly EJ, Gitlin JD. 1998. Functional expression of the Wilson disease protein reveals mislocalization and impaired copper-dependent trafficking of the common H1069Q mutation. *Proc Natl Acad Sci USA* 95:10854–10859.

Steel KP, Brown SD. 1996. The genetics of deafness. *Curr Opin Neurobiol* 6:520–525.

Straub RE, MacLean CJ, Martin RB, Ma Y, Myakishev MV, Harris-Kerr C, Webb BT, O'Neill FA, Walsh D, Kendler KS. 1998. A schizophrenia locus may be located in region 10p15-p11. *Am J Med Genet* 81:296–301.

Common Cancers

Bishop DT, Skolnick MH. 1984. Genetic epidemiology of cancer in Utah genealogies: a prelude to the molecular genetics of common cancers. *J Cell Physiol* (Suppl); 63–77.

Burt RW, Lipkin M. 1992. Gastrointestinal cancer. In King RA, Rotter JI, Motulsky AG, eds. *The Genetic Basis of Common Diseases.* New York: Oxford University Press.

Cannon-Albright LA, Skolnick MH. 1996. The genetics of familial breast cancer. *Semin Oncol* 23 (Suppl 2):1–5.

Garnick MB, Fair WR. 1996. Prostate cancer: emerging concepts. *Ann Intern Med* 125: 205–212.

Greene MH. 1997. Genetics of breast cancer. *Mayo Clin Proc* 72:54–65.

Healy B. 1997. BRCA genes—bookmaking, fortunetelling, and medical care. *N Engl J Med* 336:1448–1449.

Isaacs WB. 1995. Molecular genetics of prostate cancer. *Cancer Surv* 25:357–379.

Le Beau MM, Larson RA. 1992. Hematologic malignancies. In King RA, Rotter JI, Motulsky AG, eds. *The Genetic Basis of Common Diseases.* New York: Oxford University Press, pp. 711–731.

Newman B, Mu H, Butler LM, Millikan RC, Moorman PG, King MC. 1998. Frequency of breast cancer attributable to BRCA1 in a population-based series of American women. *JAMA* 279:915–921.

Radford DM, Zehnbauer BA. 1996. Inherited breast cancer. *Surg Clin North Am* 76:205–220.

Rowley JD. 1990. Leukaemias, lymphomas, and related disorders. In Rimoin DL, Emery AEH, Pyeritz R, eds. *Principles and Practice of Medical Genetics,* 2nd ed. Edinburgh: Churchill Livingstone, pp. 1391–1409.

Schifeling DJ, Horton J, Tafelski TJ. 1997. Common cancers—genetics, origin, prevention, screening. *Dis Mon* 43:681–742.

REPRODUCTIVE GENETICS AND PRENATAL DIAGNOSIS

■ LEARNING OBJECTIVES

1. Preconceptional planning and prenatal care are essential for every pregnancy.

2. Chronic diseases, reproductive tract anomalies, and chromosomal aberrations can cause infertility or pregnancy loss.

3. Of early pregnancy loss (0–8 weeks), 50% is attributable to chromosome aberrations.

4. Couples with recurrent spontaneous abortions should have chromosome studies to rule out the presence of balanced rearrangements.

5. Treatments for infertility include surrogate gametes, in vitro fertilization (IVF), gamete intrafallopian transfer (GIFT), and intracytoplasmic sperm injection (ICSI).

6. Artificial reproductive technologies for lowering genetic risks include sex selection by sperm fractionation or preimplantation analysis, blastomere analysis before implantation (BABI), and IVF.

7. Routine prenatal care includes education regarding substance abuse, nutritional supplementation including particularly folic acid, screening for infection, dating of pregnancy with monitoring of fetal growth, maternal serum marker screening and fetal ultrasound.

8. Indications for prenatal diagnosis include advanced maternal age (> 35 years), prior child with a chromosome aberration, parental chromosome translocations, risks for Mendelian diseases that are susceptible to DNA or enzyme diagnosis, and risks for characteristic congenital anomalies that can be detected by maternal serum markers or ultrasound.

9. Techniques for prenatal diagnosis include chorionic villus sampling (CVS) at 8–10 weeks of pregnancy, level I or level II fetal sonography, amniocentesis at 12–18 weeks of pregnancy, and cordocentesis at 20–30 weeks of pregnancy.

10. The ability to treat fetuses with vitamin-responsive aminoacidopathies or con-

genital adrenal hyperplasia foreshadows an era of fetal risk determination and therapy.

11. Ethical issues in reproductive medicine include parental–fetal conflict of autonomy and beneficence, timing of fetal humanity, confidentiality versus rights to informed choices, and equal access to expensive medical resources.

Case 15: A Low Maternal Serum Alpha-Fetoprotein Screen
A 30-year-old woman presents for counseling regarding a low value for serum alpha-fetoprotein. She and her husband are adamant about continuing the pregnancy, but wish to pursue any information that might influence the strategies for delivery or newborn care. They have a normal family history other than a prior spontaneous abortion at 12 weeks gestation.

■ 15.1. INTRODUCTION

Although the bulk of genetic disease presents to pediatric or adult medicine specialists, the growing ability to predict and determine reproductive outcomes makes genetics an essential part of perinatal medicine. Of key importance in this area is preconceptional planning that involves knowledge of the family history, recognition of genetic or medical risks, and counseling regarding possible preventive or interventive strategies. Sometimes these strategies involve special dietary or medical measures to minimize risk to the fetus or mother. At other times they involve alternative means of fertilization or implantation, an area that is rapidly expanding because of new technology. Often genetic risks may be addressed by an expanding repertoire of prenatal diagnostic options. Regardless of special concerns, all pregnancies require routine monitoring and certain routine tests that assess well-being of the fetomaternal unit. Preconceptional planning and pregnancy monitoring then joins with postnatal management to ensure continuity of

parent-infant care. The family and pregnancy history are key elements for pediatric management and reproductive planning.

Detecting genetic disease before or prior to pregnancy is a responsibility that falls upon many medical specialties and their extended allied health services. Pediatricians must recognize disease and initiate referrals that will define risks for future pregnancies. Internists must note genetic disorders in couples that can be passed on to children, and recognize women at high risk for pregnancy problems. The obstetrician must recognize signs of genetic or congenital disease in the fetus or its mother, enlisting maternal-fetal medicine specialists to participate in high-risk management. After birth, the cycle begins again with the neonatologist who must accomplish early diagnosis of unanticipated problems or manage problems that were recognized prenatally.

The development of simple preventive measures for neural tube defects or diabetes, the expansion of prenatal testing options, the chances for fetal treatment or surgery, and the improved outcomes of neonatal surgery documented in Chapter 13 all mandate a team approach toward optimal reproductive management. In addition to its expanding horizons for intervention and treatment, obstetric medicine offers a new frontier in genetics analogous to the mental institutions that supplied so many new examples of biochemical and chromosomal disease. The many discoveries made by studying embryonic mishaps in worms or fruit flies will eventually have parallels in the study of infertility and early pregnancy loss in humans.

■ 15.2. GENETIC FACTORS IN INFERTILITY AND REPRODUCTIVE FAILURE

Approximately 10% of couples do not become pregnant after a year of trying, and another 10–20% lose the pregnancy before the fetus is viable (spontaneous abortion). At least 1% of couples experience consecutive pregnancy losses, making reproductive failure an important and common medical problem. Numerous multifactorial and genetic diseases cause decreased fertility. Genetic diseases may interfere with the formation of gonads, the function of gonads to produce gametes, the travel of gametes to join in fertilization, or the content of gametes that is necessary for a viable embryo. Environmental problems such as toxins, infections, or chronic disease may also cause infertility, and some genetic diseases like galactosemia (230400) produce metabolic toxins that interfere with fertilility. Infertility and pregnancy loss is often encountered in obstetric practice, and genetic factors must be considered during preconceptional or postabortion counseling. Genetic counseling in the reproductive arena must consider risks for fertilization and fetal survival as well as the risk for genetic diseases in offspring.

Infertility in Females

The usual incidence of pregnancy in females engaging in unprotected sexual intercourse is 25% by 1 month, 63% within 6 months, and 80–90% after 1 year (Williamson and Elias, 1992). If a desired pregnancy has not occurred after 1 year of frequent intercourse (three to four times weekly), the couple is defined as infertile. The cause of infertility is equally divided among women and men, with ovulatory failure or blocked ovarian tubes each accounting for 40% of female infertility (20% overall). The remaining 10–20% of female infertility relates to anomalies or diseases affecting the reproductive tract (vagina, cervix, and uterus—Table 15.1).

Failure to ovulate occurs in genetic conditions like 45,X Turner syndrome, galactosemia (230400), androgen insensitivity syndromes (e.g., testicular feminization—313700), or congenital adrenal hyperplasias, e.g., 201710). In these conditions, the germ cells do not form properly or fail to receive normal hormonal stimulation. The Stein-Levinthal or polycystic ovary syndrome with ovarian failure, polycystic ovaries, and hirsutism is a multifactorial cause of infertility, as are a variety of disorders

with brain dysfunction (e.g., strokes, tumors) that disturb pituitary regulation of the ovarian cycle and cause infertility (Table 15.1). Numerous systemic or chronic diseases also produce female infertility by causing pituitary and/or ovarian dysfunction (e.g., systemic lupus erythematosis, cerebrovascular disease).

If the ovary is present and functional, abnormalities of the reproductive tract can occur that preclude egg migration, egg implantation, or access to the egg by sperm. More than 60 syndromes with uterine anomalies are listed by Winter and Baraitser (1998), and decreased fertility is a common accompaniment of many malformation and chromosomal syndromes. Congenital uterine anomalies include bicornuate uterus with two uterine cavities and one cervix or didelphic uterus with two uterine cavities, two cervices, and one or two vaginal openings (Table 15.1). Uterine anomalies can cause complete infertility or decreased fertility due to abnormal implantation or fetal positioning. Less severe uterine anomalies, like large leiomyomas (fibroids) of the uterus, can cause deformation of the fetus with arthrogryposis (congenital contractures). A poorly formed uterus (Müllerian aplasia or hypoplasia) exhibits some genetic predisposition with a 1–2% recurrence risk in siblings, and is associated with renal and cervical vertebral problems in the *M*üllerian, *R*enal, *C*ervical *S*omite (MURCS) association. The Rokitansky sequence of vaginal atresia, bicornuate uterus, and renal anomalies also reflects a common origin of uterus, kidneys, and upper vagina from the paramesonephric (Müllerian) duct. Reproductive tract anomalies, infertility, and cancer occur in women exposed to diethylstilbesterol (DES) while they were fetuses due to threatened abortion in their mother.

Sexually transmitted diseases exert a higher toll on female fertility than male because of scarring of the ovarian tube. Acquired abnormalities of the female reproductive tract also include endometriosis, a disease where the uterine lining (endometrium) proliferates and extends into the ovarian tubes or pelvis (Table 15.1).

■TABLE 15.1. Causes of Female Infertility

Category	Disease	Signs and Symptoms
Ovarian dysgenesis		
Chromosomal aberrations	Turner syndrome (45,X)	Short stature, webbed neck, risks for thyroid, heart problems
Congenital anomalies	46,XX gonadal dysgenesis (233300, 233400)	Isolated ovarian dysgenesis with or without deafness
Ovarian dysfunction		
Sex hormone disorders	Congenital adrenal hypoplasias	Excess androgens, cortisol and aldosterone deficiency in some
Dysplastic ovaries	Stein-Levinthal syndrome	Polycystic ovaries, hirsutism
Other endocrine disorders	Pituitary deficiencies	Deficiency in FSH, LH
Systemic disorders, chronic illnesses	Brain dysfunction, infections, strokes, autoimmune	Altered pituitary stimulation of ovarian cycles
Reproductive tract anomalies		
Uterine	Bicornuate, didelphic uterus	Altered uterine structure
	Many malformation syndromes	McKusick-Kaufman syndrome with cardiac, renal, digital anomalies (236700)
	MURCS association	Uterine, renal, cervical spine anomalies
	Rokitansky sequence	Uterine, renal anomalies
Cervical, vaginal	Cervical aplasia, vaginal septa	Cervical or vaginal anomalies
Reproductive tract inflammation		
Infectious	Gonorrhea, syphilus, chlamydia	Scarring of ovarian tubes
Endometriosis	Endometrial tissue outside of uterus	Abnormal menstruation, pelvic pain, pain during intercourse

Source: Williamson and Elias (1992).

Notes: FSH, follicle stimulating hormone; LH, luteinizing hormone.

Infertility in Males

Entanglement of the veins and spermatic ducts (varicocele) in the scrotum accounts for about 40% of male infertility, with testicular dysgenesis (14%), endocrine disturbances (9%), other types of vas deferens obstruction (8%), and undescended testes (cryptorchidism, 4%) being other defined causes (Williamson and Elias, 1992). Abnormal formation of the testis occurs when chromosomal rearrangements or molecular lesions interfere with the cascade of genetic changes from the SRY (sex determining region on the Y) to fetal testis formation to an-

drogen secretion, to androgen receptor activation to responses by the internal and external genitalia (see Chapter 13). Pure gonadal dysgenesis with an XY karyotype can produce an external female appearance, as can testicular feminization with a complete defect in the androgen receptor (Table 15.2).

Many chromosomal or malformation syndromes like 47,XXY Klinefelter syndrome exhibit abnormal testes and spermatogenesis with infertility. Disorders with incomplete masculinization (male pseudohermaphroditism) can include partial defects in the androgen receptor, inadequate androgen synthesis as

■**TABLE 15.2.** Causes of Male Infertility

Category	Disease	Signs and Symptoms
Testicular dysgenesis		
Chromosomal aberrations	Klinefelter syndrome (47,XXY)	Tall stature, thin habitus, hypoplastic testes
Inadequate masculinization (Male pseudohermaphroditism)	46,XY gonadal dysgenesis due to mutations in the SRY region	Female appearance
	Testicular feminization (313700)	Female appearance, defective androgen receptor
Congenital anomalies	Many chromosomal and Mendelian syndromes	Cryptorchidism, micropenis, abnormal spermatogenesis
Testicular dysfunction		
Sex hormone disorders	Reifenstein syndrome (313700)	Partial androgen receptor defect
	Congenital adrenal hypoplasias	Deficient androgens, cortisol and aldosterone deficiency in some
Other endocrine disorders	Kallman syndrome (308700)	Absent smell, pituitary dysfunction
Environmental agents	Mumps, hyperthermia (abdominal testis), radiation	Hypoplastic testis, abnormal sperm
Abnormal sperm	Kartagener syndrome (244400)	Absent or abnormal sperm, lung disease, situs inversus
Reproductive tract anomalies		
Vas deferens	Varicocele	Entanglement of veins with vas deferens
	Cystic fibrosis (219700)	Absent vas deferens, lung and gastrointestinal disease
Urethra	Many malformation syndromes with hypospadias, stenosis	McKusick-Kaufman syndrome with cardiac, renal, digital anomalies (236700)
Reproductive tract inflammation		
Infectious	Gonorrhea, TB, chlamydia	Scarring of vas deferens, urethra

Source: Williamson and Elias (1992).

Notes: SRY, sex determining region on the Y; TB, tuberculosis.

in several types of congenital adrenal hyperplasia (see Chapter 13), or the Kallmann syndrome of absent olfactory lobe and cryptorchidism due to mutations in the *KAL*-1 cell adhesion molecule (see Chapter 9). Environmental exposures such as radiation or chemotherapy, infections such as mumps, or chronic diseases can damage spermatogenesis and cause male infertility, including the infertility due to cryptorchidism that reflects temperature damage to the abdominal testis. Over 340 syndromes with micropenis or cryptorchidism are listed by Baraitser and Winter (1998), emphasizing the large genetic input to male infertility.

Absence or blockage of the vas deferens can occur from varicocele or Mendelian disorders such as cystic fibrosis (Table 15.2). Infections such as gonorrhea or tuberculosis can also damage the vas deferens or urethra. The requirement for sperm motility provides another category for male infertility, and defects vary from inadequate sperm production or morphology to inadequate mobility or fertilizing capacity. The Kartagener syndrome (244400) is an interesting example of amotile sperm that results from abnormal ciliary structure. Inspection of a sperm sample under the microscope may identify these abnormalities.

Early Pregnancy Loss and Spontaneous Abortion

As mentioned previously, the 90% of couples who become pregnant in timely fashion still face a 10–20% chance of spontaneous abortion. When the spontaneous abortion occurs in the embryonic period (the first 8 weeks after conception), it is referred to as early pregnancy loss. Numerous studies have documented that about 50% of early pregnancy losses involve embryos with abnormal chromosomes (Table 15.3). The chances of finding a chromosome abnormality depend on the morphology of the abortus.

Kalousek (1997) has summarized many years of work showing that early abortuses can be divided into classes of growth disorganization, focal defects, or normal morphology (Table 15.3). Those with certain types of growth disorganizaton have higher risks for chromosomal anomalies, while those with normal morphology imply abnormalities of the corpus luteum or endometrium. Early losses with focal defects can also occur because of chromosomal anomalies such as monosomy X or triploidy, but single defects of the neural tube or palate would predict multifactorial inheritance. Early losses can thus be divided into those with significant recurrence risks (balanced translocations or multifactorial defects), those with defined chromosomal aberrations but low recurrence (trisomies, triploidies), or those with luteal failure with low recurrence risk for fetal anomalies but possible need for hormonal evaluation of the mother. Luteal fail-

ure is estimated to account for about 35% of early pregnancy loss.

Some of the normal embryos may represent early pregnancy loss because of immune problems. Although no specific HLA alleles have been associated with the tendency for pregnancy loss, sharing of HLA alleles between parents has been. These shared alleles may be transmitted to the fetus, causing homozygosity that may diminish differences between fetal and maternal antigens. It is thought that some fetal antigens must be recognized by the maternal immune system as foreign so that tolerance to the fetus can develop.

Spontaneous abortions occurring after 8 weeks gestation and up to 18–20 weeks exhibit a 4–7% frequency of chromosomal aberrations if the fetal specimens are studied to exclude retention of aborted embryos (Table 15.3). These chromosomal abnormalities have more defined morphologies, and include Turner syndrome, triploidy, and common trisomies. Triploidies have a high association of placental anomalies in which the chorionic villi become swollen and cystic (complete or partial hydatidiform moles). Molar and other changes in placentas are often found in later spontaneous abortions.

Stillbirths are defined as fetuses born without a heartbeat who are greater than 20 or 28 weeks (definitions vary by jurisdiction). Maternal diseases such as diabetes mellitus or drug abuse predominate as causes of stillbirths, with nicotine, cocaine, and alcohol having prominent roles. Placental abnormalities such as abruption (premature separation of the placenta from the uterine wall) are also common. Isolated anomalies, malformation syndromes, and chromosomal aberrations are relatively frequent, requiring careful evaluation and testing of stillborn infants (Table 15.3). Abnormal placentas, fetal infection, or intrinsic genetic syndromes cause a high frequency of intrauterine growth retardation in stillborn infants, and often these pregnancies are identified before birth by ultrasound. Twins, particularly monozygotic twins with a shared amniotic cavity, are vulnerable to stillbirths because of

■ **TABLE 15.3.** Types of Pregnancy Loss

Timing (frequency, morphology)	CA (%)	Association	Implication
Early abortion (EA), 0–8 weeks	50		Usually low RR
		Trisomies (27%)	Parental studies when
Growth disorganization (GD)		Polyploidy (10%)	>3 abortions, or if
(58–70% of EA)		Sex monosomy (9%)	chromosomal
GD1 (sac, no embryo)	60	Rearrangements (2%)	rearrangement in
GD2 (embryo, no RP)	73		embryo
GD3 (embryo, RP at head)	52		
GD4 (embryo, disproportion)	37		
Normal (16–14% of EA)	20	Luteal phase defect	Low RR
		Uterine anomaly	
Focal defects (5–18% of EA)—	92	Monosomy X	Possible multifactorial
neural tube, cleft palate, limb		Triploidy	or Mendelian RR if
defects		Trisomies	normal karyotype
Later abortion, 9–18 weeks	4–7	Major anomalies	Multifactorial RR
		Monosomy X, triploidy	Low RR
		Placental anomalies	Low RR
Stillbirths, > 20–28 weeks	5–10	Maternal disease (40%)	Usually low RR
		Abruption (12–17%)	Low RR
		Major anomalies (7–21%)	Multifactorial RR
		IUGR (7–15%)	0–50% RR
		Mendelian syndromes	>20 known, 0–50% RR
		Chromosomal syndromes	Low RR
Neonatal deaths, 0–4 weeks	?2–5	Prematurity	Low RR
after birth			
		Congenital anomalies	
		Single anomalies	Multifactorial RR
		Syndromes	0–50% RR
		Infections	Low RR
		Maternal diseases	Usually Low RR
		Fetal hydrops	0–50% RR

Source: Kalousek (1997).

Notes: EA, early abortion; RP, retinal pigment; CA, chromosomal aberrations; RR, recurrence risk for abnormal fetua and/or abortion.

vascular obstructions or entanglements of the umbilical cord.

Neonatal deaths are not technically a cause of reproductive failure in the sense of infertility or pregnancy loss, but they can be even more devastating for families desiring children. Prematurity, infections revealed by inflammation of the chorion or amnion (chorioamniitis), or maternal diseases are major contributors to neonatal death that have negligible or small genetic predisposition. However, congenital anomalies with their multifactorial or Mendelian risks are the second most

common cause of neonatal death, and Kalousek (1997) lists more than 50 syndromes that can have this presentation. Fetal hydrops (Fig. 15.1) often progresses to fetal death and should be recognized as high risk for genetic problems. Hydropic fetuses are swollen to the point that surface features may be disguised, mandating chromosomal studies even if no obvious major or minor anomalies can be seen. Heart defects, chromosomal syndromes, and genetic anemias such as thalassemia are the most common causes of fetal hydrops (Fig. 15.1, Table 15.3).

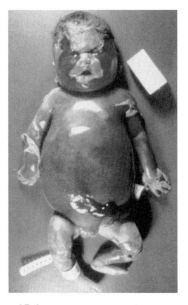

Figure 15.1. Fetal hydrops showing swollen head and neck due to subcutaneous edema. Photograph by Dr. Beverly Rogers, University of Texas Southwestern Medical Center.

An association with spontaneous abortions and stillbirths that is gaining increased attention is that with antiphospholipid antibodies. These are a group of antibodies that include an antibody mediating false positive tests for syphilis, the lupus anticoagulant that occurs in women with systemic lupus erythematosis and causes heart block in their fetuses, and an anticardiolipin antibody (Branch, 1990). The presence of antiphospholipid antibodies correlates with venous or arterial thromboses and low platelets in mothers and spontaneous abortion of infants. Branch (1990) estimates that these antibodies account for 5% of recurrent abortions. It is not known if the abortions are caused by immune reactions to fetal tissues or by the maternal blood clots and other complications.

Evaluation and Treatment of the Couple with Reproductive Problems

A key part of preconceptional planning is an adequate history concerning previous pregnan-

cies or attempts at pregnancy. Knowledge of infertility brings up the possibility of the etiologies listed in Tables 15.1 and 15.2, particularly if it is primary infertility (chronic illness or other acquired disorders may cause secondary infertility after one or more successful pregnancies). A complete history (family and medical) and physical is needed for both members of the couple, with chromosomal testing and other evaluations required if a genetic disorder like Turner syndrome is suspected. When the history and physical are normal, specialty evaluations of the endocrine system, reproductive tract and sperm analysis may be indicated. Key techniques for assessing female reproductive cycles are abdominal laparoscopy in females to visualize the ovaries and fallopian tubes, and abdominal ultrasound to assess the timing and frequency of ovulation. The details of these evaluations can be found in textbooks of reproductive medicine. Depending on the cause of infertility, strategies to induce ovulation with drugs like clomiphene or gonadotrophin hormones, insufflation of the fallopian tubes with air to improve patency, or artificial reproductive technologies with parental or surrogate gametes can be tried.

When pregnancy occurs but ends in abortion or stillbirth, examination of the aborted tissue is paramount. Embryonic tissues can be placed in sterile media for tissue culture and karyotype determination. For later spontaneous abortions and stillbirths, a detailed physical examination can decide the likelihood of a single anomaly versus a syndrome as outlined in Chapter 11. When there are multiple minor or major anomalies, then a chromosome analysis and involvement of a dysmorphologist is necessary. In outlying centers, photographs and a whole body radiograph can be enormously helpful in allowing specialists to arrive at a specific syndrome diagnosis. For stillbirths, skin biopsy for fibroblast culture or umbilical blood sampling can obtain cells for karyotyping. Many fetuses and/or placentas will provide definitive evidence of infection or vascular accident, thereby relieving the couple of genetic risk. The embryofetal examination, best performed as a formal autopsy but at least involving inspection and photographs, is vital for genetic and future preconceptual counseling.

When a couple has recurrent early pregnancy loss, or a fetus has a structural chromosome rearrangement, then chromosome studies are indicated on the parents. Rearrangements are found in only 2% of early pregnancy losses (Table 15.3), correlating with a low yield (1–2%) of chromosome aberrations found in couples with three or more spontaneous abortions. Although the high risks conferred by genetic diseases are important not to overlook, most couples will have other causes for multiple miscarriages.

Case 15 Follow-up: The prior spontaneous abortion mentioned by the couple was not examined or cultured for chromosome studies. Focal defects or congenital anomalies were not noted in the abortus.

■ 15.3. PRECONCEPTIONAL COUNSELING AND THE PRENATAL HISTORY

As stressed by Taysi (1988), most pregnant women are seen for their first prenatal visit after their second missed menstrual period at 6–8 weeks after conception. By this time, all of blastogenesis to form the germ layers and most of organogenesis to produce the major organ systems has occurred. Preventive measures commencing at 8 weeks gestation will be much less effective for the woman with alcholism, uncontrolled diabetes, phenylketonuria, or a prior history of neural tube defects. This first prenatal visit is also too late to consider new methodologies such as in vitro fertilization or preimplantation diagnosis, and reduces available counseling and preparation times for prenatal diagnostic procedures such as chorionic villus sampling. For many medical and psychosocial reasons, preconceptional evaluation and counseling is a key prelude to prenatal care. Preconceptual counseling should

occur following an abnormal outcome in a prior pregnancy or during the planning stage of a first pregnancy. It should consist of a thorough medical and family history on both prospective parents, followed by interventions directed at diagnoses that impose maternofetal risk.

Population, Family, and Age Factors

As discussed in Chapter 4, populations often differ in their frequencies of genetic diseases. Selective factors like malaria, founder effects, and genetic drift act to produce differences in allele frequencies that impose specific risks for particular ethnic groups. Table 4.2 lists disorders that must be considered for various ethnic backgrounds, including sickle cell anemia for blacks, cystic fibrosis for whites, α-thalassemia in Orientals, β-thalassemia in Italians and Greeks, and Tay-Sachs disease in Jews. All of these diseases, and an increasing number of others, have specific carrier testing that can be performed to define the recurrence risk of prospective parents.

As mentioned in Chapters 3 and 7, certain disorders increase in frequency with maternal or paternal age. Women exhibit a continuous increase in their risk for chromosomal disorders that begins at about 1 in 2000 and reaches 1 in 50 by age 45. For somewhat arbitrary reasons, the risk of about 1 in 200 at maternal age 35 is considered significant enough to justify prenatal diagnosis. Men have an increased risk for new mutations in their offspring, some of which will manifest as a new case of an autosomal dominant disorder. This risk is negligible compared to that with maternal age, and is generally considered significant above age 40.

For reasons of parental age, genetic disease, or ethnic factors, a general family history is important for all couples considering pregnancy. Although time-consuming, an adequate pedigree as outlined in Chapter 2 has greater sensitivity than routine questionnaires in ascertaining genetic risk factors (Scheuner et al., 1997). Besides the ethnic backgrounds mentioned previously, prior histories of genetic diseases, chromosomal disorders, or unusual disease presentations may trigger evaluations or requests for appropriate medical records. Once family data are gathered, medical risks for the mother and/or genetic risks for the fetus can be ascertained. With the mobility of modern society, considerable time to obtain records on family members may be required before prenatal management and diagnostic strategies can be defined. These requirements emphasize the need for a preconceptual counseling visit well before the initiation of actual pregnancy.

Disorders with Maternal Risk

Certain diseases worsen or develop complications as a result of pregnancy. Typical among them is Marfan syndrome (154700), in which the higher cardiac output of pregnancy may worsen cardiovascular lesions such as a dilated aortic valve or aorta. The risk for aortic dissection is greatest in the third trimester and during the strain of labor and delivery. Management includes a method of delivery that minimizes stress, and a trial of β-andrenergic blockade if there is progressive aortic root dilatation. Pyeritz (1993) emphasizes that women with preexisting aortic root dilation are most likely to develop complications. Ehlers-Danlos syndrome type IV also has blood vessel and connective tissue fragility, and ruptures of the aorta, intestine, or uterus have occurred during labor and delivery. The fragility of fetal membranes in Ehlers-Danlos syndromes also causes a higher rate of prematurity with its associated risks to the neonate.

A second category of disease with maternal risk is that of skeletal dysplasia. Affected women may have disfigured or smaller pelvic outlets that preclude normal deliveries. Plans for careful monitoring and dating of the fetus to allow appropriate caesarian section is important for maternal and fetal well being. Many other genetic diseases in mothers may lead to pregnancy complications, making it important to consult the appropriate references when the disease is identified during preconceptional screening.

Maternal Disorders with Risks for Fetal Well-Being

Maternal illnesses can cause problems in the fetus because of the close contact between the maternal and fetal circulations across the placental membrane. The most common problem is maternal diabetes mellitus, particularly the type II or juvenile-onset form when present prior to the onset of pregnancy. As mentioned in Chapter 13, maternal diabetes is associated with several types of anomalies in the fetus including craniospinal, cardiac, and caudal defects. The infant of the diabetic mother also has a characteristic neonatal profile, being large-for-dates, plethoric (red complexion), and unstable with risks for hypoglycemia and hypocalcemia. The degree of neonatal changes and the risk for birth defects relate to diabetic control during gestation. Poorly controlled women with long-standing diabetes can have three- to fivefold elevated risks for birth defects over the background 2–3%. Women with good control of blood sugar and insulin dosage have near normal risks for birth defects. Diabetic control must begin prior to conception so that the first critical weeks of embryogenesis are not affected.

A second area of maternal disease with grave consequences for the fetus is chemical dependency. Fetal alcohol syndrome is the disorder of greatest concern with the characteristic face (see Fig. 11.10), eye and cardiac anomalies, and mental disability. Heroin addicts can deliver drug-addicted babies that require narcotic treatment and gradual withdrawal but do not have characteristic birth defects. The effects of cocaine are still being debated, but higher risks for vascular disruptions like gastroschisis or bladder exstrophy are suggested by some studies (see Chapter 13). Although less compliant for prenatal visits, early educational and interventional programs have had success in mothers addicted to drugs or alcohol.

Mothers with epilepsy face higher risks for fetal problems that are probably related to their drug treatment. Hydantoin and trimethadione are strongly implicated as teratogens, and mothers requiring seizure control are usually shifted to phenobarbitol or tegretol. Since the hypoxia of seizures themselves is likely to be damaging to the fetus, these risks must be balanced against the use of antiepileptic agents.

Mothers with a family history of neural tube defects and those with phenylketonuria have the potential for nutritional intervention to lower fetal risks. The 2–3% risk for neural tube defects in affected mothers or in couples with a prior affected child can be decreased by at least one-third through preconceptional supplementation with folic acid (given in a simple multivitamin mixture). Mothers with phenylketonuria who are off of diet and have high phenylalanine levels can have offspring with a similar phenotype to that of fetal alcohol syndrome. Resumption of their low-phenylalanine diet, while difficult, lowers fetal risks to that of the background population.

Maternal antibodies may also attack the fetus, as discussed previously for antiphospholipid or blood group antibodies. The lupus anticoagulant antibody attacks the fetal heart and produces heart block. In severe cases, the fetus may develop hydrops and abort. Blood group incompatibilities include severe Rh disease and the presence of a "set-up"—Rh+ fetus, Rh– mother. The administration of RhoGam blocking antibody after pregnancies in Rh– women can largely avoid this problem, but some women are sensitized before their first pregnancy and require preconceptional planning of the monitoring strategy.

Many maternal diseases exhibit a maternal effect, with worsened symptoms for offspring of affected women than men. This is postulated for disorders like neurofibromatosis-1 and proven for disorders such as fragile X syndrome or myotonic dystrophy with triplet repeat expansion. Other maternal genetic diseases, along with many chronic or systemic diseases summarized in Table 15.1, increase the risk for fetal loss or malformation. These diseases, as well as others identified during the process of preconceptional counseling, may cause the pregnancy to be viewed as high risk. Women with high-risk pregnancies are often

monitored more closely, followed by specialists in maternal-fetal medicine, and presented with a variety of management or diagnostic options.

■ 15.4. OPTIONS FOR ALTERING FERTILIZATION, IMPLANTATION, OR DELIVERY

The importance of preconceptional planning is also emphasized by new options for couples with infertility or genetic risks. These include methods that provide surrogate eggs or sperm, fertilization outside of the natural reproductive tract, and testing of early embryos prior to implantation.

Surrogate Methods Without Fetal Selection

The most time-honored method for surrogate parenting is of course adoption (Table 15.4). Parents who are infertile or face high genetic risks can choose to adopt, thus avoiding the genetic risks from either parental genome. Problems that complicate adoption include the lack of a good family history, the lack of specialized evaluations of newborns that can recognize genetic disease, and the lack of adequate infantile follow-up to exclude developmental or growth problems that manifest after several months of life. Sometimes known genetic risks in the parent can complicate adoption of an infant. For example, a child at 50% risk for Huntington chorea may be at a disadvantage for adoption that cannot be rectified by DNA testing because the child is a minor. Much improvement is needed in the documentation of family history and physical problems provided by adoption agencies. This lack of information is often magnified in infants adopted from foreign countries, particularly from Third World countries with less advanced health care systems.

Of major importance in counseling prospective adoptive parents is the late manifestation of many developmental problems. A normal chromosome analysis does not guarantee

■**TABLE 15.4.** Alternative Methods for Conception

Type of Method	Alternative	Common Uses and Indications
Natural methods		
Adoption	Surrogate sperm and egg	Infertility or unacceptable genetic risks
Surrogate mothers	Surrogate egg	Maternal infertility Autosomal recessive diseases
New partners	New sperm or egg	Marital separation Autosomal recessive disease
Alternative fertilization		
Clomiphene, gonadotrophin treatment	Enhanced ovulation	Female infertility
In vitro fertilization (IVF)	New sperm	Paternal infertility Autosomal recessive diseases
In vitro fertilization (IVF) with separated X or Y sperm	Selected sperm	Risks for sex-limited diseases
Gamete intrafallopian transfer (GIFT)	New ovum and/or new sperm	Unexplained fertility
Intracytoplasmic sperm injection (ICSI)	Enhanced fertilization	Male infertility
Alternative implantation		
Blastomere analysis before implantation (BABI)	Selected, normal embryos for implantation	Couples with high genetic risks Sex selection
Polar body analysis before implantation	Selected, normal embryos for implantation	Couples with high genetic risks Sex selection
Human cloning	Selected embryos from an adult somatic cell	Consensus guidelines prohibiting use

the absence of genetic disease, and a normal examination during infancy does not guarantee the absence of later developmental and learning differences. These limitations of diagnosis are particularly important for the common adoptive scenario of infants exposed to drugs like alcohol or cocaine. Effects of such drugs on the fine tuning of brain development that occurs in the third trimester may be undetectable by MRI head scan or early developmental evaluation. Despite an externally normal appearance, such children may exhibit severe learning and behavioral problems later in childhood, with impulsivity, hyperactivity, and oppositional behaviors. On the other hand, the 3–5% general risk for abnormalities in children suggests that an optimistic outlook be

maintained for adopted children without severe histories of maternal abuse or social neglect. Overemphasis of genetic risks can impair crucial bonding between the adoptive parents and child that, with modern hormonal treatment, can include breast-feeding by adoptive mothers. The problems complicating parental versus adoptive parental rights are probably more threatening to adoption than genetic factors, as emphasized by several highly publicized and tragic cases.

The development of techniques for fertilization in the laboratory (in vitro fertilization, IVF, test-tube babies) provides other options for gamete substitution (Table 15.4). The use of abdominal laparoscopy allows eggs to be removed from the ovary and used for IVF.

The eggs may be reintroduced into the fallopian tube with the husband's sperm, a technique known as gamete intrafallopian transfer (GIFT). Pregnancy rates using the GIFT procedure for couples with unexplained infertility can reach about 30% in experienced centers as compared to 1–4% without treatment, 5–8% with clomiphene or gonadotrophin treatment, and 20% with in vitro fertilization employing sperm injection into the cervix (Guzick et al., 1998). These success rates decrease as a function of maternal age. The average cost ranges from about $10,000 for clomiphene treatment to about $50,000 for those conceived using GIFT technology.

When males have malformed sperm or low sperm counts in their ejaculate, microsurgical aspiration of sperm from the epididymus testis can be performed. The sperm nuclei can then be microinjected into oocytes to obtain a zygote containing the natural genetic material from both parents. This intracytoplasmic sperm injection (ICSI) method of artificial insemination seems to have higher risks for sex chromosome aberrations in the fetus, but may be coupled with preimplantation screening to rule out specific genetic risks as discussed below.

If parents have high genetic risks or do not respond to fertility measures using their own gametes, then egg or sperm donors can be substituted using GIFT or IVF technologies (Table 15.4). Sperm banking has been active for two decades, and fairly good screening procedures for genetic or disease risks are now in place. Many sperm banks provide matching services that allow selection of donor characteristics that are compatible with the family. Ethical problems include rights of individuals to their gametes after donation or marital separation and inappropriate methods of supplying gametes. The latter problem includes sperm banks with inadequate screening and the publicized self-supply of sperm by a male obstetrician to many women undergoing IVF.

Natural surrogate methods include adoption, surrogate mothers serving from compassion or payment, or new male partners prompted by the specter of recurrence due to autosomal recessive disease. Maternal surrogating has proved to be impractical because of the difficulties of maternal-child separation, and several states have passed laws against this practice. Paternal surrogating may be undisclosed and lead to ethical problems when prenatal diagnosis is available to define fetal status and raise the issue of nonpaternity (see problem set).

Methods Involving Fetal Selection

A rapidly evolving and controversial area of reproductive technology is the ability to select fetal characteristics without the onus of mid-pregnancy termination. The first of these methods involves sex selection by separating X and Y haploid sperm. Although timing of intercourse and particular ovulation induction methods have been claimed to alter sex ratios, it is only recently that separation of X sperm with larger amounts of nuclear DNA has been possible using flow cytometry. This technique followed by IVF allows the probability of male offspring to be reduced from about 50% to less than 10%, providing an important option for couples at 25% risk for X-linked recessive disease. On the negative side, use of this technology by couples preferring male or female offspring raises ethical concerns regarding conservation of medical resources for significant disease and a "designer child" mentality that emphasizes trivial human characters.

A more certain method for sex selection with the ability to screen for genetic disease is the technique of preimplantation diagnosis. Embryos obtained by IVF are manipulated at the morula stage to obtain a single cell for genetic analysis. The blastomere can then be analyzed for the presence of certain abnormal chromosomes or alleles and, if normal, the remaining morula can be reintroduced into the fallopian tube to allow implantation (blastomere analysis before implantation or BABI). FISH techniques using probes for chromosomes 13, 18, 21, X and Y can define fetal sex and rule out common trisomies, while PCR techniques can amplify sufficient amounts of

DNA from specific genes to allow testing for particular mutant alleles. Refinements of technique have removed the first and second polar bodies (the products of meiosis I and II) from the ovum, allowing a two-step DNA analysis without then need to remove an embryonic blastomere. A problem with the PCR technique is the tendency for some alleles not to amplify properly with the many chain reactions needed to obtain adequate DNA from a single cell. This problem of allele-dropout is being solved by coamplification of polymorphic DNA regions of the genes in question, ensuring that two repeat sizes and thus two alleles have been amplified.

The use of preimplantation diagnosis allows the reliable selection of fetal sex, selection of normal fetuses among embryos at risk for single gene disorders like Tay-Sachs disease or cystic fibrosis, and avoidance of fetuses with other DNA alterations like unstable trinucleotide repeats (fragile X, myotonic dystrophy). Substantial success rates for pregnancy have been obtained, with 86% of analyzed embryos transferred, 25–29% of pregnancies induced, and 16% yielding liveborn infants. Ethical issues include the controversies regarding the manipulation of zygotes and embryos, and the high costs ($50,000–$100,000 per pregnancy) relative to other issues of population control and improved prenatal care.

Human Cloning

In 1997, a lamb named Dolly was introduced to the public after being conceived from an adult somatic cell. Dolly was thus genetically identical to the adult ewe from which she was derived, raising the possibility that multiple offspring could be produced or cloned from the somatic cells of a single individual. Although cloning had been possible for frogs and other simpler organisms, the successful cloning of a mammal raised the possibility for cloning of humans. Such technology could avoid certain genetic risks dependent on one or both parental genomes (e.g., X-linked diseases in women or

autosomal recessive diseases where both parents are carriers). Human cloning could also provide sources for organ transplants and manufacture of scarce biological materials.

Although there is general consensus against the development of human cloning, the remarkable advances in artificial reproductive technologies have prompted considerable debate about research on human embryos. Some point to the considerable knowledge to be gained about early human development through study of these embryos, while others point to the dangers of manipulating embryonic tissues without regard to the individuals that they might become. A panel convened to study these questions presented some tentative research guidelines in 1994 (Table 15.5). Such guidelines will have an important effect on the pace of new research in reproductive medicine and the availability of these techniques to wider segments of the population. Conflicts between these research guidelines and the urge to use the ensuing technologies to help desperate couples or to make money have already caused several physicians to receive censures and other punishments (Marshall, 1997).

■ 15.5. ROUTINE PRENATAL CARE

The concept of routine prenatal care began at in the late 1800s and is now standard practice. Numerous studies have justified routine prenatal care based on cost-benefit analyses or on reduction in parental anxiety (Nagey, 1989). Prenatal care should be defined to include preconceptional counseling and planning.

Components of Prenatal Care

Although the first realization of pregnancy may be too late for some preventive measures such as diabetic control or vitamin supplementation, it does provide an opportunity to assess medical risk factors for the current pregnancy. A thorough physical examination is needed and, if not ascertained before, a complete medical and family history. The most important

■TABLE 15.5. Provisional Guidelines for Research on Human Embryos

Generally approved with case-by-case review

Research on existing, unused embryos obtained by in vitro techniques at ages up to 14 days
  post-fertilization
Creation of limited numbers of embryos for baseline data regarding artificial reproductive technology
  (ART)
Selection of blastomeres for cell extraction prior to implantation
Construction of embryonic cell lines from unused embryos
Study or induced maturation of unfertilized eggs obtained in the course of ART

Needing further consideration

Use of fetal oocytes to create embryos for research studies
Research on unused embryos between 14 and 18 days postconception[a]
Use of embryos for research obtained by monetary rewards or where the donor cannot
  be located for explicit consent

Considered unacceptable

Transfer of human embryos to animals for gestation, cross-fertilized or chimeric
  human-animal embryos
Sex selection of embryos for reasons other than risks for X-linked disease
Use of sperm, eggs, or embryos from donors who have not given explicit consent or who received more
  than usual rates of compensation
Creation of embryos solely for research purposes (e.g., for stem cells)
Transfer of embryos used for research to humans
Induction of twins through division of embryos

Source: Marshall (1994).

[a]Neural tube development representing the beginning of embryonic brain formation commences at
18 days postconception.

factors to recognize will be more common diseases such as AIDS or other sexually transmitted diseases, hypertension, morbid obesity, coronary artery disease, or diabetes mellitus, but rare disorders with maternofetal risks like Marfan syndrome must also be identified. The first prenatal visit also presents the opportunity for education and counseling regarding risk factors like alcohol or nicotine use, and allows the first estimate of gestational age. The estimated duration of pregnancy is usually dated from the last menstrual period, usually two weeks prior to conception. Because of poor recall or irregularity, independent dating of the pregnancy is often desirable by measuring palpating the height of the uterus above the umbilicus or noting the time that fetal heart tones could first be heard. Ultrasound measurements

also provide accurate gestational dating if fetal growth is normal.

Once the pregnancy is recognized and the initial prenatal visit is made, a decision is made about the magnitude of risk to mother and fetus. For most pregnancies, routine prenatal care is initiated that consists of periodic evaluation at intervals that decrease as delivery approaches (usually monthly, then weekly). When the preconceptional or prenatal evaluation reveals significant risks for mother or fetus, then the pregnancy is labeled as high-risk with more frequent and extensive evaluations. Laboratory screening tests that are clearly indicated in routine pregnancies include blood counts, urinalyses, urine cultures, blood typing, Coombs testing for isoimmunization, rubella screening, cultures for sexually transmitted diseases, and screening of blood glucose for evidence of diabetes. Higher cost screening procedures with less certain benefits include maternal serum α-fetoprotein (MSAFP) and fetal ultrasound as discussed in the following two sections (Nagey, 1989).

Other aspects of routine prenatal care include the provision of multivitamins despite the lack of controlled studies that support this recommendation. Prenatal vitamins that include folic acid do lower the risk for neural tube defects if given prior to conception. Education is also an important aspect of prenatal care, and the first prenatal visit should discuss the risks of drugs and alcohol, the importance of a balanced diet, and the significance of vaginal bleeding or labor pains. After the first visit, monitoring of maternal vital signs, maternal weight gain, fetal growth (via uterine fundal height), fetal heart tones, and the status of cervical dilation or bleeding is performed at monthly, then weekly intervals. If abnormalities are encountered, then there may be a switch to high-risk status.

Maternal Serum Alpha-Fetoprotein and Triple Testing

Early fetuses have a high concentration of α-fetoprotein (AFP) in their blood that switches to albumin during later fetal life and infancy. Radioimmunoassay to detect small amounts of AFP in amniotic fluid was first used to estimate the risk for neural tube defects. Any fetal defect that allowed leakage of fetal AFP into the amniotic fluid, including neural tube defects, abdominal wall defects, renal defects causing proteinuria, and large fetal skin defects, could produce an elevated amniotic fluid AFP. Later, the ability to detect AFP in maternal serum (MSAFP) provided a more routine test that was initially performed at 15–20 weeks of gestation. MSAFP levels were corrected for maternal factors like ethnic background, obesity, or diabetes and then averaged for particular gestational ages. Once population and gestational age norms were established, a given MSAFP value could be expressed as a multiple of the mean (MOM) for that particular mother and her gestational age. Significantly elevated MSAFP values were suggestive of neural tube defects or other AFP leakage, and confirmatory ultrasound and/or amniocentesis AFP measurements could then be offered. More than 95% of neural tube defects were detected by MSAFP screening, with only closed, skin-covered defects escaping detection.

As data accumulated on MSAFP levels relative to neural tube defects, a correlation was recognized between lower than normal MSAFP levels and fetuses with chromosome aberrations. This correlation allowed simultaneous modifications of risks for fetal neural tube defects or chromosomal anomalies based on a single MSAFP measurement. Norms were established for low MSAFP values, and significantly three values were taken as indications to offer amniocentesis for definitive detection of fetus chromosomal anomalies. Other maternal serum protein or hormone markers were then investigated, and correlation between levels of human chorionic gonadotropin or estriol and chromosomal anomalies was demonstrated. A combination of three maternal serum markers was soon established as the most sensitive indicator of fetal chromosome anomaly, and this triple test became the standard of care. The combined measurement of maternal serum AFP, chorionic gonadotropin, and estriol at 15–18 weeks gestation will detect about 70% of fetuses with chromosome anomalies (mainly Down syndrome) with a 5% false positive rate. A positive triple test screen allows the option of confirmatory amniocentesis and termination of affected fetuses within the legal limit for abortion at 22–26 weeks of gestation.

Recent developments with maternal serum screening include the evaluation of additional serum markers, trials of first trimester diagnosis, and combined risk estimates using serum marker levels plus other parameters such as maternal age or targeted ultrasound. Additional maternal serum markers include pregnancy-associated protein A or inhibin A, and ultrasound markers include increased nuchal translucency (neck folds—see following section). As discussed in Chapters 5 and 12, an increased frequency of disease will increase the positive predictive value of a screening test. Using maternal age as an independent marker for increased risk of Down syndrome can therefore increase the sensitivity of maternal serum screening. The measurement of four maternal serum markers at gestational age 16–18 weeks, coupled with ultrasound studies and maternal age corrections, has allowed detection of 90% of fetuses with Down syndrome (Yagel et al., 1998). This same strategy has been tested at 10–12 weeks of pregnancy (first trimester) with a 60–65% detection rate (Haddow et al., 1998).

Ethical problems with maternal serum screening include compromised autonomy of the couple because of inadequate counseling prior to obtaining the test. Couples may not appreciate the significant false positive (5%) and false negative (10–20%) rates, and may be confronted with prenatal diagnostic options (e.g., amniocentesis) that they had not considered. Practical problems concerning maternal serum screening include the complexity of test interpretation and the difficulty in relaying this information (risks defined by deviation from MOM, gestational age, etc.) in ways that couples can understand. There are also issues of increased cost (the volume of amniocenteses increased by 20–25% in some programs because of the need to confirm maternal serum testing) and distribution of medical resources when many women do not receive routine prenatal care.

Fetal Sonography

Routine fetal ultrasound is often performed at 8–10 weeks gestation and again at 16–18 weeks of gestation. Routine fetal sonography provides information about fetal size and growth, placental position, and single versus multiple pregnancies. It is important to realize that routine or level I ultrasound misses many congenital anomalies because of the limited time, focus, and resolution of scanning. Even low-resolution ultrasound can detect ambiguous findings such as intracranial chorionic cysts that usually resolve later in pregnancy, and these false positive findings may provoke parental anxiety and unnecessary monitoring. False negative results of routine sonography are an even greater problem, because subtle anomalies or absent anomalies in conditions such as nonspecific mental retardation yield a normal ultrasound. It is common to recommend ultrasound to families at risk for an anomaly such as a congenital heart defect only to be told that a previous ultrasound missed that anomaly in their previous child. Counseling regarding the purpose of routine level I ultrasound is thus important so couples understand its limitations. Higher resolution, level II ultrasound can identify numerous congenital anomalies, particularly when one organ is the focus of attention because of the family history (see Section 15.6).

Case 15 Follow-up: The low rather than high value for maternal serum alpha-fetoprotein is associated with chromosomal disorders, and a level II ultrasound reveals cranial and limb anomalies in the fetus. Confirmatory studies are scheduled.

■ 15.6. PRENATAL DIAGNOSIS OF GENETIC DISEASE

Once increased genetic risk is identified for a pregnancy through preconceptional counseling or prenatal screening, several options for prenatal diagnosis are available (Table 15.6). Prenatal diagnostic techniques performed early in gestation, like chorionic villus biopsy, are usually planned during preconceptional planning. Those performed later in pregnancy, like amniocentesis or percutaneous umbilical blood sampling, are often prompted by abnormal resuts of maternal serum or ultrasound screening. It is important to realize that CVS and amniocentesis are techniques for obtaining cells of fetal origin. Prenatal diagnosis using these techniques must therefore employ methods

■**TABLE 15.6.** Prenatal Diagnostic Techniques and Disease Examples

Prenatal Diagnostic Technique	Timing (weeks)[a]	Disease Examples
Preimplantation diagnosis	2 (IVF)	Common trisomies (13,18,21)
		Mendelian disorders amenable to PCR DNA diagnosis
		Adenomatous polyposis coli (175100)
		Marfan syndrome (154700)
		Cystic fibrosis (219700)
		Fragile X syndrome (309550)
Chorionic villus sampling	8–10	Chromosomal disorders detected by routine banding
Early amniocentesis	12–14	Specific microdeletion syndromes if at risk
Routine amniocentesis (Sometimes follows abnormal ultrasound or maternal serum markers)	15–18	Mendelian disorders with characterized or predominant mutant DNA alleles:
		Osteogenesis imperfecta (166240)
		Sickle cell anemia (141900)
		Medium chain CoA dehydrogenase deficiency (201450)
		Duchenne muscular dystrophy (310200)
		Mendelian disorders with characterized protein abnormalities or enzyme deficiencies
		Hurler syndrome (252800)
		Propionic acidemia (232000)
		Lesch-Nyhan syndrome (308000)
		Ornithine decarbamylase deficiency (311250)
		Blood group alleles responsible for isoimmunization
Early maternal serum markers (experimental)	10–12	Down syndrome, other chromosomal disorders
		Neural tube defects
Routine maternal serum markers (triple test)	16–18	Down syndrome, other chromosomal disorders
		Neural tube defects
Level I ultrasound (confirms pregnancy, guides PND)	10–18	Twin pregnancy, abnormal placenta, major birth defects
Level II ultrasound (for specific fetal anatomy)	14–18	Most congenital anomalies if examination focused on that organ system (e.g., heart defects, renal defects)
		Mendelian disorders with characteristic ultrasound findings (i.e., osteogenesis imperfecta with multiple fetal fractures)
Cordocentesis (Often follows abnormal ultrasound)	20–40	Fetal cytopenias
		Anemias due to blood type incompatibility
		Thrombocytopenias due to congenital infections
		Chromosomal disorders detected by routine banding
		Mendelian disorders with characterized DNA mutant alleles or enzyme deficiencies

[a]Usually defined as weeks after last menstrual period, but may be modified based on fetal measurements by examination and ultrasound.

Note: IVF, in vitro fertilization; PND, prenatal diagnosis.

that recognize cellular abnormalities like abnormal chromosomes, mutant DNA alleles, or deficient enzymes. Occasionally, exemplified by certain genetic skin disorders, tissue samples can be obtained that allow diagnosis based on tissue histology. Such prenatal diagnoses are often less reliable than those based on chromosomal, enzyme, or DNA diagnosis. The menu of prenatal diagnostic techniques, together with knowledge of genetic mechanisms, provides a list of clinical indications for prenatal diagnosis (Table 15.7). Principles of nondirective counseling mandate that families be informed about prenatal diagnostic options and allowed to reach their own decisions.

Chorionic Villus Sampling

Performed at 8–10 postmenstrual weeks, chorionic villus sampling (CVS) involves biopsy of the primitive placenta or chorion (Fig. 15.2). It should be recalled from Chapter 9 that the placenta (trophoblast) and embryo (inner cell mass) are both derived from the blastocyst—the placenta is thus representative of zygotic or fetal tissue. Fragments of the chorion can be obtained with hollow biopsy tubes inserted through the abdomen or vagina. The catheter is positioned by ultrasound, and negative pressure exerted by aspiration to deliver tissue fragments into a petri dish (Fig. 15.2). The frondlike structures of chorionic villi must be distinguished from tissues of the uterine lining or decidua; analysis of decidual tissue will yield results on the mother rather than on the fetus. Because the chorion is a rapidly dividing tissue, direct karyotype analysis can be performed by arresting chorionic cell division in metaphase. This technique yields chromosome results in 24–36 hours. Chorionic cells are also cultured to yield confirmatory results within 1–2 weeks. A tremendous advantage of CVS is that results are usually available at 10–12 weeks gestation before the woman is obviously pregnant. A prenatal diagnosis and decision about termination is thus available before the pregnancy is evident to friends and relatives.

Once concerns about separating fetal chorionic from maternal decidual tissues were addressed, prenatal diagnoses using CVS became extremely reliable. One series of 10,000 CVS procedures performed by one investigator yielded successful samples in 99.8% of transabdominal approaches (8479 cases) and 99.2% of transvaginal approaches (1521 cases—Brambati et al., 1998). These results reflect a trend toward the transabdominal approach. Fetal loss rates in this study were 2.6% by 28 weeks, a number that is viewed as similar to controls where pregnancies are identified at 8–10 weeks. Rates of premature delivery or perinatal mortality also did not differ from controls without CVS, and there was no increased risk for major birth defects (Brambati et al., 1998). These figures agree with other centers in establishing CVS as a safe and accurate technique for prenatal diagnosis. Some concern has been raised over an increased risk for limb defects after CVS, but the study by Brambati et al. (1998) and others have not supported a correlation.

One problem complicating CVS is the detection of chromosomal mosaicism in 1–3% of samples. Follow-up of these pregnancies indicates that the mosaicism is confined to the placenta in many cases. The detection of CVS mosaicism requires subsequent monitoring of the pregnancy, with additional fetal sampling through amniocentesis (fetal fibroblasts and urinary tract cells) or percutaneous umbilical blood sampling (PUBS) (fetal blood cells). If the aneuploid line found in mosaic cells is incompatible with life, as with trisomy 16, then subsequent fetal monitoring may not be indicated. However, infants born after detection of CVS mosaicism are at risk for uniparental disomy as discussed in Chapter 10. If the mosaicism arises from correction of trisomic zygotes to disomic fetuses and mosaic placentas, then one-third of these disomic fetuses will have their two chromosomes derived from one parent. Abnormal neonates born after detection of confined placental mosaicism should have DNA marker studies to ascertain the origin of that particular pair of disomic chromosomes.

■**TABLE 15.7.** Indications for Prenatal Diagnosis

Indication	Risk[a]	Available Procedures
General pregnancy screening	~ 1 in 500	Maternal serum markers (triple test) Level I ultrasound
Advanced maternal age (> 35 years)	~1 in 200	CVS, amniocentesis for routine chromosome studies
Prior child with chromosome aberration	~1 in 100	CVS, amniocentesis for routine chromosome studies
Relative with neural tube defect	~1 in 25	MSAFP, ultrasound, amniotic fluid AFP
Relative with heart defect or other characteristic single anomaly	~1 in 25	Level II ultrasound, fetal echocardiography
Parental translocation carrier	~1 in 5–10	BABI for single cell FISH chromosome studies CVS, amniocentesis for routine chromosome studies
Autosomal dominant disorder with molecular or biochemical diagnosis	~1 in 15 (GM) 1 in 2	BABI for single cell PCR and DNA analysis CVS, amniocentesis for DNA or enzyme analysis
Autosomal or X-linked recessive disorder with molecular or biochemical diagnosis	1 in 4	BABI for single cell PCR and DNA analysis CVS, amniocentesis for DNA or enzyme analysis
X-linked disorder without biochemical or molecular diagnosis	1 in 4	BABI for single cell FISH or PCR for embryonic sex CVS, amniocentesis for fetal sex
Mendelian syndrome with characteristic anomalies	1 in 2–4	Level II ultrasound

[a] for detectable disorders.

Notes: GM, germ-line mosaicism; CVS, chorionic villus sampling; MSAFP, maternal serum alpha-fetoprotein; BABI, blastomere analysis before implantation (preimplantation diagnosis).

Amniocentesis

Amniocentesis was the first definitive technique for fetal chromosome analysis and remains as the best-studied prenatal diagnostic technique (Fig. 15.3). The procedure is usually performed at 16–18 weeks of pregnancy, although improvements in technique and the advantages of ultrasound guidance have allowed amniocentesis at 12–13 weeks. A needle is introduced through the abdominal and uterine wall into the amniotic cavity under ultrasound guidance (Fig. 15.3). Gentle aspiration of 10–20 cc of amniotic fluid is performed, followed by centrifugation of the suspended fetal cells for culture. Since the fetal fibroblasts and urinary tract cells are not dividing, direct and rapid analysis of chromosomes cannot be performed unless FISH techniques are used. DNA analysis using small numbers of cells can be performed, but more reliable testing after cell culture is usually preferred. Enriched cell sus-

pensions are often incubated on small glass coverslips, allowing easy preparation of metaphase spreads by hypotonic washing, alcohol fixing, and chromosome banding treatments. These rapid culture techniques provide cytogenetic results within 7–9 days after the procedure, allowing decisions about termination by 17–19 weeks of gestation. DNA testing for diseases such as cystic fibrosis is even more rapid, while enzyme assays for diseases such as Hurler syndrome may require 2–3 weeks to obtain adequate amounts of cultured cells.

The risk of fetal loss following amniocentesis is often cited as 1 in 200–300 procedures, but is considerably lower in experienced hands. Comparisons of amniocentesis and CVS have revealed little differences in rates of pregnancy loss or fetal anomalies. Amniocentesis at the standard time of 16–18 weeks gestation had no greater risks of fetal loss than that of control pregnancies in several studies. Early amniocentesis at 12–14 weeks had similar

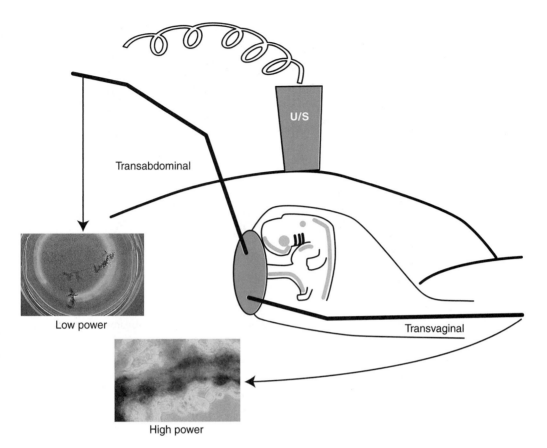

Transabdominal

U/S

Low power

High power

Transvaginal

Figure 15.2. CVS sampling showing transabdominal or transvaginal approaches and photographs of chorionic villi (inserts)—courtesy of Dr. Laird Jackson.

rates of fetal loss to CVS of 3–4% in one study (Sundberg et al., 1997), and there was an increased incidence of amniotic fluid leakage and fetal clubfoot after early amniocentesis. One advantage of second trimester amniocentesis is the ability to correlate cytogenetic or molecular findings with high-resolution ultrasound that is available on the larger fetus. These combined techniques are extremely powerful in determining the cause and prognosis of fetal anomalies, as indicated by one study demonstrating that isolated chorioid plexus cysts detected by ultrasound were never associated with abnormal chromosomes by amniocentesis (Gray et al., 1996).

Chromosomal mosaicism detected by amniocentesis is also a problem with greater significance for fetal abnormality than with CVS

mosaicism. Although the rates of mosaicism detected by amniocentesis (0.1–0.2%) is lower the 2–3% for CVS, mosaicism for lethal trisomies such as trisomy 2 or trisomy 22 predicted a 60% chance for abnormal fetal outcome—either fetal loss or an abnormal neonate. Subsequent studies such as fetal blood karyotyping through cordocentesis were not helpful in deciding the significance of amniotic fluid cell mosaicism (Kalousek, 1997).

Level II Ultrasound and Fetal Echocardiography

Once a fetus is identified as high risk for congenital anomalies, level II ultrasound becomes a potent diagnostic technique for characterizing anomalies and anomaly patterns. Defini-

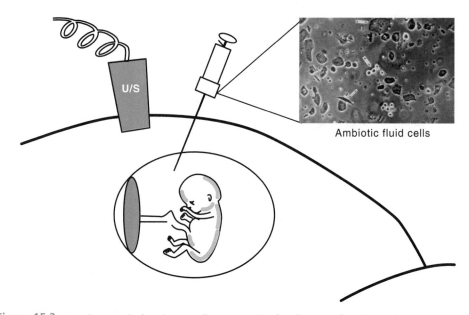

Ambiotic fluid cells

Figure 15.3. Amniocentesis showing needle penetration by ultrasound guidance; insert shows amniotic fluid with suspended fetal cells.

tive ultrasound studies are traditionally available at 16–20 weeks of gestation, but improved ultrasound machines can provide considerable information by 12–16 weeks. There is a huge difference in general level I ultrasound and level II ultrasound that is focused on particular fetal organs. By 14–16 weeks, measurements of fetal brain ventricles, detection of most skeletal anomalies, and fetal echocardiography with Doppler is available. The ability to image many fetal organs provides an extremely diverse spectrum of successful prenatal diagnoses, including most of the surgically correctable anomalies discussed in Chapter 13. Fetal ultrasound also provides a reliable method of fetal sex determination through visualization of the external genitalia.

Congenital heart defects, craniofacial defects, abdominal wall defects, limb defects, and spinal or neural tube defects can all be detected in time for decisions about termination if a focused, level II ultrasound is obtained. Such determinations are particularly valuable when maternal serum screening has suggested the possibility of neural tube defects or chromosomal abnormalities. Anencephaly and

spina bifida are easily recognized by mid-second trimester ultrasound, and detection of small, skin-covered myelomeningoceles is often successful in women at higher risk for neural tube defects. A thickened neck fold is helpful for the first trimester diagnosis of Down syndrome, as are changes in limb lengths or in shapes of the cerebral ventricles. Most major anomalies can be detected by level II ultrasound if the sonographer is alerted to their presence. Other major anomalies such as diaphragmatic hernia can be detected by routine screening, although many will be diagnosed after the period for fetal termination. As illustrated by Case 15, cordocentesis can be combined with ultrasound to diagnose chromosomal anomalies later in pregnancy so as to decide appropriate perinatal management. Ultrasound diagnosis of isolated fetal anomalies later in pregnancy also provides the opportunity for fetal surgery.

Fetoscopy

The insertion of a fetoscope into the amniotic cavity allows inspection and certain manipulations to be performed on the fetus. The technique is analogous to gastroscopy or colonoscopy that allows the visualization of internal organs in adults. A major use of fetoscopy is to sample fetal blood from the umbilical vein, as discussed for cordocentesis below. Occasionally, fetoscopy is used to obtain skin samples from fetuses at risk for genetic skin disorders such as one of the epidermolysis bullosas (e.g., 131600). The use of fetoscopy has also provided new approaches to fetal surgery by allowing access and visualization of fetal surface defects.

Fetal Blood Sampling by Cordocentesis or Maternal Blood Separation

The technique of cordocentesis or PUBS arose from the need to perform fetal transfusions because of blood group incompatibility. Once needle penetration of the amniotic cavity and fetal umbilical vein became routine, fetal blood samples could be obtained for prenatal diagnosis. As technical facility at fetal umbilical vein penetration has increased, PUBS has been performed earlier in gestation at 20–24 weeks rather than after 24 weeks to near term. Because of significant rates of fetal loss after PUBS—2.3% within 48 hours after the procedure and 0.7% within 2 weeks—PUBS is used for confirmatory or additional information after abnormal ultrasound, CVS, or amniocentesis results have been obtained (Buscaglia et al., 1996). Cordocentesis is particularly helpful when third trimester ultrasound reveals a major congenital anomaly. Chromosome analysis via PUBS can determine if the anomaly is part of a chromosomal syndrome, with subsequent pregnancy and delivery management appropriate for the diagnosis. For example, women carrying a trisomy 18 fetus would not be subjected to early cesarean section if the fetus gave evidence of stress during labor. Recognition of chromosomal syndromes by PUBS, even though after the time of possible fetal termination, also allows time for counseling, adjustment, and planning for a child with developmental anomalies.

The ability to isolate fetal cells from maternal blood samples early in gestation would provide an ideal method for prenatal diagnosis. Fetal chromosomal anomalies could be diagnosed directly rather than inferred from maternal serum screening, and DNA or enzyme diagnoses could be performed without the need for cultured cells. Many false claims have characterized this area, but the use of flow cytometry to isolate fetal nucleated cells is now yielding reliable results. One study demonstrated the recovery of more than 2000 fetal cells per 20 cc of maternal blood obtained during early pregnancy, with successful diagnosis of sex and trisomy or disomy 21 in a series of 16 pregnancies (Wachtel et al., 1996). The use of several FISH probes allowed the examination of chromosomes 13, 18, 21, X and Y in these samples, eliminating or recognizing the more common autosomal or sex chromosome aneuploidies. Separation of fetal cells from the maternal circulation is still experimental, but offers hope for less invasive means of prenatal diagnosis.

Case 15 Follow-up: The couple opted for amniocentesis after the low MSAFP value and normal ultrasound were documented. A karyotype demonstrated mosaicism for a small extra chromosome (44,XX/47,XX+fragment), and normal karyotypes are documented on the parents. The fragment resembled chromosome 22, and a diagnosis of trisomy mosaicism for the short and proximal long arm of chromosome 22 is made. FISH studies were not available at this time to confirm this diagnosis. At 30 weeks of gestation, PUBS (cordocentesis) is performed and confirms trisomy 22 mosaicism. An ultrasound study now reveals a misshapen skull with a posterior crease and an absent digit on one hand. Cesarean delivery is avoided, and a female fetus with growth retardation, cranial deformity and absent fingers is born. The cord blood karyotype confirms trisomy 22 mosaicism, and the few other children with this anomaly have had a poor outcome. Despite gastrostomy feedings, the infant died at home at age 3 months.

■ 15.7. FETAL SURGERY AND FETAL TREATMENT

Slowly the era of prenatal diagnosis with limited options is changing to an era of fetal treatment. Many fetal disorders are treated naturally by the larger metabolic mass of the mother. Interchange of fetal and maternal blood means that most fetal metabolic disorders will be corrected by maternal metabolism, and this provides a paradigm for other treatments. The administration of substances to the maternal bloodstream may reach the fetus and enhance or suppress certain gene activities. Limited knowledge of embryogenesis has prevented such therapies for birth defects, but the rapid definition of developmental genes may define ways to compensate for blocks in early signal transduction pathways (see Chapter 9). The treatment of congenital adrenal hyperplasia due to 21-hydroxylase deficiency (201910—see Chapters 12, 13) provides a preview of this approach.

Treatment by Maternal Supplementation

After couples have a child affected with 21-hydroxylase deficiency, they have a 25% recurrence risk for this autosomal recessive disorder. Affected female fetuses will be subjected to increased concentrations of androgens (see Fig. 13.5) and develop ambiguous genitalia with an enlarged clitoris (female pseudohermaphroditism). Excess androgen levels in male fetuses only enhances male genital development, so that no abnormalities are recognized until hypoglycemia or salt wasting is noted. Pregnancies at risk for 21-hydroxylase deficiency are thus treated with dexamethasone (a cortisone derivative) to suppress the manufacture of fetal adrenal steroids during early genital development (6–10 weeks). At 8–10 weeks of gestation, a CVS is performed to determine fetal sex and the staus of 21-hydoxylase activity. Dexamethasone is then stopped in male or unaffected fetuses, but continued in affected female fetuses to prevent

masculination of the external and internal genitalia. Fetal treatment thus produces a normal appearing and fertile female who still must receive injections of cortisone and mineralocorticoids. This example of birth defect prevention through control of embryonic differentiation is a model for correction of other congenital anomalies.

Another model for fetal treatment is the provision of cofactors for key enzyme reactions. Although most fetal enzyme deficiencies are corrected by maternal metabolism, vitamin-responsive disorders may require higher levels of maternal vitamins. One example of fetal treatment has involved the provision of vitamin B_{12} to a mother carrying a fetus with methylmalonic aciduria (see Chapter 12). The vitamin B_{12} supplementation decreased the amount of methylmalonic acid excreted by the mother, and presumably by the fetus, but clear benefit of prenatal versus immediate postnatal therapy is not evident (Ampola et al., 1975). Nevertheless, the ability to treat offers a future model for prenatal cofactor therapy.

Fetal Transfusion

Beginning with the treatment of erythroblastosis fetalis due to maternofetal Rh incompatibility, transfusion of blood components into the umbilical vein of mid-trimester fetuses has become an important mode of fetal therapy. Red blood cell deficiencies due to isoimmunization reactions and platelet deficiencies due to immune reactions and/or congenital infections can be treated by transfusing the appropriate blood component. Early recognition of fetuses with incompatible blood types is now possible by PCR amplification of DNA from CVS or amniocentesis samples followed by allele-specific oligonucleotide (ASO) detection of blood group alleles. The modality for introduction of blood components into fetuses also brings up the possibility of stem cell or gene therapy to correct fetal genetic disorders. Withdrawal of fetal blood, insertion of DNA vectors or stem cells, followed by transfusion of altered cells offers an approach for gene or stem cell therapy that could be used for diseases such as adenosine deaminase deficiency (102700—see Chapter 10).

Fetal Surgery

The detection of fetal anomalies that will exert deleterious effects on later fetal and neonatal development offers the opportunity for fetal therapy. Most fetal surgey has involved relatively minor procedures using catheters that puncture the abdominal wall and amnion. In fetal hydrocephalus, caused by blockage of fluid circulation through the cerebral ventricles, tubes (shunts) have been placed connecting the ventricular cavities to the external amnion. Over 80% of fetuses survived the procedure, but only 30% of the survivors had good developmental outcomes upon assessment in early childhood. The remainder had mental disabilities that were mostly in the severe range. Most disturbing was the salvage of severely affected fetuses that would normally be spontaneously aborted, allowing them to be born as severely handicapped individuals. Because of these negative outcomes in the first 40–50 cases, fetal surgery for hydrocephalus has not been pursued.

A more optimistic experience has been obtained with fetal urinary tract anomalies. After recognition of the anomaly by ultrasound, and exclusion of syndromes by ultrasound and chromosomal analysis (CVS or amniocentesis), a catheter from bladder to amniotic cavity is placed to allow drainage of urine. Relief of urinary pressure that damages the fetal kidneys is thus attained simultaneously with increased amniotic fluid that is needed to promote lung development. The fetal survival rate for such surgery is about 50%, and most children (91%) have avoided renal failure, pulmonary damage, or other chronic disorders.

Open fetal surgery, bringing the fetus outside of the uterus to be operated on, has been tried for several disorders including the repair of diaphagmatic hernia. As with all new procedures, initial results were disappointing with a high rate of fetal loss. Later operations have been successful with minimal risk to the mother. Problems with amniotic fluid leakage and uterine irritability still make open fetal surgery a high-risk procedure for premature delivery with fetal loss. If these risks can be overcome with technical advances, the improved operative access will allow operations on a wide variety of fetal anomalies.

Perinatal Management

Recognition of genetic diseases and congenital anomalies in the mother and/or fetus will have important implications for perinatal management. As mentioned previously, women with Marfan syndrome or skeletal dysplasias may require modifications of delivery that minimize stress or compensate for reduced pelvic size. Fetuses with prenatally detected anomalies may mandate management that favors the mother's health, while those with fragile bones (i.e., osteogenesis imperfecta—166240) may necessitate cesarean section to reduce the number of fractures. Neonatal evaluation will be extremely important to confirm prenatal diagnoses and to initiate proper treatments such as those required for congenital adrenal hyperplasia. The birth of an abnormal child should initiate a team approach to management as was discussed in Chapter 1. The various steps and components of this team approach, with emphasis on the roles of allied health professionals, is discussed in Chapter 16.

PROBLEM SET 15
Reproductive Genetics and Prenatal Diagnosis

Respond to the following questions with short answers, consulting Tables 15.1–15.7 or Figs. 15.1–15.3. For each clinical presentation, discuss the genetic risks and reproductive or prenatal diagnosis options for the family.

15.1. A couple in their early 30s has a child with trisomy 21.

15.2. A couple in their 20s has a child with spina bifida.

15.3. A woman is diagnosed with Turner syndrome mosaicism after an early pregnancy loss.

15.4. A couple have no children after 3 years of trying to conceive. Their family history is unremarkable.

15.5. A couple have a child with severe hydrocephalus and no other anomalies. Their family history is remarkable for a male cousin with hydrocephalus.

15.6. A man is unable to conceive children by two different marriages. He is tall and has small testes noted on physical examination.

15.7. A couple have a child who expires in the neonatal period because of a severe congenital heart defect with mitral valve dysplasia. The child has no other anomalies, and the family history is benign.

15.8. A couple in their 20s have lost three consecutive pregnancies in the first trimester.

15.9. A woman is 39 years old and wishes to have her fourth child. The other three are normal, as is her husband's medical and family history.

15.10. A couple have one child with Hurler syndrome (252800), a severe autosomal recessive disorder caused by deficiency of the enzyme L-α-iduronidase.

PROBLEM SET 15
Answers

15.1.–15.10. See Solutions

PROBLEM SET 15
Solutions

15.1. The recurrence risk after one child with a chromosome anomaly is about 1% plus the maternal age-related risk. Prenatal diagnosis can be accomplished most reliably by fetal karyotype, with level II ultrasound of the fetal head and femurs or maternal serum α-fetoprotein (MSAFP) providing risk modification for Down syndrome (Table 15.7). Because this young couple has a relatively low recurrence risk, preimplantation diagnosis would be inappropriately demanding and expensive. Chorionic villus sampling or amniocentesis would provide high diagnostic reliability with low risks (< 1 in 200) of fetal loss.

15.2. Neural tube defects such as anencephaly or spina bifida exhibit multifactorial determination with a 3–5% recurrence risk that varies slightly with ethnic background. Preconceptional counseling should be provided to lower the risk with folic acid supplementation, and level II ultrasound targeted to the craniospinal axis with MSAFP levels would provide a high likelihood of diagnosis. Amniotic fluid AFP could be used for confirmation, providing the additional advantage of a fetal karyotype.

15.3. Turner syndrome is one of many genetic disorders with infertility, and mosaicism for the 45,X chromosome abnormality increases risks for pregnancy loss or fetal chromosome abnormalities. Amniocentesis for fetal karyotyping could be offered as a safe technique unlikely to increase the prior risk for fetal loss.

15.4. An evaluation for infertility could include examination for female reproductive tract anomalies, defective ovarian function, or the presence of other medical diseases (Table 15.1). A sperm analysis and genital examination could be performed on the husband (Table 15.2). Adoption, gamete intrafallopian transfer (GIFT) with the wife's or donor oocyte, in vitro fertilization with the husband's or donor sperm, or intracytoplasmic sperm injection (ICSI) could be considered depending on whether one or both parents had reproductive abnormalities (Table 15.4).

15.5. Isolated hydrocephalus is usually a multifactorial defect with a 3–5% recurrence risk. Level II ultrasound could be employed for prenatal diagnosis at 12–16 weeks, although the hydrocephalus might not be present by that time. Although the affected male cousin is compatible with multifactorial determination, this history plus the severity of the hydrocephalus could indicate a Mendelian disorder.

If a DNA test is available for the abnormal alleles causing the Mendelian form of hydrocephalus, as in the X-linked recessive MASA syndrome (303350), then definitive prenatal diagnosis using chorionic villus sampling or amniocentesis to obtain fetal cells for DNA analysis could be performed. If the responsible mutant and normal alleles could be amplified from single cells using the polymerase chain reaction, then blastomere analysis before implantation (BABI) could be performed, with only normal embryos being implanted to continue the pregnancy. If an X-linked form of hydrocephalus were confirmed, then BABI could be used to select female embryos and avoid the risk for affected males (Table 15.7).

15.6. The man's tall stature and small testes suggest Klinefelter syndrome, and a chromosome study should be performed to document the 47,XYY karyotype. Since spermatocytes do not form in this disorder, in vitro fertilization by donor rather than intracytoplasmic sperm injection would be necessary for the couple to have children (Table 15.4).

15.7. Congenital heart defects exhibit multifactorial determination with a 3–10% recurrence risk. Level II ultrasound with fetal echocardiography should allow prenatal diagnosis of a similar heart defect by 16–18 weeks of gestation (Table 15.7).

15.8. Couples with 2–3 spontaneous abortions have a 1–2% frequency of chromosomal abnormalities. Chromosome studies could be performed followed by examination for female reproductive tract anomalies or testing for antiphospholipid or HLA antibodies.

15.9. Maternal age over 35 years is a recognized indication for prenatal diagnosis (Table 15.7). The negative family history suggests that a reliable, low-risk procedure be selected such as chorionic villus biopsy or amniocentesis.

15.10. For Mendelian disorders, prenatal diagnosis requires the ability to detect mutant alleles in the fetus through enzyme assay, protein detection, or direct DNA analsysis. The 25% recurrence risk for a severe disease would justify

preimplantation diagnosis if mutant alleles for Hurler syndrome (252800) could be amplified and detected in a single blastomere. More reliable and routine prenatal diagnosis could be offered using chorionic villus biopsy or amniecentesis followed by enzyme assay or DNA analysis of fetal cells.

BIBLIOGRAPHY

General References

Cowan BD. 1997. *Clinical Reproductive Medicine.* New York: Lippincott-Raven.

Creasy RK. 1999. *Maternal-Fetal Medicine,* 4th ed. Philadelphia: WB Saunders.

Gilbert-Barness E. 1997. *Potter's Pathology of the Fetus and Infant.* St. Louis: Mosby.

Gorlin RJ, Cohen MM Jr, Levin LS. 1990. *Syndromes of the Head and Neck.* New York: Oxford.

Isada NB. 1996. *Maternal Genetic Diseases.* Stamford, CT: Appleton & Lange.

King RA, Rotter JI, Motulsky AG. 1992. *The Genetic Basis of Common Diseases.* New York: Oxford University Press.

Kuller JA, Chescheir NC, Cefalo RC. 1996. *Prenatal Diagnosis and Reproductive Genetics.* St. Louis: Mosby.

Seibel MM. 1997. *Infertility: A Comprehensive Text,* 2nd ed. Stamford, CT: Appleton & Lange.

Winter RM, Baraitser M. 1998. *London Dysmorphology Database,* Vers. 3.0. Oxford: Oxford University Press.

Infertility

Adamson GD. 1997. Treatment of endometriosis-related infertility. *Semin Reprod Endocrinol* 15: 263–271.

Branch DW. 1990. Autoimmunity and pregnancy loss. *JAMA* 264:2453–1454.

Duncan PA, Shapiro LA, Stangel JJ. 1979. The MURCS association: Mullerian duct aplasia, renal aplasia, and cervicothoracic somite dysplasia. *J Pediatr* 95:399–402.

Guzick DS, Sullivan MW Adamson GD et al. 1998. Efficacy of treatment for unexplained infertility. *Fertil Steril* 70:207–213.

Kalousek DK. 1997. Pathology of abortion: The embryo and the previable fetus. In: Gilbert-

Barness E, ed. *Potter's Pathology of the Fetus and Infant.* St. Louis: Mosby, pp. 106–128.

Kalousek DK, Gilbert-Barness E. 1997. Causes of stillbirth and neonatal death. In Gilbert-Barness E, ed. *Potter's Pathology of the Fetus and Infant.* St. Louis: Mosby, pp. 129–163.

Meschede D, Horst J. 1997. Sex chromosome anomalies in pregnancies conceived through intracytoplasmic sperm injection: a case for genetic counseling. *Hum Reprod* 12:1125–1127.

Opitz JM. 1987. Vaginal atresia (von Mayer-Rokitansky-Kuster or MRK anomaly) in hereditary renal adysplasia (HRA). *Am J Med Genet* 26: 873–876.

Rombauts L, Dear M, Breheny S, Healy DL. 1997. Cumulative pregnancy and live birth rates after gamete intra-Fallopian transfer. *Hum Reprod* 12:1338–1342.

Simpson JL. 1992. Gynecologic disorders. In King RA, Rotter JI, Motulsky AG, eds. *The Genetic Basis of Common Diseases.* New York: Oxford University Press, pp 564–577.

Williamson RA, Elias S. 1992. Infertility and pregnancy loss. In King RA, Rotter JI, Motulsky AG, eds. *The Genetic Basis of Common Diseases.* New York: Oxford University Press, pp 577–595.

Routine Prenatal Care and Screening

Chard T, Macintosh MC. 1995. Screening for Down's syndrome. *J Perinat Med* 23:421–436.

Greenberg F. 1988. The impact of MSAFP screening on genetic services. *Am J Med Genet* 31: 223–230.

Haddow JE, Palomaki GE, Knight GJ, Williams J, Miller WA, Johnson A. 1998. Screening of maternal serum for fetal Down's syndrome in the first trimester. *N Engl J Med* 338:955–961.

Lamvu G, Kuller JA. 1997. Prenatal diagnosis using fetal cells from the maternal circulation. *Obstet Gynecol Surv* 52:433–437.

Nagey DA. 1989. The content of prenatal care. *Obstet Gynecol* 74:516–528.

Pyeritz RE. 1993. The Marfan syndrome. In Royce PM, Steinmann B, eds. *Connective Tissue and its Heritable Disorders: Molecular, Genetic, and Medical Aspects.* New York: Wiley-Liss, pp. 437–506.

Scheuner MT, Wang S-J, Raffel LJ, Larabell SK, and Rotter JI. 1997. Family history: A comprehensive genetic risk assessment method for the chronic conditions of adulthood. *Am J Med Genet* 71:315–324.

Taipale P, Hiilesmaa V, Salonen R, Ylostalo P. 1997. Increased nuchal translucency as a marker for fetal chromosomal defects. *N Engl J Med* 337: 1654–1658.

Taysi K. 1988. Preconceptional counseling. *Obstet Gynecol Clin N Am* 15:167–179.

Wald NH, Kennard A, Hackshaw A, McGuire A. 1997. Antenatal screening for Down syndrome. *J Med Screen* 4:181–246.

Yagel S, Anteby EY, Hochner-Celnikier D et al. 1998. The role of midtrimester targeted fetal organ screening combined with the "triple test" and maternal age in the diagnosis of trisomy 21: a retrospective study. *Am J Obstet Gynecol* 178: 40–44.

Prenatal Diagnosis

Buscaglia M, Ghisoni L, Bellotti M et al. 1996. Percutaneous umbilical blood sampling: indication changes and procedure loss rate in a nine year's experience. *Fetal Diagn Ther* 11:106–113.

Brambati B, Tului L, Cislaghi C, Alberti E. 1998. First 10,000 chorionic villus samplings performed on singleton pregnancies by a single operator. *Prenat Diagn* 18:255–266.

Goldberg JD, Wohlferd MM. 1997. Incidence and outcome of chromosomal mosaicism found at the time of chorionic villus sampling. *Am J Obstet Gynecol* 176:1349–1352.

Gray DL, Winborn RC, Suessen TL, Crane JP. 1996. Is genetic amniocentesis warranted when isolated choroid plexus cysts are found? *Prenat Diagn* 16:983–990.

Harper JC. 1996. Preimplantation diagnosis of inherited disease by embryo biopsy: an update of the world figures. *J Assist Reprod Genet* 13: 90–95.

Kalousek DK, Vekemans M. 1996. Confined placental mosaicism. *J Med Genet* 33:529–533.

Kaplan P, Normandin JJr, Wilson GN, Plauchu H, Lippman A, Vekemans M. 1990. Malformations and minor anomalies in children whose mothers had prenatal diagnosis: Comparison between CVS and amniocentesis. *Am J Med Genet* 37: 366–370.

Marshall E. 1994. Rules on embryo research due out. *Science* 265:1024–1026.

Marshall E. 1997. Embryologists dismayed by sanctions against geneticist. *Science* 275:472.

Rechitsky S, Strom C, Verlinsky O et al. 1998. Allele dropout in polar bodies and blastomeres. *J Assist Reprod Genet* 15:253–257.

Reubinoff BE, Schenker JG. 1996. New advances in sex preselection. *Fertil Steril* 66:343–350.

Sundberg K, Bang J, Smidt-Jensen S et al. 1997. Randomized study of risk of fetal loss related to early amniocentesis versus chorionic villus sampling. *Lancet* 350:697–703.

Verlinsky Y, Rechitsky S, Cieslak J et al. 1997. Preimplantation diagnosis of single gene disorders by two-step oocyte genetic analysis using first and second polar body. *Biochem Mol Med* 62:182–187.

Wachtel SS, Sammons D, Manley M et al. 1996. Fetal cells in maternal blood: recovery by charge flow separation. *Hum Genet* 98:162–166.

Fetal Treatment

Albanese CT, Harrison MR. 1998. Surgical treatment for fetal disease. The state of the art. *Ann NY Acad Sci* 847:74–85.

Ampola MG, Mahoney MJ, Nakamura E, Tanaka K. 1975. Prenatal therapy of a patient with vitamin B12-responsive methylmalonic acidemia. *N Engl J Med* 293:313–318.

Evans MI, Drugan A, Manning FA, Harrison MR. 1989. Fetal surgery in the 1990s. *Am J Dis Child* 143:1431–1438.

Farmer DL. 1998. Fetal surgery: a brief review. *Pediatr Radiol* 28:409–413.

Jona JZ. 1998. Advances in fetal surgery. *Pediatr Clin N Am* 45:599–604.

Quinn TM, Adzick NS. 1997. Fetal surgery. *Obstet Gynecol Clin N Am* 24:143–157.

Skupski DW, Wolf CF, Bussel JB. 1996. Fetal transfusion therapy. *Obstet Gynecol Surv* 51: 181–192.

16

GENETICS, ALLIED HEALTH, AND PREVENTIVE MANAGEMENT: THE CLINICAL GENETICS CARE PATHWAY

■ LEARNING OBJECTIVES

1. A multidisciplinary clinical genetics pathway utilizes diagnosis or diagnostic categories as a guide to preventive management.

2. The primary care physician is an ideal coordinator of the clinical genetics pathway, utilizing input from genetic specialists, genetic counselors, nurses, therapists, and social workers.

3. Nurses have many opportunities to recognize genetic disease with common presentations such as neonatal jaundice, infantile feeding problems, developmental or growth delay, predisposition to infection, school problems, delayed puberty, high-risk pregnancy, obesity, hypertension, heart disease, cancer, and mental deterioration.

4. Genetic counselors are trained to record, interpret, and educate families about their genetic risks. Acting together with genetic or other medical specialists, genetic counselors provide time-consuming

genetics education and psychosocial support.

5. Frequent developmental disabilities in genetic disorders provide many opportunies for occupational, speech, nutritional, and behavioral therapists to recognize genetic disease and initiate the clinical genetics care pathway.

6. Social workers encounter genetic disease while investigating unusual clinical problems or coordinating insurance, school, or family support issues.

7. Medical ethicists are not usual participants in clinical genetics care, but can contribute important perspective on care guidelines and on occasional cases where new technology and current practices conflict.

Case 16: ***A Newborn with Hypotonia and Unusual Facial Appearance***
After an unremarkable gestation, a term baby girl (Fig. 16.1) presents for evaluation because of low muscle tone and a facial ap-

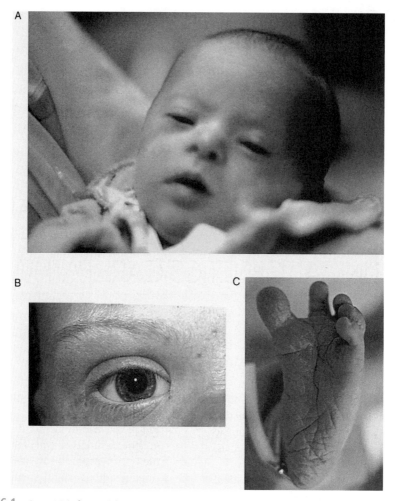

Figure 16.1. Case 16 infant with Down syndrome (*A*) and minor anomalies including epicanthal fold with Brushfield spots of the eye (*B*) or broad space between toes 1 and 2 with a deep plantar crease (*C*).

pearance resembling that of Down syndrome. The obstetrician mentions her concern to the parents and outlines the plan of evaluation. The mother becomes even more distraught when the baby is not able to breast-feed. The parents have recently moved into the state and have no family members in the vicinity.

■ 16.1. INTRODUCTION

In the modern era of health care management, emphasis has been placed on clinical pathways that optimize outcome and cost-effectiveness.

As an example, improvements in outcome for children with asthma have been demonstrated through the development of an asthma team that coordinates their medical care and education. Integral to the pathway approach is a team of health professionals that includes primary care providers, medical specialists, and allied health professionals. The team formulates guidelines oriented toward prevention of acute illness but also covering its effective treatment.

Figure 16.2 illustrates a clinical genetics care pathway that proceeds from category to specific diagnosis to preventive management based on common disease complications (Wil-

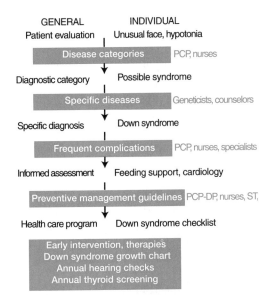

GENERAL   INDIVIDUAL
Patient evaluation   Unusual face, hypotonia

Disease categories   PCP, nurses

Diagnostic category   Possible syndrome

Specific diseases   Geneticists, counselors

Specific diagnosis   Down syndrome

Frequent complications   PCP, nurses, specialists

Informed assessment   Feeding support, cardiology

Preventive management guidelines   PCP-DP, nurses, ST,

Health care program   Down syndrome checklist

Early intervention, therapies
Down syndrome growth chart
Annual hearing checks
Annual thyroid screening

Figure 16.2. Clinical genetics care pathway. The characterization of genetic diseases and their complications translates into preventive management guidelines (center). General (left) or particular (right) application of the pathway is shown for the example of Down syndrome. Some key medical professionals are indicated (shaded). PCP, primary care provider; DP, developmental pediatrician; ST, speech therapist; OT, occupational therapist.

son and Cooley, 1999). The clinical description of a genetic disorder and the documentation of its natural history are critical steps toward providing adequate management. Through the compilation of case reports and clinical details, management guidelines can be derived that avoid major complications of disease. As shown in Figure 16.2, the scholarly process of characterizing genetic diseases is mirrored in the general approach to genetic patients (left) and for an individual patient with a particular disease like Down syndrome (right). Preventive care guidelines for patients with Down syndrome were the first to be formulated as a consensus checklist that is now accepted as a standard of care. The process shown in Figure 16.2 can be used to optimize health outcomes for any genetic disorder, pediatric or adult. The guidelines become a health-care pathway centered by a general physician and comple-

mented by other medical specialists and allied health professionals.

This book has repeatedly emphasized the importance of suspecting genetic disease when severe, unusual, or combination phenotypes are encountered. Once suspicion of genetic disease is entertained, then use of information resources and specialty referrals can lead to appropriate management without the need for detailed genetic knowledge. Primary care and allied health practitioners must suspect and recognize genetic disease so that they can assume their necessary role as coordinator of the multidisciplinary genetic care pathway. Essential ingredients of this pathway may include specialty evaluations, laboratory diagnosis, preventive care, education, rehabilitation, use of social resources, and genetic counseling. Even though patients may require continuing input from genetic specialists, as in the area of metabolic disease, the general physician can ensure integration of this care with the local essentials of immunization, emergency treatment, schooling, sports, and other community activities.

Many allied health specialties will encounter children or adults with genetic disease, and their recognition is essential for initiating the multidisciplinary care pathway. Symptoms may first be recognized by neonatal nurses, speech therapists, dieticians, or social workers, exemplified by neonatal jaundice in galactosemia (230400), nasal speech in children with the velopalatine incompetence of Shprintzen syndrome (192430), obesity in Prader-Willi syndrome (176270), or multiple fractures suggesting child abuse versus osteogenesis imperfecta (166200). Alertness for the unusually early or severe manifestations of genetic disorders is important for every allied health professional. Even common adult disorders can be ameliorated or prevented by testing for risk factors and initiation of the appropriate care pathway.

Once a genetic disorder is recognized and a diagnosis or diagnostic category provided, then the natural history and complications of that disorder establish the boundaries for a clinical care pathway (Fig. 16.2). When a specific diagnosis is unavailable, as for many children with developmental delay, the aggregate care for that categorical problem establishes an outline for preventive care. Evaluations by developmental, neurologic, and genetic specialists address etiology and possible complications such as seizures, while the general physician and ancillary health team ensure good pediatric, early intervention, and rehabilitative care. Although genetic disorders, particularly those with developmental disability, are more common in early childhood, the same approach can be used for the adult with early onset coronary artery disease or familial cancer. The clinical genetic pathway emphasizes the inescapable and necessary role of all health professionals in the care of patients with genetic disease.

■ 16.2. THE ROLE OF NURSING IN GENETICS

It is often said that nurses focus on health while doctors focus on disease. Their involvement in routine health evaluations and their emphasis on providing follow-up guidelines, gives nurses important opportunities for the recognition and preventive management of genetic disorders (Table 16.1). Nurses in the delivery room and infant nurseries may be the first to suspect congenital anomalies that affect 3–5% of children. They may notice a birth defect or symptom that mandates genetic evaluation, and set the tone for education and counseling regarding a possible genetic or congenital disorder.

Some common clinical situations where nurses can recognize genetic disease are listed in Table 16.1. Enhanced jaundice often occurs in metabolic or chromosomal disorders, and many congenital syndromes exhibit hypotonia with feeding problems. Often it is the nurse that recognizes an abnormal facial appearance in a neonate, or first answers questions regarding a congenital anomaly that presents at delivery. Developmental delays with or without hy-

potonia, chronic constipation that often occurs with hypotonia, toileting problems due to urinary tract or spinal anomalies, and school problems such as hyperactivity may all result from genetic disorders and be first encountered by nurses (Table 16.1). Other common problems in early childhood include growth problems, chronic infections, urinary tract infections, or anemias. During later childhood or adulthood, office nurses, school nurses, and public health nurses can encounter genetic disorders causing obesity, hypertension, insomnia, or memory loss (Table 16.1). Their emphasis on optimizing health-care choices allows nurses to bring the genetic patient into the multidisciplinary care pathway that enhances clinical outcome (Fig. 16.2).

A special organization called ISONG—International Society of Nurses in Genetics—has been formed to encourage the role of nurses in clinical genetics. Although traditionally neglected in nursing curricula, textbooks of genetics with nursing perspective are now available to rectify these deficiencies (Lea et al., 1998). Expansion of the roles of nurses and physician assistants in many areas of medicine, including surgeries, procedures, and unsupervised patient encounters provides another incentive for nurses to know and recognize presentations of genetic disease. In obstetrics, nurses often acquire sophistication in genetics and become primary counselors in the areas of maternal-fetal medicine and prenatal diagnosis. A blurred line between obstetric nurses and genetic counselors exist in these areas, with nurses being more familiar with clinical obstetrics and genetic counselors being more familiar with formal genetics. As with other medical specialties, a team approach involving both nurses and counselors is best for the complex and evolving area of reproductive genetics.

Once alerted to the possibility of genetic disease, the nurse can enlist the aid of general and specialty physicians to coordinate a plan for evaluation and management. When the diagnosis and management is decided, the nurse plays a key role in providing education, follow-up assessments, and anticipatory guidance.

■TABLE 16.1. Nursing Presentations of Genetic Diseases

Clinical Problem	Genetic Contributions
Enhanced neonatal jaundice, infantile feeding problems	Metabolic disorders—tyrosinemia (276700), galactosemia (230400)
	Chromosome disorders—Down syndrome, trisomy 13/18
Infantile feeding problems	Branchial arch disorders—Pierre Robin sequence, Goldenhar syndrome (141400)
	Disorders with hypotonia—SMA (253300), Prader-Willi syndrome (176270)
Neonatal congenital anomalies or unusual appearance	Mendelian—Treacher Collins (154500), Zellweger (214100) syndromes
	Chromosome disorders—Down syndrome, trisomy 13/18, others
	Isolated anomalies—Cleft palate, spina bifida
Chronic constipation, toileting problems	Disorders with hypotonia—SMA, Prader-Willi
Chronic infections, otitis, sinusitis	Chromosome disorders—Down, Turner syndrome
	Mendelian diseases—chronic granulomatous disease (306400), cystic fibrosis (219700)
Developmental delays	Chromosome disorders—most aneuploidies, microdeletions
	Mendelian disorders–fragile X syndrome (309550)
	Teratogenic disorders—fetal alcohol syndrome
Anemias	Sickle cell anemia (141900), thalassemias (273500), spherocytosis (182900)
Chronic urinary tract infections	Urinary tract anomalies, urethral stenosis
Growth problems— microcephaly	Seckel syndrome (210600), *cri-du-chat* syndrome (del 5p)
Growth problems—FTT	Cystic fibrosis, chromosomal syndromes
Growth problems—skeletal disproportion	Skeletal dysplasias—achondroplasia (100800), Stickler syndrome (108300)
Sleep apnea	Prader-Willi syndrome, Down syndrome
Delayed puberty	Turner syndrome, Down syndrome, others with disability
Obesity, overgrowth	Prader-Willi, Wiedemann-Beckwith syndrome
Hypertension	Multifactorial disorders—heart or renal defects
	Chromosome disorders—Turner syndrome (coarctation)
	Mendelian disorders—neurofibromatosis-1(162200), polycystic kidney disease (173900)
Insomnia	Manic depressive illness
Memory loss	Alzheimer disease, Huntington chorea (143100)

Note: FTT, failure to thrive with proportionate decrease in height, weight, and head circumference; SMA, spinal muscular atrophy.

Case 16 Follow-up: The nursery and obstetric nurses support the family by explaining why the physicians suspect Down syndrome. The neonatal nurses are aware of feeding risks in infants with Down syndrome and anticipate difficulties as the mother tries to breast-feed. They provide support and instruction to the mother and prevent additional stress from inadequate feeding during this anxious period. The primary physician examines the child, noting several minor anomalies that support the diagnosis of Down syndrome.

■ 16.3. THE ROLE OF GENETIC COUNSELORS

Genetic counselors acquire a master's degree in special two-year training programs that focus on genetics and psychosocial aspects of counseling. They are trained in the documentation of family histories, interpreting inheritance mechanisms and risks, and in dealing with emotional aspects of genetic risks or burdens. There is a certification examination for genetic counselors as there is for clinical geneticists, and the American Society of Genetic Counselors provides integration and leadership. Counselors also have expertise in providing access to parent support groups or genetic databases, in providing education about genetic screening or prenatal diagnostic options, and in explaining inheritance through the use of diagrams showing allele or chromosome segregation. A counseling session often lasts one hour or more until the family adequately understands the disease, its complications, and their options. Genetic counselors are extremely useful parts of the genetic care pathway, but they need clinical input from a clinical geneticist or other medical specialist.

The American Society of Human Genetics has provided the following definition of genetic counseling:

Genetic counseling is a communication process which deals with the human problems associated with the occurrence, or the risk of occurrence, of a genetic disorder in a family. This process involves an attempt by one or more appropriately trained persons to help the individual or family to (1) comprehend the medical facts, including the diagnosis, probable course of the disorder, and the available management; (2) appreciate the way heredity contributes to the disorder, and the risk of recurrence in specified relatives; (3) understand the alternatives for dealing with the risk of recurrence; (4) choose the course of action which seems to them appropriate in view of their risk, their family goals, and their ethical or religious standards, and to act in accordance with that decision; and (5) to make the best possible adjustment to the disorder in an affected family member and/or to the risk of recurrence of that disorder. (Anonymous, 1975)

The definition emphasizes genetic counseling as an educational and supportive process in which the counselor does not direct but provides information for the family to make a decision or adjustment. Accordingly, genetic counselors are most valuable in situations that require complex plans and decisions regarding genetic disease. Table 16.2 outlines some common clinical situations in which genetic counselors take leading roles. An important new role for genetic counselors has developed in the area of presymptomatic diagnosis. Because the diagnosis of genetic predisposition to Huntington chorea (143100) or hereditary breast cancer can have profound medical and psychiatric implications, it is extremely important that patients understand the impact and precision of these tests before consenting to them.

Gail Brookshire, M.S., counselor at Children's Medical Center of Dallas, Texas, points out that presymptomatic genetic testing has forced a new paradigm for medical testing. Before, tests were obtained and counseling provided only if the results were positive. Now, the period prior to testing assumes maximum importance so that the patients have opportunities for informed consent, psychiatric evaluation, and other aspects of decision making that will aid them in accepting test results. As noted for Huntington chorea in Chapter 14, even normal results for devastating diseases can provoke unanticipated reactions from patients.

Genetic counselors have major roles in three areas: adults with significant genetic predisposition where risk factors or definitive genetic tests are available; children with morphologic or metabolic diseases that involve complex tests such as karyotyping or organic acid profiles; and couples with infertility or pregnancy issues that involve interpretation and explanation of fetal DNA, chromosomal, or biochemical tests. Because genetic factors are so universal in medicine, and because risk factors or presymptomatic tests are available for many common diseases, genetic counselors

■ **TABLE 16.2.** Medical Situations Requiring Genetic Counselors

Medical Presentation	Disease Examples	Type of Information
Pediatric counseling		
Newborn with metabolic disease	Phenylketonuria (261600)	Prognosis and diet therapy 25 % RR
	Galactosemia (230400)	Carrier status
Newborn with malformation syndrome	Down syndrome	Explanation of chromosomes
	Zellweger syndrome	1–50% RR
Newborn with congenital anomaly	Cleft palate	Pedigree, risk factors,
	Spina bifida	MF 2–10% RR
New diagnosis of metabolic or morphologic disease	Marfan syndrome (154700)	Explain chromosomes, genes, pedigree, risk factors, 1–50% RR
	Wilson disease (277900)	
	OTC deficiency (311250)	
Special communities	Deaf community	Culturally sensitive counseling and education
	Jewish community	
	Black community	
Family history of genetic disorder	Sickle cell anemia (141900)	Explain genes, multifactorial determination
	Cystic fibrosis (219700)	Pedigree, risk factors, 1–50% RR
	Duchenne muscular dystrophy (310200)	
	Neural tube defects	
Prenatal counseling		
Preconception	Infertility, multiple miscarriages	Explain reproductive options, chromosome testing
Maternal serum	High or low	Explain imprecision, options for confirmatory tests
Prenatal diagnosis	CVS, amniocentesis	Explain options, risks, timing
Prenatal diagnostic results	Trisomy 18	Delivery options, grief counseling, family support
Adult counseling, presymptomatic diagnosis		
Common adult diseases	Coronary artery disease	Document pedigrees, counsel risks, coordinate risk factor testing
	Diabetes mellitus	
Neurologic disease	Huntington disease (143100)	Explain and coordinate pretest evaluation
		Explain results, 0–50% RR
Cancers	Breast cancer (BRCA1)	Explain results, 0–50% RR

Notes: OTC, ornithine transcarbamylase deficiency; CVS, chorionic villus sampling; BRCA1, breast cancer gene; RR, recurrence risk.

are not always associated with clinical geneticists. They may work with medical specialists in cancer or diabetes, with commercial chromosomal or DNA testing laboratories, or even work independently in private practice.

Every family with a chromosomal, syndromal, or metabolic disease should ideally have the opportunity to see a genetic counselor and/or clinical geneticist. Genetic diseases like cystic fibrosis (219700) or neurofibromatosis-

1 (162200) that are managed by other medical specialists may not require input from genetic counselors. However, the occurrence of unusual inheritance patterns and the utility of pedigrees in defining other genetic risk factors (Scheuner et al., 1997) favor the involvement of a genetics professional.

Case 16 Follow-up: After discharge, the chromosome results on the baby show trisomy 21. The primary physician relays these results to the family at the child's 2-week office visit and schedules a visit to the genetics clinic. A clinical geneticist examines the child and makes recommendations for ensuing care such as cardiology, audiology, and ophthalmology visits. The genetic counselor explains the difference between trisomy and translocation Down syndrome (see Chapter 7) and emphasizes the 1% recurrence risk for the parents. Referrals to the early intervention program in the family's school district are made, and a reasonable but optimistic view of developmental disabilities and medical complications in children with Down syndrome is outlined. A local parent group representative also relates their personal experience with a child with Down syndrome.

■ 16.4. THE ROLE OF SOCIAL WORKERS IN GENETICS

Social workers have diverse roles in hospitals, clinics, schools, and family services that sometimes place them in contact with genetic concerns or patients with genetic disease. For children with congenital anomalies, social workers are often part of management and discharge planning to ensure adequate home monitoring, medical equipment, and follow-up visits for the particular anomaly or syndrome. Infants exposed to alcohol or drugs during pregnancy may present for child protective service issues, requiring that social workers coordinate medical evaluations to rule out genetic disease. The question of osteogenesis imperfecta (166200) may arise during child abuse cases, rarely being the reason for fractures but routinely raised as a possibility by defending lawyers. Children with chronic diseases often have problems obtaining medical insurance, medicaid, or other social services like formula or transportation. Behavioral and school issues often arise in children with developmental disabilities, with social workers playing an important role in locating resources for evaluation and therapy. Some knowledge of genetics will be helpful to social workers in understanding the underlying diagnoses and interpreting the relevance of particular services.

Situations in which social workers can provide valuable recognition of genetic factors include adoption, child protective services, early intervention, and school behavioral services (Table 16.3). A child put up for adoption may have certain pregnancy exposures such as alcohol or cocaine, and the social worker needs some sense of the risk and type of evaluations implied by these exposures. For example, the child exposed to alcohol during gestation needs evaluation by a clinical genetics specialist to search for the pattern of minor anomalies—small eyes, thin upper lip, absent philtrum—that are characteristic (see Chapter 11). Children sustaining fractures from alleged abuse may require physical examination for the blue sclerae, prominent forehead, and bowed limbs of osteogenesis imperfecta in order to forestall defense tactics of blaming fractures on genetic disease. Sometimes neglectful parents have genetic disorders themselves that must be recognized for successful resolution. Early intervention programs may disqualify certain children based on apparent normalcy of initial evaluations, whereas the social worker must insist that diagnoses like Down syndrome require early intervention regardless of early motor performance. Children with school failures or behavioral problems may have underlying genetic causes of developmental disability that require recognition, and social workers can initiate the appropriate evaluations.

A role for social workers in the recognition of genetic diseases goes beyond their usual direction toward medical and social services.

■**TABLE 16.3.** Support and Social Issues in Genetic Disease

Age Period and Issues	Disease Examples
Infancy, early childhood	
Infant home care, insurance eligibility, early intervention services	Chromosome disorders
	Mendelian syndromes
Home or hospice care	Severe chromosome or Mendelian disorders (e.g., trisomy 18, SMA)
Special formulas, medical supplies	PKU (261600—formula low in phenylalanine)
	Spina bifida (wheelchairs, catheters)
Family supports	Chromosome disorders (Down syndrome)
	Mendelian syndromes
	Severe congenital anomalies
Childhood	
Special formulas, medical supplies, home care	Severe chronic illnesses such as osteogenesis imperfecta, Hurler syndrome (252800)
Parental compliance with child needs	PKU, galactosemia (230400)
Abuse versus genetic disease	Osteogenesis imperfecta (166200)
Parental neglect due to MD	Parents with fragile X (309550), fetal alcohol, other MD syndromes
School age	
Access to inclusive schooling	Down syndrome, other chronic conditions with MD
Access to special services (e.g., speech therapist)	Down syndrome, other chronic conditions with MD
Evaluation of behavioral problems	Down syndrome, other chronic conditions with MD
Adult	
Home care, medical equipment needs	Huntington disease (143100)
	Down syndrome
Medical insurance discrimination	Marfan syndrome (154700)
Employment discrimination	Neurosensory disorders
Job training, employment opportunities	Down syndrome, other chronic conditions with MD
Independent living	Down syndrome, other chronic conditions with MD

Notes: SMA, spinal muscular atrophy; PKU, phenylketonuria; MD, mental disability.

Knowledge of basic genetic principles and references will help them advocate for patients with genetic or congenital disorders and make them informed participants in the genetics health-care team.

Case 16 Follow-up: After genetic evaluation and counseling, the mother returns to the primary care provider when her child with Down syndrome is 4 weeks old. The mother appears fatigued with a flat affect and tear-fully complains of the long times required for feeding. The child exhibits poor weight gain and an unkempt appearance. A social worker is asked to evaluate the family, and discovers that the father's family has not accepted the child and is urging that the baby be put up for adoption. The social worker recognizes signs of depression in the mother and arranges chaplain support, a visiting nurse to continue encouragement with breast-feeding, and family counseling to include both parents and grandparents. Contact is made with the early intervention program to see if problems have been observed during their home visits. Weekly follow-up is arranged with the social worker and primary physician.

■ 16.5. THE ROLE OF NUTRITIONAL, OCCUPATIONAL, PHYSICAL, AND SPEECH THERAPISTS IN GENETICS

Genetic disorders often cause developmental, neurosensory, and/or nutritional problems in infants and children that can benefit from various types of therapy. Patients presenting to allied health professionals for treatment of one problem may actually have an underlying genetic disorder with many problems. It is therefore important that therapists, like other medical practitioners, be alert for severe or unusual problems that may indicate a genetic disorder. Appropriate evaluations may then be suggested that lead to an integrated, multidisciplinary approach to the patient through the clinical genetics care pathway illustrated in Figure 16.2.

Dieticians are often involved in the management of children with metabolic diseases because of their special dietary needs (Table 16.4). Regular dietary counseling for children with disorders such as phenylketonuria

(261600) is essential for their normal mental development, providing a graphic example of preventive management for a genetic disease. Dietary management is also benificial for adult disorders like hypercholesterolemia (143890) or diabetes mellitus, and the dietician may elicit the history of affected family members that will prompt a genetic evaluation. Besides participating in the management of recognized genetic or multifactorial disorders, dieticians often see children with early feeding problems or later obesity (Table 16.4). Suspicion and recognition of underlying genetic disorders in these children may have important implications for dietary treatment, as with the food restriction and behavioral modification necessary in Prader-Willi syndrome (176270).

Occupational and physical therapists are instrumental in treating the child with developmental delay and/or muscle weakness. Genetic disorders make a huge contribution to these two phenotypes, as indicated by Down syndrome and other chromosomal disorders or the many types of spinal muscular atrophy (253300). Recognition of children with an unusual appearance or minor anomalies can allow the therapist to initiate genetic evaluation. In disorders with congenital contractures, distinctions between genetic versus positional causes is important because positional defor-

■TABLE 16.4. Allied Health Roles in Genetic Disease

Specialist	Problems and Sample Disorders
Speech therapist	Hearing problems
	Velopalatine incompetence—Shprintzen/DiGeorge spectrum (192430)
	Oromotor problems, weak suck—Down, Prader-Willi (176270) syndromes
	Drooling—neurodegenerative disorders
	Cognitive speech delays—Down, Noonan (163950) syndromes
Occupational therapist	Motor training, activities—Down, Noonan syndromes
	Sensory integration—Williams (194050), fetal alcohol syndromes
Physical therapist	Motor training—Duchenne muscular dystrophy (310200), SMA (253300)
Dietician	Special diets—PKU (261600), galactosemia (230400), hypercholesterolemia (143890)
	Poor intake—Down, Prader-Willi syndromes
	Obesity—Down, Prader-Willi syndromes

Notes: SMA, spinal muscular atrophy; PKU, phenylketonuria.

mities often respond to therapy alone. Another example of the value of genetic recognition concerns children with Williams syndrome (194050) who have very sensitive hearing (hyperacusis). The lack of habituation (tuning out of background noise) in these children may cause extreme distractibility and interfere with learning, problems treated with the technique of sensory integration. The therapist recognizing the subtle facial differences of Williams syndrome (see Chapter 7) can make an important contribution to both therapy and genetic counseling.

Speech therapists also have numerous opportunities to treat and recognize children with underlying genetic disease. Children with hearing problems, drooling, oromotor problems, and cognitive speech delays are at high risk for genetic or multifactorial etiologies (Table 16.4). Recognition of the velopalatine incompetence of Shprintzen syndrome (192430) may suggest surgical or prosthetic approaches to the nasal speech in these children. A genetics text oriented toward speech therapy is available (Shprintzen, 1998).

Case 16 Follow-up: The primary physician and social worker follow the child with Down syndrome for several months and convince the father to participate in some health care and early intervention visits. The occupational therapist points out some simple motor exercises that allow enhanced parental interactions with the child and make them feel that they are contributing to his progress. By the age of 1 year, the mother has a more optimistic attitude and the father's parents have accepted the child.

■ 16.6. THE ROLE OF PSYCHOLOGISTS AND SCHOOL PROFESSIONALS IN GENETICS

The frequency of developmental disabilities in children with genetic disorders means that they often present to experts in developmental and psychological assessment (Table 16.5). As the child passes the 3-year age limit for early intervention, these assessments have an important influence on school placement and its accompanying IEP or individual education plan. There is a tendency for terms such as "cerebral palsy," "autism," or "pervasive developmental disorder" to be used as specific diagnoses during developmental evaluations when in fact these terms are better employed as adjectives for particular symptoms or behaviors. Specialists in developmental or psychological testing must be aware that autistic behavior can be a

■ **TABLE 16.5.** School Problems in Children with Genetic Disease

Problems manifested by affected children

Toileting problems
Impulsivity, distractibility
Hearing and vision problems
Developmental disability
Overeating, food foraging

Problems with school systems

Inappropriate or simplistic labels—autisim, PDD
Segregation of children with disabilities (no inclusion)
Lack of disability accommodations
Lack of employment training and opportunity
Life skills rather than academic curricula
Lack of social interactions to prepare for independent existence

PDD, pervasive developmental disorder.

feature of many different genetic diseases like fragile X syndrome (309550), as can the large head and unusual play behaviors of pervasive developmental disorder. Whereas these terms may be helpful in designing educational and therapeutic strategies for the child, they should not be used in place of a genetic evaluation.

Equally important to alertness for genetic etiologies in children with developmental disabilities is a positive attitude on the part of school professionals. Most such children will have mild to moderate disability like that in Down syndrome that allows reading, writing, oral presentations, and eventual training for employment. Many will also have challenging behaviors for teachers as listed in Table 16.5. Children with disabilities are greatly benefited by mixed special and normal educational environments that expose them to diverse experiences and peers. Such inclusional programs require appropriate designs with teacher assistants to prevent classroom disruption, but are preferable to segregated special educational facilities that do not provide appropriate academic and peer stimulation. A segregated environment for students with mild or moderate disabilities is reminiscent of the eugenics movement in the early part of the twentieth century that was mentioned in Chapter 1. It is important that school professionals acquire familiarity with principles of genetics and diversity so that the problems outlined in Table 16.5 do not occur.

■ 16.7. GENETIC CARE PATHWAY AND PREVENTIVE MANAGEMENT GUIDELINES

As mentioned in Chapter 11 and outlined in Figure 16.2, the diagnosis and natural history of genetic disease can provide a positive program for preventive management even when there is no cure for the disease process. Conversion of the known medical complications of a disease into a systematic flow sheet called a checklist can facilitate this preventive care, allowing primary care providers to retain their central role in the care of rare diseases. Examples of this preventive management approach is given for three types of genetic disease—a chromosomal disorder (Down syndrome), a skeletal dysplasia (achondroplasia), and a connective tissue disorder that usually presents in adults (Marfan syndrome). Each example illustrates that health-care guidelines and team management can prolong life and increase its quality for individuals with genetic disease.

Down Syndrome

As discussed in Chapter 7, Down syndrome occurs when extra chromosome 21 material present as trisomy or translocation. Trisomy 21, like other aneuploid karyotypes, implies a 1% recurrence risk for chromosomal anomalies in subsequent pregnancies. Translocations require chromosome studies on the parents to see if one of them is a balanced translocation carrier. Depending on the type of translocation, parental translocation carriers have a 5–95% recurrence risk in future pregnancies. The extra chromosome material in Down syndrome produces a wide range of medical and psychosocial problems that must be addressed by the medical care team.

Informing the parents when Down syndrome is suspected in the neonatal nursery is a critical medical event. Because of the impact of this suspicion, documentation of minor anomalies shown in Figures 11.3 and 16.1 is important in addition to the facial gestalt and low muscle tone (hypotonia). Supportive counseling is important in the initial discussion, with informative counseling provided when the karyotype results are available to confirm the diagnosis of Down syndrome. Cooley and Graham (1991), drawing upon the recommendations of Cunningham et al. (1984), emphasizes that parents be informed: (1) as soon as possible; (2) with both parents together; (3) with the baby present and addressed by name; (4) in a quiet, confidential setting; (5) in a straightforward manner with understandable language and time for questions; (6) with a balanced perspective including positive statements rather than a catalogue of problems; (7) with follow-up discussion arranged and contact information provided; (8) with provision for private time after the counseling session.

The primary care physician is often the best person to inform a family about the possibility of Down syndrome, together with nursing and genetic counseling personnel if they are avail- able. Contact with representatives of a Down syndrome parent group is the best way for par- ents to begin learning about the many psy- chosocial issues involved in raising a child with disabilities. Msall et al. (1991) empha- sizes the partnership that can be forged among families, health-care professionals, and early intervention specialists as shown in Table 16.6. Nurses will be concerned with feeding and in-

■**TABLE 16.6.** Medical Complications and Preventive Management of Down Syndrome

Category	Complications	Preventive Management
General		
Neonatal	Poor feeding	Breast-feeding education—RN
	Jaundice	Oromotor therapy—ST
		Phototherapy—GP
Genetics	Genetic disorder	Genetic counseling—G, GC
Learning	Microcephaly	Motor therapy—OT, ST
	Cognitive disability	Speech therapy—ST
	Learning differences	School inclusion, special education—SW, DP
Behavior	Hyperactivity, behavior problems	Behavior therapy—SW
Growth	Short stature	Special growth charts—RN, GP
	Obesity	Dietary counsel—RD
Cancer	Leukemia (increased 10–20-fold)	Check for anemia—RN, GP
Craniofacial		
Eye	Myopia, strabismus	Annual vision checks—RN, GP
	Nystagmus	Ophthalmology referrals
Ear	Chronic otitis	Annual hearing checks—RN, GP
	Hearing deficits	Otolaryngology referrals
Mouth	Tooth anomalies	Annual dental care
	Obstructive sleep apnea	Evaluate for sleep apnea—RN, GP
Organ Systems		
Epidermal	Dry skin, skin rashes	Check skin—RN, GP
Skeleton	Joint laxity, scoliosis	Evaluate neck, spine—GP, orthopedic specialists
	Cervical instability	Cervical spine X-rays every decade
Digestive	Constipation, GI anomalies	Check feeds, stools—RN, GP
Pulmonary	Respiratory infections	Annual influenza vaccinations—RN
	Immune dysfunction	Varicella, pneumovax vaccinations—RN
Cardiovascular	Cardiac anomalies	Neonatal echocardiogram
		Heart checks—RN, GP
		Cardiology referrals
Endocrine	Hypothyroidism	Annual thyroid testing—GP
Urogenital	Cryptorchidism, micropenis	Peer problems—GP, possible urology referral

Source: Cooley and Graham (1991).

Notes: RN, nurse; ST, speech therapist; GP, general physician; G, clinical geneticist; DP, developmental pediatrician; GC, genetic counselor; OT, occupational therapist; SW, social worker or other school/psychology professional.

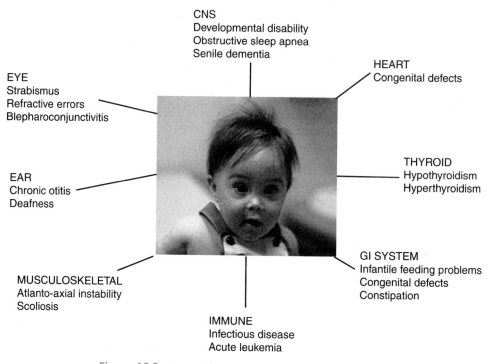

CNS
Developmental disability
Obstructive sleep apnea
Senile dementia

HEART
Congenital defects

EYE
Strabismus
Refractive errors
Blepharoconjunctivitis

THYROID
Hypothyroidism
Hyperthyroidism

EAR
Chronic otitis
Deafness

GI SYSTEM
Infantile feeding problems
Congenital defects
Constipation

MUSCULOSKELETAL
Atlanto-axial instability
Scoliosis

IMMUNE
Infectious disease
Acute leukemia

Figure 16.3. Potential complications of Down syndrome.

fant care issues in the nursery, occupational therapists with early motor therapy, and the primary physician with medical concerns like exaggerated jaundice. Social workers may address the options for adoption or foster care for parents who cannot accept a child with a handicap or who have insufficient resources. Few parents will opt to place children for adoption if they receive supportive counseling from informed professionals and parent representatives. Books to aid parents include those by Pueschel (1978) and Stray-Gunderson (1986). Institutionalization is no longer a realistic option and should be mentioned only as an example of negative and inaccurate information that may be found in the older literature on Down syndrome.

Once the initial supportive and informative counseling has been performed, attention to medical risks and preventive care should begin. The preventive measures outlined in Table 16.6 have been adapted to a checklist format that is helpful for physicians who care for children with Down syndrome. An early version of the preventive medical checklist was designed by Dr. Mary Coleman (Cohen, 1992). Rubin and Crocker (1989) have presented similar recommendations in their "Healthwatch" chart for Down syndrome (Cooley and Graham, 1991), as did Carey (1992) in his table for anticipatory guidance and health supervision. The guidelines have been formally endorsed by the Committee on Genetics (1994) of the American Academy of Pediatrics. The partnership outlined in Table 16.6 constitutes a clinical genetic care pathway for Down syndrome that should be adapted for all genetic diseases.

If no congenital anomalies are manifest in the neonate with Down syndrome, then abnormalities of the eyes, ears, teeth, heart, immune, or skeletal systems must be anticipated and screened for in later childhood (Table 16.6).

Respiratory infections are more frequent and severe in children with Down syndrome, and pneumonias or sinusitis are common. There is an increased risk for leukemia (still less than 1%), but correctable problems such as difficulty breast-feeding, constipation, hypothyroidism, chronic otitis media with hearing loss, dental anomalies, atlanto-axial (cervical spine) instability, and genital anomalies are more common. Developmental delays, learning differences, and speech problems are universal, and there is a 10% risk for psychiatric problems in older individuals with Down syndrome. Despite neuropathological changes typical of Alzheimer disease in 100% of individuals over age 35, symptomatic dementia is fortunately much less frequent (Cooley and Graham, 1991; Epstein, 1995).

Preventive care in childhood includes annual thyroid testing, monitoring of hearing and vision, and referral to ophthalmology at age 8–10 months to detect eye problems before the critical period for central acquisition of sight (age 1–2 years) expires. Sleep apnea is common in children with hypotonia, obesity, and respiratory infections and can be suspected by daytime sleepiness, growth failure, awakening with a gasp, mouth breathing, or excessive sweating. Because of their susceptibility to infection, children and adolescents with Down syndrome should receive all immunizations, including pneumococcal, varicella, and influenza vaccines in children with respiratory difficulties. Simple preventive treatments may include daily eyewash scrubs for blepharitis and nasal saline drops for sinusitis. Blepharitis is evidenced by erythema and/or swelling of the eyelids and can result in unsightly deformities of the lid or even corneal infections.

Several unproved therapies have been promoted for Down syndrome, including recent attention to the memory-enhancing drug Piracetam. This drug has been tried in European patients with Alzheimer disease, but has a minimal track record and no proven benefit in children with Down syndrome. Vitamin supplements have a long history of use in Down syndrome, despite a lack of scientific evidence for true vitamin deficiencies. Fortunately, neither Piracetam nor the common vitamin/nutrient mixtures seem to be harmful. Parents should be warned against costly biochemical analyses, "cellular" treatments by injection of animal cell mixtures, or "patterning" treatments that impose rigid schedules on families already dealing with the added stress of disability (Cooley and Graham, 1991). Plastic surgery to alter tongue size or to correct facial features is also controversial and usually not recommended.

Achondroplasia

Achondroplasia (100800) is a form of skeletal dysplasia with short limbs that is caused by mutations in the gene for the fibroblast growth receptor 3 (see Chapter 11). The incidence of achondroplasia is between 1 in 16,000 and 1 in 25,000 births. The diagnosis of achondroplasia is made by clinical examination and skeletal radiographic survey. DNA analysis could be pursued in uncertain cases but is not usually required. Patients with achondroplasia have rhizomelic (proximal) limb shortening, prominent forehead with shallow nasal bridge, and characteristic splayed or "trident" fingers. Skeletal radiographs demonstrate characteristic changes in the lumbar vertebrae and pelvis (e.g., unusual iliac wings). About 75% of achondroplastic patients represent new mutations, explaining why the majority of patients have a normal family history.

Many patients with achondroplasia are born to normal parents, provoking a crisis similar to that surrounding the birth of a child with Down syndrome. Genetic referral is essential for evaluation and counseling. Unrushed explanation of the diagnostic approach is important, followed by supportive counseling once the diagnosis seems probable. For normal parents, the recurrence risk is negligible but not zero due to the possibility of germinal mosaicism (see Chapter 10). Couples with achondroplasia have a 50% risk of having a child with achondroplasia, a 25% risk of having a child with lethal homozygous achondroplasia, and a 25%

risk of having a normal or "average-sized" child. The diagnosis of achondroplasia is increasingly made by fetal ultrasound, allowing earlier preparation and counseling of the parents.

Positive literature on achondroplasia and other dwarfing conditions is available from the Little People of America parent support group. Some parents will need time before confronting the reality forced by support groups, but the exposure to medical or psychosocial resources and the positive images promoted for their child (e.g., fashion shows at annual meetings) warrant continued encouragement to re-

alize the advantages offered by Little People of America. Most regions of the United States and Canada have local chapters.

Preventive management for achondroplasia (Table 16.7) begins with monitoring of the head circumference and neuromuscular function. Although intellectual potential is normal, a large head, flattening of the skull base (platybasia), and a small foramen magnum cause these children to be at risk for compression of the brain stem and upper spinal cord. The spinal cord compression may present as recurrent apnea, central sleep apnea, unusually severe hypotonia and developmental delay, or

■TABLE 16.7. Medical Complications and Preventive Management of Achondroplasia

Category	Complications	Preventive Management
General		
Genetics	Autosomal dominant disorder	Genetic counseling—G, GC
Development	Joint laxity, motor delays	Motor therapy—OT, PT
Growth	Short stature, obesity	Special growth charts—RN, GP
		Dietary counsel—RD
		Consider GH, endocrine referrals
Craniofacial		
Ear	Otitis media	Annual hearing checks—RN, GP
	Hearing loss	Otolaryngology referrals
Mouth	Dental crowding, malocclusion	Annual dental care
Organ Systems		
Cranium	Small foramen magnum	Monitor muscle tone—GP
	Cervical cord compression	Neurosurgery referrals
	Sudden infant death	
Skeleton	Spinal stenosis	Check spine—RN, GP
	Scoliosis	Orthopedic referrals
Limbs	Short limbs, later arthritis	Check joints—RN, GP
		Encourage exercise—RN, RD
Genital	Narrow pelvis	Monitor cycles, pregnancy—RN, GP
	Uterine fibroids, hemorrhage	Obstetric specialists, C-section
		Gynecology referrals
CNS	Hydrocephalus	Check head circumference—RN, GP
	Sleep apnea	Sleep study if symptoms
		Neurosurgery referrals

Source: Committee on Genetics (1995).

Notes: G, clinical geneticist; GC, genetic counselor; RN, nurse; OT, occupational therapist; PT, physical therapist; GP, general physician; RD, dietician; GH, growth hormone; C, cesarean.

sudden death (Pauli et al., 1995). This compression may also be associated with hydrocephalus, causing increased intracranial venous pressure from presumed constriction of jugular venous return (Table 16.7).

Skeletal problems in achondroplasia include bowing of the limbs and scoliosis (curved spine) due to ligamentous and joint laxity, and older patients may develop arthritis. Inactivity due to joint problems may exacerbate the tendency for weight gain due to short stature and decreased caloric requirement, causing a vicious cycle that needs dietary management. Other complications of achondroplasia include chronic otitis and hearing loss, uterine fibroids with menorrhagia, and a narrow pelvis in females that requires delivery by cesarean section under general anesthesia (Allanson and Hall, 1986). The clinical genetics care pathway is critical in preventing complications such as sudden death, and the roles of nurses, therapists, and dieticians in this pathway is outlined in Table 16.7. Preconceptional counseling is important for achondroplastic couples because of their high recurrence risk (some couples view their 25% risk for average-sized children as a liability) and obstetric complications. Careful monitoring of early development and evaluations for hypotonia or sleep apnea signifying spinal cord compression are essential for children with achondroplasia.

Newer therapies for dwarfism include growth hormone supplementation and surgical leg-lengthening procedures. Both are expensive, and the latter includes risks of infection or bony deformity. Growth hormone supplementation is expensive ($20,000–30,000 per year) but effective in adding several inches to the predicted adult height of $3\frac{1}{2}$–4 feet.

Marfan Syndrome

An example of preventive management for adult genetic disorders is the Marfan syndrome (154700). The condition results from mutations in the extracellular matrix protein fibrillin. Affected patients have long, narrow, hyperextensible fingers (arachnodactyly) and limbs (dolichostenomelia), optic lens dislocations, and aortic dissection due to a degenerative process affecting the blood vessels called cystic medial necrosis. Increased connective tissue laxity produces a characteristic appearance with a long face, high palate, concave chest (pectus), long limbs, and thin body build (Marfanoid habitus—see Fig. 2.2). The incidence of Marfan syndrome is about 1 in 10,000 births, and about 15% of patients represent new mutations. Diagnostic criteria have been published that require at least one major manifestation in patients with an affected first-degree relative and two major manifestations in patients with an unremarkable family history. However, Pyeritz (1993) emphasized the arbitrary and age-sensitive nature of these criteria, asserting that Marfan syndrome is one end of a continuum of connective tissue abnormality that is a challenge for molecular diagnosis and clinical delineation to resolve.

Many patients with Marfan syndrome do not present in the newborn period. Some show signs in later childhood and still others are identified as asymptomatic adults who have an affected relative. Once the diagnosis is suspected, preventive management considerations outlined in Table 16.8 should be followed. All patients should have an ophthalmologic examination and echocardiography by a cardiologist who is experienced with the condition. The aortic root diameter can be plotted against norms for the patient's age and size, allowing recognition of subclinical dilatation. Optic lens dislocation may not be obvious, and slit lamp exam with a fully dilated pupil may be needed (Pyeritz, 1993). The patients should avoid collision or highly competitive sports, as dramatized by the tragic death of Olympic star Flo Hyman.

Echocardiography is an important procedure in patients with possible or definite Marfan syndrome. If aortic dilation is found, or if other findings support the probable diagnosis of Marfan syndrome, treatment with beta-blockers such as propranolol is begun. Skeletal complications include kyphoscoliosis, pectus deformity, flat feet, and joint dislocations that

■ **TABLE 16.8.** Medical Complications and Preventive Management of Marfan Syndrome

Category	Complications	Preventive Management
General		
Genetics	Genetic disorder	Genetic counseling—G, GC
Growth	Tall stature	Special growth charts—RN, GP
	Marfanoid habitus	
Craniofacial		
Eye	Ocular anomalies	Vision checks—RN, GP
	Visual deficits	Ophthalmology referrals
	Lens dislocation	
Mouth	High or cleft palate	Annual dental visits
	Dental malocclusion	
	TMJ inflammation	
Organ systems		
Trunk	Inguinal hernia (22%)	Annual examinations—RN, GP
	Pectus excavatum (68%)	Surgery referrals
Skeleton	Joint laxity, dislocations	Annual examinations—RN, PT, GP
	Scoliosis	Orthopedic referrals
Pulmonary	Reduced vital capacity	Respiratory problems
	Pneumothorax	
	Emphysema	
Cardiovascular	Aortic, mitral insufficiency	Heart checks—RN, GP
	Aortic dissections	Cardiology referrals
	Cardiac arrythmias	Periodic echocardiograms
CNS	Sacral meningocele	Spinal examinations
	Dural ectasia	Neurology referrals

Source: Pyeritz (1993).

Notes: G, clinical geneticist; GC, genetic counselor; RN, nurse; GP, general physician; PT, physical therapist; TMJ, temporomandibular joint.

may require orthopedic input. The cardiac symptoms of adolescents and adults with Marfan syndrome can include palpitations, dyspnea, and light-headedness associated with mitral valve prolapse (not with arrythmias), and chest pain related to pneumothorax or aortic dissection. Coselli et al. (1995) stressed the need for life-long follow-up to detect complications after cardiac surgery in Marfan syndrome. Women with Marfan syndrome have more severe osteoporosis and suffer worsening cardiovascular complications during pregnancy. The prevention of sudden cardiac death, vision loss, and orthopedic deformities in Marfan syndrome testifies to the importance of care pathways and multidisciplinary management of genetic disorders.

■ 16.8. ETHICAL CONSIDERATIONS IN THE MANAGEMENT OF GENETIC DISORDERS

The medical ethicist is not a consistent member of the genetics management team, but has a growing influence on decisions made by that team. Table 16.9 lists some major areas of ethical controversy that may arise during the management of genetic disease. Most of these ethical issues concern patient autonomy or

■**TABLE 16.9.** Ethical Issues Arising in Genetic Management

Ethical Issues	Conflicts and Examples
Genetic technology	
Cloning, ART	Sanctity of human materials versus scientific advances
	e.g., IVF to provide human embryos for research
	Rights of individuals versus conservation of medical resources
	e.g., gamete selection for fetal sex in absence of disease risk
Patenting,	Company ownership versus free exchange of materials
DNA banking	e.g., patenting of human brain ESTs
	Personal ownership versus scientific fame, advancement
	e.g., reimbursement of patients for valuable materials
Individual genetic testing	
Confidentiality	Insurance discrimination versus health costs
	e.g., life insurance for individuals with risk for early death
	e.g., health insurance for persons with chronic genetic disease
	Workplace discrimination versus company efficiency and profits
	e.g., hiring of individuals with compromised work life or job efficiency
	Individual education versus overall school achievement
	e.g., inclusive education for people with disabilities
	Full disclosure versus damage to an individual
	e.g., nonpaternity, child up for adoption
Autonomy	Rights of children versus parents
	e.g., prenatal testing with abortion; postnatal testing with euthanasia
	Age of human rights and independent decision making
	e.g., prenatal testing, testing of minors
Informed consent	Widespread availability versus unrealistic time needed for counseling
	e.g., imprecise results, unanticipated choices after screening
	Free choice versus unanticipated impact of information
	e.g., depression after testing for Huntington disease (143100)
Population genetic testing (genetic screening)	
Confidentiality	Individual reproductive rights versus societal costs
	e.g., AIDS testing, sickle cell anemia (141900), or cystic fibrosis (241700) testing
Autonomy	Individual choice versus cost containment
	e.g., access to cystic fibrosis testing

confidentiality, with debate concerning the time at which a person becomes autonomous (fetal life, childhood, adolescence) or the extent of that autonomy.

With advances in genetic technology come controversies on the extent of individual choice. Guidelines concerning the limits of artificial reproductive technology (ART) were discussed in Chapter 15, with conflict over the uniqueness and rights extended to human fertilized eggs and early embryos. Societal con-cerns include the need to conserve medical costs and fair distribution of resources. The couple wishing sex selection for nonmedical reasons or the privately insured couple electing cystic fibrosis carrier testing have options not available to all in the population, and generalization of these actions would be too expensive or too unfair in a democratic society. Although confidentiality is a well-established medical principle, individuals with genetic diseases like Marfan syndrome (154700) may increase the costs to insurance companies or employers because of decreased survival or medical complications. Legislation has been passed to protect individual rights in these cases, but modifications to insure equal liabilities by competing agencies may also be needed.

Confidentiality may be a difficult issue when an individual carries a problem that may affect other family members, or when unanticipated information like nonpaternity is revealed. As discussed in Chapter 15, confidential information for the wife may be essential information to the husband, and the carrier status of one sister may be highly relevant to the reproductive risks of the other. In general, health professionals must define their patient and place their confidentiality above all others. It is generally accepted that minors should not be tested for predispositions to genetic diseases until they reach the age of consent, but this protection is not usually extended to children up for adoption or to fetuses of gestation less than 24 weeks (in most states). Neonates with genetic disorders are entitled to treatment as illustrated by the Baby Doe case, but the difference between palliative care of children with severe disabilities and passive euthanasia must often be decided on a case-by-case basis.

Ethical guidelines for equal access and quality control for genetic screening were discussed in Chapter 12, with emphasis on potential benefits and informed consent regarding the screening procedure. These principles apply to decisions about preventive management evaluations, with low-yield, high-cost testing being inadvisable. Patient autonomy also involves human and disability rights issues, with individualized school or employment programs being balanced against the general welfare. Fallacies of the eugenics movement were discussed in Chapter 2, with the rate of new mutations and the frequency of carriers counteracting prohibitions on reproduction of affected individuals for most diseases. However, valid conflicts may arise as the repertoire of genetic testing continues to increase and individuals choose to reproduce despite high risks to offspring. A preview of these conflicts occurred when a celebrity couple decided to have children despite a 50% risk for the limb defects known as ectrodactyly (183600). In Western societies, individual autonomy and confidentiality are likely to override other ethical considerations, with the health professional's first loyalty being to his or her patient.

For difficult issues, such as the transplantation of scarce organs into patients with disabilities (see problem set), hospital ethics committees are useful forums for reaching decisions. Health professionals confronting genetic issues are encouraged to take advantage of these new forums and resources for medical ethics rather than being forced into lonely and potentially costly decisions.

PROBLEM SET 16
Allied Health and Preventive Management

Respond to the following questions with short answers, consulting Tables 16.1–16.9 or Figs. 16.1–16.3. For each clinical presentation, discuss genetic risks, management issues, and the involvement of particular health professionals.

16.1. After numerous evaluations and treatments for infertility, a couple has a newborn with features of Down syndrome.

16.2. A newborn screen is positive for phenylketonuria (261600).

16.3. A teenage boy is diagnosed with Marfan syndrome (154700).

16.4. A middle-aged woman develops symptoms of Huntington disease (143100).

16.5. A newborn has short stature, a prominent forehead with shallow nasal bridge, and short limbs.

Respond to the following situations with short answers that address the key ethical issues:

16.6. A patient donates a blood sample to a research project. A cell line derived from this sample becomes a standard reagent that is sold to many research centers. The sample contains a DNA mutation that indicates a significant predisposition to cancer.

16.7. A couple wishes to adopt a child, but learn that the child's grandmother has Huntington disease (143100). They wish to have the child tested.

16.8. A commercial test pilot undergoes a routine physical and is found to have sickle cell anemia. His employer requests all results of the physical examination.

PROBLEM SET 16
Answers

16.1–16.8. See Solutions

PROBLEM SET 16
Solutions

16.1. This premium pregnancy after infertility will likely cause this couple even greater devastation when they learn about the possibility of genetic disease. Careful documentation of minor anomalies should be performed (Fig. 16.1) by the primary physician to support the possibility of Down syndrome, and care in scheduling the initial counseling session should be exercised. Provision of balanced information with both parents present in a private situation should be attempted. Contact with parent group representatives, nursing instruction to maximize feeding success, and social work involvement for grief counseling may be indicated. Following the result of chromosome analysis, genetic counseling is needed with supportive attitudes about the many capabilities of children with Down syndrome. A preventive management program with attention to hearing, vision, and other risks is then instituted, including early intervention with occupational and speech therapists (Table 16.6). A copy of the Down syndrome preventive checklist can be obtained to ensure compliance with the care guidelines.

16.2. Initial counseling by the general physician and nursing staff will include the possibil-

ity of a false positive test. If phenylketonuria (261600) is confirmed, then genetic and dietary counseling is performed to optimize compliance with a low phenylalanine diet. Monitoring of development and dietary compliance will be important for the primary physician, and a team with a clinical geneticist, genetic counselor, dietician, and social worker may be needed to follow blood phenylalanine levels, to modify the special diet, and to aid with insurance and economic issues.

16.3. The primary physician and nurse will counsel against participation in collision or high intensity sports, evaluate for skeletal changes such as scoliosis or flat feet, and coordinate referrals to eye, heart, and bone specialists (Table 16.8). Genetic counseling regarding the 50% recurrence risk and variable expressivity of autosomal dominant diseases is needed, and propranolol treatment may be indicated if the aortic artery diameter increases with age.

16.4. The primary physician and nurse will explain the nature of Huntington disease (143100) and enter the patient into a formal presymptomatic diagnosis program. After preliminary psychiatric counseling and evaluation, a DNA analysis for trinucleotide repeat expansion will be performed, and a genetic counselor will deliver news of the result with provision for follow-up family and psychosocial counseling. The primary physician and social worker may need to counteract possible insurance discrimination after a positive result, and physical therapists or nutritionists may become involved as the neurodegeneration progresses.

16.5. The primary physician and nurse must schedule an appropriate counseling session to indicate their concern about a skeletal dysplasia. If confirmatory radiography indicates a diagnosis of achondroplasia (100800), then genetic counseling regarding a probable spontaneous mutation to normal parents is needed. The primary physician initiates a preventive management program that monitors for unusual hypotonia, sleep apnea, chronic otitis, dental problems, or orthopedic problems with specialty referrals as appropriate (Table 16.7). Occupational therapists and dieticians may be helpful in dealing with hypotonia or the tendency for obesity.

16.6. Issues of patient ownership and confidentiality are raised, with conflicts between beneficence to the patient (financial rewards, predisposition to cancer) and patient autonomy through informed consent. Most consent forms for DNA banking or research studies require that the patient cede ownership to his or her DNA sample and that any results of testing will not be revealed to anyone including the patient except by their expressed consent.

16.7. The couple's autonomy prevails over the child's autonomy in that they can opt for testing on the child (e.g., AIDS testing). The DNA test for Huntington disease (143100) would not be performed by formal presymptomatic diagnosis programs since they have agreed upon guidelines that forbid testing of minors. Maleficence to the child in terms of difficulty in adoption would override beneficence since there are no benefits of early diagnosis.

16.8. The physician may release results of the physical examination to the company if the employee gave prior consent. However, legislation in many states guarantees against discrimination based on a genetic diagnosis—in this case, risks from the low oxygen of higher altitudes because of sickle cell anemia (141900). The physician should maximize patient autonomy and beneficence by informing the pilot of the diagnosis along with his employment and genetic risks.

BIBLIOGRAPHY

General References

Ahronheim JC, Moreno J, Zuckerman ID. 1994. *Ethics in Clinical Practice.* New York: Little, Brown.

Beauchamp T, Childress J. 1994. *Principles of Biomedical Ethics,* 4th ed. New York: Oxford.

Gorlin RJ, Cohen MM Jr, Levin LS. 1990. *Syndromes of the Head and Neck.* New York: Oxford.

Shprintzen RJ. 1998. *Genetics, Syndromes, and Communication Disorders.* San Diego: Singular Publishing Group, Inc.

Wilson GN, Cooley WC. 1999. *Preventive Management for Children with Congenital Anomalies and Syndromes.* Cambridge: Cambridge University Press, in press.

Nursing in Genetics

Abellah FG. 1991. The human genome initiative—implications for nurse researchers. *J Prof Nurs* 7: 332.

Fibison W. 1983. The nursing role in the delivery of genetic services. *Issues Health Care Women* 4: 1–15.

Forsman I. 1994. Evolution of the nursing role in genetics. *J Obstet Gynecol Neonat Nurs* 23: 481–486.

Lea DH, Jenkins JF, Francomano CA. 1998. *Genetics in Clinical Practice. New Directions for Nursing and Health Care.* Sudbury, MA: Jones and Bartlett.

Scanlon C, Fibison W, Forsman I, Jones S, Soeken K. 1995. *Managing Genetic Information: Implications for Nursing Practice.* Washington DC: American Nurses Publishing.

Genetic Counseling

Emery AFH, Watts MS, Clock ER. 1972. The effects of genetic counseling in Duchenne muscular dystrophy. *Clin Genet* 3:147–150.

Fraser FC. 1968. Genetic counseling and the physician. *Can Med Assoc J* 99:927–934.

Harris R. 1988. Genetic counselling and the new genetics. *Trends Genet* 4:52–55.

Leonard CO, Chase GA, Childs B. 1972. Genetic counseling: A consumer's view. *N Engl J Med* 287:433–439.

Orentlicher D, AMA Council on Ethical and Judicial Affairs. 1994. Ethical issues related to prenatal genetic testing. *Arch Fam Med* 3:633–642.

Pencarinha DF, Bell NK, Edwards JG, Best RG. 1992. Ethical issues in genetic counseling: A comparison of MS counselor and medical geneticist perspectives. *J Genet Counsel* 1:19–29.

Resta RG. 1997. Eugenics and nondirectiveness in genetic counseling. *J Genet Counsel* 6:255–258.

Scheuner MT, Wang S-J, Raffel LJ, Larabell SK, and Rotter JI. 1997. Family history: A comprehensive genetic risk assessment method for the chronic conditions of adulthood. *Am J Med Genet* 71:315–324.

Down Syndrome

Carey JC. 1992. Health supervision and anticipatory guidance for children with genetic disorders (including specific recommendations for trisomy 21, trisomy 18, and neurofibromatosis). *Pediatr Clin N Am* 39:25–53.

Cohen WI. 1992. Down syndrome preventive medical check list. *Down Syndrome Papers and Abstracts for Professionals* 15:1–7.

Committee on Genetics, American Academy of Pediatrics. 1994. Health supervision for children with Down syndrome. *Pediatr* 93:855–859.

Committee on Sports Medicine and Fitness, American Academy of Pediatrics. 1995. Atlantoaxial instability in Down syndrome: Subject review. *Pediatr* 96:151–154.

Cooley WC, Graham JM Jr. 1991. Down syndrome—an update and review for the primary pediatrician. *Clin Pediatr* 30:233–253.

Cronk C, Crocker AC, Pueschel SM et al. 1988. Growth charts for children with Down syndrome: 1 month to 18 years of age. *Pediatr* 81: 102–110.

Epstein CJ. 1995. Down syndrome (trisomy 21). In Scriver CR, Beaudet AL, Sly WS, and Valle D, eds. *The Metabolic and Molecular Bases of Inherited Disease,* 7th ed. New York: McGraw-Hill, pp. 749–794.

Msall ME, DiGaudio KM, Malone AF. 1991. Health, developmental and psychosocial aspects of Down syndrome. *Inf Young Child* 4:35–45.

Pueschel SM. 1978. *Down Syndrome. Growing and Learning.* Kansas City: Sheed Andrews & McMeel.

Rubin IL, Crocker AC. 1989. *Developmental Disabilities—Delivery of Medical Care for Children and Adults.* Philadelphia: Lea and Febiger.

Spahis J. 1994. Sleepless nights. Obstructive sleep apnea in the pediatric patient. *Pediatric Nursing* 20:469–472.

Stray-Gunderson K. 1986. *Babies with Down Syndrome: A New Parents Guide.* Kensington, MD: Woodbine House.

Achondroplasia

Allanson JE, Hall JG. 1986. Obstetric and gynecologic problems in women with chondrodystrophies. *Obstet Gynecol* 67:74–78.

Committee on Genetics 1994–5, American Academy of Pediatrics. 1995. Health supervision for children with achondroplasia. *Pediatr* 95: 443–451.

Horton WA, Rotter JI, Rimoin DL, Scott CI, Hall JG. 1978. Standard growth curves for achondroplasia. *J Pediatr* 93:435–438.

Pauli RM, Horton VK, Glinski LP, Reiser CA. 1995. Prospective assessment of risks for cervicomedullary-junction compression in infants with achondroplasia. *Am J Hum Genet* 56: 732–744.

Marfan Syndrome

Coselli JS, LeMaire SA, Buket S. 1995. Marfan syndrome: the variability and outcome of operative management. *J Vasc Surg* 21:432–443.

Grahame R, Pyeritz RE. 1995. The Marfan syndrome: joint and skin manifestations are prevalent and correlated. *Br J Rheum* 34:126–131.

Pyeritz RE. 1981. Maternal and fetal complications of pregnancy in the Marfan syndrome. *Am J Med* 71:784–790.

Pyeritz RE. 1993. Marfan syndrome. In Royce PM, Steinmann B, eds., *Connective Tissue and Its Heritable Disorders.* New York: Wiley-Liss, pp. 437–468.

Pyeritz RE, McKusick VA. 1979. The Marfan syndrome: Diagnosis and management. *New Engl J Med* 300:772–776.

Rossiter JP, Repke JT, Morales AJ, Murphy EA, Pyeritz RE. 1995. A prospective longitudinal evaluation of pregnancy in the Marfan syndrome. *Am J Obstet Gynecol* 173:1599–1606.

Salim MA, Alpert BS, Ward JC, Pyeritz RE. 1994. Effect of beta-adrenergic blockade on aortic root rate of dilation in the Marfan syndrome. *Am J Cardiol* 74:629–633.

Ethics

Annas GJ. 1993. Privacy rules for DNA databanks. Protecting coded 'future diaries.' *JAMA* 270: 2346–2350.

Asch-Goodkin J. 1998. Tough choices: What's your call? *Contemp Pediatr* 15:80–82.

Chervenak FA, Farley MA, Walters L, Hobbins JC, Mahoney MJ. 1984. When is termination of pregnancy during the third trimester morally justifiable? *N Engl J Med* 310:501–504.

Fletcher J. 1975. Abortion, euthanasia, and care of defective newborns. *N Engl J Med* 292:75–78.

Holtzman NA. 1994. Benefits and risks of emerging genetic technologies: The need for regulation. *Clin Chem* 40:1652–1657.

Orentlicher D. 1990. Genetic screening by employers. *JAMA* 263: 1005–1008.

Parent S, Shevell M. 1998. The 'first to perish.' Child euthanasia in the Third Reich. *Arch Pediatr Adolesc Med* 132:79–86.

Reilly P. 1992. ASHG statement on genetics and privacy: Testimony to United States Congress. *Am J Hum Genet* 50:640–642.

Rothenberg K, Fuller B, Rothstein M et al. 1997. Genetic information and the workplace. Legislative approaches and policy challenges. *Science* 275:1755–1757.

Wertz DC, Fletcher JC, Mulvihill JJ. 1990. Medical geneticists confront ethical dilemmas: Cross-cultural comparisons among 18 nations. *Am J Hum Genet* 46:1200–1213.

Wilfond BS. 1995. Points to consider: Ethical, legal and psychosocial implications of genetic testing in children and adolescents. *Am J Hum Genet* 57: 1233–1241.

GLOSSARY

ABO blood group locus: Genetic locus on chromosome 9 encoding enzymes that modify the H substance to produce A or B membrane antigens on red blood cells. A major contributor to transfusion reactions.

abortion: Pregnancy loss prior to the time of fetal viability (about 24 weeks), spontaneous (accidental) versus planned (elective).

acrocentric chromosome: Chromosome with small short (p) arms as opposed to metacentric chromosomes with approximately equal short and long (q) arms.

agenesis: Absence of a part of the body caused by an absent anlage.

allele: Alternative gene structure (e.g., S and A alleles of the β-globin gene).

allele association: The tendency for an allele or trait to associate with another allele more often than by expected by chance; also called *linkage disequilibrium.*

allele-specific oligonucleotides: Oligonucleotides synthesized to recognize specific normal or mutant alleles.

amniocentesis: Sampling of amniotic fluid surrounding the fetus for prenatal diagnosis.

aneuploidy: Abnormal chromosome number that is not an even multiple of the haploid karyotype, i.e., 47,XX,+21 or 90,XX.

anlage: Embryonic precursor to a tissue, organ, or region; primordium, blastema.

anomaly: Any deviation from the expected or average type in structure, form, and/or function interpreted as abnormal.

antennapedia: Fly mutation causing substitution of a limb for antenna, leading to characterization of a group of genes at the *antennapedia* locus.

anticipation: Worsening of phenotype with subsequent generations.

aplasia: The absence of a body part resulting from a failure of the anlage to develop.

apoptosis: Stereotypic sequence of cellular changes accompanying programmed cell death as separate from cell destruction due to injury (i.e., inflammation, oxygen deprivation).

arthrogryposis: Multiple joint contractures, often accompanied by dimples over the joints and webbing across the joints; has many causes including brain, nerve, or muscle dysfunction.

ASO: Allele-specific oligonucleotides used for DNA diagnosis.

association: Groups of anomalies that occur together more often than by chance, lacking the similar pattern and facial appearance of malformation syndromes.

assortative mating: Selection of mates based on shared characteristics, exemplified by couples meeting at diabetic camp.

atavism: A developmental state that is normal in phylogenetic ancestors, but abnormal in their descendants.

atrophy: Decrease in a normally developed mass of tissue(s) or organ(s) due to decrease in cell size and/or cell number.

autonomy: The right of patients to health care and to choose among health-care options.

autosomes: Those chromosomes not involved with sex differentiation (1–22 in humans).

balanced translocation: Exchange of chromosome material that creates no extra or missing DNA, usually producing a normal phenotype.

449

Barr body: Nuclear inclusion representing the inactivated X chromosome.

base pairs (bp): Adenine-thymine (A-T) or guanine-cytosine (G-C) pairing in DNA; also the basic unit for DNA strand length.

Bayes theorem, Bayesian probability: A method for modifying prior probabilities based on additional (conditional) information.

beneficence: Action to maximize good in a clinical situation.

biomarkers: Biological traits or laboratory measures that indicate predisposition to or presence of disease.

bithorax: Mutation altering fly thorax structure, leading to characterization of the *Bithorax* gene cluster.

blastogenesis: Stage of development from karyogamy and the first cell division to the end of gastrulation (stage 12, days 27–28).

brachydactyly: Short fingers and toes.

CA repeats: Polymorphisms derived from genomic regions with variable number of CA (or GT) nucleotides, providing variable DNA restriction fragments for genetic linkage studies.

candidate gene: A gene implicated in pathogenesis based on protein function, chromosomal location, or sequence homology.

cell cycle: Stereotypic cell stages between mitoses—i.e., interphase, DNA synthesis.

cell cycle checkpoints: Critical stages of the cell cycle when cells may be diverted toward replication or death.

centimorgan: Unit of measure for distance between genetic loci based on genetic linkage or recombination frequencies; each 1% of recombination equals 1 centimorgan.

central dogma: Dictum that DNA encodes RNA and RNA is translated into protein.

centromere: Portion of chromosome that holds strands together and attaches to the mitotic or meiotic spindle.

CFTR, cystic fibrosis transmembrane regulator: The gene that is mutated in cystic fibrosis to alter chloride transport.

chorionic villus sampling (CVS): Biopsy of the chorion (early placenta) to provide tissue for prenatal diagnosis.

chromosomal rearrangements: Aberration where chromosomes are broken and rejoined as opposed to numerical excess or deficiency.

chromosome imbalance: Extra or missing chromosome material.

chromosome instability (breakage): Multiple chromosome breaks and rearrangements.

chromosome jumping: Use of balanced translocations to clone fused DNA segments that are implicated in a particular disease by virtue of the translocation.

chromosome painting: Use of repetitive DNA FISH probes to fluoresce entire chromosomes or chromosome regions.

chromosome walking: Successive cloning of DNA segments along a chromosome region that has been implicated in disease by microdeletion or linkage studies.

cleft lip/palate: Congenital failure of the upper mouth (soft or hard palate) to fuse; cleft lip, cleft palate, or the combination may occur.

complementary strands or sequences: Nucleic acid segments with nucleotide sequences that complement each other and allow reassociation into duplexes (hybridization).

c-onc: Oncogenes endogenous to cells that may become activated to cause cancers; inactive alleles are known as proto-oncogenes.

concordance: Frequency with which a congenital anomaly or other trait in one twin appears in the other.

confined chorionic mosaicism: Chromosome mosaicism confined to the chorion or early placenta, with mosaic trisomy sometimes correcting to uniparental disomy.

congenital: Present at birth.

consanguinity: Relatedness or common ancestors between parents; equivalent to inbreeding.

consultand: Person requesting genetic evaluation and counseling, may be indicated by an arrow in the predigree.

contiguous gene deletions: Deletion encompassing neighboring genes to produce a composite phenotype.

coronary artery disease: Occlusion of the arteries supplying the heart muscle (coronary arteries) that can result in complete blockage (coronary thrombosis) with heart muscle injury (myocardial infarction, heart attack).

crossover: Breakage and reunion of chromosomes that realign parental loci.

cryptorchidism: Undescended testicles, frequently with an underdeveloped scrotum.

cyanosis: Bluish color to lips and fingertips due to underoxygenated blood, suggestive of anemia or cardiac disease.

cyclins: Proteins regulating the cell cycle.

cytochrome P450: Family of proteins abundant in liver that function to inactivate chemicals.

cytogenetic notation: Formal nomenclature describing karyotypes and chromosome location, i.e.:

47,XY+11: Extra chromosome 11 (Trisomy 11)

45,XY-11: Absent chromosome 11 (Monosomy 11)

46,XY,11q-: Terminal deletion of chromosome 11

46,XY,11q+: Extra material of unknown origin on 11q

46,XY,del(11p11p13): Interstitial deletion between bands p11 and p13 of chromosome 11

46,XY,dup(3q): Extra material derived from the long arm of chromosome 3

deformation: Extrinsic interference with a normally developing structure due to pressure or constraint, as with decreased amniotic fluid causing clubfoot due to uterine pressure.

developmental field defect: Anomalies deriving from a common precursor or region of the early embryo, representing a stereotypic response to different insults.

differentiation: Transformation of one cell type into another with different gene expression and functions.

diploid: The number of chromosomes (2n) typical of somatic cells of the organism.

discordance: Twins who do not share a particular trait or congenital anomaly.

disomy: Two doses of a chromosome segment—normal state for autosomes and X chromosome in females unless both chromosome segments derive from one parent (uniparental disomy).

disruption: Extrinsic interference with a normally developing structure, as with occlusion of a blood vessel supplying the structure.

dizygous twins: Twins that result from a dual fertilization, having 50% of their genes in common like siblings.

DNA bank: Repository of DNA and tissue samples from individuals of interest that can be used for current or future analysis.

DNA cloning: Isolation of a DNA segment by insertion into a simple genome (plasmid, bacteriophage) and production of multiple copies.

DNA contig: Cloned DNA segments that span a gene or chromosome region.

DNA diagnostic techniques: Use of DNA modifying enzymes, hybridization, and size separation technologies for diagnosis of identity, genetic disease, or predisposition.

DNA fingerprinting: Use of DNA polymorphisms to assess genetic relationships (i.e., paternity testing) or to match individuals with tissue samples (i.e., forensic analysis).

DNA hybridization: Rejoining (reannealing) of complementary DNA or RNA stands.

DNA library: Repository of DNA segments from an individual or tissue in the form of recombinant molecules that can be amplified for study.

DNA marker: DNA segment, often anonymous, that exhibits sufficient sequence variation to be useful in genetic linkage and DNA diagnosis.

DNA polymorphisms: Variant nucleotide sequences that produce differently sized DNA segments after restriction (VNTRs, RFLPs) or gel separation (SNPs, microsatellites).

DNA probe: DNA segment labeled with fluorescence or radioactivity used as a reagent to detect complementary sequences in tissue samples.

DNA sequence: Order of nucleotides in a DNA segment, usually displayed from the $5'$-triphosphate ($5'$ end) to the $3'$-hydroxyl ($3'$ end) nucleotides.

DNA transfection: Uptake of DNA incorporated in a recombinant virus by cultured cells.

DNA transformation: Uptake of purified DNA by cultured cells, often producing a new phenotype.

dysmorphogenesis: Abnormal development leading to abnormal shape of one or more body parts.

dysmorphology: Study of abnormal development, particularly humans with abnormal physical or morphologic traits.

dysplasia: Intrinsic developmental abnormality caused by abnormal cells or tissues, such as a hemangioma consisting of disorganized blood vessel tissue.

ecogenetics: Study of genetic variation as it affects injury from environmental agents.

emphysema: Lung disease with loss of lung (tidal) volume due to tissue damage.

empiric risks: Recurrence risks estimated by survey of affected families rather than by knowledge of genetic mechanisms and probabilities.

enhancers: DNA sequences that increase the rate of transcription.

enzyme reserve: Excess enzyme encoded by diploid gene loci such that heterozygotes with one abnormal allele will have normal metabolic rates.

erythroblastosis fetalis: Swelling (hydrops) of the fetus due to severe anemia, often caused by Rh incompatibility.

eugenics: Breeding strategies to enhance the frequency of beneficial genes and/or to decrease the frequency of detrimental genes.

exons: Portions of genes that encode protein.

expressed sequence tags: Known DNA sequences from gene segments expressed as RNA that can be used to clone and characterize these genes.

expression cassette: Gene(s) engineered for expression in host organism or cells by integrating it with appropriate transcription promoters and enhancers.

failure to thrive: Growth failure in children that can have many different causes.

familial: Present in several family members.

fetal hydrops: Swelling of fetal tissues to produce severe edema and distortion, many different causes.

FGFR3 or fibroblast growth factor receptor-3 gene: A member of the fibroblast growth factor receptor gene family responsible for achondroplasia, hypochondroplasia, and thanatophoric dwarfism.

first-degree relative: Those with 50% of genes in common (child, parent, sibs).

FISH: Fluorescent in situ hybridization, a technique by which fluorochromes are attached to DNA probes and hybridized with chromosome or cell preparations.

founder effect: Higher than expected allele frequency in a population due to inheritance of the allele from a common ancestor or group of ancestors.

framework of alleles: Association of several alleles along a contiguous chromosomal region more often than expected by chance.

fraternal twins: *See* dizygous twins.

functional cloning: Isolation of gene segments based on gene function, i.e., using antibodies to a characterized protein or expression assay where traits are deleted or restored to cultured cells.

G proteins: Proteins interacting with guanosine triphosphate (GTP), often involved in signal transduction.

gametes: Eggs and sperm with haploid chromosomes.

gametogenesis: Manufacture of eggs and sperm (gametes) through proliferation and meiosis of primary germ cells (oocytes, spermatocytes).

gene construct: Recombinant DNA containing a gene of interest surrounded by sequences engineered to promote or measure its expression.

gene flow: Changes in allele frequencies due to migration of populations.

gene map: Order of genes within a chromosome or entire genome.

genetic burden: The psychological or perceived impact of a genetic disorder.

genetic code: Mechanism for protein synthesis in which 3 bp codons in DNA specify amino acids in protein.

genetic complementation: Ability of one genetic locus to correct or override effects from another genetic locus.

genetic counseling: An educational process that discusses the mechanism, recurrence risk, prognosis, and medical options for genetic diseases or diseases that might be genetic.

genetic drift: Increase or decrease in allele frequencies due to chance differences in allele segregation, particularly applicable to small populations (bottlenecks).

genetic heterogeneity: Multiple genetic causes for the same phenotype, illustrated by autosomal dominant or X-linked Charcot-Marie-Tooth disease.

genetic hierarchy: Levels of gene expression from DNA nucleotide through gene structure, RNA transcription, RNA splicing, protein translation, protein processing, organellar and cell interaction, organ and individual function.

genetic load: Aggregate of mutations carried by an organism or species.

genetic map: Map of loci assembled by genetic linkage studies.

genetic mapping: Use of genetic linkage to produce a relative gene order based on recombination distances (centimorgans = approximately 1 megabase).

genetic risk: The probability that a gene or trait will be transmitted and/or expressed in an individual.

genetic screening: Genetic testing of individuals in a population or subgroup without regard to symptoms.

genetic transmission: Appearance of a trait in offspring of affected individuals that is assumed to be inherited or caused by genes.

genome: Complete set of genes (DNA) in an organism.

genomic DNA: DNA isolated from an organism or tissue, containing transcription signals and introns that are absent from cDNA.

genomics: The study of organismal function and disease based on a comprehensive view of gene structure and arrangement in that organism.

genotype: Genetic constitution, often with reference to particular alleles at a locus.

germinal mosaicism, germ-line mosaicism: Mosaicism within the germ line, whereby a fraction of eggs or sperm may contain a particular mutation or chromosome aberration.

guessmers: Oligonucleotides designed from amino acid sequences based on the genetic code.

gynecomastia: Enlarged breasts in a male.

Haldane's law: The rule that women having one son affected with an X-linked disorder have a 2/3 chance of being carriers for that disorder.

haploid: Half of the chromosome number of somatic cells, typically occurring in gametes.

haploinsufficiency: Deletion or inactivation of one allele to produce disease due to inadequate activity of the remaining allele.

Hardy-Weinberg law: A relationship of allele frequencies p and q specifying that the fraction of homozygotes (p^2) and (q^2) plus the fraction of heterozygotes (2pq) will account for all individuals (will equal 1).

hemizygote: Individual with a single allele at a locus, particularly in males with one X chromosome.

hemolytic anemia: Decreased numbers of red blood cells caused by increased red cell destruction (hemolysis).

heritability: Fraction of liability to disease that is determined by genetic factors.

heterochromatin: Condensed chromatin in certain chromosome regions that often exhibits individual variability and is not thought to contain actively transcribed genes.

heteroplasmy: Different mitochondrial genomes in the same cell, a mechanism by which the proportions of altered mitochondria may increase in specific tissues to cause disease.

heterozygosity: Total number of loci that are heterozygous in an individual, sometimes providing a measure of improved homeostasis and health (e.g., hybrid vigor).

heterozygote: Individual with different alleles at a locus.

histocompatibility antigens, HLA locus: Proteins on the surfaces of white blood cells encoded by a major locus (HLA locus) on chromosome 6, important for immune reactions, transplant rejection, and autoimmune disease.

holoprosencephaly: Developmental defect of the forebrain causing a spectrum of anomalies from midline cleft palate to cyclopia (single eye), all with significant mental disability due to an abnormal forebrain.

homeobox: A DNA sequence shared by several Drosophila segmentation genes.

homeostasis: A regulated internal environment that buffers internal changes or external agents to maintain a normal state.

homeotic mutations: Mutations altering segment identity in Drosophila. In a broader sense, a developmental switch analogous to that replacing one homologous insect segment with another.

homozygote: Individual with identical alleles at a locus.

horizontal transmission: Multiple affected individuals in the same sibship, producing a horizontal pattern of filled symbols in a pedigree.

hot spots: Regions of genes where mutations frequently occur.

HOX, hox: Gene clusters in humans and mice that exhibit homology to the structure and expression of Drosophila homeotic loci.

hyperglycemia: Elevated blood sugar.

hyperplasia: Overdevelopment of an organism, organ, or tissue resulting from an increased number of cells.

hypertrophy: Increase in size of cells, tissue, or organ.

hypoglycemia: Low blood sugar.

hypoplasia: Underdevelopment of an organism, organ, or tissue resulting from a decreased number of cells.

hypotrophy: Decrease in size of cells, tissue, or organ.

identical twins: *see* monozygous twins.

idiogram: Idealized diagram of chromosomes and their numbered bands.

IGF: Insulin-like growth factor.

inborn errors of metabolism: Genetic diseases that impact metabolic pathways, usually because of enzyme deficiencies. Nearly all exhibit autosomal or X-linked recessive inheritance.

incomplete penetrance: Absence of phenotypic expression in a person known from a pedigee to have an abnormal genotype.

infarction: Interrupted blood supply to tissues with oxygen starvation and cell death.

interstitial deletions: Chromosomal deletion removing regions between termini.

introns: Noncoding DNA segments between exons or protein-coding regions of genes; also called intervening sequences.

isochromosomes: Duplicate long or short chromosome arms that result in deficiency—i.e., Turner syndrome patients with i(Xq) are monosomic for Xp.

junk DNA: DNA that does not encode RNA or protein; a possible structural function is noted by the term "junk" that is collected rather than "garbage" that is disposed.

karyotype: A standard number and arrangement of chromosomes as obtained from human blood or tissue specimens. A normal karyotype is 46,XX for females and 46,XY for males.

karyotype-phenotype correlation: Matching chromosome aberrations with their clinical consequences.

kilobases (kb): Unit of DNA/RNA length = 1000 bp; megabase = 1 million bp.

L1CAM: L1 cell adhesion molecule implicated in X-linked hydrocephalus.

linkage: The tendency for neighboring genes to segregate together in families.

linkage disequilibrium: The tendency for an allele, disease, or trait to associate with another allele more often than expected by chance; also called *allele association*.

locus: Unique location of a gene on a chromosome.

LOD score: Logarithm of the odds of linkage, e.g., a LOD score of 3 indicates a 1000 to 1 likelihood that the loci are linked.

loss of heterozygosity: Loss of an allele, particularly when somatic cells lose one normal allele and become cancerous due to a remaining abnormal allele.

Lyon hypothesis: One of the two X chromosomes in females is randomly inactivated in cells of the early embryo, resulting in mixtures of cells (mosaics) with one or the other X chromosome inactivated.

major anomaly: Anomaly with cosmetic or surgical consequences.

malformation: Intrinsic abnormality of a developing structure due to altered differentiation or tissue movements.

maternal inheritance: Inheritance mechanisms that exhibit maternal transmission based on abnormal mitochondria or maternal RNAs.

meiosis: The process of germ cell division that randomly allots one chromosome from each pair to gametes and reduces the chromosome number from diploid to haploid.

Mendelian inheritance: The classical autosomal dominant, autosomal recessive, and X-linked inheritance mechanisms derived from Mendel's observations in peas.

messenger RNA (mRNA): RNA molecules transcribed from DNA and processed, provide coding segments (messages) from the nuclear genes that are translated into protein in the cytoplasm.

metabolic testing: Analysis of blood, urine, or tissue culture cells to detect abnormal levels of chemicals suggestive of biochemical (metabolic) disease.

microdeletions: Chromosome deletions requiring prometaphase banding or FISH studies for detection.

minisatellites: Repetitive DNA consisting of small numbers of repeating nucleotides exemplified by CA repeats. Used for genetic linkage and DNA fingerprinting studies.

minor anomaly: Anomaly of no medical but considerable diagnostic significance.

miscarriage: Pregnancy loss prior to the time of fetal viability (abortion is the equivalent medical term).

missense mutations: Nucleotide changes that cause a different amino acid to be incorporated into protein.

mitosis: The process of somatic cell division that produces identical genomes in daughter cells.

molecular clock: Rate of change in nucleotide or amino acid sequences among homologous genes in different organisms, allowing assessment of gene function and tracking of evolutionary lineages.

monochorionic twins: Twins sharing the same placenta, usually but not always identical (monozygous).

monosomy: Loss of a chromosome.

monozygous twins: Identical twins developing from the same fertilized egg and sharing 100% of their genes.

morphogenesis: A developmental process that includes the stages of blastogenesis and organogenesis.

morphology: Discipline of zoology that concerns itself with the form, formation, and transformation of living beings.

mosaic development: Control of cell fates during embryogenesis by segregation of protein factors within individual cell lineages.

mosaicism: Cells with different DNA sequence or karyotype within one individual.

mouse knockouts: Transgenic mice with deletion of one or both alleles at a genetic locus of interest.

MRI scan: Nuclear magnetic resonance imaging of body regions.

multifactorial determination: Occurrence of traits through the action of alleles at multiple loci plus the environment.

multipoint linkage: Linkage analysis that examines multiple traits or markers in a pedigree and orders them relative to one another.

mutation: Spontaneous change in DNA sequence or chromosome structure.

nondirective counseling: Presenting options to patients without influencing their decisions.

nondisjunction: Failure of a chromosome pair to separate during meiosis or mitosis, generating daughter cells with extra or missing chromosomes.

nonmaleficence: Action to minimize harm or adverse consequences during clinical situations.

nonsense mutations: Mutations that alter the reading frame of mRNA codons such that the translated amino acids are unrelated to the intended protein product.

normal variant: Deviation from expected or average type in structure, form, or function that is more frequent (arbitrarily > 4% of population) and more innocuous than an anomaly.

northern blot: Detection of specific RNA molecules by transfer to membranes and hybridization with DNA probes; pun on the analogous Southern blot for DNA.

obligate carrier: Carrier deduced by pedigree structure.

oligohydramnios: Decreased amniotic fluid, usually because of decreased fetal urine output or amniotic ruptures.

oligonucleotide: Short nucleotide sequence often obtained by chemical synthesis.

OMIM: On-line Mendelian Inheritance in Man, internet version of the catalogue of genetic disorders assembled by Victor A. McKusick.

oncogene: Locus that is activated in association with tumor growth; one abnormal allele is sufficient to cause tumor formation or cancer.

open reading frames: Regions of DNA that contain strings of codons that could potentially encode a protein.

organogenesis: A developmental process that extends from late stage 13 (day 28) until the end of stage 23 (day 56) when the major organs and body parts are formed.

paired box: A DNA sequence motif found in the paired gene of the fruit fly.

paired box, PAX: A shared DNA sequence region (motif) common to many genes in mice and humans.

parentalism: Violating patient autonomy by assuming or directing their medical decisions; formerly paternalism.

partial aneuploidy, partial trisomy/monosomy: Extra or missing segment(s) of chromosomes.

paternity testing: Genetic or blood group analysis to establish a probability for paternity, now often performed by DNA fingerprinting.

pattern formation: Creation of cell arrangements (structures or patterns) during embryogenesis as opposed to cell growth or differentiation.

PCR: Polymerase chain reaction by which individual gene segments are amplified through sequential cycles of polymerization, heat denaturation, and reannealing.

pedigree: A scientific diagram of genealogy using symbols to represent family members and their characteristics.

pharmacogenetics: Study of genetic variation as it pertains to drug metabolism and side effects.

phase of linkage: Combinations of alleles on parental chromosomes deduced by linkage studies.

phenocopy: Environmental effect that mimics an inherited phenotype.

phenotype: Individual traits or characters.

physical map: Gene order based on actual physical measurements in terms of chromosome bands or DNA base pairs.

pleiotropy: Multiple traits determined by a single cause, often a gene mutation.

point mutations: Single nucleotide substitutions.

polydactyly: Extra finger or toe.

polygenic inheritance: Occurrence of a trait in offspring through transmission of alleles at multiple genetic loci.

polyhydramnios: Excess amniotic fluid due to increased maternal production or decreased fetal absorption (i.e., fetal swallowing defects).

polymorphism: Multiple alleles at a locus, producing harmless amino acid or DNA sequence variants that occur in less than 1% of the population.

polypeptide chains: Proteins or, in the case of multiple subunits, components of proteins formed by peptide bonds between amino acids.

polyploidy: Abnormal chromosome number that is a multiple of the haploid karyotype, e.g., 69,XXY or 92,XXXX.

positional cloning: Isolation of gene segments based on chromosome location.

positive predictive value: Fraction of individuals testing positive who have the disease.

predisposition: Greater likelihood of disease.

primary prevention: Preventing the occurrence of disease.

primary relative: First-degree relative, i.e., those sharing 50% of genes.

primer: Oligonucleotide used to begin nucleic acid polymerization at a particular site on a DNA strand, e.g., with PCR or reverse transcriptase.

probability: Likelihood of occurrence expressed as a fraction or percentage; the likelihood that two separate events will occur may be calculated as additive (sum of individual probabilities), joint (product of individual probabilities), or conditional (probability of event B occurring given that event A has occurred).

proband: Individual bringing family to attention because of their phenotype. May be indicated by an arrow in pedigrees.

prometaphase analysis: Karyotype prepared from synchronized cells arrested in early prophase; these studies require prior notice to the laboratory.

prometaphase banding: Arrest of cells in early prophase to prepare extended chromosomes with higher resolution bands; now largely supplanted by FISH techniques.

promoter elements: Regions of DNA sequence that facilitate initiation of transcription by RNA polymerase, often upstream of genes.

propositus or proposita: Male or female affected with disease or bringing family to attention. May be indicated by an arrow in the pedigree.

protein polymorphism: Products of alternate alleles at a locus exemplified by the ABO or HLA systems.

proto-oncogenes: Genes endogenous to normal cells that may be activated to cause cancers.

Punnett square: Diagram for visualizing allele segregation.

pyloric stenosis: Congenital narrowing of the pylorus (junction of stomach and intestines) to produce vomiting.

qualitative traits: Discrete characters or phenotypes like eye color or albinism.

quantitative traits: Incremental phenotypes like height or blood pressure.

radial aplasia: Absent radius producing inward deviation of the wrist.

reciprocal translocation: Exchange of material between two chromosomes.

recombinant DNA: Chimeric DNA molecules produced by joining of segments from different species, often using the complementary "sticky ends" produced by restriction endonucleases.

recombination: Breakage and reunion of DNA strands.

recurrence risk: Probability that a relative, often a future child, will manifest a disease that has occurred in a family member.

reductionism: Breakdown of a complex process into component parts; negative connotation of characterizing a complex phenotype (i.e., an individual) by one of their parts (i.e., a mutant allele).

regulative development: Control of cell fates during embryogenesis by molecules acting on groups of cells.

repetitive DNA: DNA sequences that have multiple copies in a genome.

restriction endonuclease: A bacterial enzyme designed for defense against bacteriophage that recognizes and cleaves at specific nucleotide sequences.

restriction fragment length polymorphisms (RFLPs): DNA polymorphisms deriving from changes in nucleotides at restriction sites, yielding DNA segments of different lengths after restriction and gel electrophoresis.

restriction map: Diagram of a DNA segment indicating the positions of restriction endonuclease sites.

reverse genetics: Genetic analysis proceding from chromosomal location to cloned gene; positional cloning is now the preferred term.

Rh blood group locus: Genetic locus encoding C, D, and E antigens on the red cell membrane that are responsible for Rh incompatibility and fetal disease in humans.

risk factors: Traits, behaviors, or laboratory measures that confer increased risk (predisposition) to disease.

Robertsonian translocations: Joining of two acrocentric chromosomes at their short arms to produce a single translocation chromosome.

satellite DNA: Highly repetitive DNA that was first recognized as a separate band after DNA centrifugation.

sclerae: Whites of the eyes.

secondary prevention: Preventing a complication of disease.

segregation: Separation of genes or alleles during cell division or, for organisms, during reproduction.

selection: Change in allele frequencies due to beneficial or adverse consequences of alleles on reproduction (fitness).

sensitivity of testing: Fraction of individuals with a disease who test positive.

sequence: A cascade of primary and secondary events that are consequences of a single primary malformation or a disruption.

shotgun cloning: Construction of a recombinant DNA library that contains all DNA segments from a sample without bias toward segments of interest.

signal transduction: Interaction of signal molecules with cells (often cell membranes) to produce changes in gene expression and/or cell function.

silent mutations: Mutations that do not alter protein sequence or structure.

single copy or unique sequence DNA: DNA segments or genes present at one copy per genome.

single strand conformational polymorphisms (SSCP): Separated strands of a DNA duplex detected as individual bands by electrophoresis (a diploid locus will yield four bands, two for each allele). One of several methods allowing rapid scanning of gene segments for mutations.

sister chromatids: Replicated strands of a chromosome held together at the centromere.

SNPs, single nucleotide polymorphisms: Single nucleotide substitutions detected by DNA sequencing.

somatic cell hybridization: Fusion of somatic cells for study of gene expression from their four loci (8 alleles).

somatic mosaicism: Variation in DNA sequence or karyotype among different somatic cells of an organism.

specificity of testing: Fraction of individuals without a disease who test negative.

sporadic: Isolated case, often implying lack of inheritance or genetic causation.

staggered ends: Termini of DNA segments cleaved by certain restriction endonucleases that allow segments to join and recombine with one another.

stillbirth: Pregnancy loss and fetal death after the time of potential fetal viability.

stirpiculture: Selection of prime animals for breeding.

stop codons: Trinucleotide codons that signal termination of the amino acid chain during translation.

storage diseases: Disorders caused by the accumulation of large molecules (carbohydrates, glycoproteins, glycosaminoglycans complex lipids) in tissues, producing organ failure.

submicroscopic deletion: Small chromosome deletions that can be visualized only by DNA analysis.

supportive counseling: An educational process explaining the clinical situation with reassurance and access to suitable family or professional resources.

synapsis: Lining up of chromosomes on metaphase plate for sorting during cell division.

syndrome: Multiple anomalies thought to be pathogenetically related and not representing a sequence.

syndrome variability: Differing phenotypic manifestations among individuals with the same syndrome.

targeting sequences: Amino acid regions that direct proteins to particular cellular locations.

teratology: The study of abnormal development, particularly with regard to the disruptive influence of drugs, chemicals, and physical agents.

tertiary prevention: Ameliorating a complication of disease.

tetraploidy: Abnormal karyotype with 4 haploid genomes per cell (i.e., 92,XXYY).

tetrasomy: Four rather than the normal two doses of a chromosome segment.

threshold: A theoretical barrier at which an individual's combination of genes and environmental exposure crosses from predisposition to actual defect.

trait: A feature or characteristic of an individual.

transfusion reaction: Destruction of red blood cells and immune reaction due to incompatibility of transfused blood with host serum.

transgenic organism: Organism bred to contain an inserted DNA segment from a homologous or foreign organism.

translocation breakpoint: The region of recombination between two chromosomes.

translocation carriers: Individuals with "balanced" translocations that have no extra or missing chromosome material.

triplet repeat amplification: Increased number of tandemly repeating 3-bp units that can alter gene expression, as in Fragile X syndrome or mytonic dystrophy.

triploidy: Abnormal karyotype with three haploid genomes per cell (i.e., 69,XXY).

trisomies/monosomies: Karyotypes with extra or missing entire chromosomes.

tumor suppressor gene: Locus that prevents tumor growth when at least one allele is functional; loss of both alleles, as with a constitutional plus a somatic mutation, is associated with tumor formation or cancer.

uninformative: Genetic linkage study where parental alleles and therefore the risk for disease transmission cannot be distinguished.

uniparental disomy: Two copies of a chromosome pair in offspring derived from one parent.

variable expressivity: Variable symptoms among affected individuals in a family.

variable numbers of tandem repeats (VNTRs): DNA polymorphisms deriving from genomic regions with stretches of repeating nucleotides, yielding differently sized DNA segments after restriction and gel electrophoresis. The largest category of VNTRs are minisatellites including CA repeats.

vertical transmission: A trait present in individuals of several generations, causing a vertical pattern of filled symbols in a pedigree.

v-onc: Oncogenes discovered in tumor viruses, often related to endogenous genes (proto-oncogenes).

webbed neck (pterygium colli): Excess neck tissue representing a neck mass (cystic hygroma) in fetuses with Turner or Noonan syndromes.

western blot: Detection of specific proteins by transfer to a membrane and reaction with labeled antibodies; pun on the analogous Southern blot for DNA.

zygotic expression: Synthesis of gene products from zygotic DNA rather than maternal RNA molecules.

INDEX